## Contents

## Preface

In the fast-paced, stimuli-laden, ever-changing world of health care, it is extremely valuable for nurses to have quick access to high-quality resources. Since nurses are frequently the people administering medications, it is imperative that all nurses have current and accurate drug information. New medications are approved yearly by the FDA, who also offers yearly updates on modifications to indications, dosing, and/or warnings of adverse effects. The *2021 Lippincott Pocket Drug Guide for Nurses* is especially valuable to nurses due to its portability, efficiency, and frequent updates.

The *2021 Lippincott Pocket Drug Guide for Nurses* provides need-to-know information in an abbreviated format. Drugs are listed alphabetically. Monographs are concise. Each monograph provides the key information needed to ensure safe patient care:

- Drug class
- Pregnancy risk and Controlled Substance category
- Black box warning, if applicable
- Indications and dosages
- Dosage adjustments that also alert you, when applicable, to consult a complete drug guide or full prescription label
- Most common and most critical adverse effects
- Clinically important interactions
- Key nursing and patient teaching points to ensure safe drug use.

The pocket size makes this book easy to carry into the clinical setting for a quick check before administering the drug.

Following the drug monographs, a section on patient safety reviews the rights of medication administration, safety-oriented patient and family teaching, and other aspects of safe drug administration. Appendices cover biological agents, topical drugs, ophthalmic agents, laxatives, combination drugs, and contraceptives. To keep the book short and sweet, common abbreviations are used throughout; these are listed in the abbreviations list on pages vi–viii.

The purpose of this pocket guide is to provide critical information during the rush of a clinical setting. However, it is important to check complete facts and details as soon as time allows to ensure that the best outcomes are achieved for each patient.

I wish to recognize that this update to the *Pocket Drug Guide* is a group effort, and I am extremely grateful for the support and work of the team from Wolters Kluwer. Specifically, this edition would not have been possible without Karen Comerford (Editor), Diane Labus (Senior Managing Editor), and Collette Hendler (Editor-in-Chief). I would also like to acknowledge a deep gratitude to my family, who allow me the "quiet time" I need to edit and write. Finally, it is Amy Karch who most inspired this edition. As my mentor (and as the original author of the previous *Pocket Drug Guides*), Amy has motivated me to endeavor to produce a valuable resource for all nurses. She is missed deeply, but not forgotten.

***Rebecca G. Tucker, PhD, ACNPC, MEd, RN***

# Guide to abbreviations

***Abbreviations in headings***

| | |
|---|---|
| **BBW** | Black Box Warning |
| **CLASS** | Therapeutic/Pharmacologic Class |
| **PREG/CONT** | Pregnancy Risk Category/Controlled Substance Schedule |
| **IND & DOSE** | Indications & Dosages |
| **ADJUST DOSE** | Dosage Adjustment |
| **ADV EFF** | Adverse Effects |
| **NC/PT** | Nursing Considerations/Patient Teaching |

***Abbreviations in text***

| | |
|---|---|
| abd | abdominal |
| ABG | arterial blood gas |
| ACE | angiotensin-converting enzyme |
| ACT | activated clotting time |
| ACTH | adrenocorticotropic hormone |
| ADH | antidiuretic hormone |
| ADHD | attention-deficit hyperactivity disorder |
| adjunct | adjunctive |
| ADLs | activities of daily living |
| AHA | American Heart Association |
| AIDS | acquired immunodeficiency syndrome |
| ALL | acute lymphocytic leukemia |
| ALS | amyotrophic lateral sclerosis |
| ALT | alanine transaminase |
| a.m. | morning |
| AML | acute myelogenous leukemia |
| ANA | anti-nuclear antibodies |
| ANC | absolute neutrophil count |
| approx | approximately |
| aPTT | activated partial thromboplastin time |
| ARB | angiotensin II receptor blocker |
| ASA | acetylsalicylic acid |
| AST | aspartate transaminase |
| AV | atrioventricular |
| bid | twice a day (*bis in die*) |
| BP | blood pressure |
| BPH | benign prostatic hypertrophy |
| BSA | body surface area |
| BUN | blood urea nitrogen |
| CABG | coronary artery bypass graft |
| CAD | coronary artery disease |
| cAMP | cyclic adenosine monophosphate |
| CBC | complete blood count |
| CDAD | *Clostridium difficile*–associated diarrhea |
| CDC | Centers for Disease Control and Prevention |
| chemo | chemotherapy |
| CK | creatine kinase |
| CML | chronic myelogenous leukemia |
| CNS | central nervous system |
| combo | combination |
| conc | concentration |
| COPD | chronic obstructive pulmonary disease |
| CR | controlled-release |
| CrCl | creatinine clearance |
| CSF | cerebrospinal fluid |
| CV | cardiovascular |
| CVP | central venous pressure |
| CYP450 | cytochrome P-450 |
| d | day, days |
| $D_5W$ | dextrose 5% in water |
| DIC | disseminated intravascular coagulopathy |
| dL | deciliter (100 mL) |
| DMARD | disease-modifying antirheumatic drug |
| DR | delayed-release |
| DRESS | drug reaction w/eosinophilia and systemic symptoms |
| DVT | deep venous thrombosis |
| dx | diagnosis |
| dysfx | dysfunction |

| | |
|---|---|
| ECG | electrocardiogram |
| ED | erectile dysfunction |
| EEG | electroencephalogram |
| eGFR | epidermal growth factor receptor |
| ER | extended-release |
| ESRD | end-stage renal disease |
| ET | endotracheal |
| FDA | Food and Drug Administration |
| 5-FU | fluorouracil |
| 5-HIAA | 5-hydroxyindole acetic acid |
| FSH | follicle-stimulating hormone |
| g | gram |
| GABA | gamma-aminobutyric acid |
| GERD | gastroesophageal reflux disease |
| GFR | glomerular filtration rate |
| GGTP | gamma-glutamyl transpeptidase |
| GI | gastrointestinal |
| G6PD | glucose-6-phosphate dehydrogenase |
| GU | genitourinary |
| GVHD | graft vs. host disease |
| HBV | hepatitis B virus |
| HCG | human chorionic gonadotropin |
| Hct | hematocrit |
| HCV | hepatitis C virus |
| HDL | high-density lipoprotein |
| HER2 | human epidermal growth factor receptor-2 |
| HF | heart failure |
| Hg | mercury |
| Hgb | hemoglobin |
| Hib | *Haemophilus influenzae* type b |
| HIV | human immunodeficiency virus |
| HMG-CoA | 3-hydroxy-3-methylglutaryl coenzyme A |
| HPA | hypothalamic-pituitary axis |
| HR | hormone receptor |
| hr | hour |
| HR | heart rate |
| HSV | herpes simplex virus |
| HTN | hypertension |
| hx | history |
| IBS | irritable bowel syndrome |
| ICU | intensive care unit |
| IHSS | idiopathic hypertrophic subaortic stenosis |
| ILD | interstitial lung disease |
| IM | intramuscular |
| INR | International Normalized Ratio |
| intraop | intraoperative |
| IOP | intraocular pressure |
| IV | intravenous |
| kg | kilogram |
| L | liter |
| lb | pound |
| LDL | low-density lipoprotein |
| LFT | liver function test |
| LH | luteinizing hormone |
| LHRH | luteinizing hormone-releasing hormone |
| m | meter |
| MAC | *Mycobacterium avium* complex |
| maint | maintenance |
| MAO | monoamine oxidase |
| MAOI | monoamine oxidase inhibitor |
| max | maximum |
| mcg | microgram |
| mg | milligram |
| mgt | management |
| MI | myocardial infarction |
| min | minute |
| mL | milliliter |
| mo | month |
| MRSA | methicillin-resistant *Staphylococcus aureus* |
| MS | multiple sclerosis |
| NA | not applicable |
| neuro | neurologic |
| NG | nasogastric |
| ng | nanogram |
| NMJ | neuromuscular junction |
| NMS | neuroleptic malignant syndrome |
| NRTI | nucleoside reverse transcriptase inhibitor |
| NSAID | nonsteroidal anti-inflammatory drug |
| NSCLC | non-small-cell lung cancer |
| NSS | normal saline solution |
| n/v | nausea and vomiting |
| n/v/d | nausea, vomiting, and diarrhea |
| OCD | obsessive-compulsive disorder |
| OCT2 | organic cation transporter 2 |
| oint | ointment |
| ophthal | ophthalmic |
| OTC | over-the-counter |
| oz | ounce |

P pulse
PABA para-aminobenzoic acid
PCI percutaneous coronary intervention
PDA patent ductus arteriosus
PE pulmonary embolus
PEG percutaneous endoscopic gastrostomy
periop perioperative
PFT pulmonary function test
PG prostaglandin
P-gp P-glycoprotein
pH hydrogen ion concentration
PID pelvic inflammatory disease
PKSK9 proprotein convertase subtilism kexin type 9
p.m. evening
PMDD premenstrual dysphoric disorder
PML progressive multifocal leukoencephalopathy
PMS premenstrual syndrome
PO orally, by mouth (*per os*)
postop postoperative
preg pregnant, pregnancy
preop preoperative
PRN when required (*pro re nata*)
PSA prostate-specific antigen
pt patient
PT prothrombin time
PTCA percutaneous transluminal coronary angioplasty
PTSD post-traumatic stress disorder
PTT partial thromboplastin time
PVCs premature ventricular contractions
px prophylaxis
q every
qid four times a day (*quarter in die*)
R respiratory rate
RA rheumatoid arthritis
RBC red blood cell
RDA recommended dietary allowance
RDS respiratory distress syndrome
REMS Risk Evaluation and Mitigation Strategy
RPLS reversible posterior leukoencephalopathy syndrome
RSV respiratory syncytial virus
SA sinoatrial
SBE subacute bacterial endocarditis
sec second
SIADH syndrome of inappropriate antidiuretic hormone secretion
SJS Stevens-Johnson syndrome
SL sublingual
SLE systemic lupus erythematosus
sol solution
sp species
SR sustained-release
SSRI selective serotonin reuptake inhibitor
STD sexually transmitted disease
subcut subcutaneous
SWSD shift-work sleep disorder
s&sx signs and symptoms
sx symptoms
$T_3$ triiodothyronine
$T_4$ thyroxine (tetraiodothyronine)
TB tuberculosis
tbsp tablespoon
TCA tricyclic antidepressant
temp temperature
TIA transient ischemic attack
tid three times a day (*ter in die*)
TLS tumor lysis syndrome
TNF tumor necrosis factor
TPA tissue plasminogen activator
TPN total parenteral nutrition
TSH thyroid-stimulating hormone
tsp teaspoon
tx treatment
ULN upper limit of normal
unkn unknown
URI upper respiratory (tract) infection
USP United States Pharmacopeia
UTI urinary tract infection
UV ultraviolet
VLDL very–low-density lipoprotein
VREF vancomycin-resistant *Enterococcus faecium*
VTE venous thromboembolism
w/ with
WBC white blood cell
wk week
XR extended-release
yr year

**abacavir** (Ziagen)
**CLASS** Antiviral, NRTI
**PREG/CONT** Unkn/NA

**BBW** Risk of severe to fatal hypersensitivity reactions; increased w/ HLA-B*5701 allele. Monitor for lactic acidosis, severe hepatomegaly.
**IND & DOSE HIV infection (w/other antiretrovirals).** *Adult:* 300 mg PO bid or 600 mg/d PO. *Child 3 mo–18 yr:* 8 mg/kg PO bid or 16 mg/d PO once daily; max, 600 mg/d.
**ADJUST DOSE** Mild hepatic impairment
**ADV EFF** Fatigue, headache, insomnia, malaise, **MI**, n/v/d, rash, **severe to fatal hepatomegaly, severe to fatal lactic acidosis, severe hypersensitivity reactions,** weakness
**INTERACTIONS** Alcohol, methadone, other abacavir-containing drugs
**NC/PT** Give w/other antiretrovirals. Suggest use of barrier contraceptives; breastfeeding not advised. Monitor for s&sx of lactic acidosis, liver dysfx, hypersensitivity reactions.

**DANGEROUS DRUG**
**abaloparatide** (Tymlos)
**CLASS** Parathyroid hormone–related peptide
**PREG/CONT** High risk/NA

**BBW** Increased incidence of osteosarcoma in animal studies. Not for use w/risk of osteosarcoma; not for use longer than 2 yr during a lifetime.
**IND & DOSE Tx of postmenopausal women w/osteoporosis at high risk for fracture.** *Adult:* 80 mcg/d subcut.
**ADV EFF** Dizziness, fatigue, headache, hypercalcemia, hypercalciuria, nausea, orthostatic hypotension, palpitations, vertigo
**NC/PT** Ensure proper use of drug; calculate total dosage given. Inject into periumbilical region. Avoid use in preg/breastfeeding. Ensure of calcium/vitamin D intake. Teach pt proper preparation/administration of drug, disposal of needles/syringes; to lie down if orthostatic hypotension occurs; pt should take safety precautions w/CNS effects; report blood in urine, lower back pain, continued dizziness.

**abatacept** (Orencia)
**CLASS** Antiarthritic, immune modulator
**PREG/CONT** C/NA

**IND & DOSE Tx of adult RA.** *>100 kg:* 1,000 mg/d IV. *60–100 kg:* 750 mg/d IV. *<60 kg:* 500 mg/d IV. After initial dose, give at 2 and 4 wk, then q 4 wk. **Tx of juvenile idiopathic arthritis in child ≥6 yr.** *≥75 kg:* Use adult dose; max, 1,000 mg/d. *<75 kg:* 10 mg/kg/d IV. After initial dose, give at 2 and 4 wk. **Adult psoriatic arthritis.** *>100 kg:* 1,000 mg/d IV. *60–100 kg:* 750 mg/d IV. *<60 kg:* 500 mg/d IV. Or, 125 mg subcut/wk.
**ADV EFF** Headache, **hypersensitivity reactions and anaphylaxis, potentially serious infection**
**INTERACTIONS** Live vaccines; TNF antagonists (contraindicated)
**NC/PT** Monitor for s&sx of infection. Pretest for TB before beginning therapy. Do not give w/TNF antagonists. Do not give live vaccines during or for 3 mo after tx. Pt should avoid preg/breastfeeding; report difficulty breathing, s&sx of infection.

**abciximab** (ReoPro)
**CLASS** Antiplatelet, glycoprotein IIb/IIIa inhibitor
**PREG/CONT** C/NA

**IND & DOSE Adjunct to PCI to prevent cardiac ischemic complications in pt undergoing PCI.** *Adult:* 0.25 mg/kg by IV bolus 10–60 min before procedure, then continuous IV infusion of 0.125 mcg/kg/min for 12 hr (max, 10 mcg/min). **Unstable angina not responding to conventional therapy when PCI is planned within 24 hr,**

**w/heparin and aspirin therapy.** *Adult:* 0.25 mg/kg by IV bolus over at least 1 min, then 10 mcg/min by IV infusion for 19–24 hr, ending 1 hr after PCI.
**ADV EFF** **Bleeding,** edema, hypotension, n/v, pain, **thrombocytopenia**
**INTERACTIONS** Anticoagulants, antiplatelets, thrombolytics
**NC/PT** Provide safety measures to protect pt from bleeding and monitor for s&sx of bleeding. Monitor CBC. Give w/heparin and aspirin therapy. Clearly mark chart that pt is on drug.

## abemaciclib (Verzenio)

**CLASS** Antineoplastic, kinase inhibitor
**PREG/CONT** High risk/NA

**IND & DOSE** **Tx of HR-positive, HER2-negative advanced or metastatic breast cancer, w/fulvestrant, an aromatase inhibitor, or as monotherapy.** *Adult:* 150 mg PO bid w/ fulvestrant or aromatase inhibitor; 200 mg PO bid as monotherapy.
**ADV EFF** Abd pain, **bone marrow suppression,** decreased appetite, headache, hepatotoxicity, **ILD,** n/v/d, **thromboembolism**
**INTERACTIONS** CYP3A inhibitors, ketoconazole; avoid use
**NC/PT** Monitor blood counts/LFTs; dosage may need adjustment. Start antidiarrheal and fluid replacement at first sx of diarrhea. Pt should avoid preg (contraceptives advised)/breastfeeding; report urine/stool color changes, extreme fatigue, pain in legs/chest, diarrhea.

## abiraterone acetate (Yonsa, Zytiga)

**CLASS** Antineoplastic, CYP17 inhibitor
**PREG/CONT** X/NA

**IND & DOSE** **Tx of pts w/metastatic castration-resistant prostate cancer, w/a gonadotropin-releasing hormone analog concurrently or pts should have had a bilateral orchiectomy.** *Adult:* 1,000 mg PO once daily w/5 mg prednisone PO bid. *Yonsa,* 500 mg PO once daily w/4 mg methylprednisolone PO bid.
**ADJUST DOSE** Hepatic impairment
**ADV EFF** **Adrenocortical insufficiency,** arrhythmias, **cardiotoxicity,** cough, diarrhea, dyspepsia, dyspnea, edema, **hepatotoxicity,** hot flushes, HTN, hypokalemia, **mineralocorticoid excess**, nocturia, URI, UTI
**INTERACTIONS** CYP2D6 substrates (avoid use); CYP3A4 enzyme inducers/inhibitors; radium Ra 223 dichloride (may increase fractures/mortality)
**NC/PT** Must be taken on empty stomach w/no food 1 hr before or 2 hr after dosing; pt should swallow tablet whole and not cut/crush/chew. Not for use in preg/breastfeeding. Monitor closely for cardiotoxicity, hepatotoxicity, adrenal insufficiency, mineralocorticoid excess. Corticosteroids may be needed in stressful situations. Pt should report urine/stool color changes, chest pain.

## abobotulinumtoxinA (Dysport)

**CLASS** Neurotoxin
**PREG/CONT** Moderate risk/NA

**BBW** Dysport and all botulinum toxin products may spread from area of injection to produce s&sx consistent w/botulinum toxin effects; s&sx may include asthenia, generalized muscle weakness, diplopia, blurred vision, ptosis, dysphagia, dysphonia, dysarthria, urinary incontinence, and breathing difficulties and have been reported hrs to wks after injection. Swallowing/breathing difficulties can be life-threatening; there have been reports of death. Risk of s&sx is probably greatest in child treated for spasticity.
**IND & DOSE** **Improvement of glabellar lines.** 50 units in five equal injections q 4 mo. **Cervical dystonia.**

*Adult:* 250–1,000 units IM q 12 wk. **Tx of upper limb spasticity (excluding spasticity caused by cerebral palsy).** *Adult, child ≥2 yr:* Base dose on muscle affected, severity. Repeat not less than q 12 wk. **Tx of pediatric lower limb spasticity.** *Child ≥2 yr:* 10–15 units/kg/limb IM q 12 wk. **Tx of spasticity in adults.** 500–1,500 units IM q 12 wk.
**ADV EFF** **Anaphylactic reactions,** dizziness, headache, local reactions, **MI, spread of toxin that can lead to death**
**INTERACTIONS** Aminoglycosides, anticholinesterases, lincosamides, magnesium sulfate, NMJ blockers, polymyxin, quinidine, succinylcholine
**NC/PT** Store in refrigerator. Have epinephrine available in case of anaphylactic reactions. Do not use w/ allergy to cow's milk proteins. Effects may not appear for 1–2 d; will persist for 3–4 mo. Not for use in preg/ breastfeeding.

## acalabrutinib (Calquence)
**CLASS** Antineoplastic, Bruton tyrosine kinase inhibitor
**PREG/CONT** High risk/NA

**IND & DOSE** **Tx of pts w/mantle cell lymphoma who have received at least one prior therapy; tx of chronic lymphocytic leukemia or small lymphocytic lymphoma.** *Adult:* 100 mg PO q 12 hr.
**ADV EFF** Anemia, atrial fibrillation/ flutter, bruising, diarrhea, fatigue, headache, hemorrhage, infection, myalgia, neutropenia, second primary malignancies, thrombocytopenia
**INTERACTIONS** CYP3A inhibitors/ inducers, gastric acid–reducing agents
**NC/PT** Avoid if severe hepatic impairment. Give w/ or w/o food. Monitor for bleeding/s&sx of infection/ atrial fibrillation/flutter; monitor CBC. Drug may harm fetus. Breastfeeding not recommended during tx and for at least 3 wk after tx. Pt should swallow capsule whole w/ glass of water, use sun protection (higher risk of skin cancer).

## acamprosate calcium
(Campral)
**CLASS** Antialcoholic, GABA analog
**PREG/CONT** C/NA

**IND & DOSE** **Maint of abstinence from alcohol as part of comprehensive psychosocial tx mgt program.** *Adult:* 666 mg PO tid; begin as soon as abstinence achieved.
**ADJUST DOSE** Renal impairment
**ADV EFF** Diarrhea, **suicidality**
**INTERACTIONS** Alcohol
**NC/PT** Ensure pt is abstaining from alcohol and is in comprehensive tx program. Pt may take drug even if relapse occurs. Not for use in preg/ breastfeeding. Pt should report thoughts of suicide.

## acarbose (Precose)
**CLASS** Alpha-glucosidase inhibitor, antidiabetic
**PREG/CONT** B/NA

**IND & DOSE** **Adjunct to diet/exercise to lower blood glucose in pts w/type 2 diabetes.** *Adult:* 25 mg PO tid w/first bite of meal. Max for pt ≤60 kg, 50 mg PO tid; >60 kg, 100 mg PO tid. **Combo tx w/sulfonylureas, metformin, or insulin to enhance glycemic control.** *Adult:* Adjust dose based on blood glucose levels in combo w/dosage of other drugs used.
**ADV EFF** Abd pain, flatulence, hypoglycemia, n/v/d, **pneumatosis cystoides intestinalis**
**INTERACTIONS** Antidiabetics, celery, charcoal, coriander, dandelion root, digestive enzymes, digoxin, fenugreek, garlic, ginseng, juniper berries
**NC/PT** Give w/food. Monitor blood glucose. Pt should follow diet/exercise program and report diarrhea w/mucus discharge, rectal bleeding, constipation.

**acebutolol hydrochloride** (Sectral)
**CLASS** Antiarrhythmic, antihypertensive, beta-adrenergic blocker
**PREG/CONT** B/NA

**IND & DOSE Tx of HTN.** *Adult:* 400 mg/d PO. Maint dose, 200–1,200 mg/d PO (larger dose in two divided doses). **Mgt of PVCs.** *Adult:* 200 mg PO bid. Range to control PVCs, 600–1,200 mg/d PO. Discontinue gradually over 3 wk.
**ADJUST DOSE** Renal/hepatic impairment; elderly pts
**ADV EFF** Arrhythmias (bradycardia/tachycardia/heart block), **bronchospasm**, constipation, decreased exercise tolerance, ED, flatulence, gastric pain, HF, n/v
**INTERACTIONS** Alpha blockers, aspirin, beta blockers, bismuth subsalicylate, calcium channel blockers, clonidine, insulin, magnesium salicylate, NSAIDs, prazosin
**NC/PT** Monitor apical P; do not give if P is less than 45. May give w/food. Withdraw slowly over 3 wk after long-term therapy. Pt should report difficulty breathing.

**acetaminophen** (Acephen, Ofirmev, Tylenol, etc.)
**CLASS** Analgesic, antipyretic
**PREG/CONT** B/NA

**BBW** Risk of medication error and severe hepatotoxicity; monitor for overdose through use of multiple acetaminophen-containing products; monitor LFTs at higher end of dosage range.
**IND & DOSE Temporary reduction of fever; temporary relief of minor aches and pains caused by common cold and influenza; headache, sore throat, toothache (pts ≥2 yr); backache, menstrual cramps, minor arthritis pain, muscle aches (pts >12 yr).** *Adult, child >12 yr* (PO or rectal suppositories): 325–560 mg q 4–6 hr or 1,300 mg (ER) PO q 8 hr. *Adult, child ≥13 yr, ≥50 kg:* 1,000 mg IV q 6 hr or 650 mg IV q 4 hr; max, 1,000 mg/dose IV or 4,000 mg/d IV. *Child 13 yr, <50 kg:* 15 mg/kg IV q 6 hr or 12.5 mg/kg IV q 4 hr; max, 750 mg or 75 mg/kg/d. *Child 2–12 yr:* 15 mg/kg IV q 6 hr or 12 mg/kg IV q 4 hr; max, 75 mg/kg/d. *Child:* May repeat PO or rectal doses 4–5 ×/d; max, five doses in 24 hr or 10 mg/kg. PO doses: 11 yr, 480 mg/dose; 9–10 yr, 400 mg/dose; 6–8 yr, 320 mg/dose; 4–5 yr, 240 mg/dose; 2–3 yr, 160 mg/dose; 12–23 mo, 120 mg/dose; 4–11 mo, 80 mg/dose; 0–3 mo, 40 mg/dose. PR doses: 6–12 yr, 325 mg q 4–6 hr; 3–6 yr, 120 mg q 4–6 hr; 12–36 mo, 80 mg q 4 hr; 3–11 mo, 80 mg q 6 hr.
**ADJUST DOSE** Active liver disease, severe liver impairment, severe renal disease
**ADV EFF Hepatic failure, hepatotoxicity, myocardial damage, serious skin reactions**
**INTERACTIONS** Alcohol, anticholinergics, barbiturates, charcoal, carbamazepine, hydantoins, oral anticoagulants, rifampin, sulfinpyrazone, zidovudine
**NC/PT** Do not exceed recommended dosage. Avoid combining (many products contain acetaminophen). Monitor to assure max dose is not exceeded. Administer IV over 15 min. Not recommended for longer than 10 d. Overdose tx: acetylcysteine, possible life support. Pt should report difficulty breathing, rash.

**acetazolamide** (Diamox)
**CLASS** Antiepileptic, antiglaucoma, carbonic anhydrase inhibitor, diuretic
**PREG/CONT** C/NA

**BBW** Fatalities have occurred due to severe reactions; discontinue immediately if s&sx of serious reactions. Use caution if pt receiving high-dose

# 2021 Lippincott Pocket Drug Guide for Nurses

**Rebecca G. Tucker,** PhD, ACNPC, MEd, RN
Assistant Professor of Clinical Nursing
University of Rochester School of Nursing
Nurse Practitioner in Cardiology, Strong Memorial Hospital
Rochester, NY

Wolters Kluwer
Philadelphia • Baltimore • New York • London
Buenos Aires • Hong Kong • Sydney • Tokyo

**Chief Nurse:** Anne Dabrow Woods, DNP, RN, CRNP, ANP-BC, AGACNP-BC
**Acquisitions Editor:** Jamie Blum
**Editor-in-Chief:** Collette Hendler, RN, MS, MA, CIC
**Senior Managing Editor:** Diane Labus
**Editor:** Karen C. Comerford
**Editorial Assistant:** Linda K. Ruhf
**Marketing Manager:** Linda Wetmore
**Art Director:** Elaine Kasmer
**Design:** Joseph John Clark
**Production Project Manager:** Kim Cox
**Manufacturing Manager:** Kathleen Brown
**Production Services:** Aptara, Inc.



9 8 7 6 5 4 3 2 1

Printed in China

This work is provided "as is," and the publisher disclaims any and all warranties, express or implied, including any warranties as to accuracy, comprehensiveness, or currency of the content of this work.

This work is no substitute for individual patient assessment based upon healthcare professionals' examination of each patient and consideration of, among other things, age, weight, gender, current or prior medical conditions, medication history, laboratory data and other factors unique to the patient. The publisher does not provide medical advice or guidance and this work is merely a reference tool. Healthcare professionals, and not the publisher, are solely responsible for the use of this work including all medical judgments and for any resulting diagnosis and treatments.

Given continuous, rapid advances in medical science and health information, independent professional verification of medical diagnoses, indications, appropriate pharmaceutical selections and dosages, and treatment options should be made and healthcare professionals should consult a variety of sources. When prescribing medication, healthcare professionals are advised to consult the product information sheet (the manufacturer's package insert) accompanying each drug to verify, among other things, conditions of use, warnings and side effects and identify any changes in dosage schedule or contraindications, particularly if the medication to be administered is new, infrequently used or has a narrow therapeutic range. To the maximum extent permitted under applicable law, no responsibility is assumed by the publisher for any injury and/or damage to persons or property, as a matter of products liability, negligence law or otherwise, or from any reference to or use by any person of this work.

LPDGN21011020
ISBN-13: 978-1-9751-5889-7
ISBN-10: 1-9751-5889-X
ISSN: 2473-0602 (print)
ISSN: 2473-0610 (online)

CCS0820

aspirin; anorexia, tachypnea, lethargy, coma, death have occurred.
**IND & DOSE Open-angle glaucoma.** *Adult:* 250 mg–1 g/d PO, usually in divided doses, or 1 ER capsule bid (a.m. and p.m.). Max, 1 g/d. **Acute congestive angle-closure glaucoma.** *Adult:* 500 mg (ER) PO bid or 250 mg PO q 4 hr. **Secondary glaucoma and preoperatively.** *Adult:* 250 mg PO q 4 hr, or 250 mg PO bid, or 500 mg PO bid (ER capsules), or 500 mg PO followed by 125–250 mg PO q 4 hr. May give IV for rapid relief of increased IOP: 500 mg IV, then 125–250 mg PO q 4 hr. **Diuresis in HF.** *Adult:* 250–375 mg PO (5 mg/kg) daily in a.m. **Drug-induced edema.** *Adult:* 250–375 mg PO once q day or for 1 or 2 d alternating w/d of rest. **Epilepsy.** *Adult:* 8–30 mg/kg/d PO in divided doses. Range, 375–1,000 mg/d. **Acute altitude sickness.** *Adult, child ≥12 yr:* 500 mg–1 g/d PO in divided doses.
**ADV EFF** Urinary frequency
**INTERACTIONS** Amphetamines, lithium, procainamide, quinidine, salicylates, TCAs
**NC/PT** Do not give IM. Make oral liquid by crushing tablets and suspending in sweet syrup (do not use alcohol or glycerin). Have IOP checked periodically. May cause dizziness, increased urination. Pt should report flank pain, bleeding, weight gain of more than 3 lb/d. Name confusion between *Diamox* and *Trimox* (ampicillin).

## acetylcysteine (Acetadote)
**CLASS** Antidote, mucolytic
**PREG/CONT** B/NA

**IND & DOSE Mucolytic adjuvant therapy for abnormal, viscid, or inspissated mucus secretions in acute and chronic bronchopulmonary disease.** *Adult, child:* Nebulization w/ face mask, mouthpiece, tracheostomy: 3–5 mL of 20% sol or 6–10 mL of 10% sol tid or qid. Nebulization w/ tent, croupette: Up to 300 mL during a tx period. Direct or by tracheostomy: 1–2 mL of 10%–20% sol q 1–4 hr. Percutaneous intratracheal catheter: 1–2 mL of 20% sol or 2–4 mL of 10% sol q 1–4 hr. **To prevent/lessen hepatic injury that may occur after ingestion of potentially hepatotoxic dose of acetaminophen.** *Adult, child:* PO, 140 mg/kg loading dose, then 17 maint doses of 70 mg/kg q 4 hr, starting 4 hr after loading dose. IV, loading dose, 150 mg/kg in 200 mL IV over 60 min; maint dose 50 mg/kg in 500 mL IV over 4 hr followed by second maint dose of 100 mg/kg in 1,000 mL IV over 16 hr. Total IV dose, 300 mg/kg over 21 hr.
**ADV EFF Anaphylactoid reactions, bronchospasm,** n/v, rhinorrhea
**INTERACTIONS** (in sol) Amphotericin B, erythromycin, hydrogen peroxide, lactobionate, tetracycline
**NC/PT** Use water to remove sol from pt's face. Monitor nebulizer for buildup of drug. Have suction equipment available. May mix 20% sol w/soft drinks to concentration of 5%. Dilute oral sol w/water if using gastric tube. Warn pt of possible disagreeable odor as nebulization begins. Pt should report difficulty breathing.

## acitretin (Soriatane)
**CLASS** Antipsoriatic, retinoic acid
**PREG/CONT** X/NA

**BBW** Do not use in preg; serious fetal harm possible. Males should not father a child during and for 3 mo after tx.
**IND & DOSE Tx of severe psoriasis.** *Adult:* 25–50 mg/d PO w/main meal.
**ADV EFF Hepatotoxicity,** hypervitaminosis A, ossification abnormalities
**INTERACTIONS** Methotrexate, phenytoin, retinoids, St. John's wort, tetracyclines, vitamin D
**NC/PT** Pt must have monthly negative preg tests and agree to use two forms of contraception. Dispensed in 1-mo supply only. Must have signed pt agreement in medical record. Pt

may not donate blood for 3 yr after tx. Pt should swallow tablets whole and not cut/crush/chew them; stop drug when lesions resolve; avoid sun exposure; report urine/stool color changes.

**aclidinium bromide** (Tudorza Pressair)
**CLASS** Anticholinergic, bronchodilator
**PREG/CONT** C/NA

**IND & DOSE Long-term maint tx of bronchospasm associated w/COPD.** *Adult:* 400 mcg/actuation bid.
**ADJUST DOSE** >80 yr; <60 kg; renal/hepatic impairment
**ADV EFF** Dry mouth, glaucoma, headache, hypersensitivity reactions, nasopharyngitis, **paradoxical bronchospasm,** urine retention
**INTERACTIONS** Other anticholinergics; avoid this combo
**NC/PT** Ensure appropriate use of drug; use only w/provided inhaler. Not for acute bronchospasm; rescue inhaler should be provided. Monitor for hypersensitivity, more likely in pts w/severe hypersensitivity to milk proteins. Stop drug w/paradoxical bronchospasm. Not for use in breastfeeding. Monitor for glaucoma. Have pt void before each dose if urine retention occurs.

**acyclovir** (Sitavig, Zovirax)
**CLASS** Antiviral, purine nucleoside analog
**PREG/CONT** B/NA

**IND & DOSE Herpes genitalis.** *Adult:* 5 mg/kg IV infused over 1 hr q 8 hr for 5 d. **Herpes encephalitis.** *Adult:* 10 mg/kg IV infused over 1 hr q 8 hr for 10 d. **Herpes labialis (*Sitavig*).** *Adult:* 50-mg buccal tablet single dose 1 hr after onset of prodromal s&sx and before s&sx of lesions. **Herpes simplex** (immunocompromised pts). *Adult:* 5 mg/kg IV infused over 1 hr q 8 hr for 7 d. **Varicella zoster** (immunocompromised pts). *Adult:* 10 mg/kg IV infused over 1 hr q 8 hr for 7 d. **Initial genital herpes.** *Adult:* 200 mg PO q 4 hr five times daily (1,000 mg/d) for 10 d. **Long-term suppressive therapy.** *Adult:* 400 mg PO bid for up to 12 mo. **Recurrent therapy.** *Adult:* 200 mg IV q 4 hr five times daily for 5 d. **HSV infection.** *Child <12 yr:* 10 mg/kg IV infused over 1 hr q 8 hr for 7 d. **Varicella zoster.** *Child <12 yr:* 20 mg/kg IV over 1 hr q 8 hr for 7 d. **Shingles, HSV encephalitis.** *Child 3 mo–12 yr:* 20 mg/kg IV over 1 hr q 8 hr for 14–21 d. **Neonatal HSV.** 10 mg/kg IV infused over 1 hr q 8 hr for 10 d. *≥2 yr, ≤40 kg:* 20 mg/kg/dose PO qid (80 mg/kg/d) for 5 d. *>12 yr, >40 kg:* Give adult dose. **Ointment.** *All ages:* Apply sufficient quantity to cover all lesions 6 ×/d (q 3 hr) for 7 d. 1.25-cm (0.5-in) ribbon of ointment covers 2.5 $cm^2$ (4 $in^2$) surface area. **Cream.** *≥12 yr:* Apply enough to cover all lesions 5 ×/d for 4 d.
**ADJUST DOSE** Elderly pts, renal impairment
**ADV EFF** Inflammation or phlebitis at injection sites, n/v/d, transient topical burning w/topical use
**INTERACTIONS** Nephrotoxic drugs, probenecid, zidovudine
**NC/PT** Ensure pt well hydrated. Wear rubber glove or finger cot when applying topically. Drug not a cure and will not prevent recurrence. Pt should avoid sexual intercourse when lesions are present; use condoms to prevent spread.

**adalimumab** (Abrilada, Amjevita, Cyltezo, Hadlima, Humira, Hyrimoz)
**CLASS** Antiarthritic, TNF blocker
**PREG/CONT** B/NA

**BBW** Risk of serious infection, activation of TB; risk of lymphoma and other potentially fatal malignancies in child, adolescent.
**IND & DOSE Tx of RA, psoriatic arthritis, ankylosing spondylitis.** *Adult:* 40 mg subcut q other wk. **Crohn disease/ulcerative colitis.**

*Adult, child ≥40 kg:* Four 40-mg subcut injections in 1 day followed by 80 mg 2 wk later; 2 wk later begin 40 mg q other wk maint. *Child 17–<40 kg:* Two 40-mg subcut injections in 1 day; then 40 mg 2 wk later; then begin 20 mg subcut q other wk. **Plaque psoriasis/uveitis.** *Adult:* 80 mg subcut, then 40 mg q other wk starting 1 wk later. **Juvenile idiopathic arthritis/uveitis (≥2 yr).** *Child ≥30 kg:* 40 mg subcut q other wk. *Child 15–<30 kg:* 20 mg subcut q other wk. *Child 10–<15 kg:* 10 mg subcut q other wk. **Tx of hidradenitis suppurativa.** *Adult:* 160 mg given as four 40-mg subcut injections on day 1 or two 40-mg injections/d on days 1 and 2; second dose 2 wk later, 80 mg as two 40-mg injections in one day; third dose on day 29, 40 mg subcut, then 40 mg/wk. *Adolescents ≥12 yr, ≥60 kg:* 160 mg subcut day 1; second dose 2 wk later (day 15), 80 mg subcut; third dose (day 29) and subsequent doses, 40 mg subcut; *30–<60 kg:* 80 mg subcut day 1; second dose (day 8) and subsequent doses, 40 mg subcut q other wk.
**ADV EFF** **Anaphylaxis, bone marrow suppression, demyelinating diseases,** headache, HF, injection-site reactions, **malignancies, serious infections**
**INTERACTIONS** Anakinra, immunosuppressants, live vaccines
**NC/PT** High risk of infection; monitor pt, protect as appropriate. Monitor CNS for s&sx of demyelinating disorders. Advise pt to avoid preg. Teach proper administration/disposal of syringes. Tell pt to mark calendar for injection days, report s&sx of infection.

### adefovir dipivoxil
(Hepsera)
**CLASS** Antiviral, reverse transcriptase inhibitor
**PREG/CONT** C/NA

**BBW** Worsening hepatitis when discontinued. HIV resistance if used in undiagnosed HIV infection (test before use). Monitor for renal and hepatic toxicity. Withdraw drug and monitor if s&sx of lactic acidosis or steatosis.
**IND & DOSE** **Tx of chronic HBV.** *Adult, child ≥12 yr:* 10 mg/d PO.
**ADJUST DOSE** Renal impairment
**ADV EFF** Asthenia, elevated LFTs, **hepatitis exacerbation if discontinued, lactic acidosis, nephrotoxicity, severe hepatomegaly w/steatosis**
**INTERACTIONS** Nephrotoxic drugs; tenofovir (contraindicated)
**NC/PT** Test for HIV infection before starting tx. Monitor for renal/hepatic dysfx, lactic acidosis, steatosis. Advise against use in preg/breastfeeding. Drug does not cure disease; use precautions. Advise pt to not run out of drug (serious hepatitis can occur w/sudden stopping), report urine/stool color changes.

### adenosine (Adenocard)
**CLASS** Antiarrhythmic, diagnostic agent
**PREG/CONT** C/NA

**IND & DOSE** **Conversion to sinus rhythm from supraventricular tachycardia** *(Adenocard). Pts >50 kg:* 6 mg by IV bolus; may repeat within 1–2 min w/12-mg IV bolus up to two times. *Pts <50 kg:* 0.05–0.1 mg/kg rapid IV bolus; may repeat in 1–2 min. Max single dose, 0.3 mg/kg. **Diagnosis of suspected CAD, w/thallium.** *Adult:* 0.14 mg/kg/min IV over 6 min (total dose, 0.84 mg/kg); inject thallium at 3 min.
**ADV EFF** **Bronchoconstriction,** *facial flushing,* **fatal cardiac events, heart block, HTN, hypersensitivity reactions, hypotension, seizures, stroke**
**INTERACTIONS** Carbamazepine, digoxin, dipyridamole, theophylline, verapamil
**NC/PT** Do not refrigerate; discard unused portions. Have emergency equipment on standby and continuously monitor pt. Do not use in pts w/AV block, sinus node disease,

suspected bronchoconstrictive disease. Have methylxanthines on hand as antidote.

## ado-trastuzumab
(Kadcyla)
**CLASS** Antineoplastic, microtubular inhibitor
**PREG/CONT** High risk/NA

**BBW** Risk of hepatotoxicity, cardiac dysfx, death. Can cause fetal harm. Do not substitute for trastuzumab.
**IND & DOSE** **Tx of HER2-positive metastatic breast cancer in pts w prior tx or recurrence during or within 6 mo of tx; adjuvant tx of HER2-positive early breast cancer w/ residual invasive disease after neoadjuvant taxane- and trastuzumab-based tx.** *Adult:* 3.6 mg/kg as IV infusion q 3 wk until disease progression or toxicity. Do not exceed 3.6 mg/kg.
**ADV EFF** Constipation, fatigue, headache, **hemorrhage, hepatotoxicity, infusion reactions, left ventricular impairment,** musculoskeletal pain, neurotoxicity, **pulmonary toxicity,** thrombocytopenia
**INTERACTIONS** Strong CYP3A4 inhibitors; avoid this combo. Do not use w/5% dextrose solutions
**NC/PT** Ensure proper use; HER2 testing required. Do not substitute for trastuzumab. Rule out preg before starting tx (contraceptives advised); not for use in breastfeeding. Monitor LFTs, platelet count (before and periodically during tx), cardiac output, neuro/respiratory function. Infusion reaction may require slowing or interrupting infusion. Pt should mark calendar for infusion dates; take safety precautions w/neurotoxicity; report difficulty breathing, dark urine, yellowing of skin/eyes, abd pain, swelling, dizziness, unusual bleeding.

**DANGEROUS DRUG**

## afatinib (Gilotrif)
**CLASS** Antineoplastic, kinase inhibitor
**PREG/CONT** High risk/NA

**IND & DOSE** **First-line tx of pts w/ metastatic NSCLC whose tumors have eGFR exon 19 deletions or exon 21 substitution; tx of metastatic squamous NSCLC progressing after platinum-based tx.** *Adult:* 40 mg/d PO at least 1 hr before or 2 hr after meal.
**ADJUST DOSE** Renal impairment
**ADV EFF** Abd pain, **bullous/exfoliative skin disorders,** dehydration, **diarrhea, GI perforation, hepatotoxicity, ILD,** keratitis, n/v/d, rash, stomatitis, weight loss
**INTERACTIONS** P-gp inducers/ inhibitors
**NC/PT** Ensure proper dx. Monitor renal function/LFTs. Risk of dehydration. Pt should avoid preg/breastfeeding; perform proper mouth care; eat small, frequent meals; take drug at least 1 hr before or 2 hr after meal; report rash, difficulty breathing; severe n/v/d; urine/stool color changes.

## aflibercept (Eylea)
**CLASS** Fusion protein, ophthal agent
**PREG/CONT** Moderate risk/NA

**IND & DOSE** **Tx of pts w/neovascular (wet) age-related macular degeneration.** *Adult:* 2 mg (0.05 mL) by intravitreal injection q 4 wk for first 3 mo, then 2 mg once q 8 wk. **Tx of macular edema after retinal vein occlusion.** *Adult:* 2 mg by intravitreal injection q 4 wk. **Tx of diabetic macular edema/ diabetic retinopathy.** *Adult:* 2 mg by intravitreal injection q 4 wk for five injections, then once q 8 wk
**ADV EFF** Cataract, endophthalmitis, eye infections, eye pain, increased IOP, intraocular infection, retinal detachment, **thrombotic events,** vision changes, vitreous floaters

**NC/PT** Monitor pt closely during and immediately after injection. Contraception advised during and for 3 mo after tx; breastfeeding not advised during tx. Advise pt to immediately report eye redness, sensitivity to light, sudden vision changes.

## agalsidase beta

(Fabrazyme)
**CLASS** Enzyme
**PREG/CONT** B/NA

**IND & DOSE** **Tx of Fabry disease.** *Adult:* 1 mg/kg IV q 2 wk at no more than 0.25 mg/min.
**ADV EFF** **Anaphylaxis, potentially serious infusion reactions** (chills, fever, dyspnea, n/v, flushing, headache, chest pain, tachycardia, facial edema, rash)
**NC/PT** Ensure appropriate supportive measures available during infusion. Premedicate w/antipyretics; immediately discontinue if infusion reaction. Pt should report difficulty breathing, chest pain.

**DANGEROUS DRUG**

## albiglutide (Tanzeum)

**CLASS** Antidiabetic, GLP-1 receptor agonist
**PREG/CONT** C/NA

**BBW** Risk of thyroid C-cell tumors, including medullary thyroid carcinoma; not for use w/hx or family hx of thyroid cancer or multiple endocrine neoplasia syndrome type 2. Risk of acute renal injury.
**IND & DOSE** **Adjunct to diet/exercise to improve glycemic control in pts w/type 2 diabetes.** *Adult:* 30 mg subcut in abdomen, thigh, upper arm wkly; max, 50 mg/wk subcut.
**ADV EFF** Hypersensitivity reactions, hypoglycemia, injection-site reactions, n/v/d, **pancreatitis,** renal impairment
**INTERACTIONS** Oral medications (delays gastric emptying)
**NC/PT** Ensure proper use; not a first-line tx. Inject into abdomen, thigh, upper arm; rotate injection sites. Monitor glucose, renal function. May be combined w/other antidiabetics. Not for use in preg/breastfeeding, type 1 diabetes, ketoacidosis, preexisting GI disease. Pt should continue diet/exercise program; properly dispose of needles/syringes; report hypoglycemia episodes, severe abd pain, injection-site reactions.

## albumin (human)

(Albuminex, Kedbumin)
**CLASS** Blood product, plasma protein
**PREG/CONT** C/NA

**IND & DOSE** **Plasma volume expansion related to shock/burns/nephrosis, etc.** *Adult:* 5%—500 mL by IV infusion as rapidly as possible; additional 500 mg in 15–30 min; 20% or 25%—maintain plasma albumin conc at 2.5 ± 0.5 g/100 mL. *Child:* 0.6–1 g/kg, 25 g/d IV of 20% or 25%.
**ADV EFF** BP changes, chills, fever, flushing, HF, n/v, rash
**NC/PT** Monitor BP during infusion; discontinue if hypotension occurs. Stop infusion if headache, fever, BP changes occur; treat w/antihistamine. Adjust infusion rate based on pt response.

## albuterol sulfate

(AccuNeb, Proventil HFA, Ventolin HFA, VoSpire ER)
**CLASS** Antiasthmatic, beta agonist, bronchodilator, sympathomimetic
**PREG/CONT** C/NA

**IND & DOSE** **Relief, px of bronchospasm in COPD.** *Adult:* 2–4 mg PO tid–qid or 4–8 mg ER tablets q 12 hr. *Child 6–12 yr:* 2 mg PO 3–4 ×/d or 4 mg ER tablet PO q 12 hr. *Child 2–5 yr:* 0.1 mg/kg PO tid; max, 4 mg PO tid. **Acute bronchospasm.**

*Adult:* 1–2 inhalations q 4–6 hr; max, 12 inhalations/d; 2.5 mg tid–qid by nebulization. *Child 2–12 yr, >15 kg:* 2.5 mg bid–tid by nebulization; *<15 kg:* 0.5% sol tid–qid by nebulization over 5–15 min. **Exercise-induced bronchospasm.** *Adult, child ≥4 yr:* 2 inhalations 15–30 min before exercise.
**ADJUST DOSE** Elderly pts, pts sensitive to beta-adrenergic stimulation
**ADV EFF** Anxiety, apprehension, **bronchospasm, cardiac arrhythmias,** fear, flushing, n/v, pallor, sweating
**INTERACTIONS** Aminophylline, beta-adrenergics, digoxin, insulin, linezolid, QT-prolonging drugs, sympathomimetics
**NC/PT** Do not exceed recommended doses. Have beta blocker on standby. Pt should not cut/crush/chew tablets; should use caution (dizziness may occur), use inhalation for acute bronchospasm, report worsening of condition.

**DANGEROUS DRUG**

**aldesleukin** (Proleukin)
**CLASS** Antineoplastic, immune modulator (interleukin-2 product)
**PREG/CONT** C/NA

**BBW** Restrict use in pts w/abnormal pulmonary or cardiac tests or hx of pulmonary or cardiac disease. Risk of capillary leak syndrome, disseminated infections (antibiotic px recommended). Withhold if severe lethargy or somnolence.
**IND & DOSE Tx of metastatic renal carcinoma/metastatic melanoma.** *Adult:* 600,000 international units/kg IV q 8 hr over 15 min for total of 14 doses; 9 d of rest, then repeat. Max, 28 doses/course.
**ADV EFF Bone marrow suppression, cardiac arrhythmias, cardiotoxicity, hepatotoxicity, hypotension,** n/v/d, **nephrotoxicity, pulmonary toxicity**
**INTERACTIONS** Bone marrow suppressants, cardiotoxic drugs, CNS depressants, dexamethasone, hepatotoxic drugs, nephrotoxic drugs
**NC/PT** Obtain baseline ECG. Protect pt from infection (antibiotic px). Ensure proper mouth care. Pt should avoid preg/breastfeeding; report s&sx of bleeding, infection, severe lethargy.

**alectinib** (Alecensa)
**CLASS** Antineoplastic, kinase inhibitor
**PREG/CONT** High risk/NA

**IND & DOSE Tx of pts w/anaplastic lymphoma kinase-positive, metastatic NSCLC.** *Adult:* 600 mg PO bid w/food.
**ADV EFF Bradycardia,** constipation, edema, fatigue, **hepatotoxicity, interstitial pneumonitis, severe myalgia and CK elevation,** renal impairment.
**NC/PT** Ensure proper dx. Perform LFTs before and q 2 wk for first 2 mo, then periodically during use; dose adjustment may be needed. Monitor CK levels q 2 wk during first mo and w/complaints of muscle pain/weakness. Monitor lungs/HR regularly; adjust dose as needed. Not for use in preg (contraceptives advised)/breastfeeding. Pt should take daily w/food; report difficulty breathing, shortness of breath, muscle pain/weakness, urine/stool color changes.

**alemtuzumab** (Campath, Lemtrada)
**CLASS** Monoclonal antibody, MS drug
**PREG/CONT** C/NA

**BBW** *Campath:* Serious, including fatal, cytopenias, infusion reactions, infections, can occur. Limit doses to 30 mg (single) and 90 mg (cumulative wkly); higher doses increase risk of pancytopenia. Withhold for serious infusion reactions. Give px for *Pneumocystis jiroveci* pneumonia/herpes virus. Monitor during infusion. *Lemtrada:* Risk of serious to fatal autoimmune conditions and serious to life-threatening infusion reactions; monitor pt at least 2 hr postinfusion. Increased risk of malignancies. Ensure proper use; monitor pt closely. Serious/life-threatening stroke has been reported within 3 d of administration. Instruct pt to seek immediate care for stroke s&sx. Only available through restricted distribution program.

**IND & DOSE** **Tx of relapsing, remitting MS in pts intolerant to other tx (*Lemtrada*).** *Adult:* 12 mg/d IV over 4 hr on 5 consecutive d, then 12 mg/d on 3 consecutive d 12 mo after first tx course. **Tx of B-cell chronic lymphocytic leukemia (*Campath*):** 30 mg/d once, then increase to recommended dose of 30 mg/d 3 ×/wk IV for 12 wk if safe for pt. Premedicate w/oral antihistamine and acetaminophen.

**ADV EFF** **Autoimmune cytopenias, cancer development, hypersensitivity reactions, infusion reaction,** n/v/d, thyroid disorders, URI, urticaria

**NC/PT** Limit use to pts w/inadequate response to two or more other drugs. Premedicate w/corticosteroids, antivirals for herpes px. Monitor CBC monthly during and for 48 mo after last infusion. Monitor thyroid function q 3 mo until 48 mo after last infusion. Monitor pt closely during infusion; reaction can occur after infusion ends. Not for use in preg/breastfeeding. Protect pt from infection; ensure standard cancer screening. Do not administer live vaccines. Pt should take small, frequent meals; report fever, s&sx of infection, difficulty breathing.

## alendronate sodium

(Binosto, Fosamax)

**CLASS** Bisphosphonate, calcium regulator

**PREG/CONT** C/NA

**IND & DOSE** **Tx of postmenopausal osteoporosis; men w/osteoporosis.** *Adult:* 10 mg/d PO or 70 mg PO once a wk. **Px of osteoporosis.** *Adult:* 5 mg/d PO or 35 mg PO once wkly. **Tx of Paget disease.** *Adult:* 40 mg/d PO for 6 mo; may retreat after 6-mo tx-free period. **Tx of glucocorticoid-induced osteoporosis.** *Adult:* 5 mg/d PO (10 mg/d PO for postmenopausal women not on estrogen).

**ADJUST DOSE** Renal impairment

**ADV EFF** Bone pain, esophageal erosion, femur fractures, GI irritation, headache, hypocalcemia, n/v/d, osteonecrosis of jaw

**INTERACTIONS** Antacids, aspirin, calcium, iron, NSAIDs, ranitidine

**NC/PT** Give w/full glass of water or dissolve effervescent tablet in ½ glass water, wait 5 min, stir, then have pt swallow in a.m. at least 30 min before other food or medication; have pt stay upright for 30 min and until first food of day. Monitor serum calcium level; ensure pt has adequate calcium and vitamin D intake. Consider limiting use to 3–5 yr to decrease risk of long-bone fractures. Pt should report difficulty swallowing, bone pain.

## alfuzosin hydrochloride

(Uroxatral)

**CLASS** Alpha-adrenergic blocker, BPH drug

**PREG/CONT** B/NA

**IND & DOSE** **Tx of s&sx of BPH.** *Adult:* 10 mg/d PO after same meal each day.

**ADJUST DOSE** Hepatic impairment

**ADV EFF** Dizziness, intraop floppy iris syndrome, orthostatic hypotension, prolonged QT

**INTERACTIONS** Adrenergic blockers, antihypertensives, itraconazole, ketoconazole, nitrates, phosphodiesterase inhibitors, protease inhibitors, QT-prolonging drugs, ritonavir

**NC/PT** Ensure pt does not have prostate cancer. Monitor for orthostatic hypotension. Advise pt to change positions slowly, take safety precautions for dizziness; store tablets in dry place, protected from light. Pt should not cut/crush/chew tablets.

## alglucosidase alfa
(Lumizyme, Myozyme)
**CLASS** Enzyme, Pompe disease drug
**PREG/CONT** B/NA

**BBW** Risk of life-threatening anaphylactic reactions; have medical support readily available. Potential for rapid disease progression. Risk of cardiorespiratory failure; monitor pts w/ cardiorespiratory disorders carefully.
**IND & DOSE To increase ventilator-free survival in pts w/infantile-onset Pompe disease (*Myozyme*); tx of pts ≥8 yr w/Pompe disease (*Lumizyme*).** *Adult, child:* 20 mg/kg IV infusion over 4 hr q 2 wk.
**ADV EFF Anaphylaxis, cardiopulmonary failure,** chest discomfort, dyspnea, flushing, neck pain, **rapid progression of disease,** rash, urticaria, v/d
**NC/PT** Have medical support readily available during administration. Begin infusion at 1 mg/kg/hr; increase by 2 mg/kg/hr to reach desired dose, carefully monitoring pt response. *Lumizyme* available only by limited access program. Monitor for disease progression.

## alirocumab (Praluent)
**CLASS** PCSK9 inhibitor antibody
**PREG/CONT** Moderate risk/NA

**IND & DOSE Adjunct to diet/exercise to reduce risk of MI/stroke/ unstable angina; adjunct to diet, alone or w/other lipid-lowering tx, in pts w/primary hyperlipidemia to reduce LDL cholesterol.** *Adult:* 75 mg subcut once q 2 wk; max, 150 mg subcut once q 2 wk; or 300 mg subcut once q 4 wk.
**ADV EFF** Flulike sx, **hypersensitivity reactions,** injection-site reactions, nasopharyngitis
**NC/PT** Monitor LDL at baseline and periodically. Monitor for severe hypersensitivity reaction; stop drug, provide supportive care. Use caution in preg/breastfeeding. Ensure use of diet/exercise program. Teach proper administration/disposal of needles/ syringes and not to reuse or share syringe/pen. Pt should rotate injection sites w/each use, mark calendar for injection days, review information w/each prescription; report difficulty breathing, rash, injection-site pain/ inflammation.

## aliskiren (Tekturna)
**CLASS** Antihypertensive, renin inhibitor
**PREG/CONT** D/NA

**BBW** Use during preg can cause fetal injury or death.
**IND & DOSE Tx of HTN, alone or w/ other antihypertensives.** *Adult:* 150–300 mg/d PO. *Child >50 kg:* adult doses; *20–50 kg:* 75–150 mg/d PO; *<20 kg:* not recommended.
**ADJUST DOSE** Severe renal impairment
**ADV EFF Angioedema w/respiratory sx,** cough, diarrhea, dizziness, dyspepsia, fatigue, GERD, headache, hyperkalemia, hypotension, impaired renal function, URI
**INTERACTIONS** ACE inhibitors, ARBs, cyclosporine, furosemide, itraconazole, NSAIDs, thiazides
**NC/PT** Rule out preg; not for use in breastfeeding. Monitor potassium level, renal function tests. Store drug in dry place at room temp. Other drugs may also be needed to control BP; do not combine w/other drugs affecting renin system. Pt should report difficulty breathing, neck swelling, dizziness.

## allopurinol (Aloprim, Zyloprim)
**CLASS** Antigout, purine analog
**PREG/CONT** C/NA

**IND & DOSE Gout/hyperuricemia.** *Adult:* 100–800 mg/d PO in divided

doses. **Hyperuricosuria.** *Adult:* 200–300 mg/d PO. **Px of acute gouty attacks.** *Adult:* 100 mg/d PO; increase by 100 mg/d at wkly intervals until uric acid is 6 mg/dL or less. **Px of uric acid nephropathy in certain malignancies.** *Adult:* 600–800 mg/d PO for 2–3 d w/high fluid intake. *Child 6–10 yr:* 300 mg/d PO. *Child <6 yr:* 150 mg/d PO. **Recurrent calcium oxalate stones.** *Adult:* 200–300 mg/d PO. **Parenteral use.** *Adult:* 200–400 mg/m²/d IV to max of 600 mg/d as continuous infusion or at 6-, 8-, 12-hr intervals. *Child:* 200 mg/m²/d IV as continuous infusion or at 6-, 8-, 12-hr intervals.
**ADJUST DOSE** Elderly pts, renal impairment
**ADV EFF** Drowsiness, headache, n/v/d, **serious to fatal skin reactions**
**INTERACTIONS** ACE inhibitors, amoxicillin, ampicillin, anticoagulants, cyclophosphamide, theophylline, thiazides, thiopurines
**NC/PT** Give after meals; encourage 2.5–3 L/d fluid intake. Check urine alkalinity. Pt should discontinue at first sign of rash; avoid OTC medications.

## almotriptan malate (Axert)

**CLASS** Antimigraine, serotonin selective agonist, triptan
**PREG/CONT** C/NA

**IND & DOSE** **Tx of acute migraines w/ or w/o aura.** *Adult, child 12–17 yr:* 6.25–12.5 mg PO as single dose at first sign of migraine; may repeat in 2 hr. Max, two doses/24 hr.
**ADJUST DOSE** Hepatic/renal impairment
**ADV EFF** BP changes, dizziness, dry mouth, medication-overuse headache, **MI,** nausea, potentially fatal cerebrovascular events, pressure in chest, **serotonin syndrome**
**INTERACTIONS** Antifungals, antivirals, ergots, ketoconazole, macrolides, MAOIs, nefazodone, SSRIs
**NC/PT** For acute migraine, not px. Ensure pt has not used ergots within 24 hr. Not for use in preg. Pt should not take more than two doses/24 hr; discontinue if s&sx of angina; monitor environment. Drug overuse headache may require detoxification. Pt should report GI problems, numbness/tingling, chest pain.

## alogliptin (Nesina)

**CLASS** Antidiabetic, DPP-4 inhibitor
**PREG/CONT** B/NA

**IND & DOSE** **Adjunct to diet/exercise to improve glycemic control in type 2 diabetes.** *Adult:* 25 mg/d PO.
**ADJUST DOSE** Renal impairment
**ADV EFF** Headache, **hepatotoxicity, HF, hypersensitivity reactions,** hypoglycemia, nasopharyngitis, **pancreatitis, potentially debilitating arthralgia**, URI
**NC/PT** Ensure continued diet/exercise program. Not for use in type 1 diabetes. Monitor blood glucose; heart, renal, liver, pancreatic function. May give w/other antidiabetics. Pt should continue diet/exercise program, report severe joint pain (drug should be discontinued), abnormal swelling, chest pain, difficulty breathing, uncontrolled blood glucose, all herbs/other drugs used.

## alosetron (Lotronex)

**CLASS** 5-$HT_3$ antagonist, IBS drug
**PREG/CONT** B/NA

**BBW** Only indicated for women w/severe diarrhea-dominant IBS who have failed to respond to conventional tx. Ensure pt understands risks of use and warning signs to report. Discontinue immediately at s&sx of constipation, ischemic colitis.
**IND & DOSE** **Tx of severe diarrhea-predominant IBS in women w/ chronic IBS, no anatomic or**

**biochemical abnormalities of GI tract, and who have failed to respond to conventional therapy.** *Adult:* 0.5–1 mg PO bid.
**ADJUST DOSE** Elderly pts, mild to moderate hepatic impairment
**ADV EFF** Constipation, **ischemic colitis**
**INTERACTIONS** Cimetidine, clarithromycin, fluoroquinolones, fluvoxamine, GI motility drugs, itraconazole, ketoconazole, telithromycin, voriconazole
**NC/PT** Ensure pt has signed physician-pt agreement. Give w/ or w/o food. Monitor for s&sx of constipation. Not for use in preg. Regular follow-up required. Pt should report constipation.

**▶NEW DRUG**

**alpelisib** (Piqray)
**CLASS** Antineoplastic; kinase inhibitor
**PREG/CONT** High risk/NA

**IND & DOS** **Tx of HR-positive, HER2-negative, PIK3CA-mutated, advanced or metastatic breast cancer as detected by FDA-approved test after progression on or after an endocrine-based regimen in combo w/fulvestrant.** *Postmenopausal women/men:* 300 mg PO daily w/food.
**ADV EFF** Blood count decreases, diarrhea, fatigue, hyperglycemia, hypersensitivity, n/v, **pneumonitis**, rash, **severe cutaneous reactions**
**INTERACTIONS** BCRP inhibitors, CYP2C9 substrates, CYP3A4 inducers
**NC/PT** Continue tx until disease progression or unacceptable toxicity. Monitor for hypersensitivity reactions including severe cutaneous reactions, worsening respiratory sx, severe diarrhea. Monitor glucose level. Stress potential for embryo-fetal toxicity. Pt should avoid preg (contraception during tx and for 1 wk after tx advised); swallow whole w/ food.

**alpha$_1$-proteinase inhibitor** (Aralast NP, Glassia, Prolastin-C, Zemaira)
**CLASS** Blood product
**PREG/CONT** C/NA

**IND & DOSE** **Chronic replacement tx for pts w/congenital alpha$_1$-antitrypsin deficiency; tx of pts w/ early evidence of panacinar emphysema.** *Adult:* 60 mg/kg IV once wkly (*Aralast NP, Prolastin*). **Chronic augmentation and maint therapy of pts w/alpha$_1$-proteinase inhibitor deficiency w/emphysema.** *Adult:* 0.08 mL/kg/min IV over 15 min once/wk (*Zemaira*) or 60 mg/kg IV once/wk no faster than 0.04 mg/kg/min (*Glassia*).
**ADV EFF** Dizziness, fever, flulike sx, headache, light-headedness
**NC/PT** Do not mix w/other agents or diluting sols. Warn pt that this is a blood product and can carry risk of blood-borne diseases. Discontinue if s&sx of hypersensitivity. Pt should report fever, chills, joint pain.

**ALPRAZolam** (Xanax, Xanax XR)
**CLASS** Anxiolytic, benzodiazepine
**PREG/CONT** D/C-IV

**IND & DOSE** **Mgt of anxiety disorders; short-term relief of anxiety sx; anxiety associated w/depression.** *Adult:* 0.25–0.5 mg PO tid; adjust to max 4 mg/d in divided doses. **Panic disorder.** *Adult:* 0.5 mg PO tid; increase at 3- to 4-day intervals to 1–10 mg/d or 0.5–1 mg/d ER tablets. Range, 3–6 mg/d.
**ADJUST DOSE** Elderly pts, advanced hepatic disease, debilitation
**ADV EFF** Anger, apathy, confusion, constipation, crying, **CV collapse**, diarrhea, disorientation, drowsiness (initially), drug dependence (withdrawal syndrome when drug is discontinued), dry mouth, fatigue, hostility, lethargy, light-headedness,

mild paradoxical excitatory reactions during first 2 wk of tx, restlessness, sedation
**INTERACTIONS** Alcohol, carbamazepine, cimetidine, digoxin, disulfiram, grapefruit juice, hormonal contraceptives, isoniazid, kava, ketoconazole, levodopa, omeprazole, valerian root, valproic acid
**NC/PT** Taper gradually when discontinuing. Pt should avoid alcohol/grapefruit juice; take safety measures w/CNS effects; not cut/crush/chew ER tablet. Name confusion w/*Xanax* (alprazolam), *Celexa* (citalopram), and *Cerebyx* (fosphenytoin), and between alprazolam and lorazepam.

## alprostadil (Caverject, Caverject Impulse, Edex, Muse, Prostin VR Pediatric)
**CLASS** Prostaglandin
**PREG/CONT** Unkn/NA

**BBW** Apnea occurs in 10%–12% of neonates treated w/alprostadil, particularly those <2 kg. Monitor respiratory status continuously; have ventilatory assistance readily available. Move neonate often during first hr of infusion.
**IND & DOSE** **Tx of ED.** *Adult:* Intracavernous injection, 0.2–60 mcg using 0.5-in, 27–30G needle; may repeat up to 3 ×/wk. Urogenital system, 125–250 mcg; max, 2 systems/24 hr. **Palliative tx to temporarily maintain patency of ductus arteriosus.** *Child:* 0.025–0.05 mcg/kg/min IV infusion; max, 0.4 mcg/kg/min if needed.
**ADV EFF** **Apnea, bleeding,** bradycardia, **cardiac arrest,** flushing, hypotension, respiratory distress, tachycardia; w/intracavernous injection: **penile fibrosis,** priapism
**NC/PT** Constantly monitor arterial pressure and blood gases w/IV use. Use extreme caution. Teach pt injection technique/proper disposal of needles/syringes. Be aware of possible needle breakage (*Caverject Impulse*). Name confusion w/*Prostin VR Pediatric* (alprostadil), *Prostin* $F_2$ (dinoprost— available outside US), *Prostin* $E_2$ (dinoprostone), and *Prostin 15M* (carboprost in Europe).

**DANGEROUS DRUG**

## alteplase recombinant
(Activase, Cathflo Activase)
**CLASS** Thrombolytic enzyme, TPA
**PREG/CONT** C/NA

**IND & DOSE** **Acute MI.** *Adult>67 kg:* 100 mg as 15-mg IV bolus followed by 50 mg infused over 30 min; then 35 mg over next 60 min. *Adult≤67 kg:* 15-mg IV bolus followed by 0.75 mg/kg infused over 30 min (max, 50 mg); then 0.5 mg/kg over next 60 min (max, 35 mg). For 3-hr infusion, 60 mg in first hr (6–10 mg as bolus); 20 mg over second hr; 20 mg over third hr. Pts <65 kg should receive 1.25 mg/kg over 3 hr. **PE.** *Adult:* 100 mg IV infusion over 2 hr, followed immediately by heparin therapy when PTT or thrombin time returns to twice normal or less. **Acute ischemic stroke.** *Adult:* 0.9 mg/kg (max, 90 mg total dose) infused over 60 min w/10% given as IV bolus over first min. **Restoration of function of central venous access devices.** *Adult:* 2 mg (*Cathflo Activase*) in 2 mL sterile water for injection; may repeat after 2 hr.
**ADV EFF** **Bleeding, cardiac arrhythmias, intracranial hemorrhage,** n/v, urticaria
**INTERACTIONS** Anticoagulants, aspirin, dipyridamole
**NC/PT** Discontinue heparin and alteplase if serious bleeding occurs. Monitor coagulation studies; apply pressure or pressure dressings as needed to control bleeding. Type and cross-match blood. Initiate tx within first 6 hr of MI, within 3 hr of stroke.

DANGEROUS DRUG

## altretamine (Hexalen)

**CLASS** Antineoplastic
**PREG/CONT** D/NA

**BBW** Must be used under supervision of oncologist. Monitor blood counts regularly; monitor neuro exams regularly for neurotoxicity.
**IND & DOSE Palliative tx of pts w/ persistent or recurrent ovarian cancer after first-line therapy w/cisplatin and/or alkylating agent–based combo.** *Adult:* 260 mg/m$^2$/d PO for 14 or 21 consecutive d of 28-d cycle w/meals or at bedtime.
**ADV EFF Bone marrow depression, neurotoxicity,** n/v/d
**INTERACTIONS** Antidepressants, cimetidine, MAOIs, pyridoxine
**NC/PT** Not for use in preg/breastfeeding. Monitor blood counts regularly. Perform neuro exam before and regularly during tx. Give antiemetic if n/v severe. Pt should report s&sx of infection, numbness/tingling.

## aluminum hydroxide gel (generic)

**CLASS** Antacid
**PREG/CONT** Unkn/NA

**IND & DOSE Hyperacidity, symptomatic relief of upset stomach associated w/hyperacidity.** *Adult:* Tablets/capsules, 500–1,500 mg 3–6 ×/d PO between meals and at bedtime. Liquid, 5–10 mL between meals and at bedtime. *Child:* 5–15 mL PO q 3–6 hr or 1–3 hr after meals and at bedtime. **Px of GI bleeding in critically ill infants.** 2–5 mL/dose PO q 1–2 hr.
**ADV EFF** Constipation, **intestinal obstruction**
**INTERACTIONS** Benzodiazepines, corticosteroids, diflunisal, digoxin, fluoroquinolones, iron, isoniazid, oral drugs, penicillamine, phenothiazines, ranitidine, tetracyclines
**NC/PT** Do not give oral drugs within 1–2 hr of this drug. Monitor serum phosphorus levels w/long-term therapy. Advise pt to chew tables thoroughly and follow w/water. Constipation may occur.

## alvimopan (Entereg)

**CLASS** Peripheral mu-opioid receptor antagonist
**PREG/CONT** B/NA

**BBW** For short-term use in hospitalized pts only; risk of MI. Only available via restricted program for 15 doses.
**IND & DOSE To accelerate time to upper and lower GI recovery after partial large or small bowel resection surgery w/primary anastomosis.** *Adult:* 12 mg 30 min–5 hr before surgery, then 12 mg PO bid for up to 7 d. Max, 15 doses.
**ADJUST DOSE** Renal/hepatic impairment
**ADV EFF** Anemia, back pain, constipation, dyspepsia, flatulence, hypokalemia, **MI**, urine retention
**NC/PT** Not for use w/severe hepatic or renal dysfx. For short-term, in-hospital use only. Recent use of opioids may lead to increased adverse effects. Pt should report chest pain, urine retention.

## amantadine (Gocovri, Osmolex ER)

**CLASS** Antiparkinsonian, antiviral
**PREG/CONT** C/NA

**IND & DOSE Influenza A virus px or tx.** *Adult:* 200 mg/d PO or 100 mg PO bid for 10 d. *Child 9–12 yr:* 100 mg PO bid. *Child 1–9 yr:* 4.4–8.8 mg/kg/d PO in one or two divided doses; max, 150 mg/d. **Parkinsonism tx.** *Adult:* 100 mg PO bid (up to 400 mg/d). *Gocovri:* 137 mg PO daily at bedtime; after a week increase to 274 mg PO daily at bedtime. *Osmolex ER:* Initially, 129 mg PO daily; may increase wkly

to max 322 mg PO daily. **Drug-induced extrapyramidal reactions.** *Adult:* 100 mg PO bid, up to 300 mg/d in divided doses. *Osmolex ER:* Initially, 129 mg PO daily; may increase wkly to max 322 mg PO daily.
**ADJUST DOSE** Elderly pts, seizure disorders, renal disease
**ADV EFF** Dizziness, insomnia, n/d
**INTERACTIONS** Anticholinergics, hydrochlorothiazide, QT-prolonging drugs, triamterene
**NC/PT** Do not discontinue abruptly w/Parkinson disease. Dispense smallest amount possible. Pt should take safety precautions if dizziness occurs.

## ambrisentan (Letairis)

**CLASS** Antihypertensive, endothelin receptor antagonist
**PREG/CONT** High risk/NA

**BBW** Rule out preg before starting tx; may cause fetal harm. Pt should use two forms of contraception.
**IND & DOSE Tx of pulmonary arterial HTN to improve exercise ability and delay clinical worsening.** *Adult:* 5–10 mg/d PO.
**ADV EFF** Abd pain, anemia, constipation, decreased Hgb/sperm count, edema, fluid retention, flushing, **hepatic impairment,** nasal congestion, nasopharyngitis, sinusitis
**ADJUST DOSE** Hepatic impairment; not recommended
**INTERACTIONS** Cyclosporine
**NC/PT** Available only through restricted access program. May be combined w/tadalafil. Measure Hgb at start, at 1 mo, then periodically. Not for use in preg/breastfeeding; negative preg test, use of two forms of contraception required. Pt should report swelling, difficulty breathing; not cut/crush/chew tablets.

**▶NEW DRUG**

## amifampridine (Ruzurgi), amifampridine phosphate (Firdapse)

**CLASS** Cholinergic agonist, potassium channel blocker, orphan
**PREG/CONT** Unkn (Ruzurgi); moderate risk (Firdapse)/NA

**IND & DOSE Tx of Lambert-Eaton myasthenic syndrome in adult (*Firdapse*), child 6–16 yr (*Ruzurgi*).** *Adult:* Initially, 15–30 mg/d PO in three to four divided doses. Max single dose, 20 mg; max daily dose, 80 mg. *Child 6–16 yr, ≥45 kg:* Initially, 15–30 mg/d PO in two to three divided doses. Max single dose, 30 mg; max daily dose, 100 mg. *Child–16 yr, <45 kg:* Initially 7.5–15 mg/d PO in two to three divided doses. Max single dose, 15 mg; max daily dose, 50 mg.
**ADV EFF** Abd/back pain, diarrhea, dizziness, dyspepsia, headache, HTN, **hypersensitivity reactions,** muscle spasms, nausea, paresthesia/dysesthesia, **seizures,** URI
**INTERACTIONS** Drugs that lower seizure threshold or have cholinergic effects
**NC/PT** Start w/low dose; then titrate up. Use lowest recommended dose in renal/hepatic impairment or if known N-acetyltransferase 2 poor metabolism. May divide tablets and give via feeding tube in suspension form if needed. Give w/o regard to food. Watch for sx of hypersensitivity and seizures.

## amifostine (Ethyol)

**CLASS** Cytoprotective
**PREG/CONT** C/NA

**IND & DOSE To reduce cumulative renal toxicity associated w/cisplatin therapy in pts w/advanced ovarian cancer; to reduce incidence of moderate to severe xerostomia in pts w/ postop radiation for head/neck cancer.** *Adult:* 910 mg/$m^2$ IV daily over

15 min before chemo, over 3 min before radiation therapy.
**ADJUST DOSE** Elderly pts, CV disease
**ADV EFF** **Cutaneous reactions,** dizziness, hypocalcemia, hypotension, n/v
**INTERACTIONS** Cyclosporine
**NC/PT** Premedicate w/antiemetic, dexamethasone. Monitor BP carefully during tx. Discontinue at s&sx of cutaneous reaction. Pt should take safety precautions w/dizziness.

## amikacin sulfate (generic)
**CLASS** Aminoglycoside
**PREG/CONT** D/NA

**BBW** Monitor for nephrotoxicity, ototoxicity w/baseline and periodic renal function and neuro exams. Risk of serious toxicity, including neuromuscular blockade and respiratory paralysis.
**IND & DOSE** **Short-term tx of serious infections caused by susceptible strains of *Pseudomonas* sp, *Escherichia coli*, indole-positive and indole-negative *Proteus* sp, *Providencia* sp, *Klebsiella* sp, *Enterobacter* sp, *Serratia* sp, *Acinetobacter* sp, suspected gram-negative infections before susceptibility is known; initial tx of staphylococcal infection if penicillin contraindicated.** *Adult, child:* 15 mg/kg/d IM or IV in two–three equal doses at equal intervals, not to exceed 1.5 g/d, for 7–10 d. **UTIs.** *Adult, child:* 250 mg IM or IV bid.
**ADJUST DOSE** Elderly pts, renal failure
**ADV EFF** Anorexia, **nephrotoxicity,** n/v/d, ototoxicity, pain at injection site, superinfections
**INTERACTIONS** Hetastarch in IV sol, NMJ blockers, ototoxic drugs, penicillin
**NC/PT** Culture before tx. Monitor renal function, length of tx. Ensure pt well hydrated. Give IM dose by deep injection. Pt should report loss of hearing. Name confusion between amikacin and anakinra.

## aMILoride hydrochloride
(Midamor)
**CLASS** Potassium-sparing diuretic
**PREG/CONT** B/NA

**BBW** Monitor pt for hyperkalemia.
**IND & DOSE** **Adjunct tx for edema of HF or HTN; to prevent hypokalemia in pts at risk.** *Adult:* Add 5 mg/d PO to usual antihypertensive dose; may increase dose to 10–20 mg/d w/ careful electrolyte monitoring.
**ADV EFF** Anorexia, ED, n/v/d, weakness
**INTERACTIONS** ACE inhibitors, digoxin, potassium supplements, spironolactone, triamterene
**NC/PT** Give early in day w/food. Monitor weight, edema, serum electrolytes. Advise pt to take early in day (so increased urination will not disturb sleep) and avoid foods high in potassium.

## amino acids (Aminosyn, FreAmine, HepatAmine, ProcalAmine, etc)
**CLASS** Calorie agent, protein substrate
**PREG/CONT** C/NA

**IND & DOSE** **To provide nutrition to pts in negative nitrogen balance and unable to maintain in other ways.** *Adult:* 1–1.5 g/kg/d amino acid injection IV into peripheral vein; 250–500 mL/d amino acid injection IV mixed w/appropriate dextrose, vitamins, and electrolytes as part of TPN sol. Must be individualized. **Hepatic encephalopathy.** *Adult:* 80–120 g amino acid/d; 500 mL *HepatAmine* w/500 mL 50% dextrose and electrolyte sol IV over 8–12 hr/d. **Child w/renal failure.** 0.5–1 g/kg/d amino acid IV mixed w/dextrose as appropriate. **Amino acids replacement.** *Adult, child ≥16 yr:* 1.5 g/kg/d IV. *Child 13–15 yr:* 1.7 g/kg/d IV. *Child 4–12 yr:* 2 g/kg/d IV. *Child 1–3 yr:* 2–2.5 g/kg/d IV.

**ADV EFF** Dizziness, headache, infection, n/v, pain at infusion site, **pulmonary edema**
**INTERACTIONS** Tetracyclines
**NC/PT** Use strict aseptic technique in preparation/administration. Individualize dose based on lab values. Replace all IV apparatus daily. Infuse slowly; monitor closely. Pt should report difficulty breathing.

## aminocaproic acid
(Amicar)
**CLASS** Systemic hemostatic
**PREG/CONT** C/NA

**IND & DOSE** **Tx of excessive bleeding due to systemic hyperfibrinolysis/urinary fibrinolysis.** *Adult:* Initially, 5 g PO or IV followed by 1–1.25 g q hr to produce and sustain plasma levels of 0.13 mg/mL; do not give more than 30 g/d. **Acute bleeding.** *Adult:* 4–5 g IV in 250 mL diluent during first hr of infusion; then continuous infusion of 1 g/hr in 50 mL diluent. Continue for 8 hr or until bleeding stops. **Px of recurrence of subarachnoid hemorrhage.** *Adult:* 36 g/d PO or IV in six divided doses.
**ADV EFF** Abd cramps, dizziness, headache, malaise, n/v/d, **PE,** tinnitus
**INTERACTIONS** Estrogen, hormonal contraceptives
**NC/PT** Pt on oral therapy may need up to 10 tablets first hr and around-the-clock dosing. Orient/support pt if CNS effects occur. Monitor for s&sx of clotting.

## aminolevulinic acid hydrochloride (Gleolan, Levulan)
**CLASS** Photosensitizer
**PREG/CONT** C/NA

**IND & DOSE** **Tx of nonkeratotic actinic keratosis of face and scalp w/light therapy.** *Adult:* 20% sol applied directly to lesions, followed by light therapy within next 14–18 hr (scalp or face) or 3 hr (upper extremities); once q 8 wk if needed. **Adjunct for visualization of malignant tissue during surgery (*Gleolan*).** 20 mg/kg PO 3 hr before anesthesia.
**ADV EFF** Local crusting, local erosion, itching, photosensitivity, scaling, transient amnesia
**NC/PT** Clean and dry area; break ampule and apply directly to lesions. May repeat in 8 wk. Pt should avoid sunlight due to extreme photosensitivity, report amnestic episodes.

**DANGEROUS DRUG**

## amiodarone hydrochloride (Nexterone, Pacerone)
**CLASS** Adrenergic blocker, antiarrhythmic
**PREG/CONT** D/NA

**BBW** Reserve use for life-threatening arrhythmias; serious toxicity, including arrhythmias, pulmonary toxicity, possible.
**IND & DOSE** **Tx of life-threatening recurrent ventricular arrhythmias.** *Adult:* Loading dose, 800–1,600 mg/d PO in divided doses for 1–3 wk; reduce dose to 600–800 mg/d PO in divided doses for 1 mo; if rhythm stable, reduce dose to 400 mg/d PO in one to two divided doses for maint dose. Or, 1,000 mg IV over 24 hr: 150 mg IV loading dose over 10 min, followed by 360 mg IV over 6 hr at 1 mg/min, then 540 mg IV at 0.5 mg/min over next 18 hr. After first 24 hr, maint infusion of 0.5 mg/min (720 mg/24 hr) or less IV can be cautiously continued for 2–3 wk. Switch to PO form as soon as possible. Convert to PO dose based on duration of IV therapy: Less than 1 wk, initial PO dose is 800–1,600 mg; 1–3 wk, initial PO dose is 600–800 mg; more than 3 wk, initial PO dose is 400 mg.
**ADV EFF** Anorexia, ataxia, **cardiac arrest, cardiac arrhythmias,** constipation, corneal microdeposits, fatigue, **hepatotoxicity,** hyperthyroidism,

hypothyroidism, n/v, photosensitivity, **pulmonary toxicity**
**INTERACTIONS** Azole antifungals, beta blockers, calcium channel blockers, digoxin, ethotoin, fluoroquinolones, grapefruit juice, macrolide antibiotics, phenytoin, quinidine, ranolazine, simvastatin, thioridazine, trazodone, vardenafil, warfarin, ziprasidone
**NC/PT** Monitor cardiac rhythm continually and pulmonary function w/periodic chest X-ray. Regular blood tests and serum-level checks needed. Obtain baseline ophthal exam, then periodically. Not for use in preg. Pt should avoid grapefruit juice, report vision/breathing changes.

## amitriptyline hydrochloride (generic)

**CLASS** Antidepressant, TCA
**PREG/CONT** D/NA

**BBW** Increased risk of suicidality in child, adolescent, young adult; monitor carefully.
**IND & DOSE Relief of sx of depression (endogenous).** *Adult, hospitalized pts:* Initially, 100 mg/d PO in divided doses; gradually increase to 200–300 mg/d as needed. *Outpt:* Initially, 75 mg/d PO in divided doses; may increase to 150 mg/d. Maint dose, 40–100 mg/d (may give as single bedtime dose). *Child ≥12 yr:* 10 mg PO tid, then 20 mg at bedtime. **Chronic pain.** *Adult:* 75–150 mg/d PO.
**ADJUST DOSE** Elderly pts
**ADV EFF** Anticholinergic effects, confusion, constipation, disturbed concentration, dry mouth, **MI**, orthostatic hypotension, photosensitivity, sedation, **stroke**
**INTERACTIONS** Anticholinergics, barbiturates, cimetidine, clonidine, disulfiram, ephedrine, epinephrine, fluoxetine, furazolidone, hormonal contraceptives, levodopa, MAOIs, methylphenidate, nicotine, norepinephrine, phenothiazines, QT-prolonging drugs, thyroid medication
**NC/PT** Restrict drug access in depressed or suicidal pts; give major portion at bedtime. Pt should be aware of sedative effects and avoid driving, etc; not mix w/other sleep-inducing drugs; avoid prolonged exposure to sun or sunlamps; report thoughts of suicide.

## amLODIPine besylate

(Norvasc)
**CLASS** Antianginal, antihypertensive, calcium channel blocker
**PREG/CONT** C/NA

**IND & DOSE Tx of chronic stable angina/Prinzmetal angina; to reduce angina risk and need for revascularization procedures in pts w/CAD w/o HF; tx of essential HTN.** *Adult:* Initially, 5 mg/d PO; may gradually increase dose over 7–14 d to max 10 mg/d PO. **Tx of HTN.** *Child 6–17 yr:* 2.5–5 mg/d PO.
**ADJUST DOSE** Elderly pts, hepatic impairment
**ADV EFF Angina,** dizziness, fatigue, flushing, headache, hypotension, lethargy, light-headedness, MI, nausea, peripheral edema
**INTERACTIONS** Anticholinergics, barbiturates, cimetidine, clonidine, disulfiram, ephedrine, epinephrine, fluoxetine, furazolidone, hormonal contraceptives, levodopa, MAOIs, methylphenidate, nicotine, norepinephrine, phenothiazines, QT-prolonging drugs, simvastatin, thyroid medication
**NC/PT** Monitor closely when adjusting dose; monitor BP w/hx of nitrate use. Monitor cardiac rhythm during initiation and periodically during tx. Not for use in breastfeeding. Name confusion between *Norvasc* (amlodipine) and *Navane* (thiothixene).

## ammonium chloride
(generic)
**CLASS** Electrolyte, urine acidifier
**PREG/CONT** C/NA

**IND & DOSE Tx of hypochloremic states and metabolic alkalosis; urine acidification.** *Adult:* Dosage determined by pt's condition and tolerance. Monitor dosage rate and amount by repeated serum bicarbonate determinations. IV infusion should not exceed conc of 1%–2% of ammonium chloride
**ADV EFF Ammonia toxicity, hepatic impairment,** pain at injection site
**INTERACTIONS** Amphetamine, chlorpropamide, dextroamphetamine, ephedrine, flecainide, methadone, methamphetamine, mexiletine, pseudoephedrine
**NC/PT** Give IV slowly. Monitor for possible fluid overload, acidosis; have sodium bicarbonate or sodium lactate available in case of overdose.

## amoxapine (generic)
**CLASS** Anxiolytic, TCA
**PREG/CONT** C/NA

**BBW** Increased risk of suicidality in child, adolescent, young adult; monitor carefully.
**IND & DOSE Relief of sx of depression; tx of depression w/anxiety or agitation.** *Adult:* Initially, 50 mg PO bid–tid; gradually increase to 100 mg PO bid–tid by end of first wk if tolerated; increase above 300 mg/d only if dosage ineffective for at least 2 wk. Usual effective dose, 200–300 mg/d.
**ADJUST DOSE** Elderly pts
**ADV EFF** Anticholinergic effects, confusion, constipation, disturbed concentration, dry mouth, **MI,** orthostatic hypotension, photosensitivity, sedation, **stroke**
**INTERACTIONS** Anticholinergics, barbiturates, cimetidine, clonidine, disulfiram, ephedrine, epinephrine, fluoxetine, furazolidone, hormonal contraceptives, levodopa, MAOIs, methylphenidate, nicotine, norepinephrine, phenothiazines, QT-prolonging drugs, thyroid medication
**NC/PT** Restrict drug access in depressed or suicidal pts; give major portion at bedtime. Pt should be aware of sedative effects and avoid driving, etc; should not mix w/other sleep-inducing drugs; should avoid prolonged exposure to sun or sunlamps; report thoughts of suicide.

## amoxicillin (Amoxil, Moxatag)
**CLASS** Antibiotic, penicillin-type
**PREG/CONT** B/NA

**IND & DOSE Tx of tonsillitis/pharyngitis caused by *Streptococcus pyogenes* (ER tablet); infections due to susceptible strains of *Haemophilus influenzae, Escherichia coli, Proteus mirabilis, Neisseria gonorrhoeae, Streptococcus pneumoniae, Enterococcus faecalis,* streptococci, non–penicillinase-producing staphylococci, *Helicobacter pylori* infection in combo w/other agents; postexposure px against *Bacillus anthracis.*** *Adult, child >40 kg:* URIs, GU, skin and soft-tissue infections, 250 mg PO q 8 hr or 500 mg PO q 12 hr; severe infection, 500 mg PO q 8 hr or 875 mg PO q 12 hr; postexposure anthrax px, 500 mg PO tid to complete 60-day course after 14–21 d of a fluoroquinolone or doxycycline; lower respiratory infection, 500 mg PO q 8 hr or 875 mg PO bid; uncomplicated gonococcal infections, 3 g amoxicillin PO as single dose; *C. trachomatis* in preg, 500 mg PO tid for 7 d or 875 mg PO bid; tonsillitis/pharyngitis, 775 mg/d PO for 10 d w/food (ER tablet); *H. pylori* infection, 1 g PO bid w/clarithromycin 500 mg PO bid and lansoprazole030 mg PO bid for 14 d. *Child ≥3 mo, <40 kg:* URIs, GU infections, skin and soft-tissue infections, 20 mg/kg/d PO in divided doses q 8 hr or 25 mg/kg/d PO in divided doses q 12 hr; severe infection, 40 mg/kg/d PO in divided doses q 8 hr or 45 mg/kg/d

PO in divided doses q 12 hr; postexposure anthrax px, 80 mg/kg/d PO divided in three doses to complete 60-day course after 14–21 d of fluoroquinolone or doxycycline tx. *Child ≥3 mo:* Mild to moderate URIs, GU infections, skin infections, 20 mg/kg PO daily in divided doses q 8 hr or 25 mg/kg PO in divided doses q 12 hr; acute otitis media, 80–90 mg/kg/d PO for 10 d (severe cases) or 5–7 d (moderate cases); gonorrhea in prepubertal child, 50 mg/kg PO w/25 mg/kg probenecid PO as single dose; lower respiratory infections/severe URI, GU, and skin infections, 40 mg/kg PO daily in divided doses q 8 hr or 45 mg/kg PO daily in divided doses q 12 hr. *Child up to 12 wk:* 30 mg/kg PO daily in divided doses q 12 hr.
**ADJUST DOSE** Renal impairment
**ADV EFF** Abd pain, **anaphylaxis,** fever, gastritis, glossitis, n/v/d, sore mouth, superinfections, wheezing
**INTERACTIONS** Chloramphenicol, hormonal contraceptives, probenecid, tetracyclines
**NC/PT** Culture before tx. Monitor for superinfections; n/v/d may occur. Pt should not cut/crush/chew ER tablets; should continue until at least 2 d after s&sx resolve; complete full course.

---

**amphetamine** (Adzenys XR-ODT, Evekeo, Mydayis)
**CLASS** CNS stimulant
**PREG/CONT** High risk/C-II

**BBW** High risk of abuse and dependence; select pt accordingly/monitor closely.
**IND & DOSE Tx of ADHD in pts ≥6 yr.** *Adult:* 12.5 mg/d PO in a.m. *Adult, child ≥13 yr:* 12.5 mg/d PO (*Mydayis*); titrate to max 50 mg/d (adult), 25 mg/d (child). *Child 6–17 yr:* 6.3 mg/d PO in a.m. (*Adzenys XR-ODT*). Max: 12.5 mg/d for child 13–17 yr, 18.8 mg/d for child 6–12 yr. *Child ≥6 yr:* 5 mg/d or bid PO based on response (*Evekeo*). *Child 3–5 yr:* 2.5 mg/d PO (*Evekeo*). **Tx of narcolepsy.** *Adult:* 5–60 mg/d PO (*Evekeo*). **Tx of exogenous obesity.** *Adult, child >12 yr:* Up to 30 mg/d PO in divided doses (*Evekeo*).
**ADJUST DOSE** Renal impairment (*Mydayis*)
**ADV EFF** Abd pain, agitation, anorexia, growth suppression, HTN, nervousness, n/v/d, peripheral vascular disease, psychiatric adverse reactions, **sudden cardiac death,** tachycardia, weight loss. *Mydayis:* **CV reactions,** decreased appetite, irritability, seizures, serotonin syndrome
**INTERACTIONS** Acidifying, alkalinizing agents, MAOIs (*Mydayis*), serotonergic agents
**NC/PT** Ensure proper dx/baseline ECG. Include as part of team approach to tx. Do not substitute for other amphetamine-containing products; dosages vary. Monitor BP/P regularly. Monitor growth/weight in child. Evaluate for bipolar disorder before use. Arrange for periodic breaks to evaluate need for drug. Pt must allow tablet to dissolve in saliva on the tongue (*Adzenys*), then swallow; take once daily in a.m.; secure drug (a controlled substance). Pt should take drug first thing in a.m.; take consistently w/or w/out food; avoid preg (contraceptives advised)/breastfeeding; be aware of abuse/dependence potential; report insomnia, numbness/tingling, chest pain, significant weight loss, abnormal thoughts, palpitations.

---

**DANGEROUS DRUG**

**amphotericin B; amphotericin B cholesteryl sulfate; amphotericin B, liposome** (Abelcet, AmBisome)
**CLASS** Antifungal
**PREG/CONT** B/NA

**BBW** Reserve systemic use for progressive or potentially fatal infections. Not for use in noninvasive disease; toxicity can be severe.

**IND & DOSE Tx of potentially fatal, progressive fungal infections not responsive to other tx.** *Adult, child:* 5 mg/kg/d IV as single infusion at 2.5 mg/kg/hr (*Abelcet*). **Aspergillosis.** *Adult, child:* 3 mg/kg/d IV over more than 2 hr (*AmBisome*). **Presumed fungal infection in febrile neutropenic pts.** *Adult, child:* 3 mg/kg/d IV (*AmBisome*). **Cryptococcal meningitis in HIV pts.** *Adult, child:* 6 mg/kg/d IV (*AmBisome*). **Leishmaniasis.** *Adult, child:* 3 mg/kg/d IV, days 1–5, 14, and 21 for immunocompetent pts; 4 mg/kg/d IV, days 1–5, 10, 17, 24, 31, and 38 for immunocompromised pts (*AmBisome*).
**ADV EFF** Cramping, dyspepsia, electrolyte disturbances, n/v/d, pain at injection site, **renal toxicity**
**INTERACTIONS** Antineoplastics, corticosteroids, cyclosporine, digitalis, nephrotoxic drugs, thiazide diuretics, zidovudine
**NC/PT** Dose varies among brand names; check carefully. Culture before tx. Monitor injection sites, electrolytes, kidney function. Use antihistamines, aspirin, antiemetics, meperidine to improve comfort, drug tolerance.

## ampicillin (generic)
**CLASS** Antibiotic, penicillin
**PREG/CONT** B/NA

**IND & DOSE Tx of bacterial infections caused by susceptible strains; tx of GU infections.** *Adult:* 500 mg IM, IV, PO q 6 hr. **Tx of respiratory tract infections.** *Adult:* 250 mg IM, IV, PO q 6 hr. **Tx of digestive system infections.** *Adult:* 500 mg PO q 6 hr for 48–72 hr after pt asymptomatic or eradication evident. **Tx of STDs in pts allergic to tetracycline.** *Adult:* 3.5 g ampicillin PO w/1 g probenecid. **Px of bacterial endocarditis for dental, oral, or upper respiratory procedures in pts at high risk.** *Adult:* 2 g ampicillin IM or IV within 30 min of procedure. *Child:* 50 mg/kg ampicillin IM or IV within 30 min of procedure. Six hr later, 25 mg/kg ampicillin IM or IV or 25 mg/kg amoxicillin PO. **Tx of respiratory and soft-tissue infections.** *Adult, child ≥40 kg:* 250–500 mg IV or IM q 6 hr. *<40 kg:* 25–50 mg/kg/d IM or IV in equally divided doses at 6- to 8-hr intervals. *20–40 kg:* 250 mg PO q 6 hr. *<20 kg:* 50 mg/kg/d PO in equally divided doses q 6–8 hr. **Tx of GI and GU infections, including women w/*N. gonorrhoeae*.** *Adult, child >40 kg:* 500 mg IM or IV q 6 hr. *≤40 kg:* 50 mg/kg/d IM or IV in equally divided doses q 6–8 hr. *20–40 kg:* 500 mg PO q 6 hr. *<20 kg:* 100 mg/kg/d PO in equally divided doses q 6–8 hr. **Tx of bacterial meningitis.** *Adult, child:* 150–200 mg/kg/d by continuous IV drip, then IM injections in equally divided doses q 3–4 hr. **Tx of septicemia.** *Adult, child:* 150–200 mg/kg/d IV for at least 3 d, then IM q 3–4 hr.
**ADJUST DOSE** Renal impairment
**ADV EFF** Abd pain, **anaphylaxis,** fever, gastritis, glossitis, n/v/d, sore mouth, superinfections, wheezing
**INTERACTIONS** Atenolol, chloramphenicol, hormonal contraceptives, probenecid, tetracyclines
**NC/PT** Culture before tx. Give on empty stomach. Do not give IM injections in same site. Check IV site for thrombosis. Monitor for superinfections. Pt should use second form of contraception while on drug. May experience n/v/d.

## anagrelide (Agrylin)
**CLASS** Antiplatelet
**PREG/CONT** C/NA

**IND & DOSE Tx of essential thrombocythemia secondary to myeloproliferative disorders to reduce elevated platelet count and risk of thrombosis; to improve associated s&sx, including thrombohemorrhagic events.** *Adult:* Initially, 0.5 mg PO qid or 1 mg PO bid; do not increase by more than 0.5 mg/d each wk. Max, 10 mg/d or 2.5 mg as single dose. *Child:* Initially, 0.5 mg/d PO; do not increase by more than 0.5 mg/d each wk. Max, 10 mg/d or 2.5 mg in single dose.

**ADJUST DOSE** Moderate hepatic impairment
**ADV EFF** Abd pain, asthenia, **bleeding, complete heart block,** headache, **HF, MI,** n/v/d, palpitations, **pancreatitis, prolonged QT,** thrombocytopenia
**INTERACTIONS** Aspirin, drugs that affect bleeding, grapefruit juice, NSAIDs
**NC/PT** Pretreatment ECG; assess for cardiopulmonary disease. Obtain platelet count q 2 d for first wk, then wkly. Provide safety measures. Monitor for bleeding; mark chart for alert in invasive procedures. Not for use in preg. Pt should take on empty stomach; avoid grapefruit juice; report bleeding, chest pain, swelling. Name confusion between *Agrylin* and *Aggrastat* (tirofiban).

## anakinra (Kineret)

**CLASS** Antiarthritic, interleukin-1 receptor antagonist
**PREG/CONT** B/NA

**IND & DOSE To reduce s&sx and slow progression of moderately to severely active RA in pts who have failed on one or more DMARDs.** *Adult ≥18 yr:* 100 mg/d subcut at about same time each day. **Tx of neonatal-onset multisystem inflammatory disease.** *Child:* 1–2 mg/kg/d subcut to max 8 mg/kg/d.
**ADJUST DOSE** Renal impairment, elderly pts
**ADV EFF** Hypersensitivity reactions, infections, injection-site reactions, sinusitis, URI
**INTERACTIONS** Etanercept; immunizations; TNF blockers (increased risk of serious infection; combo not recommended)
**NC/PT** Store refrigerated, protected from light. Obtain neutrophil count regularly. Not for use in preg. Rotate inject sites. Other antiarthritics may also be needed. Pt should dispose of needles/syringes appropriately, report s&sx of infection. Name confusion between anakinra and amikacin.

**DANGEROUS DRUG**

## anastrozole (Arimidex)

**CLASS** Antiestrogen, antineoplastic, aromatase inhibitor
**PREG/CONT** X/NA

**IND & DOSE Tx of advanced breast cancer in postmenopausal women w/disease progression after tamoxifen tx; first-line tx of postmenopausal women w/hormone receptor (HR)–positive or HR–unkn locally advanced or metastatic breast cancer; adjuvant tx of postmenopausal women w/HR–positive early breast cancer.** *Adult:* 1 mg/d PO.
**ADV EFF** Asthenia, back pain, bone pain, CV events, decreased bone density, fractures, hot flashes, insomnia, n/v, pharyngitis
**INTERACTIONS** Estrogens, tamoxifen
**NC/PT** Monitor lipid levels periodically, bone density. Use analgesics for pain. Not for use in preg.

## angiotensin II (Giapreza)

**CLASS** Vasoconstrictor
**PREG/CONT** Unkn/NA

**IND & DOSE To increase BP in pts w/ septic or other distributive shock.** *Adult:* 20 ng/kg/min IV; titrate as frequently as q 5 min by increments of up to 15 ng/kg/min. Max dose: no greater than 80 ng/kg/min during first 3 hr. Maint dose: not over 40 ng/kg/min.
**ADV EFF** **Acidosis, delirium,** fungal infection, hyperglycemia, **peripheral ischemia,** tachycardia, **thromboembolic events.**
**INTERACTIONS** ACE inhibitors, ARBs
**NC/PT** Dilute in NSS before use. Discard diluted sol after 24 hr.

## anidulafungin (Eraxis)

**CLASS** Antifungal, echinocandin
**PREG/CONT** Unkn/NA

**IND & DOSE Tx of candidemia/ other *Candida* infections.** *Adult:* 200 mg

by IV infusion on day 1, then 100 mg/d by IV infusion; generally for minimum of 14 d. **Tx of esophageal candidiasis.** *Adult:* 100 mg by IV infusion on day 1, then 50 mg/d by IV infusion for minimum of 14 d.
**ADV EFF** **Liver toxicity,** n/v/d
**NC/PT** Culture before tx. Monitor LFTs. Not for use in preg/breastfeeding. Pt should maintain fluid/food intake, report urine/stool color changes.

## antihemophilic factor
(Advate, Hemofil M, Humate-P, ReFacto, Wilate, Xyntha)
**CLASS** Antihemophilic
**PREG/CONT** C/NA

**IND & DOSE** **Tx of hemophilia A; short-term px (*ReFacto*) to reduce frequency of spontaneous bleeding; surgical or invasive procedures in pts w/von Willebrand disease in whom desmopressin is ineffective or contraindicated.** *Adult, child:* Dose depends on weight, severity of deficiency, severity of bleeding; monitor factor VIII levels to establish dose needed. Follow tx carefully w/factor VIII level assays. Formulas used as dosage guide:

$$\text{Expected Factor VIII increase (\% of normal)} = \frac{\text{AHF/IU given} \times 2}{\text{weight in kg}}$$

$$\text{AHF/IU required} = \text{weight (kg)} \times \text{desired factor VIII increase (\% of normal)} \times 0.5$$

**ADV EFF** **AIDS** (from repeated use of blood products), **bronchospasm, hemolysis, hepatitis,** stinging at infusion site, tachycardia
**NC/PT** Monitor factor VIII levels regularly. Monitor P. Reduce infusion rate w/significant tachycardia. Pt should wear or carry medical alert information.

## antihemophilic factor (factor VIII) (recombinant)
(Kovaltry, Novoeight, Nuwiq)
**CLASS** Clotting factor
**PREG/CONT** Unkn/NA

**IND & DOSE** **Tx/control of bleeding episodes, periop bleeding mgt in pts w/hemophilia A.** *Adult, child:* Dose per calculations on FDA label **Px to reduce bleeding episodes in hemophilia A.** *Adult, child 12–17 yr:* 30–40 international units/kg IV q other day. *Child 2–11 yr:* 25–50 international units/kg q other day or 3 ×/wk.
**ADV EFF** Back pain, dry mouth, headache, **hypersensitivity reactions,** factor VIII antibody production, injection-site reaction, vertigo
**NC/PT** Ensure dx; not for tx of von Willebrand disease. For acute use, refer to guidelines for usual dosage; use formula to determine actual dose. Use caution in preg/breastfeeding. For px, teach proper storage/administration/reconstitution, disposal of needles/syringes; recommend med-alert identification. Pt should report difficulty breathing, chest pain, numbness/tingling, continued bleeding.

## antihemophilic factor (recombinant) Fc fusion protein (Eloctate)
**CLASS** Antihemophilic
**PREG/CONT** Unkn/NA

**IND & DOSE** **Tx of congenital hemophilia A (for bleeding episodes, periop use).** *Adult, child:* Given IV:

$$\text{Expected Factor VIII increase (\% of normal)} = \frac{\text{AHF/IU given} \times 2}{\text{weight in kg}}$$

$$\text{AHF/IU required} = \text{weight (kg)} \times \text{desired factor VIII increase (\% of normal)} \times 0.5$$

**Routine px of bleeding in congenital hemophilia A.** 50 international units/kg

IV q 4 d; based on response, range 25–65 international units/kg q 3–5 d.
**ADV EFF** **Anaphylaxis,** arthralgia, myalgia
**NC/PT** Monitor factor VIII levels regularly. Monitor P. Reduce infusion rate w/significant tachycardia. Use caution in preg. Pt should wear or carry medical alert information.

## antihemophilic factor (recombinant) porcine sequence (Obizur)

**CLASS** Antihemophilic
**PREG/CONT** C/NA

**IND & DOSE** **Tx of bleeding episodes in adults w/acquired hemophilia A.** *Adult:* 200 units/kg IV; titrate based on response and factor VIII recovery.
**ADV EFF** **Anaphylaxis,** inhibitory antibody production
**NC/PT** Monitor factor VIII levels and pt closely during infusion. Pt should wear or carry medical alert information; use caution in preg.

## antithrombin, recombinant (ATryn)

**CLASS** Coagulation inhibitor
**PREG/CONT** C/NA

**IND & DOSE** **Px of periop and peripartum thromboembolic events in pts w/hereditary antithrombin deficiency.** *Adult:* Individualize dose based on antithrombin level; loading dose over 15 min IV followed by maint dose to keep antithrombin activity levels 80%–120% of normal. Surgical pts, use formula 100 – baseline antithrombin activity ÷ 2.3 × body wt; maint, divide by 10.2. Preg pt, 100 – baseline antithrombin activity ÷ 1.3 × body wt; maint, divide by 5.4.
**ADV EFF** **Hemorrhage,** infusion-site reactions
**INTERACTIONS** Heparin, low-molecular-weight heparin
**NC/PT** Not for use w/allergy to goats or goat products. Follow clotting studies closely.

## antithrombin III (Thrombate III)

**CLASS** Coagulation inhibitor
**PREG/CONT** C/NA

**IND & DOSE** **Tx of pts w/hereditary antithrombin III deficiency in connection w/surgical or obstetrical procedures or when suffering from thromboembolism; replacement tx in congenital antithrombin III deficiency.** *Adult:* Dosage units = desired antithrombin level (%) – baseline antithrombin level (%) × body wt (kg) ÷ 1.4 q 2–8 d IV.
**ADV EFF** **Hemorrhage,** infusion-site reactions
**INTERACTIONS** Heparin, low-molecular-weight heparin
**NC/PT** Frequent blood tests required. Dosage varies widely. Monitor for bleeding. Human blood product; slight risk of blood-transmitted diseases.

## apalutamide (Erleada)

**CLASS** Androgen receptor inhibitor
**PREG/CONT** High risk/NA

**IND & DOSE** Tx of metastatic and nonmetastatic castration-resistant prostate cancer. *Adult:* 240 mg (four 60-mg tablets) PO daily.
**ADV EFF** Arthralgia, **CV events,** decreased appetite, diarrhea, fall, fatigue, fracture, hot flush, HTN, nausea, peripheral edema, rash, **seizures,** weight loss
**INTERACTIONS** Substrates of BCRP, CYP2C9, CYP2C19, CYP3A4, OATP1B1, P-gp, UGT; may decrease effectiveness of these drugs
**NC/PT** Pt should receive a gonadotropin-releasing hormone analog concurrently or should have had bilateral orchiectomy. Assess pt fall/fracture risk before starting drug; warn

pt of increased fall/fracture risk, increased risk of seizures. Not indicated for females; warn males about high embryo-fetal risk (contraceptives during tx and for at least 3 mo after tx advised). Pt may take drug w/ or w/o food.

**DANGEROUS DRUG**

## apixaban (Eliquis)

**CLASS** Anticoagulant, direct thrombin inhibitor
**PREG/CONT** B/NA

**BBW** Premature discontinuation increases risk of thrombotic events; consider coverage w/another anticoagulant if discontinued for reasons other than pathological bleeding. Risk of epidural/spinal hematomas if used in pts w/spinal puncture of anesthesia.
**IND & DOSE** **To reduce stroke, embolism in pts w/nonvalvular atrial fibrillation.** *Adult:* 5 mg PO bid; reduce to 2.5 mg PO bid if age >80 yr, weight >60 kg, serum creatinine >1.5 mg/dL. **Px of DVT after hip/knee replacement.** *Adult:* 2.5 mg PO bid. **Tx of DVT/PE.** *Adult:* 10 mg PO bid for 7 d, then 5 mg PO bid. **To reduce risk of recurrent DVT/PE.** *Adult:* 2.5 mg PO bid.
**ADJUST DOSE** Elderly pts, severe renal impairment
**ADV EFF** **Bleeding, rebound thrombotic events w/discontinuation, severe hypersensitivity reactions**
**INTERACTIONS** Carbamazepine, clarithromycin, itraconazole, ketoconazole, other drugs that increase bleeding, phenytoin, rifampin, ritonavir, St. John's wort
**NC/PT** Not for use w/artificial heart valves or antiphospholipid syndrome. Reversal agent is available. Monitor for bleeding; do not stop suddenly. Pt should avoid preg/breastfeeding, OTC drugs that affect bleeding; not stop drug suddenly; take safety precautions to avoid injury; report increased bleeding, chest pain, headache, dizziness.

## apomorphine (Apokyn)

**CLASS** Antiparkinsonian, dopamine agonist
**PREG/CONT** C/NA

**IND & DOSE** **Intermittent tx of hypomobility "off" episodes caused by advanced Parkinson disease.** *Adult:* 2 mg subcut; increase slowly to max of 6 mg. Give 300 mg trimethobenzamide PO tid for 3 d before starting to completion of 2 mo of tx.
**ADV EFF** Chest pain, compulsive behaviors, dizziness, dyskinesia, edema, **fibrotic complications,** flushing, hallucinations, **hepatic impairment,** hypotension, **hypersensitivity,** loss of impulse control, n/v, **renal impairment,** rhinorrhea, sedation, somnolence, **syncope,** sweating, yawning
**INTERACTIONS** Antihypertensives, dopamine antagonists, 5-$HT_3$ antagonists (granisetron, ondansetron, etc), QT-prolonging drugs, vasodilators
**NC/PT** Give subcut injection in stomach, upper arm, or leg; rotate sites. Protect pt when CNS effects occur. Teach proper administration/disposal of needles/syringes. Many CNS effects possible; pt should take safety precautions w/CNS changes, hypotension.

## apremilast (Otezla)

**CLASS** Antiarthritic, phosphodiesterase-4 inhibitor
**PREG/CONT** C/NA

**IND & DOSE** **Tx of active psoriatic arthritis, moderate to severe plaque psoriasis, oral ulcers associated w/ Behçet disease.** *Adult:* 30 mg PO bid. Titrate as follows: Day 1, 10 mg PO in a.m.; day 2, 10 mg PO in a.m. and p.m.; day 3, 10 mg PO in a.m. and 20 mg PO in p.m.; day 4, 20 mg in a.m. and p.m.; day 5, 20 mg in a.m. and 30 mg in p.m.; day 6 and thereafter, 30 mg PO bid.
**ADJUST DOSE** Renal disease

**ADV EFF** Depression, headache, n/v/d (possibly severe), weight loss
**INTERACTIONS** Carbamazepine, phenobarbital, phenytoin, rifampin
**NC/PT** Titrate dose to effective level to decrease GI effects. Give small, frequent meals. May need to decrease dose or stop drug if severe n/v/d. Monitor weight loss; stop drug if significant. Watch for depression, possible suicidality. Pt should take daily as directed, report severe GI upset, significant weight loss, thoughts of suicide, increasing depression.

## **aprepitant** (Cinvanti, Emend), **fosaprepitant** (Emend for Injection)

**CLASS** Antiemetic, substance P and neurokinin 1 receptor antagonist
**PREG/CONT** Low risk/NA

**IND & DOSE W/other antiemetics for prevention of acute and delayed n/v associated w/initial and repeat courses of moderately or highly emetogenic cancer chemo.** *Adult:* Aprepitant, 125 mg PO 1 hr before chemo (day 1) and 80 mg PO once daily in a.m. on days 2 and 3 w/ dexamethasone or ondansetron; or *Cinvanti,* 130 mg IV (single-dose regimen) or 100 mg IV (3-day regimen) w/ other antiemetics; or fosaprepitant, 115 mg IV 30 min before chemo on day 1 of antiemetic regimen; infuse over 15 min. *Child ≥12 yr or <12 yr weighing ≥30 kg:* 115 mg IV 30 min before chemo infused over 15 min on day 1 of antiemetic regimen; 125 mg/d PO days 2 and 3. **Postop n/v.** *Adult:* 40 mg PO within 3 hr before anesthesia induction.
**ADV EFF** Alopecia, anorexia, constipation, diarrhea, dizziness, fatigue
**INTERACTIONS** Docetaxel, etoposide, hormonal contraceptives, ifosfamide, imatinib, irinotecan, paclitaxel, pimozide, vinblastine, vincristine, vinorelbine, warfarin
**NC/PT** Give first dose w/dexamethasone 1 hr before start of chemo; give additional doses of dexamethasone and ondansetron as indicated as part of antiemetic regimen. Give within 3 hr before anesthesia induction if used to prevent postop n/v. Provide safety precautions, analgesics as needed. Pt should use caution w/dizziness, drowsiness.

## **arformoterol tartrate** (Brovana)

**CLASS** Bronchodilator, long-acting beta agonist
**PREG/CONT** C/NA

**IND & DOSE Long-term maint tx of bronchoconstriction in pts w/COPD.** *Adult:* 15 mcg bid (a.m. and p.m.) by nebulization. Max, 30 mcg total daily dose.
**ADV EFF Asthma-related deaths, paradoxical bronchospasm**
**INTERACTIONS** Beta-adrenergic blockers, diuretics, MAOIs, QT-prolonging drugs, TCAs
**NC/PT** Not for use in acute bronchospasm; not indicated to treat asthma. Ensure pt continues other drugs to manage COPD, especially long-term control drugs and inhaled corticosteroids. Not for use in preg/breastfeeding. Teach proper use of nebulizer. Pt should have periodic evaluation of respiratory status.

**DANGEROUS DRUG**

## **argatroban** (Argatroban)

**CLASS** Anticoagulant
**PREG/CONT** Low risk/NA

**IND & DOSE Px or tx of thrombosis in pts w/heparin-induced thrombocytopenia, including pts at risk undergoing PCI.** *Adult:* 2 mcg/kg/min IV; PCI, bolus of 350 mcg/kg IV over 3–5 min, then 25 mcg/kg/min IV.
**ADV EFF Bleeding, cardiac arrest,** chest pain, dyspnea, fever, headache, hypotension, n/v/d

**INTERACTIONS** Heparin, thrombolytics, warfarin
**NC/PT** Monitor for s&sx of bleeding.

## ARIPiprazole (Abilify, Abilify Discmelt, Abilify Maintena, Aristada)

**CLASS** Atypical antipsychotic, dopamine/serotonin agonist and antagonist
**PREG/CONT** High risk/NA

**BBW** Elderly pts w/dementia-related psychosis have increased risk of death if given atypical antipsychotics; not approved for this use. Risk of suicidal ideation increases w/antidepressant use, especially in child, adolescent, young adult; monitor accordingly.
**IND & DOSE** Oral sol may be substituted on mg-to-mg basis up to 25 mg of tablet. Pts taking 30-mg tablets should receive 25 mg if switched to sol. **Tx of schizophrenia.** *Adult:* 10–15 mg/d PO. Increase dose q 2 wk to max of 30 mg/d. Or 441 mg IM in deltoid muscle q 4 wk or 662–882 mg IM in gluteal muscle q 4–6 wk (*Aristada*). *Child 13–17 yr:* Initially, 2 mg/d PO. Adjust to 5 mg/d after 2 d, then to target dose of 10 mg/d; max, 30 mg/d. **Tx of bipolar disorder.** *Adult:* 15 mg/d PO as one dose; maint, 15–30 mg/d PO. *Child 10–17 yr:* Initially, 2 mg/d PO; titrate to 5 mg/d after 2 d, then to 10 mg/d after another 2 d. Target dose, 10 mg/d; max, 30 mg/d. **Adjunct tx of major depressive disorder.** *Adult:* Initially, 2–5 mg/d PO; maint, 2–15 mg/d as adjunct therapy. **Tx of agitation.** *Adult:* 5.25–15 mg IM; usual dose, 9.75 mg IM. May give cumulative doses of up to 30 mg/d PO. **Irritability associated w/autistic disorder.** *Child 6–17 yr:* 2 mg/d PO; titrate to maint dose of 5–15 mg/d. **Tx of Tourette disorder.** *≥50 kg:* 2 mg/d PO; titrate to 10–20 mg/d PO. *<50 kg:* 2 mg/d PO; titrate to 5–10 mg/d.
**ADV EFF** **Akathisia,** bone marrow suppression, cognitive/motor impairment, compulsive disorders (including pathological gambling), dyslipidemia, hyperglycemia, **NMS,** orthostatic hypotension, **seizures** (potentially life-threatening), suicidality, tardive dyskinesia, weight gain
**INTERACTIONS** Alcohol, carbamazepine, CNS depressants, CYP2D6 inhibitors (fluoxetine, paroxetine, quinidine), CYP3A4 inhibitors (ketoconazole), lorazepam
**NC/PT** Dispense least amount possible to suicidal pts. Ensure pt well hydrated. Switch to oral sol w/difficulty swallowing. Adjust ER injection dose based on current oral use; see manufacturer's guideline. Not for use in preg/breastfeeding. Monitor weight; assess for hyperglycemia. May react w/many medications; monitor drug regimen. Pt should take safety precautions for cognitive/motor impairment, be alert to possibility of pathological compulsive disorders. Confusion between aripiprazole and proton pump inhibitors; use extreme caution.

## armodafinil (Nuvigil)

**CLASS** CNS stimulant, narcoleptic
**PREG/CONT** C/C-IV

**IND & DOSE** **To improve wakefulness in pts w/excessive sleepiness associated w/obstructive sleep apnea/hypopnea syndrome; narcolepsy.** *Adult:* 150–250 mg/d PO as single dose in a.m. **Shift work sleep disorder.** *Adult:* 150 mg/d PO taken 1 hr before start of work shift.
**ADJUST DOSE** Elderly pts, severe hepatic impairment
**ADV EFF** Angioedema, **anaphylaxis,** dizziness, headache, insomnia, nausea, psychiatric sx, **SJS**
**INTERACTIONS** Cyclosporine, ethinyl estradiol, hormonal contraceptives, midazolam, omeprazole, phenytoin, TCAs, triazolam, warfarin

**NC/PT** Rule out underlying medical conditions; not intended for tx of obstruction. Should be part of comprehensive program for sleep. Provide safety measures if CNS effects occur. Stop drug if psychiatric sx occur. Not for use in preg/breastfeeding. Pt should use barrier contraceptives, avoid alcohol, take safety precautions w/CNS effects.

**DANGEROUS DRUG**

## arsenic trioxide (Trisenox)

**CLASS** Antineoplastic
**PREG/CONT** High risk/NA

**BBW** Extremely toxic and carcinogenic; monitor blood counts, electrolytes. Prolonged QT, arrhythmias; monitor ECG.
**IND & DOSE Induction and remission of acute promyelocytic leukemia (APL) in pts refractory to retinoid or anthracycline chemo or w/ tretinoin for tx of pts w/low-risk APL w/t(15:17) translocation or PML/ RAR-alpha gene expression.** *Adult:* Induction, 0.15 mg/kg/d IV until bone marrow remission; max, 60 doses. Consolidation, 0.15 mg/kg/d IV 5 d/wk during wk 1–4 or 8-wk cycle for total of four cycles in combo w/tretinoin.
**ADJUST DOSE** Severe hepatic impairment
**ADV EFF** Abd pain, **APL differentiation syndrome, cancer, complete heart block,** cough, dizziness, dyspnea, edema, **encephalopathy,** fatigue, headache, hepatotoxicity, **hyperleukocytosis,** leukocytosis, n/v/d, **prolonged QT**
**INTERACTIONS** Cyclosporine, ethinyl estradiol, hormonal contraceptives, midazolam, omeprazole, phenytoin, TCAs, triazolam, warfarin
**NC/PT** Monitor CBC, ECG, LFTs, electrolytes closely. Provide comfort measures for GI effects, safety measures for CNS effects. Not for use in preg/breastfeeding.

## asenapine (Saphris, Secuado)

**CLASS** Atypical antipsychotic, dopamine/serotonin antagonist
**PREG/CONT** High risk/NA

**BBW** Elderly pts w/dementia-related psychosis have increased risk of death if given atypical antipsychotics; not approved for this use. Risk of suicidal ideation increases w/antidepressant use, especially in child, adolescent, young adult; monitor accordingly.
**IND & DOSE Tx of schizophrenia.** *Adult:* 5–10 mg SL bid. Initially, 3.8 mg/d transdermal. May increase to 5.7 or 7.6 mg/d after 1 week (*Secuado*). **Acute tx of manic or mixed episodes associated w/bipolar I disorder; adjunct tx w/lithium or valproate for acute tx of manic or mixed episodes associated w/bipolar I disorder.** *Adult:* 5–10 mg SL bid; may decrease to 5 mg/d if needed. **Tx of manic or mixed episodes w/bipolar I disorder.** *Child 10–17 yr:* 2.5–10 mg SL bid.
**ADJUST DOSE** Severe hepatic impairment
**ADV EFF** Akathisia, bone marrow suppression, cognitive/motor impairment, dizziness, dyslipidemia, extrapyramidal sx, hyperglycemia, **NMS,** orthostatic hypotension, **prolonged QT,** somnolence, **suicidality,** weight gain
**INTERACTIONS** Alcohol, antihypertensives, CNS depressants, fluvoxamine, QT-prolonging drugs
**NC/PT** Monitor ECG periodically. Provide safety measures for CNS effects. Monitor weight gain/blood glucose. Apply *Secuado* transdermal system q 24 hr to either hip, abdomen, upper arm, or upper back. Not for use in preg/breastfeeding. Pt should not swallow tablet but place under tongue (where it will dissolve within sec) and not eat or drink for 10 min; change positions slowly; take safety measures w/CNS effects; report thoughts of suicide.

## asfotase alfa (Strensiq)

**CLASS** Alkaline phosphatase
**PREG/CONT** Low risk/NA

**IND & DOSE Tx of perinatal, juvenile-onset hypophosphatasia.** *Adult, child:* 2 mg/kg subcut 3 ×/wk or 1 mg/kg subcut 6 ×/wk; max, 3 mg/kg 3 ×/wk.
**ADV EFF** Ectopic calcifications (eye, kidneys), hypersensitivity reactions, lipodystrophy
**NC/PT** Ensure proper dx. Monitor phosphate level. Rotate injection sites; do not give in inflamed, swollen areas. Teach caregiver proper administration/disposal of needles/syringes.

**DANGEROUS DRUG**

## asparaginase Erwinia chrysanthemi (Erwinaze)

**CLASS** Antineoplastic
**PREG/CONT** High risk/NA

**IND & DOSE Tx of pts w/ALL who have developed sensitivity to asparaginase or pegaspargase.** *Adult, child:* 25,000/$m^2$ international units IM for each scheduled dose of pegaspargase or asparaginase; limit volume to 2 mL/injection.
**ADV EFF Anaphylaxis,** arthralgia, **coagulation disorders, hyperglycemia,** n/v, **pancreatitis,** rash, **seizures,** thrombotic events, urticaria
**NC/PT** Monitor for severe reaction, hyperglycemia, pancreatitis, coagulation disorders. Not for use in preg. Prepare calendar to keep track of appointments. Pt should have regular blood tests.

## aspirin (Bayer, Bufferin, Heartline, Norwich, St. Joseph's, etc)

**CLASS** Analgesic, antiplatelet, antipyretic, salicylate
**PREG/CONT** D/NA

**IND & DOSE Tx of mild to moderate pain, fever.** *Adult:* 325–1,000 mg PO q 4–6 hr; max, 4,000 mg/d. SR tablets, 1,300 mg PO, then 650–1,300 mg q 8 hr; max, 3,900 mg/d. Suppositories, 1 rectally q 4 hr. *Child:* 10–15 mg/kg/dose PO q 4 hr, up to 60–80 mg/kg/d. Do not give to pts w/chickenpox or flu sx. **Arthritis.** *Adult:* Up to 3 g/d PO in divided doses. *Child:* 90–130 mg/kg/24 hr PO in divided doses at 6- to 8-hr intervals. Maintain serum level of 150–300 mcg/mL. **Ischemic stroke, TIA.** *Adult:* 50–325 mg/d PO. **Angina, recurrent MI prevention.** *Adult:* 75–325 mg/d PO. **Suspected MI.** *Adult:* 160–325 mg PO as soon as possible; continue daily for 30 d. **CABG.** *Adult:* 325 mg PO 6 hr after procedure, then daily for 1 yr. **Acute rheumatic fever.** *Adult:* 5–8 g/d PO; modify to maintain serum salicylate level of 15–30 mg/dL. *Child:* Initially, 100 mg/kg/d PO, then decrease to 75 mg/kg/d for 4–6 wk. Therapeutic serum salicylate level, 150–300 mcg/mL. **Kawasaki disease.** *Child:* 80–100 mg/kg/d PO divided q 6 hr; after fever resolves, 1–5 mg/kg/d once daily.
**ADV EFF Acute aspirin toxicity,** bleeding, dizziness, difficulty hearing, dyspepsia, epigastric discomfort, nausea, occult blood loss, tinnitus
**INTERACTIONS** Alcohol, alkalinizers, antacids, anticoagulants, corticosteroids, furosemide, nitroglycerin, NSAIDs, urine acidifiers
**NC/PT** Do not use in child w/chickenpox or flu sx. Monitor dose for use in child. Give w/full glass of water. Pt should not cut/crush/chew SR preparations; should check OTC products for aspirin content to avoid overdose; report ringing in ears, bloody stools.

## atazanavir sulfate (Reyataz)

**CLASS** Antiretroviral, protease inhibitor
**PREG/CONT** Low risk/NA

**IND & DOSE W/other antiretrovirals for tx of HIV-1 infection.** *Adult:*

Therapy-naïve, 300 mg/d PO w/100 mg ritonavir PO once daily; if unable to tolerate ritonavir, can give 400 mg PO once daily; therapy-experienced, 300 mg/d PO w/100 mg ritonavir PO taken w/food. *Child 3 mo and at least 10 kg–<18 yr:* Therapy-naïve, base dose on weight, 150–300 mg/d atazanavir PO w/80–100 mg ritonavir daily PO; therapy-experienced, base dose on weight, 200–300 mg/d atazanavir PO w/100 mg ritonavir PO. Must be taken w/food.
**ADJUST DOSE** Hepatic/renal impairment
**ADV EFF** Cardiac conduction problems, headache, liver enzyme elevation, nausea, phenylketonuria (w/oral powder in pts w/phenylketonuria), rash, **severe hepatomegaly w/ steatosis** (sometimes fatal)
**INTERACTIONS** Antacids, bosentan, indinavir, irinotecan, lovastatin, proton pump inhibitors, rifampin, sildenafil, simvastatin, St. John's wort, warfarin. Contraindicated w/ergot derivatives, midazolam, pimozide, triazolam
**NC/PT** Ensure HIV testing has been done. Monitor LFTs. Ensure pt takes drug w/other antiretrovirals. Withdraw drug at s&sx of lactic acidosis. Not for use in preg/breastfeeding. Does not cure disease. Oral powder only for child between 10 and 25 kg. Must be taken w/ritonavir and food. Pt should avoid St. John's wort, report use of this drug and all other drugs to all health care providers.

## atenolol (Tenormin)
**CLASS** Antianginal, antihypertensive, $beta_1$-adrenergic blocker
**PREG/CONT** D/NA

**BBW** Do not discontinue drug abruptly after long-term therapy; taper drug gradually over 2 wk w/ monitoring; risk of MI, arrhythmias.
**IND & DOSE HTN.** *Adult:* 50 mg PO once/d; after 1–2 wk, may increase to 100 mg/d. **Angina pectoris.** *Adult:* Initially, 50 mg/d PO; up to 200 mg/d may be needed. **Acute MI.** *Adult:* 100 mg/d PO or 50 mg PO bid for 6–9 d or until discharge.
**ADJUST DOSE** Elderly pts, renal impairment
**ADV EFF** Bradycardia, **bronchospasm,** cardiac arrhythmias, ED, exercise tolerance decrease, flatulence, gastric pain, **laryngospasm,** n/v/d
**INTERACTIONS** Ampicillin, anticholinergics, aspirin, bismuth subsalicylate, calcium salts, clonidine, hormonal contraceptives, insulin, lidocaine, prazosin, quinidine, verapamil
**NC/PT** Do not stop suddenly; taper over 2 wk. Pt should take safety precautions w/CNS effects, report difficulty breathing.

## atezolizumab (Tecentriq)
**CLASS** Antineoplastic, programmed death-ligand blocking antibody
**PREG/CONT** High risk/NA

**IND & DOSE Tx of locally advanced or metastatic urothelial carcinoma; as single agent for metastatic NSCLC.** *Adult:* 840 mg IV q 2 wk, 1,200 mg IV q 3 wk, or 1,680 mg IV q 4 wk over 60 min. **Tx of metastatic NSCLC in combo w/ or w/o bevacizumab, w/ paclitaxel and carboplatin for first line or tx w/progression of NSCLC after platinum-based tx.** *Adult:* 1,200 mg IV over 60 min q 3 wk. **Tx of pts w/metastatic triple-negative breast cancer whose tumors express PD-L1, w/paclitaxel.** *Adult:* 840 mg IV on days 1 and 15 of 28-d cycle followed by 100 mg/m$^2$ paclitaxel protein-bound on days 1, 8, and 15 of 28-d cycle. **Tx of small cell lung cancer.** *Adult:* 1,200 mg IV q 3 wk before chemo followed by carboplatin and etoposide. Maint: 840 mg IV q 2 wk, 1,200 mg IV q 3 wk, or 1,680 mg IV q 4 wk.

**ADV EFF** Constipation, decreased appetite, fatigue, fever; **immune-related colitis, endocrinopathies, hepatitis, myasthenic syndrome, pancreatitis, pneumonitis;** infection, infusion reaction, nausea, UTI
**NC/PT** Monitor respiratory, thyroid, CNS function; LFTs, glycemic control, pancreatic enzymes, vision changes. Watch for severe diarrhea, s&sx of infection. Regulate infusion rate; slow w/any infusion reaction, stop w/severe reaction. Pt should avoid preg (contraceptives advised)/breastfeeding; report difficulty breathing, numbness/tingling, severe diarrhea, vision changes.

## atoMOXetine hydrochloride (Strattera)

**CLASS** Selective norepinephrine reuptake inhibitor
**PREG/CONT** C/NA

**BBW** Increased risk of suicidality in child, adolescent. Monitor closely; alert caregivers of risk.
**IND & DOSE Tx of ADHD as part of total tx program.** *Adult, child >70 kg:* 40 mg/d PO; increase after minimum of 3 d to target total daily dose of 80 mg PO. Max, 100 mg/d. *Child ≥6 yr, ≤70 kg:* 0.5 mg/kg/d PO; increase after minimum of 3 d to target total daily dose of about 1.2 mg/kg/d PO. Max, 1.4 mg/kg or 100 mg/d, whichever is less.
**ADJUST DOSE** Hepatic impairment
**ADV EFF** Aggressive behavior/hostility, constipation, cough, dry mouth, insomnia, n/v, priapism, **sudden cardiac death, suicidality**
**INTERACTIONS** CYP3A4 substrates, fluoxetine, MAOIs (do not give within 14 d of atomoxetine), paroxetine, quinidine
**NC/PT** Ensure proper dx; part of comprehensive tx program. Rule out cardiac abnormalities; baseline ECG suggested. Monitor growth. Provide drug vacation periodically. Give before 6 p.m. to allow sleep. Not for use in preg. Pt should avoid OTC drugs/herbs that may be stimulants.

## atorvastatin calcium (Lipitor)

**CLASS** Antihyperlipidemic, HMG-CoA inhibitor
**PREG/CONT** X/NA

**IND & DOSE Adjunct to diet to lower total cholesterol, serum triglycerides, LDL and increase HDL in pts w/ primary hypercholesterolemia, mixed dyslipidemia, familial hypercholesterolemia, elevated serum triglycerides; to prevent MI, CV disease in pts w/many risk factors; to reduce risk of MI and CV events in pts w/hx of CAD.** *Adult:* 10–20 mg PO once daily w/o regard to meals; maint, 10–80 mg/d PO. *Child 10–17 yr:* 10 mg PO daily; max, 20 mg/d.
**ADV EFF** Abd pain, constipation, cramps, flatulence, headache, **liver failure, rhabdomyolysis w/renal failure, stroke**
**INTERACTIONS** Antifungals, cimetidine, clarithromycin, cyclosporine, digoxin, diltiazem, erythromycin, fibric acid derivatives, grapefruit juice, hormonal contraceptives, nefazodone, niacin, protease inhibitors, tacrolimus
**NC/PT** Obtain baseline and periodic LFTs. Withhold drug in acute or serious conditions. Give in p.m. Ensure pt is using diet/exercise program. Not for use in preg (contraceptives advised). Pt should report muscle pain. Name confusion between written orders for *Lipitor* (atorvastatin) and *Zyrtec* (cetirizine).

## atovaquone (Mepron)

**CLASS** Antiprotozoal
**PREG/CONT** C/NA

**IND & DOSE Px and acute oral tx of mild to moderate *Pneumocystis jiroveci* pneumonia in pts intolerant of trimethoprim-sulfamethoxazole.** *Adult, child 13–16 yr:* Px of *P. jiroveci* pneumonia, 1,500 mg PO daily w/meal.

Tx of *P. jiroveci* pneumonia, 750 mg PO bid w/food for 21 d.
**ADJUST DOSE** Elderly pts
**ADV EFF** Dizziness, fever, headache, insomnia, n/v/d
**INTERACTIONS** Rifampin
**NC/PT** Give w/meals. Ensure drug is taken for 21 d for tx. Pt should report severe GI reactions.

## atropine sulfate (AtroPen, Isopoto Atropine)

**CLASS** Anticholinergic, antidote, belladonna
**PREG/CONT** C/NA

**IND & DOSE** **Antisialagogue; tx of parkinsonism, bradycardia, pylorospasm, urinary bladder relaxation, uterine relaxation.** *Adult:* 0.4–0.6 mg PO, IM, IV, subcut. *Child:* Base dose on weight, 0.1–0.4 mg PO, IM, IV, subcut. **Bradyarrhythmia.** *Adult:* 0.4–1 mg (max, 2 mg) IV q 1–2 hr as needed. *Child:* 0.01–0.03 mg/kg IV. **Antidote for cholinergic drug overdose, organophosphorus insecticides; initial tx for nerve agent poisoning.** *Adult:* 2–3 mg parenterally; repeat until s&sx of atropine intoxication appear. Use of auto-injector recommended. **Ophthal sol for eye refraction.** *Adult:* 1–2 drops into eye 1 hr before refracting. **Ophthal sol for uveitis.** *Adult:* 1–2 drops into eye tid.
**ADJUST DOSE** Elderly pts
**ADV EFF** Altered taste perception, bradycardia, decreased sweating, dry mouth, n/v, palpitations, **paralytic ileus,** predisposition to heat prostration, urinary hesitancy, urine retention
**INTERACTIONS** Anticholinergics, antihistamines, haloperidol, MAOIs, phenothiazines, TCAs
**NC/PT** Ensure adequate hydration. Provide temp control. Monitor HR. Pt should empty bladder before taking if urine retention occurs. Sugarless lozenges may help dry mouth.

## auranofin (Ridaura)

**CLASS** Antirheumatic, gold salt
**PREG/CONT** C/NA

**BBW** Discontinue at first sign of toxicity. Severe bone marrow depression, renal toxicity, diarrhea possible.
**IND & DOSE** **Mgt of pts w/active classic RA w/insufficient response to NSAIDs.** *Adult:* 3 mg PO bid or 6 mg/d PO; after 6 mo may increase to 3 mg PO tid. Max, 9 mg/d.
**ADV EFF** **Angioedema, bone marrow suppression, diarrhea,** eye changes, **GI bleeding,** gingivitis, **interstitial pneumonitis,** peripheral neuropathy, photosensitivity, rash, **renal failure,** stomatitis
**NC/PT** Monitor blood counts; renal/lung function. Corticosteroids may help w/mild reactions. Pt should avoid ultraviolet light, use sunscreen or protective clothes.

## avanafil (Stendra)

**CLASS** ED drug, phosphodiesterase-5 inhibitor
**PREG/CONT** Low risk/NA

**IND & DOSE** **Tx of ED.** *Adult:* 100 mg PO 15 min before sexual activity; range, 50–200 mg no more than once/d.
**ADJUST DOSE** Severe renal/hepatic impairment
**ADV EFF** Back pain, dyspepsia, flushing, headache, **MI,** nasal congestion, nasopharyngitis, nonarteritic ischemic optic neuropathy, sudden hearing loss, vision changes
**INTERACTIONS** Alcohol, alpha blockers, amprenavir, antihypertensives, aprepitant, diltiazem, fluconazole, fosamprenavir, grapefruit juice, guanylate cyclase inhibitors, itraconazole, ketoconazole, nitrates, ritonavir, verapamil
**NC/PT** Ensure proper dx. Does not prevent STDs; does not work in absence of sexual stimulation. Pt should not use w/nitrates, antihypertensives,

grapefruit juice, alcohol; should report sudden loss of vision or hearing, erection lasting over 4 hr.

**avatrombopag** (Doptelet)
**CLASS** Colony-stimulating factor, hematopoietic agent, thrombopoietic agent, thrombopoietin receptor agonist
**PREG/CONT** Moderate risk/NA

**IND & DOSE Tx of pts w/chronic liver disease who are scheduled for a procedure.** *Adult w/platelet count <40 × 10⁹/L:* 60 mg PO daily for 5 d. *Adult w/platelet count 40–<50 × 10⁹/L:* 40 mg PO daily for 5 d. Tx of pts w/ chronic immune thrombocytopenia w/insufficient response to previous tx. *Adult:* Initially, 20 mg PO daily to maintain platelet count ≥50 × 10⁹/L. Max, 40 mg PO daily.
**ADV EFF** Abd pain, fatigue, fever, headache, nausea, peripheral edema, **thromboembolic complications including portal vein thrombosis**
**NC/PT** Begin dosing 10–13 d before procedure; pt should undergo procedure within 5–8 d after final dose. Monitor platelet count before dosing and before procedure. Pt should take w/food.

**avelumab** (Bavencio)
**CLASS** Antineoplastic, programmed death ligand-1 (PD-L1) blocking antibody
**PREG/CONT** High risk/NA

**IND & DOSE Tx of metastatic Merkel cell carcinoma; tx of advanced or metastatic urothelial carcinoma; tx of advanced renal cell carcinoma, w/axitinib.** *Adult, child ≥12 yr:* 800 mg IV q 2 wk.
**ADV EFF CV events,** decreased appetite; fatigue; **immune-mediated pneumonitis, hepatitis, colitis, nephritis, endocrinopathies;** infusion reactions, n/v/d
**NC/PT** Premedicate w/antihistamine and acetaminophen before first four infusions and before subsequent doses if needed. Infuse slowly; stop and discontinue drug w/infusion reactions. Monitor LFTs, pulmonary/renal function; watch for diarrhea. Withhold drug or provide support as needed. Pt should mark calendar for infusion days; avoid preg (contraceptives advised)/breastfeeding; report difficulty breathing, urine/stool color changes, severe diarrhea.

**DANGEROUS DRUG**

**axicabtagene ciloleucel** (Yescarta)
**CLASS** Antineoplastic
**PREG/CONT** Unkn/NA

**BBW** Cytokine release syndrome (CRS) can occur, including fatal or life-threatening reactions. Do not give axicabtagene ciloleucel to pt w/active infection or inflammatory disorder. Treat severe or life-threatening CRS w/tocilizumab alone or tocilizumab and corticosteroids. Neurotoxicities, including fatal or life-threatening reactions, have occurred. Monitor for neurotoxicities; provide supportive care and/or corticosteroids as needed. Drug only available via Yescarta REMS program.
**IND & DOSE Tx of large B-cell lymphoma (relapsed or refractory).** *Adult:* Target dose: $2 \times 10^6$ CAR-positive viable T cells/kg body weight; max dose, $2 \times 10^8$ CAR-positive viable T cells. Dose adjustment may be needed due to toxicity.
**ADV EFF** Aphasia, capillary leak syndrome, cardiac arrhythmia/failure, chills, cough, **CRS, cytopenia,** dehydration, delirium, dizziness, dyspnea, edema, fatigue, fever, headache, hypoxia, **HBV reactivation,** HTN, hypotension, **infection,** limb/back pain, motor dysfx, **neurotoxicity,** pleural effusion, renal insufficiency, **secondary malignancy,** tachycardia, thrombosis, tremor, weight loss
**NC/PT** Rule out preg (contraceptives advised). Ensure tocilizumab/

emergency equipment on hand before infusion, during recovery. Premedicate w/acetaminophen 650 mg PO and diphenhydramine 12.5 mg IV or PO about 60 min before infusion. Avoid prophylactic systemic corticosteroids. Monitor high-risk pt w/pulse oximetry, continuous cardiac telemetry.

**axitinib** (Inlyta)
**CLASS** Antineoplastic, kinase inhibitor
**PREG/CONT** D/NA

**IND & DOSE** **Tx of advanced renal cell cancer after failure of one prior systemic therapy.** *Adult:* 5 mg PO bid 12 hr apart w/full glass of water.
**ADJUST DOSE** Hepatic impairment
**ADV EFF** Anorexia, asthenia, cardiac failure, constipation, diarrhea, dysphonia, fatigue, hand-foot syndrome, **GI perforation/fistula, hemorrhage, hepatic injury,** HTN, **hypertensive crisis, hypothyroidism, proteinuria, RPLS, thrombotic events,** vomiting, weight loss
**INTERACTIONS** Strong CYP3A4/5 inhibitors/inducers (carbamazepine, dexamethasone, ketoconazole, phenobarbital, phenytoin, rifabutin, rifampin, rifapentine, St. John's wort); avoid these combos
**NC/PT** Monitor closely for adverse reactions; have supportive measures readily available. Stop at least 24 hr before scheduled surgery. Can cause fetal harm; not for use in preg (contraceptives advised). Pt should take w/full glass of water; report s&sx of bleeding, severe headache, severe GI effects, urine/stool changes, swelling, difficulty breathing; avoid St. John's wort.

**azaCITIDine** (Vidaza)
**CLASS** Antineoplastic, nucleoside metabolic inhibitor
**PREG/CONT** High risk/NA

**IND & DOSE** **Tx of myelodysplastic syndrome, including refractory anemias and chronic myelomonocytic leukemia.** *Adult:* 75 mg/m²/d subcut or IV for 7 d q 4 wk; may increase to 100 mg/m²/d after two cycles if no response. Pt should have at least four–six cycles.
**ADJUST DOSE** Hepatic impairment
**ADV EFF** **Bone marrow suppression,** fever, **hepatic impairment,** injection-site reactions, n/v/d, pneumonia, **renal impairment, TLS**
**NC/PT** Not for use in preg. Men on drug should not father a child. Monitor CBC, LFTs, renal function. Premedicate w/antiemetic. Pt should report s&sx of infection, bleeding.

**azaTHIOprine** (Azasan, Imuran)
**CLASS** Immunosuppressant
**PREG/CONT** D/NA

**BBW** Monitor blood counts regularly; severe hematologic effects may require stopping drug. Increases risk of neoplasia; alert pt accordingly.
**IND & DOSE** **Px of rejection w/renal homotransplantation.** *Adult:* 3–5 mg/kg/d PO as single dose on day of transplant; maint, 1–3 mg/kg/d PO. **Tx of classic RA unresponsive to other tx.** *Adult:* 1 mg/kg PO as single dose or bid. May increase at 6–8 wk and thereafter by steps at 4-wk intervals; max, 2.5 mg/kg/d.
**ADJUST DOSE** Elderly pts, renal impairment
**ADV EFF** **Carcinogenesis, hepatotoxicity,** leukopenia, macrocytic anemia, n/v, **serious infection,** thrombocytopenia
**INTERACTIONS** Allopurinol, NMJ blockers
**NC/PT** Monitor blood counts carefully. Give w/food if GI upset a problem. Protect from infection.

## azilsartan medoxomil
(Edarbi)
**CLASS** Antihypertensive, ARB
**PREG/CONT** D/NA

**BBW** Rule out preg before starting tx. Suggest use of barrier contraceptives during tx; fetal injury and death have been reported.
**IND & DOSE Tx of HTN, alone or w/other antihypertensives.** *Adult:* 80 mg/d PO. For pts on high-dose diuretics or who are volume-depleted, consider starting dose of 40 mg/d; titrate if tolerated.
**ADV EFF** Diarrhea, hyperkalemia, renal impairment
**INTERACTIONS** ARBs, lithium, NSAIDs, renin blockers
**NC/PT** Rule out preg (barrier contraceptives advised). Not for use in breastfeeding. Monitor in situations that could lead to lower BP. Mark chart if pt is going to surgery; possible volume problems after surgery.

## azithromycin (AzaSite, Zithromax, Zmax)
**CLASS** Macrolide antibiotic
**PREG/CONT** B/NA

**IND & DOSE Tx of mild to moderate acute bacterial exacerbations of COPD, pneumonia, pharyngitis/tonsillitis (as second-line), uncomplicated skin/skin-structure infections.** *Adult:* 500 mg PO as single dose on first day, then 250 mg PO daily on days 2–5 for total dose of 1.5 g or 500 mg/d PO for 3 d. **Tx of nongonococcal urethritis, genital ulcer disease, cervicitis due to *Chlamydia trachomatis*.** *Adult:* Single 1-g PO dose. **Tx of gonococcal urethritis/cervicitis, mild to moderate acute bacterial sinusitis, community-acquired pneumonia.** *Adult:* Single 2-g PO dose. *Child ≥6 mo:* 10 mg/kg/d PO for 3 d. **Disseminated MAC infections.** *Adult:* Prevention, 1,200 mg PO once wkly. Tx, 600 mg/d PO w/ethambutol. **Tx of acute sinusitis.** *Adult:* 500 mg/d PO for 3 d or single 2-g dose of *Zmax*. Tx of community-acquired pneumonia. *Adult, child ≥16 yr:* 500 mg IV daily for at least 2 d, then 500 mg PO for 7–10 d. *Child 6 mo–15 yr:* 10 mg/kg PO as single dose on first day, then 5 mg/kg PO on days 2–5, or 60 mg/kg *Zmax* as single dose. **Tx of mild community-acquired pneumonia.** *Adult:* 500 mg PO on day 1, then 250 mg PO for 4 d. **Tx of PID.** *Adult:* 500 mg IV daily for 1–2 d, then 250 mg/d PO for 7 d. **Tx of otitis media.** *Child ≥6 mo:* 10 mg/kg PO as single dose, then 5 mg/kg PO on days 2–5, or 30 mg/kg PO as single dose, or 10 mg/kg/d PO for 3 d. **Tx of pharyngitis/tonsillitis.** *Child ≥2 yr:* 12 mg/kg/d PO on days 1–5; max, 500 mg/d. **Tx of bacterial conjunctivitis.** *Adult, child:* 1 drop to affected eye bid for 2 d; then 1 drop/d for 5 d.
**ADV EFF** Abd pain, **angioedema**, diarrhea, **prolonged QT**, superinfections
**INTERACTIONS** Aluminum- and magnesium-containing antacids, QT-prolonging drugs, theophylline, warfarin
**NC/PT** Culture before tx. Give on empty stomach 1 hr before or 2 hr after meals. Prepare sol by adding 60 mL water to bottle and shaking well; pt should drink all at once. Superinfections possible.

## aztreonam (Azactam, Cayston)
**CLASS** Monobactam antibiotic
**PREG/CONT** B/NA

**IND & DOSE Tx of UTIs.** *Adult:* 500 mg–1 g IV or IM q 8–12 hr. **Tx of moderately severe systemic infection.** *Adult:* 1–2 g IV or IM q 8–12 hr. *Child ≥9 mo:* 30 mg/kg IV or IM q 8 hr. **Tx of severe systemic infection.** *Adult:* 2 g IV or IM q 6–8 hr. *Child ≥9 mo:* 30 mg/kg IV or IM q 8 hr. **Tx of cystic fibrosis pts w/*Pseudomonas aeruginosa* infections.** *Adult, child ≥7 yr:* 75 mg inhalation using *Altera Nebulizer*

*System* tid for 28 d; space doses at least 4 hr apart. Then 28 d off.
**ADJUST DOSE** Renal impairment
**ADV EFF** **Anaphylaxis,** injection-site reactions, n/v/d, pruritus, rash
**NC/PT** Culture before tx. Discontinue, provide supportive tx if anaphylaxis occurs. Monitor for injection-site reactions. Use inhaled form only w/ provided nebulizer system. Pt should report difficulty breathing.

## bacitracin (Baci-IM)
**CLASS** Antibiotic
**PREG/CONT** C/NA

**BBW** Monitor renal function tests daily w/IM tx; risk of serious renal toxicity.
**IND & DOSE** **Pneumonia, empyema caused by susceptible strains of staphylococci in infants.** *>2.5 kg:* 1,000 units/kg/d IM in two–three divided doses. *<2.5 kg:* 900 units/kg/d IM in two–three divided doses. **Px of minor skin abrasions; tx of superficial skin infections.** *Adult, child:* Apply topical ointment to affected area 1–3 ×/d; cover w/sterile bandage if needed. Do not use longer than 1 wk. **Superficial infections of conjunctiva or cornea.** *Adult, child:* Dose varies by product; see package insert.
**ADV EFF** Contact dermatitis (topical), **nephrotoxicity,** pain at injection site, superinfections
**INTERACTIONS** Aminoglycosides, NMJs
**NC/PT** Culture before tx. Reconstituted IM sol stable for 1 wk. Ensure adequate hydration. Monitor renal function closely (IM). Pt should report s&sx of infection.

## baclofen (Gablofen, Lioresal, Ozobax)
**CLASS** Centrally acting skeletal muscle relaxant
**PREG/CONT** C/NA

**BBW** Taper gradually to prevent rebound spasticity, hallucinations, possible psychosis, rhabdomyolysis, other serious effects; abrupt discontinuation can cause serious reactions.
**IND & DOSE** **Alleviation of s&sx of spasticity from MS or spinal cord injuries** (intrathecal). *Adult:* Testing usually done w/50 mcg/mL injected into intrathecal space over 1 min. Pt is observed for 4–8 hr, then 75 mcg/1.5 ml is given; pt is observed for 4–8 hr; final screening bolus of 100 mcg/2 ml is given 24 hr later if response still inadequate. Maint for spasticity of cerebral origin, 22–1,400 mcg/d; maint for spasticity of spinal cord origin, 12–2,003 mcg/d. **Spinal cord injuries, other spinal cord diseases** (oral). *Adult:* 5 mg PO tid for 3 d; 10 mg PO tid for 3 d; 15 mg PO tid for 3 d; 20 mg PO tid for 3 d. Thereafter, additional increases may be needed. Max, 80 mg/d.
**ADJUST DOSE** Elderly pts, renal impairment
**ADV EFF** Confusion, dizziness, drowsiness, fatigue, headache, hypotension, insomnia, urinary frequency, weakness
**INTERACTIONS** CNS depressants
**NC/PT** Use caution if spasticity needed to stay upright. Monitor implantable intrathecal delivery site/ system. Do not inject directly into pump catheter access port; risk of life-threatening infection. Taper slowly if discontinuing. Not for use in preg. Pt should avoid OTC sleeping drugs and alcohol; take safety precautions w/CNS effects.

## baloxavir marboxil (Xofluza)
**CLASS** Antiviral, endonuclease inhibitor
**PREG/CONT** No data for humans; no risk in animal studies/NA

**IND & DOSE** **Tx of acute uncomplicated influenza in pts ≥12 yr w/s&sx for no more than 48 hours.** *≥80 kg:* 80 mg PO once. *40–79 kg:* 40 mg PO once.

**ADV EFF** Bronchitis, diarrhea, headache, hypersensitivity, nasopharyngitis, nausea
**INTERACTIONS** Avoid giving w/ polyvalent cation-containing laxatives/antacids/oral supplements (eg, calcium, iron, magnesium, selenium, zinc); live attenuated influenza vaccines may be less effect
**NC/PT** Give at first appearance of influenza sx. Pt should take w/ or w/o food, but NOT w/dairy products, calcium-fortified beverages, or drugs/ supplements containing calcium, iron, magnesium, selenium, or zinc; consult prescriber before receiving a live attenuated influenza vaccine after taking Xofluza.

## balsalazide disodium (Colazal)

**CLASS** Anti-inflammatory
**PREG/CONT** B/NA

**IND & DOSE Tx of mildly to moderately active ulcerative colitis.** *Adult:* Three 750-mg capsules PO tid (total daily dose, 6.75 g) for up to 12 wk. Or, three 1.1-g tablets PO bid (total daily dose 6.6 g) for up to 8 wk. *Child 5–17 yr:* Three 750-mg capsules PO tid (6.75 g/d) for 8 wk, or one 750-mg capsule PO tid (2.25 g/d) for up to 8 wk.
**ADV EFF** Abd pain, cramps, depression, fatigue, flatulence, flulike sx, n/v/d, renal impairment
**NC/PT** Serious effects; use extreme caution. Not for use in pts w/salicylate hypersensitivity. Maintain hydration. Observe for worsening of ulcerative colitis. Drug is high in sodium; monitor sodium intake. Pt should take w/ meals, continue all restrictions and tx used for ulcerative colitis. Name confusion between *Colazal* (balsalazide) and *Clozaril* (clozapine).

## basiliximab (Simulect)

**CLASS** Immunosuppressant
**PREG/CONT** B/NA

**BBW** Only physicians experienced in immunosuppressive therapy and mgt of organ transplant pts should prescribe. Pts should be managed in facilities equipped and staffed w/ adequate lab and supportive medical resources.
**IND & DOSE Px of acute rejection in renal transplant pts, w/other immunosuppressants.** *Adult:* Two doses of 20 mg IV—first dose 2 hr before transplant, second dose on day 4 posttransplant.
**ADV EFF** Abd pain, cramps, HTN, **hypersensitivity reactions, infections,** n/v/d, pain
**NC/PT** Not for use in preg/breastfeeding. Monitor for hypersensitivity reactions; protect pt from infections.

## BCG intravesical (Tice BCG)

**CLASS** Antineoplastic
**PREG/CONT** C/NA

**BBW** Use precautions when handling. Contains live mycobacteria; infections can occur.
**IND & DOSE Intravesical use in tx/ px of carcinoma in situ of urinary bladder; px of primary or recurrent stage Ta and/or T1 papillary tumors after transurethral resection.** *Adult:* 1 ampule in 50 mL diluent instilled via catheter into bladder by gravity.
**ADV EFF Bone marrow suppression,** chills, cystitis, dysuria, hematuria, infections, malaise, n/v, urinary urgency, UTI
**INTERACTIONS** Antibiotics, isoniazid
**NC/PT** Monitor for infection/local reactions. Pt should avoid fluids 4 hr before tx; empty bladder before instillation; lie down for first hr (turning side to side), then upright for 1 hr; try to retain fluid in bladder for 2 hr;

empty bladder, trying not to splash liquid; disinfect urine w/bleach; avoid contact w/urine; increase fluid intake over next few hours; report s&sx of infection, blood in urine.

## beclomethasone dipropionate (QNASL, QVAR, QVAR REDIHALER), beclomethasone dipropionate monohydrate (Beconase AQ)

**CLASS** Corticosteroid
**PREG/CONT** C/NA

**IND & DOSE Maint, control, px of asthma.** *Adult, child ≥12 yr:* 40–160 mcg by inhalation bid; max, 320 mcg /bid. Titrate to response: "Low" dose: 80–240 mcg/d; "medium" dose: 240–480 mcg/d; "high" dose: >480 mcg/d. *Child 5–11 yr:* 40 mcg bid; max, 80 mcg bid. **Relief of s&sx of seasonal or perennial and nonallergic rhinitis; px of recurrence of nasal polyps after surgical removal.** *Adult, child ≥12 yr:* 1–2 inhalations (42–84 mcg) in each nostril bid (total, 168–336 mcg/d). *Child 6–12 yr:* 1 inhalation in each nostril bid (total, 168 mcg ).
**ADV EFF Cushing syndrome,** epistaxis, headache, local irritation, nausea rebound congestion
**NC/PT** Taper oral steroids slowly in switching to inhaled forms. If using nasal spray, use nose decongestant to facilitate penetration of drug. If using other inhalants, use several min before using this drug. If using respiratory inhalant, allow at least 1 min between puffs. Pt should rinse mouth after each inhalation, report worsening of asthma.

## bedaquiline (Sirturo)

**CLASS** Antimycobacterial, antituberculotic
**PREG/CONT** B/NA

**BBW** Increased risk of death; reserve for pts resistant to other effective therapy. Prolonged QT, risk of serious to fatal arrhythmias. Monitor ECG; avoid other QT-prolonging drugs.
**IND & DOSE Tx of pts w/multidrug-resistant pulmonary TB, w/other antituberculotics when effective TB program cannot be provided.** *Adult, child (2–<18 yr weighing at least 30 kg):* 400 mg/d PO for 2 wk; then 200 mg/d PO 3 ×/wk for 22 wk, w/other antituberculotics.
**ADJUST DOSE** Hepatic impairment, severe renal impairment
**ADV EFF** Arthralgia, headache, **hepatic impairment,** nausea, **prolonged QT**
**INTERACTIONS** Ketoconazole, lopinavir, QT-prolonging drugs, rifampin, ritonavir
**NC/PT** Obtain baseline ECG; monitor periodically. Monitor LFTs. Ensure proper use of drug and use w/other antituberculotics; must give using directly observed therapy. Not for use in breastfeeding. Pt should mark calendar for tx days; swallow capsule whole and not cut/crush/chew it; ensure also taking other drugs for TB; avoid alcohol; report urine/stool color changes, abnormal heartbeat.

## belatacept (Nulojix)

**CLASS** T-cell costimulation blocker
**PREG/CONT** C/NA

**BBW** Increased risk of posttransplant lymphoproliferative disorder involving CNS, more likely without immunity to Epstein-Barr virus. Increased risk of cancers and serious infections.
**IND & DOSE Px of organ rejection in pts w/renal transplants, w/other immunosuppressants.** *Adult:* Days 1 and 5, 10 mg/kg IV over 30 min; repeat end of wk 2, 4, 8, 12. Maint starting at wk 16 and q 4 wk thereafter, 5 mg/kg IV over 30 min. Must be given w/basiliximab, mycophenolate, and corticosteroids.
**ADV EFF** Anemia, constipation, cough, edema, graft dysfx, headache, hyperkalemia, hypokalemia, **infections**

(potentially fatal), **malignancies, PML, posttransplant lymphoproliferative disorder,** UTI
**INTERACTIONS** Live vaccines
**NC/PT** Not for use in liver transplants. Not for use in preg/breastfeeding. Use only provided silicone-free syringe to prepare drug. Ensure use of concomitant drugs. Monitor blood counts, s&sx of infection, orientation, mood. Protect from infection. Encourage cancer screening exams.

## belimumab (Benlysta)
**CLASS** B-cell activating factor inhibitor
**PREG/CONT** C/NA

**IND & DOSE Tx of pts w/active, antibody-positive SLE, w/standard tx.** *Adult:* 200 mg subcut once/wk. *Adult, child ≥5 yr:* 10 mg/kg IV over 1 hr at 2-wk intervals for first three doses, then at 4-wk intervals.
**ADV EFF** Bronchitis, **death, depression/suicidality, hypersensitivity reactions, malignancies,** migraine, n/v/d, pain, pharyngitis, PML, **serious to fatal infections**
**INTERACTIONS** Live vaccines
**NC/PT** Not for use in preg/breastfeeding. Premedicate w/antihistamines, corticosteroids. Do not use w/acute infection; monitor for infections. Encourage cancer screening. Protect pt w/suicidal thoughts.

## belinostat (Beleodaq)
**CLASS** Antineoplastic, histone deacetylase inhibitor
**PREG/CONT** D/NA

**IND & DOSE Tx of relapsed/ refractory peripheral T-cell lymphoma.** *Adult:* 1,000 mg/m$^2$/d IV over 30 min on days 1–5 of 21-day cycle; repeat until disease progression or unacceptable toxicity.
**ADV EFF Bone marrow suppression,** fatigue, fever, **hepatotoxicity,** n/v/d, **serious to fatal infection, TLS**
**NC/PT** Rule out preg. Monitor bone marrow, LFTs, TLS; modify dose, support pt as needed. Not for use in preg (contraceptives advised)/ breastfeeding. Protect from infection; encourage cancer screening. Advise small, frequent meals; rest periods. Pt should report urine/stool color changes, unusual bleeding, severe n/v/d.

## benazepril hydrochloride (Lotensin)
**CLASS** ACE inhibitor, antihypertensive
**PREG/CONT** D/NA

**BBW** Rule out preg; fetal abnormalities and death have occurred if used during second or third trimester. Encourage contraceptive measures.
**IND & DOSE Tx of HTN, alone or as part of combo tx.** *Adult:* 10 mg PO daily. Maint, 20–40 mg/d PO; max, 80 mg/d. *Child ≥6 yr:* 0.1–0.6 mg/kg/d; max, 40 mg/d.
**ADJUST DOSE** Renal impairment
**ADV EFF** Cough, hepatotoxicity, hyperkalemia, renal toxicity, **SJS**
**INTERACTIONS** Allopurinol, ARBs, capsaicin, indomethacin, lithium, NSAIDs, potassium-sparing diuretics, renin inhibitors
**NC/PT** Use caution before surgery; mark chart. Protect pt w/decreased fluid volume. Not for use in preg. Cough may occur. Pt should change position slowly if dizzy, light-headed; report rash.

**DANGEROUS DRUG**

## bendamustine hydrochloride (Bendeka, Treanda)
**CLASS** Alkylating agent, antineoplastic
**PREG/CONT** D/NA

**IND & DOSE Chronic lymphocytic leukemia.** *Adult:* 100 mg/m$^2$ IV over 30 min (*Treanda*), 10 min (*Bendeka*) on days 1 and 2 of 28-day cycle for up

to six cycles. **Indolent non–B cell Hodgkin lymphoma.** *Adult:* 120 mg/m² IV over 60 min (*Treanda*), 10 min (*Bendeka*) on days 1 and 2 of 21-day cycle for up to eight cycles.
**ADJUST DOSE** Hepatic/renal impairment
**ADV EFF** Extravasation injury, fatigue, fever, infections, infusion reaction, **malignancies, myelosuppression,** n/v/d, **rash to toxic skin reactions, TLS**
**INTERACTIONS** Ciprofloxacin, fluvoxamine, nicotine, omeprazole
**NC/PT** Monitor blood counts closely; dosage adjustment may be needed. Protect pt from infection, bleeding. Monitor pt closely during infusion; note infusion times for specific drug being used. Premedicate w/antihistamines, antipyretics, corticosteroids. Assess skin regularly. Not for use in preg/breastfeeding. Pt may feel very tired; should plan activities accordingly.

## benznidazole (generic)
**CLASS** Nitroimidazole antimicrobial
**PREG/CONT** High risk/NA

**IND & DOSE Tx of Chagas disease in child.** *Child 2–12 yr:* 5–8 mg/kg PO in two divided doses approx 12 hr apart for 60 d.
**ADV EFF** Abd pain, bone marrow depression, decreased appetite/weight, nausea, **paresthesia, peripheral neuropathy,** pruritus, skin reactions
**INTERACTIONS** Alcohol, disulfiram
**NC/PT** Monitor skin/blood counts. Watch for neuro sx. Pt should avoid preg (contraceptives advised)/ breastfeeding; report numbness/ tingling, rash, fever, marked weight loss.

## benzonatate (Tessalon, Zonatuss)
**CLASS** Antitussive
**PREG/CONT** C/NA

**IND & DOSE Sx relief of nonproductive cough.** *Adult, child ≥10 yr:* 100–200 mg PO tid; max, 600 mg/d.
**ADV EFF** Constipation, dizziness, headache, nausea, rash, sedation
**NC/PT** Pt should not cut/crush/chew capsules; must swallow capsule whole; use caution if CNS effects occur.

## benztropine mesylate (Cogentin)
**CLASS** Anticholinergic, antiparkinsonian
**PREG/CONT** C/NA

**IND & DOSE Adjunct to tx of parkinsonism.** *Adult:* Initially, 0.5–1 mg PO at bedtime; total daily dose, 0.5–6 mg at bedtime or in two–four divided doses; may give IM or IV at same dose. **Control of drug-induced extrapyramidal disorders.** *Adult:* 1–2 mg IM (preferred) or IV to control condition, then 1–4 mg PO daily or bid to prevent recurrences. **Extrapyramidal disorders occurring early in neuroleptic tx.** *Adult:* 2 mg PO bid to tid. Withdraw drug after 1 or 2 wk to determine continued need.
**ADJUST DOSE** Elderly pts
**ADV EFF** Blurred vision, constipation, decreased sweating, dry mouth, tachycardia, urinary hesitancy, urine retention
**INTERACTIONS** Alcohol, anticholinergics, haloperidol, phenothiazines, TCAs
**NC/PT** Pt should discontinue if dry mouth makes swallowing or speaking difficulty, use caution in hot weather when decreased sweating could lead to heat prostration, avoid alcohol and OTC drugs that could cause serious CNS effects, empty bladder before

each dose if urine retention a problem, use caution if CNS effects occur.

**beractant** (natural lung surfactant) (Survanta)
**CLASS** Lung surfactant
**PREG/CONT** Unkn/NA

**IND & DOSE Px for infants at risk for RDS.** Give first dose of 100 mg phospholipids/kg birth weight (4 mL/kg) intratracheally soon after birth, preferably within 15 min. After determining needed dose, inject ¼ of dose into ET tube over 2–3 sec; may repeat no sooner than 6 hr after dose. **Rescue tx of premature infants w/RDS.** Give 100 mg phospholipids/kg birth weight (4 mL/kg) intratracheally. Give first dose as soon as possible within 8 hr of birth after RDS diagnosis is made and pt is on ventilator; may repeat after 6 hr from previous dose.
**ADV EFF Bradycardia, hypotension, intraventricular hemorrhage,** nonpulmonary infections, patent ductus arteriosus, sepsis
**NC/PT** Monitor ECG and $O_2$ saturation continuously during and for at least 30 min after administration. Ensure ET tube is correctly placed. Suction immediately before dosing; do not suction for 1 hr after dosing.

**betamethasone** (generic), **betamethasone dipropionate** (Diprolene AF, Maxivate), **betamethasone sodium phosphate and acetate** (Celestone Soluspan), **betamethasone valerate** (Beta-Val, Luxiq)
**CLASS** Corticosteroid
**PREG/CONT** C/NA

**IND & DOSE Tx of primary or secondary adrenocortical insufficiency; hypercalcemia w/cancer; short-term mgt of inflammatory and allergic disorders; thrombocytopenia purpura; ulcerative colitis; MS exacerbations; trichinosis w/neuro or cardiac involvement.** *Adult:* Oral (betamethasone), initially, 0.6–7.2 mg/d. IM (betamethasone sodium phosphate, betamethasone sodium phosphate and acetate), initially, 0.5–9 mg/d. Intrabursal, intra-articular, intradermal, intralesional (betamethasone sodium phosphate and acetate), 1.5–12 mg intra-articular (depending on joint size), 0.2 mL/cm$^3$ intradermally (max, 1 mL/wk); 0.25–1 mL at 3- to 7-day intervals for foot disorders. Topical dermatologic cream, ointment (betamethasone dipropionate), apply sparingly to affected area daily or bid.
**ADV EFF** Aggravation of infection, headache, immunosuppression, increased appetite, local stinging and burning, masking of infection, vertigo, weight gain
**INTERACTIONS** Live vaccines
**NC/PT** Give oral dose at 9 a.m. Taper dosage when discontinuing. Pt should avoid overusing joints after injection; be cautious w/occlusive dressings; not stop drug suddenly; wear medical alert tag; apply sparingly if using topically; avoid exposure to infection; monitor blood glucose w/long-term use.

**betaxolol hydrochloride valerate** (Betoptic S)
**CLASS** Antiglaucoma drug, antihypertensive, beta-selective blocker
**PREG/CONT** C/NA

**IND & DOSE HTN, alone or w/other antihypertensives.** *Adult:* 10 mg PO daily, alone or added to diuretic therapy. **Tx of ocular HTN/open-angle glaucoma, alone or w/other antiglaucoma drugs.** *Adult*: 1 or 2 drops ophthal sol bid to affected eye(s).
**ADJUST DOSE** Elderly pts, severe renal impairment, dialysis pts
**ADV EFF** Allergic reactions, bradycardia, cardiac arrhythmias, decreased exercise tolerance, dizziness, HF, n/v/d, ocular itching/tearing (ophthal)

**INTERACTIONS** Anticholinergics, aspirin, hormonal contraceptives, insulin, prazosin, salicylates, verapamil
**NC/PT** Do not discontinue abruptly; taper over 2 wk. Protect eyes or joints from injury after dosing. Give eyedrops as instructed to avoid systemic absorption.

## bethanechol chloride (Urecholine)

**CLASS** Cholinergic, parasympathomimetic
**PREG/CONT** C/NA

**IND & DOSE** **Acute postop and postpartum nonobstructive urine retention; neurogenic atony of urinary bladder w/retention.** *Adult:* 10–50 mg PO 3–4 ×/d.
**ADV EFF** Abd discomfort, **cardiac arrest**, flushing, n/v/d, sweating
**INTERACTIONS** Cholinergics, ganglionic blockers
**NC/PT** Give on empty stomach 1 hr before or 2 hr after meals. Keep atropine on hand for severe response. Safety precautions if CNS effects occur.

## betrixaban (Bevyxxa)

**CLASS** Anticoagulant, factor Xa inhibitor
**PREG/CONT** Moderate risk/NA

**BBW** Risk of epidural or spinal hematoma in pt w/spinal anesthesia or spinal puncture; may result in long-term or permanent paralysis.
**IND & DOSE** **Px of VTE in hospitalized pts at risk due to restricted mobility or other risk factors.** *Adult:* 160 mg PO followed by 80 mg/d for 35–42 d.
**ADJUST DOSE** Hepatic impairment (avoid use), renal impairment
**ADV EFF** **Bleeding, renal impairment**
**INTERACTIONS** P-gp inhibitors, other anticoagulants
**NC/PT** Monitor LFTs, renal function, bleeding. Not for use w/artificial heart valve. Pt should avoid preg/breastfeeding, drugs that interfere w/clotting; report s&sx of bleeding/bruising, urine/stool color changes, coughing or vomiting blood, dizziness, headache, swelling.

**DANGEROUS DRUG**

## bevacizumab (Avastin, Mvasi, Zirabev)

**CLASS** Antineoplastic, monoclonal antibody
**PREG/CONT** High risk/NA

**IND & DOSE** **Tx of metastatic cancer of colon/rectum, w/5-FU.** *Adult:* 5–10 mg/kg IV q 14 d until progression; first infusion over 90 min, second over 60 min, then over 30 min. **Tx of metastatic, unresectable or locally advanced nonsquamous NSCLC.** *Adult:* 15 mg/kg IV q 3 wk. **Tx of glioblastoma.** *Adult:* 10 mg/kg IV q 2 wk. **Tx of metastatic renal cell carcinoma.** *Adult:* 10 mg/kg IV q 2 wk w/interferon alfa. **Tx of resistant, metastatic, or recurrent cervical cancer.** *Adult:* 15 mg/kg IV q 3 wk w/other drugs. **Tx of platinum-resistant epithelial ovarian, fallopian tube, or primary peritoneal cancer.** *Adult:* 10 mg/kg IV q 2 wk w/paclitaxel, doxorubicin, or wkly topotecan, or 15 mg/kg q 3 wk w/topotecan q 3 wk. **Tx of platinum-sensitive epithelial ovarian, fallopian tube, or primary peritoneal cancer.** *Adult:* 15 mg/kg IV q 3 wk w/carboplatin and gemcitabine for 6–10 cycles, then 15 mg/kg q 3 wk alone.
**ADV EFF** **Arterial thrombotic events**, back pain, epistaxis, exfoliative dermatitis, headache, HTN, **infusion reactions, non-GI fistula formation, proteinuria, ovarian failure, rectal hemorrhage, RPLS**, rhinitis
**NC/PT** Do not initiate within 28 d of major surgery and until surgical wound is completely healed. Do not give as IV push or bolus. Monitor BP, wounds (for healing issues), during infusion (for infusion reactions). Not for use in preg (risk of embryo-fetal

toxicity)/breastfeeding. Possible risk of HF. Pt should report rectal bleeding, high fever, changes in neuro function.

DANGEROUS DRUG

**bexarotene** (Targretin)
**CLASS** Antineoplastic
**PREG/CONT** High risk/NA

**BBW** Not for use in preg; fetal harm can occur.
**IND & DOSE** **Cutaneous manifestations of cutaneous T-cell lymphoma in pts refractory to other tx.** *Adult:* 300 mg/m²/d PO; may adjust to 200 mg/m²/d PO, then 100 mg/m²/d PO.
**ADV EFF** Abd pain, asthenia, dry skin, headache, **hepatic impairment,** hyperlipidemia, hypothyroidism, lipid abnormalities, nausea, **pancreatitis,** photosensitivity, rash
**INTERACTIONS** Atorvastatin, carboplatin, gemfibrozil, paclitaxel, tamoxifen
**NC/PT** Rule out preg before start of tx; ensure pt is using contraceptives. Monitor LFTs, amylase, lipids, thyroid function. Protect pt from exposure to sunlight. Not for use in breastfeeding. Pt should swallow capsules whole, not cut/crush/chew them; take once/d w/meal; report urine/stool color changes.

**bezlotoxumab** (Zinplava)
**CLASS** Monoclonal antibody
**PREG/CONT** Unkn/NA

**IND & DOSE** **To reduce risk of recurrence of *Clostridium difficile* infection in pts taking antibacterial drugs who are at high risk for recurrence.** *Adult:* 10 mg/kg IV over 60 min as single dose, given during antibacterial drug tx.
**ADV EFF** Fever, headache HF, nausea
**NC/PT** Not for tx of *C. difficile* infection; must be given w/antibacterial tx. Monitor pts w/known HF. Use caution in preg/breastfeeding. Pt should continue antibacterial tx of CDAD; report swelling, difficulty breathing.

DANGEROUS DRUG

**bicalutamide** (Casodex)
**CLASS** Antiandrogen
**PREG/CONT** X/NA

**IND & DOSE** **Tx of stage D2 metastatic carcinoma of prostrate, w/ LHRH.** *Adult:* 50 mg/d PO a.m. or p.m.
**ADJUST DOSE** Hepatic/renal impairment
**ADV EFF** Anemia, asthenia, constipation, diarrhea, dyspnea, edema, gynecomastia, hematuria, hot flashes, nausea, nocturia, pain, **severe hepatic injury to fatal hepatic failure**
**INTERACTIONS** CYP3A4 substrates, midazolam, warfarin
**NC/PT** Used w/LHRH only. Monitor LFTs regularly, PSA, glucose. Not for use in preg/breastfeeding. Pt should report trouble breathing, blood in urine, yellowing of eyes or skin.

**bismuth subsalicylate** (Kaopectate, Pepto-Bismol, Pink Bismuth)
**CLASS** Antidiarrheal
**PREG/CONT** C (1st, 2nd trimesters); D (3rd trimester)/NA

**IND & DOSE** **To control diarrhea/gas/upset stomach/indigestion/heartburn/nausea; to reduce number of bowel movements and help firm stool.** *Adult, child ≥12 yr:* 2 tablets or 30 mL (524 mg) PO; repeat q 30 min–1 hr as needed (max, eight doses/24 hr). *Child 9–11 yr:* 1 tablet or 15 mL PO. *Child 6–8 yr:* 2/3 tablet or 10 mL PO. *Child 3–5 yr:* 1/3 tablet or 5 mL PO. **Tx of traveler's diarrhea.** *Adult, child ≥12 yr:* 1 oz (524 mg) PO q 30 min for total of eight doses.
**ADV EFF** Darkening of stool
**INTERACTIONS** Antidiabetics, aspirin, methotrexate, sulfinpyrazone, tetracyclines, valproic acid

**NC/PT** Shake liquid well. Have pt chew tablets (not swallow whole). Pt should not take w/drugs containing aspirin. Pt should report ringing in ears; stools may be dark.

## bisoprolol fumarate (generic)

**CLASS** Antihypertensive, beta-selective adrenergic blocker
**PREG/CONT** C/NA

**IND & DOSE Mgt of HTN, alone or w/other antihypertensives.** *Adult:* 5 mg PO daily, alone or added to diuretic therapy; 2.5 mg may be appropriate. Max, 20 mg PO daily.
**ADJUST DOSE** Renal/hepatic impairment
**ADV EFF** Bradycardia, **bronchospasm,** cardiac arrhythmias, constipation, decreased exercise tolerance, ED, fatigue, flatulence, headache, n/v/d
**INTERACTIONS** Anticholinergics, hormonal contraceptives, insulin, NSAIDs, prazosin, salicylates
**NC/PT** Do not discontinue abruptly; taper over 2 wk. Controversial need to stop before surgery. If diabetic pt, monitor glucose levels regularly. Pt should avoid OTC drugs.

**DANGEROUS DRUG**

## bivalirudin (Angiomax)

**CLASS** Anticoagulant, thrombin inhibitor
**PREG/CONT** B/NA

**IND & DOSE Pts w/unstable angina undergoing PTCA.** *Adult:* 0.75 mg/kg IV, then 1.75 mg/kg/hr during procedure. **Tx/px of heparin-induced thrombocytopenia in pts undergoing PTCA.** *Adult:* 0.75 mg/kg IV bolus, then 1.75 mg/kg/hr during procedure; may continue for up to 4 hr, then 0.2 mg/kg/hr for up to 20 hr if needed.
**ADJUST DOSE** Renal impairment
**ADV EFF Bleeding,** fever, headache, hypotension, thrombocytopenia
**INTERACTIONS** Heparin, thrombolytics, warfarin
**NC/PT** Used w/aspirin therapy. Monitor for bleeding; could indicate need to discontinue.

**DANGEROUS DRUG**

## bleomycin sulfate (BLM)

**CLASS** Antibiotic, antineoplastic
**PREG/CONT** D/NA

**BBW** Monitor pulmonary function regularly and chest X-ray wkly or biwkly for onset of pulmonary toxicity. Be alert for rare, severe idiosyncratic reaction, including fever, chills, HTN, in lymphoma pts.
**IND & DOSE Palliative tx of squamous cell carcinoma/lymphomas/testicular carcinoma, alone or w/other drugs.** *Adult:* 0.25–0.5 unit/kg IV, IM, or subcut once or twice wkly. **Tx of malignant pleural effusion.** *Adult:* 60 units dissolved in 50–100 mL NSS via thoracotomy tube.
**ADJUST DOSE** Renal impairment
**ADV EFF** Chills, dyspnea, fever, hair loss, hyperpigmentation, idiosyncratic reactions to **anaphylaxis,** pneumonitis, **pulmonary fibrosis,** stomatitis, striae, vesiculation, vomiting
**INTERACTIONS** Digoxin, oxygen, phenytoin
**NC/PT** Label reconstituted sol and use within 24 hr. Monitor LFTs, renal function tests, pulmonary function regularly; consult physician immediately if s&sx of toxicity. Not for use in preg. Pt should mark calendar for injection dates, cover head w/temp extremes (hair loss possible).

## blinatumomab (Blincyto)

**CLASS** Antineoplastic, monoclonal antibody
**PREG/CONT** High risk/NA

**BBW** Life-threatening cytokine-release syndrome (CRS) and neurotoxicities possible. Monitor closely; interrupt or stop as recommended.

**IND & DOSE Tx of Philadelphia chromosome–negative relapsed or refractory B-cell precursor ALL.** *Adult at least 45 kg:* Cycle 1, 28 mcg/d as continuous IV on days 1–28, tx free for 14 d; repeat for two to four cycles. *<45 kg:* 15 mcg/m²/d (not to exceed 28 mcg/d) for days 1–28, tx free for 14 d; repeat for two to four cycles.
**ADV EFF CNS toxicity,** constipation, **CRS,** edema, fever, hypokalemia, infections, nausea, pancreatitis, rash
**NC/PT** Hospitalize for first 9 d of cycle 1, first 2 d of cycle 2. Follow reconstitution directions carefully. Premedicate w/dexamethasone 20 mg IV 1 hr before first dose or if interrupting for 4 or more hr. Administer using infusion pump to ensure constant flow rate; carefully check dose and timing. Monitor for infection, pancreatitis. Not for use in preg/breastfeeding. Pt should take safety precautions w/CNS effects; mark calendar for tx days; report difficulty breathing, dizziness, edema, rash.

**DANGEROUS DRUG**

## bortezomib (Velcade)

**CLASS** Antineoplastic, proteasome inhibitor
**PREG/CONT** High risk/NA

**IND & DOSE Tx of multiple myeloma; tx of mantle cell lymphoma in pts who have received at least one other tx.** *Adult:* 1.3 mg/m² as 3–5 sec IV bolus or subcut for nine 6-day cycles (days 1, 4, 8, 11), then 10 d of rest, then days 22, 25, 29, 32; may repeat tx for multiple myeloma if 6 mo since failed tx.
**ADJUST DOSE** Hepatic impairment
**ADV EFF** Anemia, anorexia, asthenia, constipation, HF, hypotension, leukopenia, neutropenia, n/v/d, **peripheral neuropathies, pulmonary infiltrates,** thrombocytopenia, TLS
**INTERACTIONS** Ketoconazole, omeprazole, ritonavir, St. John's wort
**NC/PT** Monitor for neuro changes. Dose individualized to prevent overdose. Monitor CBC. Try to maintain hydration if GI effects are severe. Not for use in preg/breastfeeding. Diabetic pts, pts w/CV disease require close monitoring. Pt should use care when driving or operating machinery until drug's effects are known; report s&sx of infection, difficulty breathing.

## bosentan (Tracleer)

**CLASS** Endothelin receptor antagonist, pulmonary antihypertensive
**PREG/CONT** X/NA

**BBW** Rule out preg before tx; ensure pt is using two forms of contraception during tx and for 1 mo after tx ends. Verify preg status monthly. Obtain baseline then monthly liver enzyme levels. Dose reduction or drug withdrawal indicated if liver enzymes elevated; liver failure possible. Available only through restricted access program.
**IND & DOSE Tx of pulmonary arterial HTN in pts w/WHO class II–IV sx.** *Adult, child >12 yr:* 62.5 mg PO bid for 4 wk. Then, for pts 40 kg or more, maint dose is 125 mg PO bid. For pts <40 kg but >12 yr, maint dose is 62.5 mg PO bid.
**ADJUST DOSE** Hepatic impairment
**ADV EFF** Decreased Hgb/hematocrit, decreased sperm count, edema, flushing, headache, hypotension, **liver injury,** nasopharyngitis
**INTERACTIONS** Atazanavir, cyclosporine A, glyburide, hormonal contraceptives, ritonavir (serious toxicity), statins
**NC/PT** Available only through restricted access program. Obtain baseline Hgb, at 1 and 3 mo, then q 3 mo. Monitor LFTs. Do not use w/ cyclosporine or glyburide. Taper if discontinuing. Not for use in preg (barrier contraceptives advised)/ breastfeeding. Pt should keep chart of activity tolerance to monitor drug's effects; report urine/stool color changes.

**bosutinib** (Bosulif)
**CLASS** Antineoplastic, kinase inhibitor
**PREG/CONT** High risk/NA

**IND & DOSE Tx of chronic, accelerated, or blast phase Philadelphia chromosome–positive (Ph+) CML w/resistance or intolerance to other tx.** *Adult:* 500 mg/d PO, up to 600 mg/d if complete hematologic response does not occur by wk 12 and no serious adverse effects. Adjust dose based on toxicity. **Tx of newly diagnosed chronic phase Ph+ CML.** *Adult:* 400 mg/d PO w/food.
**ADJUST DOSE** Hepatic impairment
**ADV EFF** Abd pain, anemia, **cardiac failure,** edema, fatigue, fever, **fluid retention, GI toxicity, hepatotoxicity, myelosuppression,** n/v/d, rash, renal toxicity
**INTERACTIONS** CYP3A inhibitors/inducers (carbamazepine, dexamethasone, ketoconazole, phenobarbital, phenytoin, rifabutin, rifampin, rifapentine, St. John's wort), P-gp inhibitors; avoid these combos. Proton pump inhibitors
**NC/PT** Monitor closely for bone marrow suppression, GI toxicity; monitor renal function. Not for use in preg/breastfeeding. Pt should take once a day, report s&sx of bleeding, severe GI effects, urine/stool color changes, swelling.

**▶NEW DRUG**

**bremelanotide** (Vyleesi)
**CLASS** Melanocortin receptor agonist
**PREG/CONT** Unkn/NA

**IND & DOSE Tx of premenopausal women w/acquired, generalized hypoactive sexual desire disorder as characterized by low sexual desire that causes marked distress/interpersonal difficulty and is NOT due to coexisting medical/psychiatric condition, relationship problems, or drug effect.** *Adult:* 1.75 mg subcut 45 min before anticipated sexual performance. Not more than one dose within 24 hr.
**ADV EFF** BP increase, focal hyperpigmentation, hr decrease, injection site reactions, nausea
**INTERACTIONS** May slow absorption of PO drugs due to slower gastric emptying; may decrease exposure to naltrexone
**NC/PT** Before tx, consider CV risk, due to possible BP/HR changes. Pt should use contraceptives during tx, stop drug if preg, report drug exposure to preg exposure registry.

**brentuximab** (Adcetris)
**CLASS** Monoclonal antibody
**PREG/CONT** High risk/NA

**BBW** Risk of potentially fatal PML.
**IND & DOSE Tx of Hodgkin lymphoma for immediate use and after failure of autologous stem-cell transplant or if high risk of relapse or progression; tx of systemic anaplastic large-cell lymphoma (sALCL); tx of primary cutaneous anaplastic large-cell lymphoma or CD30-expressing mycosis fungoides.** *Adult:* 1.8 mg/kg IV over 30 min q 3 wk for max of 16 cycles. **Tx of untreated Stage III or IV classical Hodgkin lymphoma, w/doxorubicin, vinblastine, and dacarbazine.** *Adult:* 1.2 mg/kg up to 120 mg q 2 wk for max of 12 doses. **Tx of untreated sALCL or other CD30-expressing peripheral T-cell lymphomas (PTCL), including angioimmunoblastic T-cell lymphoma and PTCL not otherwise specified, w/cyclophosphamide, doxorubicin, and prednisone.** *Adult:* 1.8 mg/kg up to max of 180 mg q 3 wk for six–eight doses.
**ADV EFF Anaphylactic reactions,** chills, cough, dyspnea, fever, hematologic toxicities, **hepatotoxicity,** infections, infusion reactions, nausea, neutropenia, **peripheral neuropathy, PML, pulmonary toxicity, SJS, TLS**

**INTERACTIONS** Bleomycin, ketoconazole, rifampin
**NC/PT** Monitor pt during infusion. Monitor neutrophil count, LFTs, pulmonary function; dose adjustment may be needed. Protect pt w/peripheral neuropathies. Not for use in preg/breastfeeding. Pt should report mood or behavior changes, changes in vision or walking, weakness, rash, infections, difficulty breathing.

**▶NEW DRUG**
**DANGEROUS DRUG**

## brexanolone (Zulresso)

**CLASS** Antidepressant, $GABA_A$ receptor modulator
**PREG/CONT** Unkn/Pending DEA review

**BBW** Drug causes excessive sedation/sudden loss of consciousness. Must monitor pt w/continuous pulse oximetry. Pt must be accompanied during interactions w/child. Only available through restricted
**IND & DOSE** **Tx of postpartum depression.** *Adult:* Initially, 30 mcg/kg/hr IV, titrated up per dosing
**ADV EFF** Dry mouth, hot flush, **sedation/loss of consciousness, suicidal thoughts/behaviors**
**NC/PT** Health care provider must be on site to monitor/intervene during infusion. Avoid use in pts w/ESRD. Fetal harm possible based on animal studies. Stop infusion if excessive sedation until sx resolve; then resume at lower dose. Do not mix other drugs in infusion bag.

## brexpiprazole (Rexulti)

**CLASS** Atypical antipsychotic, dopamine/serotonin agonist/antagonist
**PREG/CONT** High risk/NA

**BBW** Elderly pts w/dementia-related psychosis have increased risk of death if given atypical antipsychotics; not approved for this use. Risk of suicidal ideation increases w/antidepressant use, especially in child, adolescents, young adults; monitor accordingly. Not approved for use in child.
**IND & DOSE** **Tx of schizophrenia.** *Adult:* 1 mg/d PO; max, 4 mg/d. **Adjunct tx for major depressive disorder.** *Adult:* 0.5–1 mg/d PO; max, 3 mg/d.
**ADV EFF** **Akathisia,** bone marrow suppression, cognitive/motor impairment, dyslipidemia, hyperglycemia, **NMS,** orthostatic hypotension, **seizures** (potentially life-threatening), suicidality, syncope, tardive dyskinesia, weight gain
**INTERACTIONS** Alcohol, carbamazepine, CNS depressants, CYP2D6 inhibitors (fluoxetine, paroxetine, quinidine), CYP3A4 inhibitors (ketoconazole), lorazepam
**NC/PT** Dispense least amount possible to suicidal pts. Not for use in preg (risk of abnormal muscle movements, withdrawal)/breastfeeding. Monitor weight; assess for hyperglycemia. May react w/many drugs; monitor regimen. Take safety precautions for cognitive/motor impairment; use cautiously if low BP possible; ensure hydration. Caution pt about potential for compulsive gambling/behavior. Pt should report suicidal thoughts, s&sx of infection, abnormal muscle movements. Confusion between brexpiprazole and proton pump inhibitors; use extreme caution.

## brigatinib (Alunbrig)

**CLASS** Antineoplastic, tyrosine kinase inhibitor
**PREG/CONT** High risk/NA

**IND & DOSE** **Tx of pts w/anaplastic lymphoma kinase (ALK)-positive metastatic NSCLC who have progressed on or are intolerant to crizotinib.** *Adult:* 90 mg PO q d for first 7 d; if tolerated, increase to 180 mg PO q d.
**ADV EFF** **Bradycardia,** cough, diarrhea, fatigue, headache, **HTN,** hyperglycemia, **ILD/pneumonitis,** nausea,

**pancreatic enzyme elevation,** visual disturbance
**INTERACTIONS** CYP3A inhibitors/inducers and substrates
**NC/PT** May give w/ or w/o food. Monitor HR, BP, CK, lipase/amylase/glucose; watch for new/worsening respiratory s&sx; consider dose reduction for concerning findings. Women should use nonhormonal contraception during tx and for at least 4 mo after tx. Men should use contraception during tx and for at least 3 mo after tx. Pt should not breastfeed during and for at least 1 wk after tx; report visual changes; inform prescriber of all concomitant medications, including prescription/OTC drugs, vitamins/herbs; avoid grapefruit/grapefruit juice.

## brivaracetam (Briviact)

**CLASS** Antiepileptic
**PREG/CONT** High risk/NA

**IND & DOSE Adjunct tx of partial-onset seizures in pts ≥4 yr.** *Adult, child >16 yr:* 50 mg PO bid; may adjust to 25 mg bid or up to 100 mg bid based on response. IV form available for temporary use for pt ≥16 yr. *Child 4–<16 yr:* PO doses bid based on body weight.
**ADJUST DOSE** Hepatic impairment
**ADV EFF Angioedema, bronchospasm,** dizziness, fatigue, n/v, psychiatric reactions, somnolence, **suicidality**
**INTERACTIONS** Carbamazepine, levetiracetam, phenytoin, rifampin
**NC/PT** Monitor response to adjust dose; taper when discontinuing. Use injectable form only temporarily. Pt should avoid preg (contraceptives advised)/breastfeeding; avoid driving/operating hazardous machinery if CNS effects; not stop drug suddenly (must be tapered); report difficulty breathing, unusual swelling, thoughts of suicide, changes in behavior.

## brodalumab (Siliq)

**CLASS** Interleukin antagonist, monoclonal antibody
**PREG/CONT** Moderate risk/NA

**BBW** Suicidal ideation and suicide have occurred; be alert for changes in behavior. Available only through restricted program.
**IND & DOSE Tx of moderate to severe plaque psoriasis in pts who are candidates for systemic therapy or phototherapy who have failed or lost response to systemic therapy.** *Adult:* 210 mg subcut at weeks 0, 1, and 2; then 210 mg subcut q 2 wk.
**ADV EFF** Arthralgia, **Crohn disease,** diarrhea, fatigue, headache, injection-site reactions, myalgia, **potentially serious infections, suicidality,** TB
**INTERACTIONS** Live vaccines
**NC/PT** Do not use w/Crohn disease. Use caution in preg/breastfeeding. Mark calendar w/injections dates. Pt should avoid exposure to infection; report s&sx of infection, severe diarrhea, thoughts of suicide.

## bromocriptine mesylate (Cycloset, Parlodel)

**CLASS** Antidiabetic, antiparkinsonian, dopamine receptor agonist
**PREG/CONT** B/NA

**IND & DOSE Tx of postencephalitic or idiopathic Parkinson disease.** *Adult, child ≥15 yr:* 11.25 mg PO bid. Assess q 2 wk, and adjust dose; max, 100 mg/d. **Tx of hyperprolactinemia.** *Adult, child ≥15 yr:* 1.25–2.5 mg PO daily; range, 2.5–15 mg/d. **Tx of acromegaly.** *Adult, child ≥15 yr:* 1.25–2.5 mg PO for 3 d at bedtime; add 1.25–2.5 mg as tolerated q 3–7 d until optimal response. Range, 20–30 mg/d. **Tx of type 2 diabetes.** *Adult:* 0.8 mg/d PO in a.m. within 2 hr of waking; increase by 1 tablet/wk to max 6 tablets (4.8 mg) daily (*Cycloset* only).

**ADV EFF** Abd cramps, constipation, dyspnea, fatigue, n/v/d, orthostatic hypotension
**INTERACTIONS** Erythromycin, phenothiazines, sympathomimetics
**NC/PT** Ensure proper dx before starting tx. Taper dose if used in parkinsonism. Not for use in preg/breastfeeding. Pt should take drug for diabetes once a day in a.m., use safety precautions if dizziness/orthostatic hypotension occur.

**brompheniramine maleate** (BroveX, J-Tan, Lo-Hist 12, Respa-AR)
**CLASS** Antihistamine
**PREG/CONT** C/NA

**IND & DOSE** **Relief of sx of seasonal rhinitis, common cold; tx of nonallergic pruritic sx.** *Adult, child ≥12 yr:* Products vary. ER tablets, 6–12 mg PO q 12 hr. Chewable tablets, 12–24 mg PO q 12 hr (max, 48 mg/d). ER capsules, 12–24 mg/d PO. Oral suspension (*BroveX*), 5–10 mL (12–24 mg) PO q 12 hr (max, 48 mg/d). Oral liquid, 10 mL (4 mg) PO 4 ×/d. Oral suspension 5 mL PO q 12 hr (max, two doses/d). *Child 6–12 yr:* ER tablets, 6 mg PO q 12 hr. Chewable tablets, 6–12 mg PO q 12 hr (max, 24 mg/d). ER capsules, 12 mg/d PO. Oral liquid, 5 mL (2 mg) PO 4 ×/d. Oral suspension (*BroveX*), 5 mL (12 mg) PO q 12 hr (max, 24 mg/d). Oral suspension, 2.5 mL PO q 12 hr (max, 5 mL/d). *Child 2–6 yr:* Chewable tablets, 6 mg PO q 12 hr (max, 12 mg/d). Oral liquid, 2.5 mL (1 mg) PO 4 ×/d. Oral suspension (*BroveX*), 2.5 mL (6 mg) PO q 12 hr up (max, 12 mg/d). Oral suspension 1.25 mL PO q 12 hr (max, 2.5 mg/d). *Child 12 mo–2 yr:* Oral suspension, 1.25 mL (3 mg) PO q 12 hr (max, 2.5 mL [6 mg]/d). Oral liquid, titrate dose based on 0.5 mg/kg/d PO in equally divided doses 4 ×/d.
**ADJUST DOSE** Elderly pts
**ADV EFF** **Anaphylactic shock**, disturbed coordination, dizziness, drowsiness, faintness, thickening bronchial secretions
**INTERACTIONS** Alcohol, anticholinergics, CNS depressants
**NC/PT** Double-check dosages; products vary widely. Pt should not cut/crush/chew ER tablets; should avoid alcohol, take safety precautions if CNS effects occur.

**budesonide** (Entocort EC, Ortikos, Pulmicort Flexhaler, Pulmicort Respules, Rhinocort, Uceris)
**CLASS** Corticosteroid
**PREG/CONT** B (inhalation); high risk (oral)/NA

**IND & DOSE** **Nasal spray mgt of allergic rhinitis sx.** *Adult, child ≥6 yr:* 64 mcg/d as 1 spray (32 mcg) in each nostril once daily. Max for pts >12 yr, 256 mcg/d as 4 sprays per nostril once daily. Max for pts 6–<12 yr, 128 mcg/d (given as 2 sprays per nostril once daily). **Maint tx of asthma as prophylactic therapy.** *Adult, child ≥12 yr:* 360 mcg by inhalation bid; max, 720 mcg bid. "Low" dose, 180–600 mcg/d; "medium" dose, 600–1,200 mcg/d; "high" dose, >1,200 mcg/d. *Child 5–11 yr:* 180 mcg by inhalation bid; max, 360 mcg bid. "Low" dose, 180–400 mcg/d; "medium" dose, 400–800 mcg/d; "high" dose, >800 mcg/d. *Child 0–11 yr:* 0.5–1 mg by inhalation once daily or in two divided doses using jet nebulizer. Max, 1 mg/d. "Low" dose, 0.25–0.5 mg/d (0–4 yr), 0.5 mg/d (5–11 yr); "medium" dose, 0.5–1 mg/d (0–4 yr), 1 mg/d (5–11 yr); "high" dose, >1 mg/d (0–4 yr), 2 mg/d (5–11 yr). **Tx/maint of clinical remission for up to 3 mo of mild to moderate active Crohn disease involving ileum/ascending colon.** *Adult:* 9 mg/d PO in a.m. for up to 8 wk. May retreat recurrent episodes for 8-wk periods. Maint, 6 mg/d PO for up

to 3 mo, then taper until cessation complete.
**ADJUST DOSE** Hepatic impairment
**ADV EFF** Back pain, cough, dizziness, fatigue, headache, lethargy, nasal irritation, pharyngitis
**INTERACTIONS** Erythromycin, grapefruit juice, indinavir, itraconazole, ketoconazole, ritonavir, saquinavir
**NC/PT** Taper systemic steroids when switching to inhaled form. Ensure proper administration technique for nasal spray/inhalation. Monitor for potential hypercorticism. Pt should not cut/crush/chew PO tablets; should take once/d in a.m.; avoid grapefruit juice; take safety precautions w/CNS effects.

## bumetanide (Bumex)

**CLASS** Loop diuretic
**PREG/CONT** C/NA

**BBW** Monitor electrolytes/hydration/hepatic function w/long-term tx; water and electrolyte depletion possible.
**IND & DOSE** **Tx of edema associated w/HF, renal and hepatic diseases.** *Adult:* Oral, 0.5–2 mg/d PO; may repeat at 4- to 5-hr intervals. Max, 10 mg/d. Intermittent therapy, 3–4 d on, then 1–2 off. Parenteral, 0.5–1 mg IV/IM over 1–2 min; may repeat in 2–3 hr; max, 10 mg/d.
**ADJUST DOSE** Elderly pts, renal impairment
**ADV EFF** Anorexia, asterixis, drowsiness, headache, hypokalemia, nocturia, n/v/d, orthostatic hypotension, pain at injection site, polyuria
**INTERACTIONS** Aminoglycosides, cardiac glycosides, cisplatin, NSAIDs, probenecid
**NC/PT** Switch to PO as soon as possible. Monitor electrolytes. Give early in day to avoid disrupting sleep. Pt should eat potassium-rich diet, check weight daily (report loss/gain of >3 lb/d).

**DANGEROUS DRUG**

## buprenorphine hydrochloride (Belbuca, Buprenex, Butrans Transdermal, Probuphine)

**CLASS** Opioid agonist-antagonist analgesic
**PREG/CONT** Moderate risk; high risk (implantable form)/C-III

**BBW** Risk of addiction, abuse, misuse; life-threatening respiratory depression; accidental exposure to child; neonatal opioid withdrawal syndrome. Secure drug, limit access. Not for use in preg.
**IND & DOSE** **Relief of moderate to severe pain** (parenteral). *Adult:* 0.3 mg IM or by slow (over 2 min) IV injection. May repeat once, 30–60 min after first dose; repeat q 6 hr. *Child 2–12 yr:* 2–6 mcg/kg body weight IM or slow IV injection q 4–6 hr. **Tx of opioid dependence** (oral). *Adult:* 8 mg on day 1, 16 mg on day 2 and subsequent induction days (can be 3–4 d). Maint, 12–16 mg/d SL (*Suboxone*). **Mgt of moderate to severe chronic pain in pts needing continuous, around-the-clock opioid analgesic for extended period** (transdermal and buccal). *Adult:* Initially, 5 mcg/hr, intended to be worn for 7 d; max, 20 mcg/hr. If opioid-naive, 75 mcg SL once or twice/d, as tolerated. May increase after 4 d. See conversion table for switching from other opioids (*Belbuca*). **Maint tx of opioid dependence in pts w/prolonged clinical stability on low doses of transdermal buprenorphine.** *Adult:* 1 implant (80 mg) inserted subdermally in upper arm for 6 mo; remove at end of 6th mo (*Probuphine*).
**ADJUST DOSE** Elderly, debilitated pts
**ADV EFF** Dizziness, headache, hypotension, hypoventilation, miosis, n/v, **respiratory depression**, sedation, sweating, vertigo
**INTERACTIONS** Barbiturates, benzodiazepines, general anesthetics, opioid analgesics, phenothiazines, sedatives
**NC/PT** Have opioid antagonists, facilities for assisted respiration on

hand. Taper as part of comprehensive tx plan. Use implant only in pts chronically stabilized on low transdermal doses. Implant must be inserted and removed by trained professionals; monitor wkly for potential adverse effects; one-time use only; do not reinsert. Not for use in preg/breastfeeding. Pt should place translingual tablet under tongue until dissolved, then swallow; apply transdermal patch to clean, dry area, leave for 7 d (remove old patch before applying new one and do not repeat use of site for 3 wk); use safety precautions w/CNS effects.

**DANGEROUS DRUG**

### buPROPion hydrobromide (Aplenzin), buPROPion hydrochloride (Forfivo XL, Wellbutrin SR, Wellbutrin XL, Zyban)

**CLASS** Antidepressant, smoking deterrent

**PREG/CONT** Moderate risk/NA

**BBW** Monitor response and behavior; suicide risk in depressed pts, child, adolescent, young adult. Serious mental health events possible, including changes in behavior, depression, and hostility. *Aplenzin* not indicated for smoking cessation; risk of serious neuropsychiatric events, including suicide, when used for this purpose.

**IND & DOSE** **Tx of major depressive disorder.** *Adult:* 300 mg PO as 100 mg tid; max, 450 mg/d. SR, 150 mg PO bid. ER, 150 mg/d PO. *Aplenzin,* 174–348 mg/d PO; max, 522 mg/d. **Smoking cessation.** *Adult:* 150 mg (*Zyban*) PO daily for 3 d; increase to 300 mg/d in two divided doses at least 8 hr apart. Treat for 7–12 wk. **Tx of seasonal affective disorder.** *Adult:* 150 mg (*Wellbutrin XL*) PO daily in a.m.; max, 300 mg/d. Begin in autumn; taper off (150 mg/d for 2 wk before discontinuation) in early spring. *Aplenzin,* 174–348 mg/d PO; continue through winter season.

**ADJUST DOSE** Renal/hepatic impairment

**ADV EFF** Agitation, constipation, depression, dry mouth, headache, migraine, **suicidality**, tachycardia, tremor, weight loss

**INTERACTIONS** Alcohol, amantadine, cyclophosphamide, levodopa, MAOIs, paroxetine, sertraline

**NC/PT** Check labels carefully; dose varies among *Wellbutrin* forms. Avoid use w/hx of seizure disorder. Discuss risk in preg/breastfeeding before use. Monitor hepatic/renal function. Smoking cessation: Pt should quit smoking within 2 wk of tx. May be used w/ transdermal nicotine. Pt should avoid alcohol; take safety precautions for CNS effects; report thoughts of suicide.

### burosumab-twza (Crysvita)

**CLASS** Anti-FGF23 monoclonal antibody

**PREG/CONT** Unkn/NA

**IND & DOSE** **Tx of X-linked hypophosphatemia in adult/child ≥6 mo.** *Adult:* 1 mg/kg body weight rounded to nearest 10 mg, up to max of 90 mg subcut q 4 wk. *Child >10 kg:* 0.8 mg/kg rounded to nearest 10 mg subcut q 2 wk, to max 90 mg. *Child <10 kg:* 1 mg/kg rounded to nearest 1 mg subcut q 2 wk.

**ADV EFF** Constipation, decreased vitamin D, dizziness, fever, headache, **hypersensitivity,** increased phosphorus, injection-site reactions, restless legs syndrome, tooth infection, vomiting

**INTERACTIONS** Active vitamin D analog, oral phosphate

**NC/PT** Contraindicated if serum phosphorus within normal or higher; in pts w/severe renal impairment or hypersensitivity reactions. Pt should notify provider for rash, hives, worsening restless legs syndrome.

**busPIRone** (generic)
**CLASS** Anxiolytic
**PREG/CONT** B/NA

**IND & DOSE Mgt of anxiety disorders; short-term relief of anxiety sx.** *Adult:* 15 mg/d PO; may increase slowly to optimum therapeutic effect. Max, 60 mg/d.
**ADV EFF** Abd distress, dizziness, dry mouth, headache, insomnia, light-headedness, n/v/d
**INTERACTIONS** Alcohol, CNS depressants, erythromycin, fluoxetine, grapefruit juice, haloperidol, itraconazole, MAOIs
**NC/PT** Suggest sugarless lozenges for dry mouth, analgesic for headache. Pt should avoid OTC sleeping drugs, alcohol, grapefruit juice; take safety measures for CNS effects.

**DANGEROUS DRUG**

**busulfan** (Busulfex, Myleran)
**CLASS** Alkylating agent, antineoplastic
**PREG/CONT** High risk/NA

**BBW** Arrange for blood tests to evaluate bone marrow function before tx, wkly during, and for at least 3 wk after tx ends. Severe bone marrow suppression possible. Hematopoietic progenitor cell transplantation required to prevent potentially fatal complications of prolonged myelosuppression.
**IND & DOSE Palliative tx of chronic myelogenous leukemia; bone marrow transplantation** (oral). *Adult:* Remission induction, 4–8 mg or 60 mcg/kg PO. Maint, resume tx w/induction dosage when WBC count reaches 50,000/mm$^3$; if remission shorter than 3 mo, maint of 1–3 mg PO daily advised to control hematologic status. *Child:* May give 60–120 mcg/kg/d PO, or 1.8–4.6 mg/m$^2$/d PO for remission induction. **W/cyclophosphamide as conditioning regimen before allogenic hematopoietic progenitor cell transplant for CML** (parenteral). *Adult:* 0.8 mg/kg IV of ideal body weight or actual body weight, whichever is lower, as 2-hr infusion q 6 hr for 4 consecutive d; total of 16 doses.
**ADJUST DOSE** Hepatic impairment
**ADV EFF** Amenorrhea, anemia, hyperpigmentation, leukopenia, menopausal sx, n/v/d, ovarian suppression, **pancytopenia, pulmonary dysplasia, seizures, SJS**
**NC/PT** Arrange for respiratory function test before and periodically during tx; monitor CBC. Reduce dose w/bone marrow suppression. Ensure pt is hydrated. Give IV through central venous catheter. Premedicate for IV tx w/ phenytoin, antiemetics. Not for use in preg (barrier contraceptives advised)/ breastfeeding. Pt should drink 10–12 glasses of fluid each day; report difficulty breathing, severe skin reactions.

**DANGEROUS DRUG**

**butorphanol tartrate** (generic)
**CLASS** Opioid agonist-antagonist analgesic
**PREG/CONT** C (preg); D (labor & delivery)/C-IV

**IND & DOSE Relief of moderate to severe pain; preop or preanesthetic medication; to supplement balanced anesthesia.** *Adult:* 2 mg IM q 3–4 hr or 1 mg IV q 3–4 hr; range, 0.5–2 mg IV q 3–4 hr. *During labor:* 1–2 mg IV/ IM at full term during early labor; repeat q 4 hr. **Relief of moderate to severe pain** (nasal spray). 1 mg (1 spray/nostril); repeat in 60–90 min if adequate relief not achieved; may repeat two-dose sequence q 3–4 hr.
**ADJUST DOSE** Elderly pts; hepatic/ renal impairment
**INTERACTIONS** Barbiturate anesthetics
**ADV EFF** Nausea, sedation, slow shallow respirations
**NC/PT** Ensure ready access to respiratory assist devices when giving IV/IM. Protect from falls; sedation. Visual disturbances possible. Pt should not drive or perform other tasks requiring alertness.

## C1-inhibitor (human)
(Berinert, Cinryze)
**CLASS** Blood product, esterase inhibitor
**PREG/CONT** C/NA

**IND & DOSE Px of angioedema attacks in adult, adolescent, child ≥6 yr w/hereditary angioedema.** *Adult, adolescent:* 1,000 units IV at 1 mL/min over 10 min q 3–4 d. Or, 20 IU/kg IV at 4 mL/min (*Berinert*). *Child (6–11 yr):* 500 units IV at 1 mL/min over 5 min q 3–4 d.
**ADV EFF Blood-related infections,** headache, **hypersensitivity reactions,** n/v, rash, **thrombotic events**
**NC/PT** Have epinephrine available in case of severe hypersensitivity reactions. Slight risk of blood-related diseases. Not for use in preg/breastfeeding. Pt should report difficulty breathing, hives, chest tightness.

## C1-inhibitor (recombinant)
(Ruconest)
**CLASS** Blood product, esterase inhibitor
**PREG/CONT** C/NA

**IND & DOSE Tx of acute angioedema attacks in adults, adolescents w/hereditary angioedema.** *Adult, adolescent ≥84 kg:* 4,200 international units IV over 5 min. No more than two doses/24 hr. *<84 kg:* 50 international units/kg IV over 5 min.
**ADV EFF** Headache, **hypersensitivity reactions,** n/d, **serious thrombotic events**
**NC/PT** Have epinephrine available in case of severe hypersensitivity reactions. Use in preg/breastfeeding only if clearly needed. Teach pt/significant other how to prepare, administer drug at onset of attack, proper disposal of needles/syringes. Pt should report difficulty breathing, chest tightness.

## C1 esterase inhibitor (subcut, IV) (Cinryze, Haegarda)
**CLASS** Blood product derivative, C1 esterase inhibitor
**PREG/CONT** High risk/NA

**IND & DOSE Px of hereditary angioedema attacks.** *Adult, adolescent w/Haegarda:* 60 units/kg/dose subcut q 3–4 d. *≥12 yr w/Cinryze:* 1,000–2,500 units IV q 3–4 d. *6–11 yr w/Cinryze:* 500 units IV q 3–4 d; adjust dose based on individual response, up to 1,000 units q 3–4 d.
**ADV EFF** Dizziness, fever, headache, **hypersensitivity,** injection-site reaction, nasopharyngitis, nausea, **thrombosis**, vomiting
**INTERACTIONS** Androgens, estrogen derivatives, progestins
**NC/PT** Monitor for hypersensitivity/thrombotic events. Teach pt proper administration technique (subcut). Instruct pt on common and life-threatening adverse effects.

## cabazitaxel (Jevtana)
**CLASS** Antineoplastic, microtubular inhibitor
**PREG/CONT** High risk/NA

**BBW** Severe hypersensitivity reactions possible; prepare to support pt. Severe neutropenia, deaths have occurred; monitor blood counts closely. Not for use w/hx of severe reactions to cabazitaxel or polysorbate 80.
**IND & DOSE W/oral prednisone for tx of pts w/hormone-refractory metastatic prostate cancer previously treated w/docetaxel.** *Adult:* 25 mg/m² IV over 1 hr q 3 wk.
**ADJUST DOSE** Elderly pts, hepatic impairment
**ADV EFF** Abd pain, alopecia, anorexia, arthralgia, asthenia, **bone marrow suppression,** constipation, cough, dysgeusia, dyspnea, fever, **hepatic impairment, hypersensitivity**

**reactions, interstitial pneumonitis, neutropenia,** n/v/d, **renal failure**
**INTERACTIONS** Strong CYP3A inhibitors, inducers
**NC/PT** Not indicated for use in females. Premedicate w/antihistamine, corticosteroid, and $H_2$ antagonist; antiemetic if needed. Always give w/ oral prednisone. Drug requires two dilutions before administration. Monitor blood count; dose adjustment needed based on neutrophil count; do not administer if neutrophil count <1,500/mm³. Monitor LFTs, renal function, respiratory status. Ensure hydration; tx w/antidiarrheals may be needed. May need to delay/discontinue if severe GI disorder. Not for use in preg/breastfeeding. Protect from infection. Pt should mark calendar w/ dates for tx, try to maintain food and liquid intake; report difficulty breathing, rash, s&sx of infection.

## cabozantinib (Cabometyx, Cometriq)
**CLASS** Antineoplastic, kinase inhibitor
**PREG/CONT** High risk/NA

**IND & DOSE Tx of progressive, metastatic medullary thyroid cancer.** *Adult:* 140 mg/d PO. **Tx of advanced renal cell carcinoma; tx of hepatocellular carcinoma in pts who have been treated w/sorafenib.** *Adult:* 60 mg/d PO (*Cabometyx*).
**ADJUST DOSE** Hepatic impairment
**ADV EFF** Abd pain, anorexia, constipation, fatigue, **GI perforation/fistulas,** hair color change, **hemorrhage, HTN,** n/v/d, **osteonecrosis of jaw, palmar-plantar erythrodysesthesia syndrome, proteinuria, RPLS, thromboembolic events,** weight loss, **wound complications**
**INTERACTIONS** Strong CYP3A4 inducers/inhibitors, grapefruit juice; avoid these combos
**NC/PT** Do not substitute *Cometriq* capsules w/*Cabometyx* tablets. Monitor for s&sx of bleeding, GI perforation, drug interactions. Not for use in preg/breastfeeding. Pt should take as directed on empty stomach and not eat at least 2 hr before and 1 hr after taking drug; swallow capsule whole and not cut/crush/chew it; avoid grapefruit juice; report s&sx of bleeding (bruising, coughing up blood, tarry stools, bleeding that will not stop); acute stomach pain; choking, difficulty swallowing; swelling/pain in mouth or jaw; chest pain; acute leg pain; difficulty breathing.

## caffeine (Caffedrine, Enerjets, NoDoz, Vivarin), caffeine citrate (Cafcit)
**CLASS** Analeptic, CNS stimulant, xanthine
**PREG/CONT** C/NA

**IND & DOSE Aid in staying awake; adjunct to analgesic preparations.** *Adult:* 100–200 mg PO q 3–4 hr as needed. **Tx of respiratory depression associated w/CNS depressant overdose.** *Adult:* 500 mg–1 g caffeine and sodium benzoate (250–500 mg caffeine) IM; max, 2.5 g/d. May give IV in severe emergency. **Short-term tx of apnea of prematurity in infants between 28 and 33 wk gestation.** *Premature infants:* 20 mg/kg IV over 30 min followed 24 hours later by 5 mg/kg/d IV over 10 min or PO as maint (*Cafcit*).
**ADV EFF** Diuresis, excitement, insomnia, restlessness, tachycardia, withdrawal syndrome (headache, anxiety, muscle tension)
**INTERACTIONS** Cimetidine, ciprofloxacin, clozapine, disulfiram, ephedra, guarana, hormonal contraceptives, iron, ma huang, mexiletine, theophylline
**NC/PT** Ensure parental support w/ premature infant use. Pt should avoid foods high in caffeine; not stop drug abruptly (withdrawal sx possible); avoid dangerous activities if CNS effects occur.

**▶NEW DRUG**

## calaspargase pegol-mknl (Asparlas)

**CLASS** Amino acid enzyme, antineoplastic, orphan
**PREG/CONT** Unkn/NA

**IND & DOSE Tx of acute lymphoblastic leukemia as component of multiagent chemo regimen.** *Adult, child ≥1 mo:* 2,500 units/m² IV no more than every 21 d.
**ADV EFF Bleeding, hepatotoxicity, hypersensitivity, pancreatitis, thrombosis**
**INTERACTIONS** Oral contraceptives
**NC/PT** Monitor bilirubin/transaminases wkly during and for 6 wk after tx. Give in setting w/resuscitation equipment to treat anaphylaxis; monitor for hypersensitivity reactions during and for 1 hr after administration. Potential for embryo-fetal toxicity; obtain preg test before tx. Pt should use nonoral contraception during and for 3 mo after tx.

## calcitonin, salmon (Miacalcin)

**CLASS** Calcium regulator, hormone
**PREG/CONT** Unkn/NA

**IND & DOSE Tx of Paget disease.** *Adult:* 100 units/d IM or subcut. **Tx of postmenopausal osteoporosis when other tx not suitable.** *Adult:* 100 units/d IM or subcut. **Tx of hypercalcemia.** *Adult:* 4 units/kg q 12 hr IM or subcut. If response unsatisfactory after 1–2 d, increase to 8 units/kg q 12 hr; if response still unsatisfactory after 2 more d, increase to 8 units/kg q 6 hr.
**ADV EFF** Flushing of face or hands, hypocalcemia, **hypersensitivity reactions,** local inflammatory reactions at injection site, **malignancy,** n/v, rash, urinary frequency
**INTERACTIONS** Lithium
**NC/PT** Before use, give skin test to pt w/hx of allergies; give w/calcium carbonate (1.5 g/d) and vitamin D (400 units/d). Monitor for hypocalcemia. Monitor serum alkaline phosphatase and urinary hydroxyproline excretion before and during first 3 mo of therapy, then q 3–6 mo. Inject doses of more than 2 mL IM, not subcut. Teach pt proper technique/disposal of needles/syringes. Pt should report difficulty breathing, facial edema, chest discomfort.

## calcium salts: calcium acetate (Eliphos, Phoslyra), calcium carbonate (Caltrate, Chooz, Tums), calcium chloride, calcium citrate (Cal-Cee, Cal-Citrate), calcium glubionate (Calcionate, Calciquid), calcium gluconate (generic), calcium lactate (Cal-Lac)

**CLASS** Antacid, electrolyte
**PREG/CONT** C/NA

**IND & DOSE RDA** (carbonate or lactate). *Adult >50 yr:* 1,200 mg/d PO. *Adult 19–50 yr:* 1,000 mg/d PO. *Child 14–18 yr:* 1,300 mg/d PO. *Child 9–13 yr:* 1,300 mg/d PO. *Child 4–8 yr:* 800 mg/d PO. *Child 1–3 yr:* 500 mg/d PO. *Child 7–12 mo:* 270 mg/d PO. *Child 0–6 mo:* 210 mg/d PO. *Preg/breastfeeding, 19–50 yr:* 1,000 mg/d PO. *Preg/breastfeeding, 14–18 yr:* 1,300 mg/d PO. **Dietary supplement** (carbonate or lactate). *Adult:* 500 mg–2 g PO bid–qid. **Antacid.** *Adult:* 0.5–2 g PO calcium carbonate as needed. **Tx of hypocalcemic disorders.** *Adult:* 500 mg–1 g calcium chloride IV at intervals of 1–3 d. *Child:* 2.7–5 mg/kg or 0.027–0.05 mL/kg calcium chloride IV q 4–6 hr, or 200–500 mg/d IV (2–5 mL of 10% sol); for infants, no more than 200 mg IV (2 mL of 10% sol) in divided doses (calcium gluconate). **Tx of**

**magnesium intoxication.** *Adult:* 500 mg calcium chloride IV promptly. **Tx of hyperphosphatemia.** *Adult:* 2,001–2,668 mg PO w/each meal (calcium acetate). **Cardiac resuscitation.** *Adult:* 500 mg–1 g IV or 200–800 mg calcium chloride into ventricular cavity.
**ADV EFF** Anorexia, bradycardia, constipation, hypercalcemia, hypotension, irritation at injection site, n/v, peripheral vasodilation, rebound hyperacidity, tingling
**INTERACTIONS** Fluoroquinolones, quinidine, salicylates, tetracyclines, thyroid hormone, verapamil
**NC/PT** Do not give oral drugs within 1–2 hr of antacid. Avoid extravasation of IV fluid; tissue necrosis possible. Monitor serum phosphate periodically. Monitor cardiac response closely w/parenteral tx. Pt should take drug between meals and at bedtime; chew antacid tablets thoroughly before swallowing and follow w/glass of water; not take w/other oral drugs; space at least 1–2 hr after antacid.

## calfactant (natural lung surfactant) (Infasurf)

**CLASS** Lung surfactant
**PREG/CONT** Unkn/NA

**IND & DOSE Px of infants at risk for developing RDS; rescue tx of premature infants up to 72 hr old who have developed RDS.** Instill 3 mL/kg of birth weight in two doses of 1.5 mL/kg each intratracheally. Repeat doses of 3 mL/kg (to total of three doses) given 12 hr apart.
**ADV EFF Bradycardia,** hyperbilirubinemia, **hypotension, intraventricular hemorrhage,** nonpulmonary infections, **patent ductus arteriosus,** sepsis
**NC/PT** Monitor ECG and $O_2$ saturation continuously during and for at least 30 min after administration. Ensure ET tube correctly placed; suction immediately before dosing. Do not suction for 1 hr after dosing. Maintain appropriate interventions for critically ill infant.

## canagliflozin (Invokana)

**CLASS** Antidiabetic, sodium-glucose cotransporter 2 inhibitor
**PREG/CONT** High risk/NA

**BBW** Risk of lower limb amputations in pts w/risk of CV disease or lower limb infections/ulcers.
**IND & DOSE W/diet/exercise to improve glycemic control or to reduce risk of major CV events in pts w/type 2 diabetes; to reduce risk of ESRD, CV death, and HF hospitalization in pts w/type 2 diabetes and diabetic nephropathy w/albuminuria.** *Adult:* 100 mg/d before first meal of day; max, 300 mg/d.
**ADJUST DOSE** Severe hepatic/renal impairment or hypersensitivity reactions (contraindicated)
**ADV EFF** Bone fracture, dehydration, diabetic ketoacidosis, genital yeast infections, hypoglycemia, hypotension, hyperkalemia, hyperlipidemia, increased LDL, lower-limb amputation, polyuria, UTI, urosepsis
**INTERACTIONS** Celery, coriander, dandelion root, digoxin, fenugreek, garlic, ginger, juniper berries, phenobarbital, phenytoin, rifampin
**NC/PT** Not for use w/type 1 diabetes, diabetic ketoacidosis, preg/breastfeeding. Monitor blood glucose, $HbA_{1c}$, BP periodically; also monitor for UTI, genital infections, bone loss. Pt should continue diet/exercise program, other antidiabetics as ordered; take safety measures w/dehydration; report sx of UTI/genital infections.

## canakinumab (Ilaris)

**CLASS** Interleukin blocker
**PREG/CONT** Moderate risk/NA

**IND & DOSE Tx of cryopyrin-associated periodic syndromes, including familial cold autoinflammatory syndrome and Muckle-Wells**

**syndrome.** *Adult, child ≥4 yr:* >40 kg, 150 mg subcut; 15–<40 kg, 2 mg/kg subcut; 15–40 kg w/inadequate response, 3 mg/kg subcut. Injections given q 8 wk. **Tx of TNF receptor-associated periodic syndrome, hyperimmunoglobulin D syndrome, familial Mediterranean fever.** *Adult, child >40 kg:* 150 mg subcut q 4 wk; max, 300 mg subcut q 4 wk. *≤40 kg:* 2 mg/kg subcut q 4 wk; max, 4 mg/kg subcut q 4 wk. **Tx of juvenile RA.** *Adult, child ≥2 yr:* 4 mg/kg subcut q 4 wk.
**ADV EFF** Diarrhea, flulike sx, headache, nasopharyngitis, nausea, **serious infections**
**INTERACTIONS** Immunosuppressants, live vaccines
**NC/PT** Use extreme caution in pts w/ infections; monitor for infections. Not for use in preg/breastfeeding. Pt should report s&sx of infection.

## candesartan cilexetil (Atacand)

**CLASS** Antihypertensive, ARB
**PREG/CONT** D/NA

**BBW** Rule out preg before starting tx. Suggest barrier birth control; fetal injury and deaths have occurred. If preg detected, discontinue as soon as possible.
**IND & DOSE Tx of HTN.** *Adult:* 16 mg PO daily; range, 8–32 mg/d. *Child 6–<17 yr:* >50 kg, 8–16 mg/d PO; range, 4–32 mg/d PO; <50 kg, 4–8 mg/d PO; range, 4–16 mg/d PO. *Child 1–<6 yr:* 0.20 mg/kg/d oral suspension; range, 0.05–0.4 mg/kg/d. **Tx of HF.** *Adult:* 4 mg/d PO; may be doubled at 2-wk intervals. Target dose, 32 mg/d PO as single dose.
**ADJUST DOSE** Volume depletion
**ADV EFF** Abd pain, diarrhea, dizziness, headache, hyperkalemia, hypotension, renal impairment, URI sx
**INTERACTIONS** ARBs, lithium, NSAIDs, renin inhibitors
**NC/PT** If BP not controlled, can add other antihypertensives. Use caution if pt goes to surgery; volume depletion possible. Monitor renal function, potassium. Not for use in preg (barrier contraception advised)/breastfeeding. Pt should use care in situations that could lead to fluid volume loss; monitor fluid intake.

## cangrelor (Kengreal)

**CLASS** Platelet inhibitor
**PREG/CONT** Unkn/NA

**IND & DOSE Adjunct to PCI to reduce risk of periprocedural MI, repeat revascularization, stent thrombosis in pts who have not received platelet inhibitors.** *Adult:* 30 mcg/kg as IV bolus before procedure; then 4 mcg/kg/min IV infusion for at least 2 hr or for duration of procedure (whichever longer).
**ADV EFF Bleeding, hypersensitivity reactions**
**INTERACTIONS** Clopidogrel, prasugrel; do not coadminister
**NC/PT** Monitor for bleeding. Administer by dedicated IV line. Switch to oral ticagrelor, prasugrel, or clopidogrel after infusion ends to maintain platelet inhibition. Use caution in preg/breastfeeding. Pt should report difficulty breathing, chest pain.

**DANGEROUS DRUG**

## capecitabine (Xeloda)

**CLASS** Antimetabolite, antineoplastic
**PREG/CONT** D/NA

**BBW** Increased risk of excessive bleeding, even death, if combined w/ warfarin; avoid this combo. If combo must be used, monitor INR and PT closely; adjust anticoagulant dose as needed. Bleeding is seen more often in pts >60 yr w/cancer, within days and up to months after initiation; may occur within 1 mo of stopping drug.
**IND & DOSE Tx of metastatic breast and colorectal cancer; adjuvant postop Dukes C colon cancer.** *Adult:* 2,500 mg/m$^2$/d PO in two divided

doses 12 hr apart within 30 min after meal for 2 wk, followed by 1 wk rest. Given as 3-wk cycles for eight cycles (24 wk); adjuvant tx for total of 6 mo. If used w/docetaxel, 1,250 PO bid a.m. and p.m. within 30 min after meal for 2 wk, combined w/docetaxel 75 mg/m² IV over 1 hr q 3 wk.
**ADJUST DOSE** Elderly pts; renal impairment (contraindicated w/severe renal impairment)
**ADV EFF** Anorexia, **cardiomyopathy, coagulopathy,** constipation, dehydration, dermatitis, hand-and-foot syndrome, hyperbilirubinemia, leukopenia, **mucocutaneous toxicity, myelosuppression, MI,** n/v/d, **renal impairment, SJS,** stomatitis
**INTERACTIONS** Antacids, docetaxel, leucovorin (risk of severe toxicity, death), phenytoin, warfarin
**NC/PT** Obtain baseline and periodic renal function tests, CBC; monitor for s&sx of toxicity. Monitor nutritional status, fluid intake. Give frequent mouth care; correct dehydration. Not for use in preg (barrier contraceptives advised)/breastfeeding. Pt should mark calendar for tx days; avoid exposure to infection; report s&sx of infection, rash, chest pain, severe diarrhea.

**▶NEW DRUG**

## caplacizumab-yhdp (Cablivi)

**CLASS** Anti-von Willebrand factor, immunomodulator, orphan
**PREG/CONT** Unkn/NA

**IND & DOSE Tx of acquired thrombotic thrombocytopenic purpura (aTTP) w/plasma exchange and immunosuppressants.** *Adult:* Day 1, 11-mg bolus IV 15 min before plasma exchange; then 11 mg subcut after plasma exchange. Then 11 mg subcut daily after each plasma exchange and for 30 d beyond last plasma exchange.
**ADV EFF Bleeding,** headache
**INTERACTIONS** Anticoagulants
**NC/PT** First IV dose given by health care provider. If after initial tx course, sx of persistent underlying disease, such as suppressed ADAMTS13 activity levels, remain, may extend tx for max of 28 d. Discontinue if pt experiences more than two recurrences of aTTP while on drug. Withhold 7 d before elective surgery/ dental procedures.

## capreomycin (Capastat Sulfate)

**CLASS** Antibiotic, antituberculotic
**PREG/CONT** C/NA

**BBW** Arrange for audiometric testing and assessment of vestibular function, renal function tests, and serum potassium before and regularly during tx; severe risk of renal failure, auditory damage. Drug's safety not established in child or preg women.
**IND & DOSE Tx of pulmonary TB unresponsive to first-line antituberculotics, as part of combo therapy.** *Adult:* 1 g daily (max, 20 mg/kg/d) IM or IV for 60–120 d, followed by 1 g IM 2–3 ×/wk for 12–24 mo.
**ADJUST DOSE** Elderly pts, renal impairment
**ADV EFF** Nephrotoxicity, ototoxicity
**INTERACTIONS** Nephrotoxic drugs, NMJ blockers
**NC/PT** Culture and sensitivity before tx. Use w/other antituberculotics. Give by deep IM injection. Obtain audiometric testing regularly. Monitor renal function, potassium regularly. Pt should report hearing changes.

## captopril (generic)

**CLASS** ACE inhibitor, antihypertensive
**PREG/CONT** D/NA

**BBW** Rule out preg; fetal abnormalities and death have occurred if used during second or third trimester. Encourage use of contraceptive measures.

**IND & DOSE Tx of HTN, alone or as part of combo therapy.** *Adult:* 25 mg PO bid or tid. Range, 25–150 mg bid–tid; max, 450 mg/d. **Tx of HF.** *Adult:* 6.25–12.5 mg PO tid. Maint, 50–100 mg PO tid; max, 450 mg/d. **Left ventricular dysfx after MI.** *Adult:* 6.25 mg PO, then 12.5 mg PO tid; increase slowly to 50 mg PO tid starting as early as 3 d post-MI. **Tx of diabetic nephropathy.** *Adult:* Reduce dosage; suggested dose, 25 mg PO tid.
**ADJUST DOSE** Elderly pts, renal impairment
**ADV EFF Agranulocytosis,** aphthous ulcers, cough, dysgeusia, **HF,** hyperkalemia, **MI, pancytopenia,** proteinuria, rash, tachycardia
**INTERACTIONS** ACE inhibitors, allopurinol, ARBs, indomethacin, lithium, probenecid, renin inhibitors
**NC/PT** Use caution before surgery; mark chart. Monitor renal function, potassium. Give 1 hr before meals. Protect pt in situations of decreased fluid volume. Not for use in preg. Cough may occur. Pt should change position slowly if dizzy, light-headed; avoid OTC preparations; consult prescriber before stopping drug.

## carBAMazepine
(Carbatrol, Epitol, Equetro, TEGretol, TEGretol-XR)
**CLASS** Antiepileptic
**PREG/CONT** High risk/NA

**BBW** Risk of aplastic anemia and agranulocytosis; obtain CBC, including platelet/reticulocyte counts, and serum iron determination before starting tx; repeat wkly for first 3 mo and monthly thereafter for at least 2–3 yr. Discontinue if evidence of marrow suppression. Increased risk of suicidality; monitor accordingly. Risk of serious to fatal dermatologic reactions, including SJS, in pts w/ HLA-B*1502 allele w/*Tegretol.* Pts at risk should be screened for this allele.
**IND & DOSE Refractory seizure disorders.** *Adult:* 200 mg PO bid on first day. Increase gradually by up to 200 mg/d in divided doses q 6–8 hr, or 100 mg PO qid suspension; range, 800–1,200 mg/d. *Child 6–12 yr:* 100 mg PO bid on first day. Increase gradually by adding 100 mg/d at 6- to 8-hr intervals until best response achieved; max, 1,000 mg/d. *Child <6 yr:* Optimal daily dose, <35 mg/kg/d PO. **Tx of trigeminal neuralgia.** *Adult:* 200 mg/d PO on first day. May increase by up to 200 mg/d, using 100-mg increments q 12 hr as needed. Range, 200–1,200 mg/d; max, 1,200 mg/d. **Tx of bipolar 1 disorder.** *Adult:* 400 mg/d PO in divided doses; max, 1,600 mg/d (*Equetro* only).
**ADJUST DOSE** Elderly pts
**ADV EFF Bone marrow suppression, CV complications,** dizziness, drowsiness, **hepatic cellular necrosis w/total loss of liver tissue, hepatitis, HF,** n/v, **SJS,** unsteadiness
**INTERACTIONS** Barbiturates, charcoal, cimetidine, danazol, doxycycline, erythromycin, isoniazid, lithium, MAOIs, NMJ blockers, phenytoin, primidone, valproic acid, verapamil, warfarin
**NC/PT** Use only for indicated uses. Taper dose if withdrawing; abrupt removal can precipitate seizures. Obtain baseline and frequent LFTs, monitor CBC; dose adjustment made accordingly. Evaluate for therapeutic serum levels (usually 4–12 mcg/mL). Not for use in preg (barrier contraceptives advisable)/breastfeeding. Pt may open *Equetro* capsule and sprinkle contents over food (should not chew capsules/beads); should swallow ER tablets whole, wear medical alert tag, avoid CNS depressants (alcohol), report s&sx of infection, rash.

## carbinoxamine maleate
(Karbinal ER)
**CLASS** Antihistamine
**PREG/CONT** C/NA

**IND & DOSE Tx of seasonal/perennial allergic rhinitis;**

**vasomotor rhinitis; allergic conjunctivitis; allergic skin reactions; dermatographism; anaphylactic reactions; allergic reactions to blood/ blood products.** *Adult, child ≥12 yr:* 6–16 mg PO q 12 hr. *Child 6–11 yr:* 6–12 mg PO q 12 hr. *Child 4–5 yr:* 3–8 mg PO q 12 hr. *Child 2–3 yr:* 3–4 mg PO q 12 hr.
**ADV EFF** Dizziness, drowsiness, dry mouth, epigastric distress, rash, thickened secretions, urine retention
**INTERACTIONS** CNS depressants, MAOIs; avoid this combo
**NC/PT** Ensure pt can tolerate anticholinergic effects; suggest increased fluids, humidifier. Not for use in preg/ breastfeeding. Pt should measure drug using mL measure provided; take safety measures w/CNS effects; use humidifier, increase fluid intake; report difficulty breathing, fainting.

DANGEROUS DRUG

## CARBOplatin (generic)

**CLASS** Alkylating agent, antineoplastic
**PREG/CONT** D/NA

**BBW** Evaluate bone marrow function before and periodically during tx; do not give next dose if marked bone marrow depression. Consult physician for dosage. Ensure epinephrine, corticosteroids, antihistamines readily available in case of anaphylactic reactions, which may occur within min of administration.
**IND & DOSE** **Initial, palliative tx of pts w/advanced ovarian cancer.** *Adult:* As single agent, 360 mg/m$^2$ IV over at least 15 min on day 1 q 4 wk; based on blood counts.
**ADJUST DOSE** Elderly pts, renal impairment
**ADV EFF** Abd pain, alopecia, asthenia, **anaphylactic reactions, bone marrow suppression, bronchospasm, cancer,** constipation, electrolyte abnormalities, n/v/d, peripheral neuropathies, renal impairment
**INTERACTIONS** Aluminum (in sol)
**NC/PT** Antiemetic may be needed. Obtain CBC regularly; dose adjustment may be needed. Ensure emergency equipment available in case of anaphylactic reaction. Not for use in preg. Hair loss, GI effects possible. Pt should report s&sx of infection, difficulty breathing.

## carboprost tromethamine (Hemabate)

**CLASS** Abortifacient, prostaglandin
**PREG/CONT** C/NA

**IND & DOSE** **Termination of preg 13–20 wk from first day of last menstrual period; evacuation of uterus in missed abortion or intrauterine fetal death.** *Adult:* 250 mcg (1 mL) IM; give 250 mcg IM at 1.5- to 3.5-hr intervals. Max, 12 mg total dose. **Tx of postpartum hemorrhage.** *Adult:* 250 mcg IM as one dose; may use multiple doses at 15- to 90-min intervals. Max, 2 mg (eight doses).
**ADV EFF** Diarrhea, flushing, hypotension, nausea, **perforated uterus, uterine rupture**
**NC/PT** Pretreat w/antiemetics and antidiarrheals. Give by deep IM injection. Ensure abortion complete; monitor for infection. Ensure adequate hydration. Several IM injections may be needed.

## carfilzomib (Kyprolis)

**CLASS** Antineoplastic, proteasome inhibitor
**PREG/CONT** D/NA

**IND & DOSE** **Tx of relapsed or refractory multiple myeloma in pts w/disease progression after at least one or more prior therapies, as monotherapy or in combo w/lenalidomide and dexamethasone.** *Adult:* 20/70 mg/m$^2$ IV once wkly over 30 min w/dexamethasone, or 20/56 mg/m$^2$ IV twice wkly over 30 min w/dexamethasone or alone, or 20/27 mg/m$^2$ IV twice wkly over 10 min w/lenalidomide

and dexamethasone or alone. Tx administered in specific cycled doses
**ADV EFF** Anemia, dyspnea, fatigue, fever, **hepatotoxicity, HF/ischemia, infusion reactions, liver failure,** n/v/d, **pulmonary complications, pulmonary HTN,** renal failure, **RPLS,** thrombocytopenia, **TLS, venous thrombosis**
**INTERACTIONS** Fatal/serious toxicities in combo w/melphalan and prednisone in newly diagnosed transplant-ineligible pts
**NC/PT** Premedicate w/ dexamethasone; hydrate before/after tx. Monitor for potentially severe adverse reactions; arrange for supportive measures, dose adjustment. Not for use in preg. Pt should mark calendar for tx days; report difficulty breathing, swelling, urine/stool color changes, chest pain, vision changes.

## carglumic acid (Carbaglu)

**CLASS** Carbamoyl phosphate synthetase I activator
**PREG/CONT** C/NA

**IND & DOSE Tx of acute hyperammonemia.** *Adult, child:* 100–250 mg/kg/d PO in divided doses; may be made into sol and given through NG tube. Titrate based on plasma ammonia level and clinical sx. **Tx of chronic hyperammonemia.** *Adult, child:* 10–100 mg/kg/d in two–four divided doses. Titrate to target normal plasma ammonia level for age.
**ADV EFF** Abd pain, anemia, fever, headache, infections, nasopharyngitis, n/v/d
**NC/PT** Monitor ammonia levels during tx; dose adjustment may be needed. Restrict protein intake until ammonia level regulated. Not for use in preg/breastfeeding. Store in refrigerator until opened, then room temp. Date bottle; discard after 1 mo. Pt should report s&sx of infection.

## cariprazine (Vraylar)

**CLASS** Atypical antipsychotic, dopamine/serotonin agonist and antagonist
**PREG/CONT** High risk/NA

**BBW** Elderly pts w/dementia-related psychosis have increased risk of death if given atypical antipsychotics; not approved for this use. Risk of suicidal ideation increases w/antidepressant use, especially in child, adolescent, young adult; monitor accordingly; not approved for use in child.
**IND & DOSE Tx of schizophrenia; tx of manic or mixed episodes of bipolar 1 disorder.** *Adult:* 1.5–6 mg/d PO. **Tx of depressive episodes associated w/bipolar 1 disorder.** *Adult:* 1.5–3 mg/d PO.
**ADV EFF Akathisia,** bone marrow suppression, cognitive/motor impairment, dyslipidemia, hyperglycemia, **NMS,** orthostatic hypotension, **seizures** (potentially life-threatening), suicidality, syncope, tardive dyskinesia, weight gain
**INTERACTIONS** Alcohol, carbamazepine, CNS depressants, CYP2D6 inhibitors (fluoxetine, paroxetine, quinidine), CYP3A4 inhibitors (ketoconazole), lorazepam
**NC/PT** Dispense least amount possible to suicidal pts. Not for use in preg (risk of abnormal muscle movements, withdrawal)/breastfeeding. Monitor weight; assess for hyperglycemia. May react w/many drugs; monitor regimen. Take safety precautions for cognitive/motor impairment; use cautiously if low BP possible; ensure hydration. Pt should report thoughts of suicide, s&sx of infection, abnormal muscle movements.

## carisoprodol (Soma)

**CLASS** Centrally acting skeletal muscle relaxant
**PREG/CONT** C/NA

**IND & DOSE Relief of discomfort associated w/acute, painful**

**musculoskeletal conditions, as adjunct.** *Adult, child >16 yr:* 250–350 mg PO tid–qid. Pt should take last dose at bedtime for max of 2–3 wk.
**ADJUST DOSE** Hepatic/renal impairment
**ADV EFF** **Allergic/idiosyncratic reaction,** agitation, **anaphylactoid shock,** ataxia, dizziness, drowsiness, irritability, tremor, vertigo
**NC/PT** Monitor for idiosyncratic reaction, most likely w/first dose. Provide safety measures w/CNS effects. May become habit-forming; use caution. Pt should avoid other CNS depressants, report difficulty breathing.

**DANGEROUS DRUG**

## carmustine (BCNU) (BiCNU, Gliadel)

**CLASS** Alkylating agent, antineoplastic
**PREG/CONT** D/NA

**BBW** Do not give more often than q 6 wk because of delayed bone marrow toxicity. Evaluate hematopoietic function before, wkly during, and for at least 6 wk after tx to monitor for bone marrow suppression. Monitor for pulmonary/delayed toxicity, which can occur yrs after therapy; death possible. Cumulative doses of 1,400 mg/m$^2$ increase risk.
**IND & DOSE** **Palliative tx alone or w/other agents (injection) for brain tumors, Hodgkin lymphoma, non-Hodgkin lymphoma, multiple myeloma.** *Adult, child:* 150–200 mg/m$^2$ IV q 6 wk as single dose or in divided daily injections (75–100 mg/m$^2$ on 2 successive d); adjust dose based on CBC. **Adjunct to surgery for tx of recurrent glioblastoma as implantable wafer (w/prednisone); tx of newly diagnosed high-grade malignant glioma** (wafer). *Adult, child:* Wafers implanted in resection cavity as part of surgical procedure; up to 8 wafers at a time.
**ADV EFF** **Bone marrow suppression** (may be delayed 4–6 wk), **cancer,** hepatotoxicity, local burning at injection site, **pulmonary fibrosis,** pulmonary infiltrates, **renal failure,** stomatitis
**INTERACTIONS** Cimetidine, digoxin, mitomycin, phenytoin
**NC/PT** Monitor CBC before and wkly during tx. Do not give full dose within 2–3 wk of radiation or other chemo. Monitor pulmonary function; toxicity can be delayed. Monitor LFTs, renal function, injection site for local reaction. Premedicate w/antiemetic. Not for use in preg. Pt should try to maintain fluid intake/nutrition; report difficulty breathing, s&sx of infection.

## carvedilol (Coreg)

**CLASS** Alpha and beta blocker, antihypertensive
**PREG/CONT** C/NA

**IND & DOSE** **Mgt of HTN, alone or w/other drugs.** *Adult:* 6.25 mg PO bid; maintain for 7–14 d, then increase to 12.5 mg PO bid. Max, 50 mg/d. **Tx of mild to severe HF.** *Adult:* 3.125 mg PO bid for 2 wk, then may increase to 6.25 mg PO bid. Max, 25 mg/d if <85 kg, 50 mg if >85 kg. **Tx of left ventricular dysfx after MI.** *Adult:* 6.25 mg PO bid; increase after 3–10 d to 25 mg PO bid. **Converting to once-daily CR capsules.** 3.125 mg bid, give 10 mg CR; 6.25 mg bid, give 20 mg CR; 12.5 mg bid, give 40 mg CR; 25 mg bid, give 80 mg CR.
**ADJUST DOSE** Hepatic impairment
**ADV EFF** Bradycardia, bronchospasm, constipation, diabetes, diarrhea, dizziness, fatigue, flatulence, gastric pain, **hepatic injury, HF,** hypotension, rhinitis, tinnitus, vertigo
**INTERACTIONS** **Amiodarone,** antidiabetics, clonidine, cyclosporine, digoxin, diltiazem, hypotensives, rifampin, verapamil
**NC/PT** Do not discontinue abruptly; taper when discontinuing (risk of CAD

exacerbation). Use caution if surgery planned. Use care in conversion to CR capsules. Monitor for orthostatic hypotension. Monitor LFTs. Not for use in preg/breastfeeding. Provide safety measures. Pt should not cut/crush/chew CR capsules; should take w/food, change position slowly if lowered BP occurs; if diabetic, should use caution and monitor glucose carefully.

## caspofungin acetate
(Cancidas)
**CLASS** Antifungal, echinocandin
**PREG/CONT** C/NA

**IND & DOSE** **Tx of invasive aspergillosis; tx of esophageal candidiasis; tx of candidemia/other *Candida* infections; empirical tx when fungal infection suspected in neutropenic pts.** *Adult:* Loading dose, 70 mg IV, then 50 mg/d IV infusion for at least 14 d. *Child 3 mo–17 yr:* Loading dose, 70 mg/m$^2$ IV, then 50 mg/m$^2$ IV daily for 14 d.
**ADJUST DOSE** Hepatic impairment, concurrent rifampin or inducers of drug clearance
**ADV EFF** Decreased serum potassium, diarrhea, fever, **hepatic damage,** hypersensitivity reactions, hypotension, increased liver enzymes
**INTERACTIONS** Cyclosporine, rifampin
**NC/PT** Monitor for IV complications. Monitor potassium; monitor LFTs before and during tx. Not for use in preg/breastfeeding. Pt should report difficulty breathing, swelling, rash.

## cefadroxil (generic)
**CLASS** Cephalosporin
**PREG/CONT** B/NA

**IND & DOSE** **Tx of pharyngitis/tonsillitis caused by susceptible bacteria strains.** *Adult:* 1 g/d PO in single dose or two divided doses for 10 d. *Child:* 30 mg/kg/d PO in single or two divided doses; continue for 10 d. **Tx of UTIs caused by susceptible bacteria strains.** *Adult:* 1–2 g/d PO in single dose or two divided doses for uncomplicated lower UTIs. For all other UTIs, 2 g/d in two divided doses. *Child:* 30 mg/kg/d PO in divided doses q 12 hr. **Tx of skin/skin-structure infections caused by susceptible bacteria strains.** *Adult:* 1 g/d PO in single dose or two divided doses. *Child:* 30 mg/kg/d PO in divided doses.
**ADJUST DOSE** Elderly pts, renal impairment
**ADV EFF** Abd pain, **anaphylaxis,** anorexia, **bone marrow depression, colitis,** flatulence, n/v/d, rash, superinfections
**INTERACTIONS** Aminoglycosides, bacteriostatic agents, probenecid
**NC/PT** Culture before tx. Give w/meals to decrease GI discomfort; give oral vancomycin for serious colitis. Refrigerate suspension. Pt should not cut/crush/chew ER tablets; should complete full course of therapy; report diarrhea w/blood or mucus, difficulty breathing.

## cefdinir (generic)
**CLASS** Cephalosporin
**PREG/CONT** B/NA

**IND & DOSE** **Tx of community-acquired pneumonia, uncomplicated skin/skin-structure infections.** *Adult, adolescent:* 300 mg PO q 12 hr for 10 d. **Tx of acute exacerbation of chronic bronchitis, acute maxillary sinusitis, pharyngitis/tonsillitis.** *Adult, adolescent:* 300 mg PO q 12 hr for 10 d or 600 mg PO q 24 hr for 10 d. **Tx of otitis media, acute maxillary sinusitis, pharyngitis/tonsillitis.** *Child 6 mo–12 yr:* 7 mg/kg PO q 12 hr or 14 mg/kg PO q 24 hr for 10 d; max, 600 mg/d. **Tx of skin/skin-structure infections.** *Child 6 mo–12 yr:* 7 mg/kg PO q 12 hr for 10 d.
**ADJUST DOSE** Renal impairment

**ADV EFF** Abd pain, **anaphylaxis,** anorexia, **colitis,** flatulence, n/v/d, rash, superinfections
**INTERACTIONS** Aminoglycosides, antacids, oral anticoagulants
**NC/PT** Culture before tx. Give w/ meals to decrease GI discomfort; give oral vancomycin for serious colitis. Arrange for tx of superinfections. Store suspension at room temp; discard after 10 d. Pt should complete full course of tx; report diarrhea w/ blood or mucus, difficulty breathing.

## cefepime hydrochloride
(Maxipime)
**CLASS** Cephalosporin
**PREG/CONT** B/NA

**IND & DOSE** **Tx of mild to moderate UTI.** *Adult:* 0.5–1 g IM or IV q 12 hr for 7–10 d. **Tx of severe UTI.** *Adult:* 2 g IV q 12 hr for 10 d. **Tx of moderate to severe pneumonia.** *Adult:* 1–2 g IV q 12 hr for 10 d. **Tx of moderate to severe skin infections.** *Adult:* 2 g IV q 12 hr for 10 d. **Empiric therapy for febrile neutropenic pts.** *Adult:* 2 g IV q 8 hr for 7 d. **Tx of complicated intra-abd infections.** *Adult:* 2 g IV q 12 hr for 7–10 d. *Child >2 mo, <40 kg:* 50 mg/kg/d IV or IM q 12 hr for 7–10 d depending on infection severity. If treating febrile neutropenia, give q 8 hr (max, 2 g/d).
**ADJUST DOSE** Elderly pts, renal impairment
**ADV EFF** Abd pain, **anaphylaxis,** anorexia, **colitis,** disulfiram reaction w/alcohol, flatulence, **hepatotoxicity,** n/v/d, phlebitis, rash, superinfections
**INTERACTIONS** Alcohol, aminoglycosides, oral anticoagulants
**NC/PT** Culture before tx. Administer IV over 30 min. Have vitamin K available if hypoprothrombinemia occurs. Pt should avoid alcohol during and for 3 d after tx; report diarrhea w/blood or mucus, difficulty breathing, rash.

## cefotaxime sodium
(Cefotaxime)
**CLASS** Cephalosporin
**PREG/CONT** B/NA

**IND & DOSE** **Tx of lower respiratory tract, skin, intra-abd, CNS, bone/joint infections; UTIs; peritonitis caused by susceptible bacteria.** *Adult:* 2–8 g/d IM or IV in equally divided doses q 6–8 hr; max, 12 g/d. *Child 1 mo–12 yr <50 kg:* 50–180 mg/kg/d IV or IM in four to six divided doses. *Child 1–4 wk:* 50 mg/kg IV q 8 hr. *Child 0–1 wk:* 50 mg/kg IV q 12 hr. **Tx of gonorrhea.** *Adult:* 0.5–1 g IM in single injection. **Disseminated infection.** *Adult:* 1–2 g V q 8 hr. **Periop px.** *Adult:* 1 g IV or IM 30–90 min before surgery. **Cesarean section.** *Adult:* 1 g IV after cord is clamped, then 1 g IV or IM at 6 and 12 hr.
**ADJUST DOSE** Elderly pts, renal impairment
**ADV EFF** Abd pain, **anaphylaxis,** anorexia, **bone marrow depression, colitis,** disulfiram reaction w/alcohol, flatulence, **hepatotoxicity,** n/v/d, phlebitis, rash, superinfections
**INTERACTIONS** Alcohol, aminoglycosides, oral anticoagulants
**NC/PT** Culture before tx. Ensure no hx of hypersensitivity to penicillin/other cephalosporins; have epinephrine and emergency equipment on standby in pts w/hx of type 1 allergic reactions. Give IV slowly. Pt should avoid alcohol during and for 3 d after tx; report diarrhea w/blood or mucus, difficulty breathing.

## ceFOXitin sodium
(generic)
**CLASS** Cephalosporin
**PREG/CONT** B/NA

**IND & DOSE** **Tx of lower respiratory tract, skin, intra-abd, CNS, bone/joint infections; UTIs, peritonitis caused by susceptible bacteria.** *Adult:* 2–8 g/d IM or IV in equally divided

doses q 6–8 hr. *Child ≥3 mo:* 80–160 mg/kg/d IM or IV in divided doses q 4–6 hr. Max, 12 g/d. **Tx of gonorrhea.** *Adult:* 2 g IM w/1 g oral probenecid. **Uncomplicated lower respiratory tract infections, UTIs, skin infections.** *Adult:* 1 g q 6–8 hr IV. **Moderate to severe infections.** *Adult:* 1 g q 4 hr IV to 2 g q 6–8 hr IV. **Severe infections.** *Adult:* 2 g q 4 hr IV or 3 g q 6 hr IV. **Periop px.** *Adult:* 2 g IV or IM 30–60 min before initial incision, q 6 hr for 24 hr after surgery. **Cesarean section.** *Adult:* 2 g IV as soon as cord clamped, then 2 g IM or IV at 4 and 8 hr, then q 6 hr for up to 24 hr. **Transurethral prostatectomy.** *Adult:* 1 g before surgery, then 1 g q 8 hr for up to 5 d.
**ADJUST DOSE** Elderly pts, renal impairment
**ADV EFF** Abd pain, **anaphylaxis,** anorexia, **bone marrow depression, colitis,** disulfiram reaction w/alcohol, flatulence, **hepatotoxicity,** n/v/d, phlebitis, rash, superinfections
**INTERACTIONS** Alcohol, aminoglycosides, oral anticoagulants
**NC/PT** Culture before tx. Give IV slowly. Have vitamin K available for hypoprothrombinemia. Pt should avoid alcohol during and for 3 d after tx; report diarrhea w/blood or mucus, difficulty breathing.

## cefpodoxime proxetil

(generic)
**CLASS** Cephalosporin
**PREG/CONT** B/NA

**IND & DOSE** **Tx of upper/lower respiratory tract infections, skin/skin-structure infections, UTIs, otitis media caused by susceptible strains; STD caused by *Neisseria gonorrhoeae.*** *Adult:* 100–400 mg PO q 12 hr depending on infection severity for 5–14 d. *Child:* 5 mg/kg/dose PO q 12 hr; max, 100–200 mg/dose for 10 d. **Tx of acute otitis media.** *Child:* 10 mg/kg/d PO divided q 12 hr; max, 400 mg/d for 5 d.
**ADJUST DOSE** Elderly pts, renal impairment
**ADV EFF** Abd pain, **anaphylaxis,** anorexia, **bone marrow depression, colitis,** flatulence, **hepatotoxicity,** n/v/d, phlebitis, rash, superinfections
**INTERACTIONS** Aminoglycosides, oral anticoagulants
**NC/PT** Culture before tx. Refrigerate suspension. Give oral vancomycin for serious colitis. Pt should take w/food; complete full course of tx; report diarrhea w/blood or mucus, difficulty breathing.

## cefprozil (generic)

**CLASS** Cephalosporin
**PREG/CONT** B/NA

**IND & DOSE** **Tx of upper/lower respiratory tract infections, skin/skin-structure infections, otitis media, acute sinusitis caused by susceptible strains.** *Adult:* 250–500 mg PO q 12–24 hr for 10 d. **Tx of acute otitis media, sinusitis.** *Child 6 mo–12 yr:* 7.5–15 mg/kg PO q 12 hr for 10 d. **Tx of pharyngitis/tonsillitis.** *Child 2–12 yr:* 7.5 mg/kg PO q 12 hr for 10 d. **Tx of skin/skin-structure infections.** *Child 2–12 yr:* 20 mg/kg PO once daily for 10 d.
**ADJUST DOSE** Elderly pts, renal impairment
**ADV EFF** Abd pain, **anaphylaxis,** anorexia, **bone marrow depression, colitis,** flatulence, **hepatotoxicity,** n/v/d, phlebitis, rash, superinfections
**INTERACTIONS** Aminoglycosides, oral anticoagulants
**NC/PT** Culture before tx. Refrigerate suspension. Give oral vancomycin for serious colitis. Pt should take w/food; complete full course of tx; report diarrhea w/blood or mucus, difficulty breathing.

## ceftaroline fosamil

(Teflaro)
**CLASS** Cephalosporin
**PREG/CONT** Unkn/NA

**IND & DOSE** **Tx of acute bacterial skin/skin-structure infections;**

**community-acquired pneumonia caused by susceptible strains.** *Adult:* 600 mg by IV infusion over 1 hr q 12 hr for 5–14 d (skin/skin-structure infections) or 5–7 d (community-acquired pneumonia). *Child 2 yr–<18 yr:* >33 kg: 400 mg IV q 8 hr or 600 mg q 12 hr over 5–60 min. ≤33 kg: 12 mg/kg IV q 8 hr over 5–60 min. *Child 2 mo–<2 yr:* 8 mg/kg IV q 8 hr over 5–60 min. *Child gestational age 34 wk and postnatal ≥12 d to <2 mo:* 6 mg/kg IV q 8 hr over 30–60 min (acute bacterial infections).
**ADJUST DOSE** Renal impairment
**ADV EFF** CDAD, dizziness, **hemolytic anemia, hypersensitivity reactions,** injection-site reactions, rash, **renal failure**
**NC/PT** Culture before tx. Small/frequent meals may help GI effects. Monitor injection site, CBC. Not for use in preg/breastfeeding. Pt should report severe diarrhea, difficulty breathing.

## cefTAZidime (Fortaz, Tazicef)

**CLASS** Cephalosporin
**PREG/CONT** B/NA

**IND & DOSE** **Tx of lower respiratory, skin/skin-structure, intra-abd, CNS, bone/joint infections; UTIs, septicemia caused by susceptible strains, gynecologic infections caused by *Escherichia coli*.** *Adult:* Usual dose, 1 g (range, 250 mg–2 g) q 8–12 hr IM or IV; max, 6 g/d. *Child 1 mo–12 yr:* 30 mg/kg IV q 12 hr. *Child 0–4 wk:* 30 mg/kg IV q 12 hr. **Tx of UTIs caused by susceptible bacteria strains.** *Adult:* 250–500 mg IV or IM q 8–12 hr. **Tx of pneumonia, skin/skin-structure infections caused by susceptible bacteria strains.** *Adult:* 500 mg–1 g IV or IM q 8 hr. **Tx of bone/joint infections caused by susceptible bacteria strains.** *Adult:* 2 g IV q 12 hr. **Tx of gynecologic, intra-abd, life-threatening infections; meningitis.** *Adult:* 2 g IV q 8 hr.
**ADJUST DOSE** Elderly pts, renal impairment
**ADV EFF** Abd pain, **anaphylaxis,** anorexia, **bone marrow depression, CDAD, colitis,** disulfiram-like reaction w/alcohol, flatulence, injection-site reactions, n/v/d, pain, phlebitis, superinfections
**INTERACTIONS** Aminoglycosides, alcohol, oral anticoagulants
**NC/PT** Culture before tx. Do not mix in sol w/aminoglycosides. Have vitamin K available if hypoprothrombinemia occurs. Pt should avoid alcohol during and for 3 d after tx; report diarrhea w/blood or mucus, difficulty breathing.

## cefTRIAXone sodium

(generic)
**CLASS** Cephalosporin
**PREG/CONT** B/NA

**IND & DOSE** **Tx of lower respiratory tract, intra-abd, skin/structure, bone/joint infections; acute bacterial otitis media, UTIs, septicemia caused by susceptible strains.** *Adult:* 1–2 g/d IM or IV as one dose or in equal divided doses bid; max, 4 g/d. *Child:* 50–75 mg/kg/d IV or IM in divided doses q 12 hr; max, 2 g/d. **Tx of gonorrhea and PID caused by *Neisseria gonorrhoeae*.** *Adult:* Single 250-mg IM dose. **Tx of meningitis.** *Adult:* 1–2 g/d IM or IV as one dose or in equal divided doses bid for 4–14 d; max, 4 g/d. Loading dose of 100 mg/kg may be used. **Periop px.** *Adult:* 1 g IV 30–120 min before surgery.
**ADV EFF** Abd pain, **anaphylaxis,** anorexia, **bone marrow depression, colitis,** disulfiram-like reactions w/alcohol, flatulence, **hepatotoxicity,** n/v/d, pain, superinfections
**INTERACTIONS** Aminoglycosides, alcohol, oral anticoagulants
**NC/PT** Culture before tx. Give w/meals. Protect drug from light. Have vitamin K available if hypoprothrombinemia occurs. Do not mix w/other antimicrobials. Arrange tx for superinfections. Pt should avoid

alcohol during and for 3 d after tx; complete full course of tx; report diarrhea w/blood or mucus, difficulty breathing.

**cefuroxime axetil** (generic), **cefuroxime sodium** (Zinacef)
**CLASS** Cephalosporin
**PREG/CONT** B/NA

**IND & DOSE** **Tx of upper respiratory tract, skin/skin-structure infections; acute bacterial otitis media, uncomplicated gonorrhea, bacterial sinusitis, UTIs, early Lyme disease caused by susceptible strains.** *Adult, child ≥12 yr:* 250 mg PO bid. For severe infections, may increase to 500 mg PO bid. Treat for up to 10 d. Or 750 mg–1.5 g IM or IV q 8 hr, depending on infection severity, for 5–10 d. *Child >3 mo:* 50–100 mg/kg/d IM or IV in divided doses q 6–8 hr. **Tx of acute otitis media.** *Child 3 mo–12 yr:* 250 mg PO bid for 10 d. **Tx of pharyngitis/tonsillitis.** *Child 3 mo–12 yr:* 125 mg PO q 12 hr for 10 d. **Tx of acute sinusitis.** *Child 3 mo–12 yr:* 250 mg PO bid for 10 d. **Tx of impetigo.** *Child 3 mo–12 yr:* 30 mg/kg/d (max, 1 g/d) in two divided doses for 10 d. **Uncomplicated gonorrhea.** *Adult:* 1.5 g IM (at two different sites) w/1 g oral probenecid. **Periop px.** *Adult:* 1.5 g IV 30–60 min before initial incision, then 750 mg IV or IM q 8 hr for 24 hr after surgery. **Tx of bacterial meningitis.** *Child:* 200–240 mg/kg/d IV in divided doses q 6–8 hr.
**ADJUST DOSE** Elderly pts, impaired renal function
**ADV EFF** Abd pain, **anaphylaxis**, anorexia, **bone marrow depression**, CDAD, **colitis**, disulfiram-like reactions w/alcohol, flatulence, **hepatotoxicity**, n/v/d, pain, superinfections
**INTERACTIONS** Aminoglycosides, alcohol, oral anticoagulants
**NC/PT** Culture before tx. Give w/meals. Have vitamin K available for hypoprothrombinemia. Do not mix w/other antimicrobials. Arrange for tx of superinfections. Use oral suspension for child who cannot swallow tablets. Pt should avoid alcohol during and for 3 d after tx; complete full course of tx; report diarrhea w/blood or mucus, difficulty breathing.

**celecoxib** (CeleBREX)
**CLASS** Cox-2 specific inhibitor, NSAID
**PREG/CONT** C (1st, 2nd trimesters); D (3rd trimester)/NA

**BBW** Increased risk of CV thrombotic events; contraindicated in CABG surgery, GI bleeding. Monitor accordingly.
**IND & DOSE** **Tx of acute pain, dysmenorrhea; mgt of RA.** *Adult:* 100 mg PO bid; may increase to 200 mg/d PO bid as needed. **Tx of osteoarthritis.** *Adult:* 200 mg/d PO. **Tx of ankylosing spondylitis.** *Adult:* 200 mg/d PO; after 6 wk, may try 400 mg/d for 6 wk. **Tx of juvenile RA.** *Child ≥2 yr:* >25 kg, 100 mg capsule PO bid; 10–≤25 kg, 50 mg capsule PO bid.
**ADJUST DOSE** Hepatic/renal impairment
**ADV EFF** **Agranulocytosis, anaphylactoid reactions**, dizziness, dyspepsia, edema, headache, HF, insomnia, **MI**, rash to serious dermatologic effects, **renal toxicity**, somnolence, **stroke**
**INTERACTIONS** Alcohol, drugs affecting hemostasis, lithium, nicotine, warfarin
**NC/PT** Avoid use in pts w/severe HF, third trimester of preg, pts w/aspirin-sensitive asthma. Give w/food if GI upset occurs. Use comfort measures to help relieve pain, safety measures if CNS effects occur. Pt should report difficulty breathing, chest pain, swelling, rash. Name confusion w/*Celebrex* (celecoxib), *Celexa* (citalopram), *Xanax* (alprazolam), and *Cerebyx* (fosphenytoin).

**cemiplimab-rwlc** (Libtayo)
**CLASS** Antineoplastic, anti-PD-1 monoclonal antibody, immune checkpoint inhibitor
**PREG/CONT** High risk/NA

**IND & DOSE** **Tx of pts w/metastatic cutaneous squamous cell carcinoma (CSCC) or locally advanced CSCC who are not candidates for curative surgery or curative radiation.** *Adult:* 350 mg IV over 30 min q 3 wk.
**ADV EFF** Diarrhea, fatigue, **infusion-related reactions**, rash, **severe and fatal immune-mediated reactions, including pneumonitis, colitis, hepatitis, endocrinopathies, nephritis w/renal dysfx**
**NC/PT** Warn pt about and monitor for immune-mediated adverse reactions/infusion-related reactions. Advise pt of potential for embryo-fetal toxicity.

**▶NEW DRUG**

**cenobamate** (Xcopri)
**CLASS** Antiepileptic
**PREG/CONT** Unkn/Pending DEA review

**IND & DOSE** **Tx of partial-onset seizures.** *Adult:* Initially, 12.5 mg PO daily, titrated up to 200 mg PO daily; max, 400 mg daily.
**ADV EFF** Diplopia, dizziness, **DRESS**, fatigue, headache, **QT shortening, suicidal**
**INTERACTIONS** Carbamazepine, clobazam, CNS depressants, lamotrigine, oral contraceptives, phenobarbital, phenytoin
**NC/PT** Start w/low dose and titrate up. Use lowest recommended dose if renal/hepatic impairment; not recommended if severe impairment. Gradually withdraw to minimize risk of increased seizure frequency. Drug may cause fetal harm; pt should use nonhormonal contraception.

**cephalexin** (Keflex)
**CLASS** Cephalosporin
**PREG/CONT** B/NA

**IND & DOSE** **Tx of respiratory tract infections, acute bacterial otitis media, bone infections, UTIs caused by susceptible strains.** *Adult:* 1–4 g/d in divided doses; usual dose, 250 mg PO q 6 hr. *Child:* 25–50 mg/kg/d PO in divided doses. **Tx of skin/skin-structure infections, uncomplicated cystitis, streptococcal pharyngitis.** *Adult:* 500 mg PO q 12 hr. May need larger doses in severe cases; max, 4 g/d. *Child:* Divide usual daily dose; give q 12 hr. **Tx of otitis media.** *Child:* 75–100 mg/kg/d PO in four divided doses.
**ADV EFF** Abd pain, **anaphylaxis**, anorexia, **bone marrow depression, colitis**, disulfiram-like reactions w/alcohol, flatulence, **hepatotoxicity**, n/v/d, pain, superinfections
**INTERACTIONS** Aminoglycosides, alcohol, oral anticoagulants
**NC/PT** Culture before tx. Give w/ meal. Pt should avoid alcohol during and for 3 d after tx; report diarrhea w/ blood or mucus, difficulty breathing.

**ceritinib** (Zykadia)
**CLASS** Antineoplastic, kinase inhibitor
**PREG/CONT** High risk/NA

**IND & DOSE** **Tx of metastatic NSCLC in pts whose tumors are anaplastic lymphoma kinase–positive.** *Adult:* 450 mg/d PO w/food.
**ADV EFF** Bradycardia, constipation, GI toxicity, **hepatotoxicity**, hyperglycemia, n/v/d, pancreatitis, **prolonged QT, serious to fatal pneumonitis**
**INTERACTIONS** CYP3A inducers/ inhibitors, grapefruit juice, QT-prolonging drugs
**NC/PT** Ensure pt has been tested for appropriate sensitivity. Monitor LFTs, pulmonary function, glucose (in diabetics). Pt should avoid preg

(contraceptives advised)/breastfeeding, grapefruit juice; take w/food; report difficulty breathing, urine/stool color changes, severe diarrhea.

## cerliponase alfa (Brineura)

**CLASS** Hydrolytic lysosomal N-terminal tripeptidyl peptidase
**PREG/CONT** Unkn/NA

**IND & DOSE To slow loss of ambulation in symptomatic child ≥3 yr w/ late infantile neuronal cord lipofuscinosis type 2.** *Child:* 300 mg q other week by intraventricular infusion, followed by intraventricular electrolytes over 4½ hr.
**ADV EFF** Bradycardia, device-related infections including meningitis, fever, headache, hematoma, hypotension, hypersensitivity reactions, irritability
**NC/PT** Use aseptic technique during preparation/administration. Monitor device for leakage/infection; contraindicated if sx or localized infection around device, w/CNS infection, or in pt w/ventriculoperitoneal shunt. Monitor ECG during/after infusion. Observe for potential hypersensitivity reactions. Teach caregivers s&sx of device infection and hypersensitivity, including anaphylaxis, and to report fever, slow HR, vomiting, difficulty breathing.

## certolizumab (Cimzia)

**CLASS** Immune modulator, TNF blocker
**PREG/CONT** C/NA

**BBW** Risk of serious infections, cancer, CNS demyelinating disorders. Prescreen for TB and HBV; monitor pt carefully. Lymphoma/other malignancies reported in child and adolescent treated w/TNF blockers; not indicated for child.
**IND & DOSE To reduce s&sx of Crohn disease; tx of moderately to severely active RA, active psoriatic arthritis, ankylosing spondylitis; tx of active nonradiographic axial spondyloarthritis w/inflammation; tx of plaque psoriasis.** *Adult:* 400 mg subcut (given as two 200-mg injections) repeated at 2 wk and 4 wk (all uses). Maint, 400 mg q 4 wk. For pt ≤90 kg, may consider 200 mg q other wk after initial doses of 400 at wk 2 and 4 (plaque psoriasis).
**ADV EFF Anaphylaxis,** HBV reactivation, **HF, lupuslike syndrome, malignancies, serious to fatal infections,** rash, URIs, UTIs
**INTERACTIONS** Abatacept, anakinra, live vaccines, natalizumab, rituximab
**NC/PT** Monitor carefully for s&sx of allergic reaction/infection. Not for use in preg. Pt should report s&sx of infection, difficulty breathing, swelling.

## cetirizine hydrochloride (Quzyttir, Zyrtec Allergy)

**CLASS** Antihistamine
**PREG/CONT** B/NA

**IND & DOSE Mgt of seasonal and perennial allergic rhinitis; tx of chronic, idiopathic urticaria.** *Adult, child≥6 yr:* 10 mg/d PO or 5 mg PO bid; max, 10 mg. *Child 6–11 yr:* 5 or 10 mg PO daily. *Child 2–6 yr:* 2.5 mg PO once daily; max, 5 mg/d. **Tx of acute urticaria** (*Quzyttir*). *Adult, adolescent ≥12 yr:* 10 mg/d IV. *Child 6–11 yr:* 5 or 10 mg/d IV. *Child 6 mo–5 yr:* 2.5 mg/d IV.
**ADJUST DOSE** Elderly pts; renal/hepatic impairment
**ADV EFF** Bronchospasm, sedation, somnolence
**NC/PT** Provide syrup or chewable tablets for child. Pt should maintain intake of fluids, use humidifier if secretions thicken; take safety precautions if sedation occurs; report difficulty breathing. Name confusion between *Zyrtec* (cetirizine) and *Zyprexa* (olanzapine) and between *Zyrtec* (cetirizine) and *Zantac* (ranitidine).

## cetrorelix acetate
(Cetrotide)
**CLASS** Fertility drug
**PREG/CONT** X/NA

**IND & DOSE Inhibition of premature LH surges in women undergoing controlled ovarian stimulation.** *Adult:* 3 mg subcut. If HCG not given within 4 d, continue 0.25 mg/kg/d subcut until HCG is given.
**ADV EFF** Headache, **hypersensitivity reactions,** injection-site reactions, nausea, ovarian overstimulation
**NC/PT** Part of comprehensive fertility program; many follow-up tests will be needed. Pt should learn proper administration/disposal of needles/syringes; report difficulty breathing.

**DANGEROUS DRUG**

## cetuximab (Erbitux)
**CLASS** Antineoplastic, monoclonal antibody
**PREG/CONT** High risk/NA

**BBW** Serious to fatal infusion reactions, cardiac arrest, and sudden death have occurred. Closely monitor serum electrolytes during and after tx.
**IND & DOSE Tx of advanced colorectal cancer; *K-Ras* wild-type, EGFR-expressing colorectal cancer; advanced squamous cell carcinoma of head/neck w/radiation or as monotherapy after failure of platinum therapy.** *Adult:* 400 mg/m$^2$ IV loading dose over 120 min, then 250 mg/m$^2$ IV over 60 min wkly.
**ADV EFF Cardiac arrest, dermatologic toxicity,** diarrhea, headache, **hypomagnesemia,** increased tumor progression, increased death w/*Ras*-mutant mCRC, infections, **infusion reactions, pulmonary toxicity,** rash, pruritus
**NC/PT** Premedicate w/$H_1$ antagonist IV 30–60 min before first dose. Base future doses on clinical response. Do not infuse faster than 10 mg/min. Have emergency equipment on hand. Monitor electrolytes; assess lungs and skin for s&sx of toxicity; discontinue if serious infusion reactions. Males/females should use contraception during and for 6 mo after tx; females should not breastfeed during or for 2 mo after tx. Pt should report s&sx of infection, difficulty breathing, rash.

## cevimeline hydrochloride (Evoxac)
**CLASS** Parasympathomimetic
**PREG/CONT** C/NA

**IND & DOSE Tx of dry mouth in pts w/Sjögren syndrome.** *Adult:* 30 mg PO tid w/food.
**ADV EFF Cardiac arrhythmias, bronchial narrowing,** dehydration, dyspepsia, excessive sweating, headache, n/v/d, URIs, visual blurring
**INTERACTIONS** Beta-adrenergic antagonists
**NC/PT** Give w/meals. Monitor for dehydration. Pt should take safety precautions if visual changes occur.

## charcoal, activated
(Actidose-Aqua, Liqui-Char)
**CLASS** Antidote
**PREG/CONT** C/NA

**IND & DOSE Emergency tx in poisoning by most drugs/chemicals.** *Adult:* 50–60 g or 1 g/kg PO, or approx 8–10 times by volume amount of poison ingested, as oral suspension. Give as soon as possible after poisoning. W/gastric dialysis, 20–40 g PO q 6 hr for 1–2 d for severe poisonings; for optimum effect, give within 30 min of poisoning. *Child 1–12 yr:* >32 kg, 50–60 g PO; 16–32 kg, 25–30 g PO; <16 kg and <1 yr, not recommended.
**ADV EFF** Black stools, constipation, diarrhea, vomiting
**INTERACTIONS** Laxatives, milk products, oral medications
**NC/PT** For use w/conscious pts only. Take steps to prevent aspiration; have

life-support equipment readily available. Pt should drink 6–8 glasses of liquid/d to avoid constipation. Name confusion between *Actidose* (charcoal) and *Actos* (pioglitazone).

## **chenodiol** (generic)

**CLASS** Gallstone solubilizer
**PREG/CONT** X/NA

**BBW** Highly toxic to liver. Reserve use for select pts where benefit clearly outweighs risk.
**IND & DOSE Tx of selected pts w/ radiolucent gallstones when surgery not an option.** *Adult:* 250 mg PO bid for 2 wk, then 13–16 mg/kg/d in two divided doses a.m. and p.m. for up to 6–9 mo.
**ADV EFF Colon cancer,** diarrhea, **hepatotoxicity,** neutropenia
**INTERACTIONS** Clofibrate, warfarin
**NC/PT** Ensure correct selection of pt. Monitor LFTs carefully. Not for use in preg (barrier contraceptives advised). Long-term therapy requires frequent tests. Diarrhea will occur. Pt should report urine/stool color changes.

**DANGEROUS DRUG**

## **chlorambucil** (Leukeran)

**CLASS** Antineoplastic, nitrogen mustard
**PREG/CONT** D/NA

**BBW** Arrange for blood tests to evaluate hematopoietic function before and wkly during tx. Severe bone marrow suppression possible. Drug is carcinogenic; monitor pt regularly. Rule out preg before starting tx. Encourage use of barrier contraceptives; drug is teratogenic. May cause infertility.
**IND & DOSE Palliative tx of chronic lymphocytic leukemia (CLL); malignant lymphoma, including lymphosarcoma; giant follicular lymphoma; Hodgkin lymphoma.** *Adult:* Initial dose and short-course therapy, 0.1–0.2 mg/kg/d PO for 3–6 wk; may give single daily dose. CLL alternative regimen, 0.4 mg/kg PO q 2 wk, increasing by 0.1 mg/kg w/each dose until therapeutic or toxic effect occurs. Maint, 0.03–0.1 mg/kg/d PO; max, 0.1 mg/kg/d.
**ADV EFF Acute leukemia,** alopecia, **bone marrow depression**
**NC/PT** Monitor CBC regularly. Rule out preg. Do not give full dose within 4 wk of radiation or other chemo. Divide dose w/severe n/v; maintain hydration. Sterility can occur. Hair loss is common; alert pt of possibility. Pt should report s&sx of infection. Name confusion w/*Leukeran* (chlorambucil), *Myleran* (busulfan), *Alkeran* (melphalan), and leucovorin.

## **chloramphenicol sodium succinate** (generic)

**CLASS** Antibiotic
**PREG/CONT** C/NA

**BBW** Severe, sometimes fatal blood dyscrasias (in adults) and severe, sometimes fatal gray syndrome (in newborns, premature infants) possible. Restrict use to situations in which no other antibiotic effective. Monitor serum levels at least wkly to minimize toxicity risk (therapeutic conc: peak, 10–20 mcg/mL; trough, 5–10 mcg/mL).
**IND & DOSE Severe infections caused by susceptible strains.** *Adult:* 50 mg/kg/d IV in divided doses q 6 hr up to 100 mg/kg/d in severe cases. **Severe infections and cystic fibrosis regimen.** *Child:* 50–100 mg/kg/d IV in divided doses q 6 hr. Neonate, child w/immature metabolic processes, 25 mg/kg/d IV; individualize doses at 6-hr intervals.
**ADJUST DOSE** Elderly pts; hepatic/renal impairment
**ADV EFF Anaphylaxis, bone marrow depression, gray baby syndrome, n/v/d,** superinfections
**INTERACTIONS** Bone marrow suppressants, glipizide, glyburide, phenytoins, tolazamide, tolbutamide, vitamin $B_{12}$, warfarin

**NC/PT** Culture before tx. Do not give IM. Monitor serum levels. Monitor CBC carefully. Change to another antibiotic as soon as possible.

## chlordiazepoxide (Librium)

**CLASS** Anxiolytic, benzodiazepine
**PREG/CONT** D/C-IV

**IND & DOSE** **Mgt of anxiety disorders.** *Adult:* 5 or 10 mg PO, up to 20 or 25 mg, tid–qid. *Child >6 yr:* Initially, 5 mg PO bid–qid; may increase to 10 mg bid–tid. **Preop apprehension.** *Adult:* 5–10 mg PO tid–qid on days preceding surgery. **Alcohol withdrawal.** *Adult:* 50–100 mg PO, then repeated doses as needed (max, 300 mg/d).
**ADJUST DOSE** Elderly pts, debilitating disease
**ADV EFF** Apathy, confusion, constipation, **CV collapse,** depression, diarrhea, disorientation, drowsiness, drug dependence w/withdrawal, fatigue, incontinence, lethargy, light-headedness, restlessness, urine retention
**INTERACTIONS** Alcohol, aminophylline, cimetidine, disulfiram, dyphylline, hormonal contraceptives, smoking, theophylline
**NC/PT** Monitor LFTs, renal function, CBC periodically during long-term therapy. Taper gradually after long-term use. Not for use in preg (barrier contraceptives advised); use caution w/breastfeeding. Pt should take safety precautions w/CNS effects.

## chloroquine phosphate (generic)

**CLASS** Amebicide, 4-aminoquinoline, antimalarial
**PREG/CONT** C/NA

**IND & DOSE** **Tx of extraintestinal amebiasis.** *Adult:* 1 g (600 mg base)/d PO for 2 d, then 500 mg (300 mg base)/d for 2–3 wk. **Px/tx of acute malaria attacks caused by susceptible strains.** *Adult:* Suppression, 300 mg base PO once a wk on same day for 2 wk before exposure, continuing until 8 wk after exposure; acute attack, 600 mg base PO initially, then 300 mg 6–8 hr, 24 hr, and 48 hr after initial dose for total dose of 1.5 g in 3 d. *Child:* Suppression, 5 mg base/kg PO once a wk on same day for 2 wk before exposure, continuing until 8 wk after exposure; acute attack, 10 mg base/kg PO initially; then 5 mg base/kg 6 hr later; then third dose 18 hr later; then last dose 24 hr after third dose. Max, 10 mg base/kg/d or 300 mg base/d.
**ADV EFF** **N/v/d, permanent retinal changes,** visual distortion
**INTERACTIONS** Cimetidine
**NC/PT** Double-check child doses; child very susceptible to overdose. Give w/food if GI effects. Arrange for ophthal exam before and during long-term tx. Pt should take safety measures if vision changes.

## chlorothiazide (Diuril), chlorothiazide sodium (generic)

**CLASS** Thiazide diuretic
**PREG/CONT** C/NA

**IND & DOSE** **Adjunct tx for edema; tx of HTN.** *Adult:* 0.5–2 g daily PO or IV. *Child:* Generally, 10–20 mg/kg/d PO in single dose or two divided doses. *Child 2–12 yr:* 375 mg–1 g PO in two divided doses. *Child 6 mo–2 yr:* 125–375 mg PO in two divided doses. *Child <6 mo:* Up to 30 mg/kg/d PO in two doses.
**ADV EFF** **Agranulocytosis,** anorexia, **aplastic anemia,** constipation, ED, n/v/d, nocturia, polyuria, vertigo
**INTERACTIONS** Alcohol, antidiabetics, cholestyramine, corticosteroids, diazoxide, digoxin, lithium, opioids
**NC/PT** Do not give IM or subcut. Monitor and record weight daily. Pt should take w/food if GI upset, take early in day so sleep will not be disturbed. Increased urination will occur; pt should plan day accordingly.

**chlorpheniramine maleate** (Aller-Chlor, Allergy, Chlor-Trimeton Allergy)
**CLASS** Antihistamine
**PREG/CONT** C/NA

**IND & DOSE Symptomatic relief of s&sx associated w/perennial and seasonal allergic rhinitis; vasomotor rhinitis; common cold; allergic conjunctivitis.** *Adult, child >12 yr:* 4 mg PO q 4–6 hr; max, 24 mg in 24 hr (tablets, syrup). ER tablets, 16 mg w/liquid PO q 24 hr. SR tablets, 8–12 mg PO at bedtime or q 8–12 hr during day. ER capsules, 12 mg/d PO; max, 24 mg/d. Caplets, 8–12 mg/d PO q 12 hr. *Child 6–12 yr:* 2 mg q 4–6 hr PO; max, 12 mg in 24 hr (tablets, syrup).
**ADJUST DOSE** Elderly pts
**ADV EFF Anaphylactic shock, aplastic anemia,** bronchial secretion thickening, disturbed coordination, dizziness, drowsiness, epigastric distress, sedation
**INTERACTIONS** Alcohol, CNS depressants
**NC/PT** Periodic CBC w/long-term tx. Pt should take w/food; not cut/crush/chew SR/ER forms; avoid alcohol; take safety precautions w/CNS effects.

**chlorproMAZINE hydrochloride** (generic)
**CLASS** Antiemetic, antipsychotic, anxiolytic, dopamine blocker, phenothiazine
**PREG/CONT** C/NA

**BBW** Risk of death in elderly pts w/dementia-related psychoses; not approved for this use.
**IND & DOSE Tx of excessive anxiety/agitation.** *Adult:* 25 mg IM; may repeat in 1 hr w/25–50 mg IM. Increase gradually in inpts, up to 400 mg q 4–6 hr. Switch to oral dose as soon as possible, 10 mg PO tid–qid; increase to 25 mg PO bid–tid. 25–50 mg PO tid for outpts; up to 2,000 mg/d PO for inpatients. *Child 6 mo–12 yr, outpts:* 0.5 mg/kg PO q 4–6 hr; 1 mg/kg rectally q 6–8 hr; 0.55 mg/kg IM q 6–8 hr; max, 40 mg/d (up to 5 yr) or 75 mg/d (5–12 yr). *Child, inpts:* 50–100 mg/d PO; max, 40 mg/d IM (up to 5 yr), 75 mg/d IM (5–12 yr). **Preop/postop anxiety.** *Adult:* Preop, 25–50 mg PO 2–3 hr before surgery or 12.5–25 mg IM 1–2 hr before surgery; intraop, 12.5 mg IM repeated in 30 min or 2 mg IV repeated q 2 min (up to 25 mg total) to control vomiting (if no hypotension occurs); postop, 10–25 mg PO q 4–6 hr or 12.5–25 mg IM repeated in 1 hr (if no hypotension occurs). *Child 6 mo–12 yr:* Preop, 0.55 mg/kg PO 2–3 hr before surgery or 0.55 mg/kg IM 1–2 hr before surgery; intraop, 0.25 mg/kg IM or 1 mg (diluted) IV, repeated at 2-min intervals up to total IM dose; postop, 0.55 mg/kg PO q 4–6 hr or 0.55 mg/kg IM, repeated in 1 hr (if no hypotension occurs). **Tx of acute intermittent porphyria.** *Adult:* 25–50 mg PO or 25 mg IM tid–qid until pt can take oral tx. **Adjunct tx of tetanus.** *Adult:* 25–50 mg IM tid–qid, usually w/barbiturates, or 25–50 mg IV diluted and infused at 1 mg/min. *Child:* 0.55 mg/kg IM q 6–8 hr or 0.5 mg/min IV; max, 40 mg/d (up to 23 kg), 75 mg/d (23–45 kg). **Antiemetic.** *Adult:* 10–25 mg PO q 4–6 hr, or 50–100 mg rectally q 6–8 hr, or 25 mg IM. If no hypotension, give 25–50 mg q 3–4 hr. Switch to oral dose when vomiting ends. *Child:* 0.55 mg/kg PO q 4–6 hr, or 0.55 mg/kg IM q 6–8 hr. Max IM dose, 75 mg/d (5–12 yr), 40 mg/d (up to 5 yr). **Tx of intractable hiccups.** *Adult:* 25–50 mg PO tid–qid. If sx persist for 2–3 d, give 25–50 mg IM; if inadequate response, give 25–50 mg IV in 500–1,000 mL saline.
**ADJUST DOSE** Elderly pts
**ADV EFF Anaphylactoid reactions, aplastic anemia,** blurred vision, **bronchospasm, cardiac arrest, cardiomegaly,** drowsiness, dry mouth, extrapyramidal syndromes, **HF,** hypotension, **laryngospasm,** n/v/d, **NMS,** orthostatic hypotension, photophobia,

**pulmonary edema,** urine retention, urticaria, vertigo
**INTERACTIONS** Alcohol, anticholinergics, barbiturate anesthetics, beta blockers, epinephrine, meperidine, norepinephrine
**NC/PT** Do not give by subcut injection; give slowly by deep IM injection into upper outer quadrant of buttock. If giving drug via continuous infusion for intractable hiccups, keep pt flat in bed; avoid skin contact w/parenteral drug sol; monitor renal function, CBC; withdraw slowly after high-dose use. Aspiration risk w/loss of cough reflex. Pt should avoid alcohol, take safety measures if CNS effects occur, protect from sun exposure. Name confusion between chlorpromazine, chlorpropamide, and clomipramine.

## chlorzoxazone (generic)

**CLASS** Centrally acting skeletal muscle relaxant
**PREG/CONT** C/NA

**IND & DOSE Relief of discomfort associated w/acute, painful musculoskeletal conditions as adjunct to rest, physical therapy, other measures.** *Adult:* 250 mg PO tid–qid; may need 500 mg PO tid–qid. Max, 750 mg tid–qid.
**ADV EFF Anaphylaxis,** dizziness, drowsiness, GI disturbances, **hepatic impairment,** light-headedness, orange to red urine
**INTERACTIONS** Alcohol, CNS depressants
**NC/PT** Use other measures to help pain. Pt should avoid alcohol and sleep-inducing drugs, take safety measures if CNS effects occur, be aware that urine color will change.

## cholestyramine (Prevalite)

**CLASS** Bile acid sequestrant, antihyperlipidemic
**PREG/CONT** C/NA

**IND & DOSE Adjunct to reduce elevated serum cholesterol in pts w/primary hypercholesterolemia; pruritus associated w/partial biliary obstruction.** *Adult:* 4 g PO once to twice a day; w/constipation, start w/4 g once a day; maint, 8–16 g/d divided into two doses. Max, 6 packets or scoopfuls (24 g/d). *Child:* 240 mg/kg/d PO in two–three divided doses; max, 8 g/d.
**ADV EFF** Constipation to fecal impaction, hemorrhoid exacerbation, increased bleeding tendencies
**INTERACTIONS** Corticosteroids, digitalis, diuretics, fat-soluble vitamins, thiazide preparations, thyroid medication, warfarin
**NC/PT** Mix packet contents w/water, milk, fruit juice, noncarbonated beverages, soup, applesauce, pineapple; do not give in dry form. Monitor for constipation, which could be severe. Pt should take w/meals, take other oral drugs 1 hr before or 4–6 hr after this drug; avoid preg/breastfeeding.

## cholic acid (Cholbam)

**CLASS** Bile acid
**PREG/CONT** Unkn/NA

**IND & DOSE Tx of bile acid synthesis disorders; adjunct tx of peroxisomal disorders.** *Adult, child:* 10–15 mg/kg/d PO; w/concomitant familial hypertriglyceridemia, use 11–17 mg/kg/d PO.
**ADV EFF** Abd pain, **hepatotoxicity,** intestinal polyps, malaise, n/v/d, peripheral neuropathies, reflux esophagitis, skin lesions, UTI
**INTERACTIONS** Aluminum-containing antacids, bile acid resins, bile salt efflux inhibitors, cyclosporine
**NC/PT** Monitor LFTs before, q mo for 3 mo; then at 3, 6, 9 mo; then q 6 mo for 3 yr; then annually. Give w/food. Pt should not cut/crush/chew capsule (capsule may be opened and contents sprinkled on drink/food); should allow 4–6 hr between aluminum-based antacids/bile acid resins and this drug; take safety precaution w/CNS effects; eat small meals for GI

problems; enroll in preg registry if preg occurs.

**choline magnesium trisalicylate** (Tricosal)
**CLASS** NSAID, salicylate
**PREG/CONT** C/NA

**IND & DOSE** **Tx of osteoarthritis/RA.** *Adult:* 1.5–2.5 g/d PO; max, 4.5 g/d in divided doses. **Tx of pain/fever.** *Adult:* 2–3 g/d PO in divided doses. *Child:* 217.5–652.5 mg PO q 4 hr as needed.
**ADV EFF** **Anaphylactoid reactions,** dizziness, drowsiness, GI bleeding, headache, heartburn, indigestion, n/v, sweating
**INTERACTIONS** ACE inhibitors, antidiabetics, carbonic anhydrase inhibitors, corticosteroids, insulin, meglitinide, methotrexate, valproic acid
**NC/PT** Pt should take w/full glass of water and not lie down for 30 min after taking; take w/food if GI effects are severe; use safety precautions if CNS effects occur; report difficulty breathing.

**chorionic gonadotropin** (Pregnyl)
**CLASS** Hormone
**PREG/CONT** X/NA

**BBW** Drug has no known effect on fat metabolism and is not for tx of obesity.
**IND & DOSE** **Tx of prepubertal cryptorchidism not due to anatomic obstruction.** *Adult, child >4 yr:* 4,000 USP units IM 3 ×/wk for 3 wk; then 5,000 USP units IM q second day for four injections; then 15 injections of 500–1,000 USP units over 6 wk; then 500 USP units 3 ×/wk for 4–6 wk. If unsuccessful, start another course 1 mo later, giving 1,000 USP units/injection. **Tx of hypogonadotropic hypogonadism in males.** *Adult, child >4 yr:* 500–1,000 USP units IM 3 ×/wk for 3 wk; then same dose twice/wk for 3 wk; then 1,000–2,000 USP units IM 3 ×/wk; then 4,000 USP units 3 ×/wk for 6–9 mo. Reduce dose to 2,000 USP units 3 ×/wk for additional 3 mo. **Induction of ovulation and preg.** *Adult:* 5,000–10,000 units IM 1 day after last menotropins dose.
**ADV EFF** Gynecomastia, headache, irritability, **ovarian cancer, ovarian hyperstimulation,** pain at injection site
**NC/PT** Must give IM. Prepare calendar of tx schedule. Discontinue if s&sx of ovarian overstimulation. Provide comfort measures for headache, pain at injection site.

**chorionic gonadotropin alfa** (Ovidrel)
**CLASS** Fertility drug
**PREG/CONT** X/NA

**IND & DOSE** **Ovulation induction in infertile women.** *Adult:* 250 mcg subcut 1 day after last FSH dose.
**ADV EFF** Abd pain, injection-site pain, multiple births, n/v, ovarian enlargement, **ovarian hyperstimulation; pulmonary, vascular thromboembolic events**
**NC/PT** Part of comprehensive fertility program. Inject into abdomen. Risk of multiple births. Pt should report difficulty breathing, sudden abd or leg pain.

**cidofovir** (generic)
**CLASS** Antiviral
**PREG/CONT** C/NA

**BBW** Risk of severe renal impairment; monitor renal function closely. Risk of neutropenia; monitor CBC closely. Cancer, impaired fertility, tetragenic effects reported.
**IND & DOSE** **Tx of CMV retinitis in AIDS pts.** *Adult:* 5 mg/kg IV over 1 hr for 2 wk, then 5 mg/kg IV q 2 wk.
**ADV EFF** Decreased IOP, dyspnea, fever, infection, n/v, neutropenia, pneumonia, proteinuria, **renal failure**

**NC/PT** Use only for stated indication; not for other diseases. Give w/ PO probenecid (2 g before each dose, then 1 g at 2 and 8 hr after each dose). Monitor renal function, CBC. Protect pt from infection. Not for use in preg/ breastfeeding. Mark calendar for tx days.

## cilostazol (generic)

**CLASS** Antiplatelet, phosphodiesterase III inhibitor
**PREG/CONT** C/NA

**BBW** Do not give to pts w/HF; decreased survival reported.
**IND & DOSE** **To reduce s&sx of intermittent claudication, allowing increased walking distance.** *Adult:* 100 mg PO bid at least 30 min before or 2 hr after breakfast and dinner; may not notice response for 2–12 wk.
**ADJUST DOSE** Administration w/ CYP3A4, CYP2C19 inhibitors
**ADV EFF** Bleeding, diarrhea, dizziness, dyspepsia, flatulence, headache, **HF**, nausea, rhinitis
**INTERACTIONS** Azole antifungals, diltiazem, grapefruit juice, high-fat meal, macrolide antibiotics, omeprazole, smoking
**NC/PT** Not for use in preg (barrier contraceptives advised). Pt should take on empty stomach 30 min before or 2 hr after breakfast and dinner, take safety precautions to prevent injury, avoid grapefruit juice, continue tx for up to 12 wk to see results.

## cimetidine (Tagamet HB)

**CLASS** Histamine$_2$ antagonist
**PREG/CONT** B/NA

**IND & DOSE** **Tx of heartburn/acid indigestion.** *Adult:* 200 mg PO as s&sx occur; max, 400 mg/24 hr for max of 2 wk. **Tx of active duodenal ulcer.** *Adult:* 800 mg PO at bedtime or 300 mg PO qid w/meals and at bedtime or 400 mg PO bid; continue for 4–6 wk. Intractable ulcers, 300 mg IM or IV q 6–8 hr. Maint, 400 mg PO at bedtime. **Tx of active benign gastric ulcer.** *Adult:* 300 mg PO qid w/meals and at bedtime or 800 mg at bedtime for 8 wk. **Tx of pathologic hypersecretory syndrome.** *Adult:* 300 mg PO qid w/meals and at bedtime or 300 mg IV or IM q 6 hr. Individualize doses as needed; max, 2,400 mg/d. **Tx of erosive GERD.** *Adult:* 1,600 mg PO in divided doses bid–qid for 12 wk. **Px of upper GI bleeding.** *Adult:* 50 mg/hr continuous IV infusion for up to 7 d.
**ADJUST DOSE** Elderly pts, renal impairment
**ADV EFF** **Cardiac arrhythmias,** confusion, diarrhea, dizziness, hallucinations, ED
**INTERACTIONS** Alcohol, alkylating agents, benzodiazepines, beta-adrenergic blockers, carbamazepine, chloroquine, lidocaine, nifedipine, pentoxifylline, phenytoin, procainamide, quinidine, smoking, theophylline, TCAs
**NC/PT** Give w/meals and at bedtime. Give IM undiluted into large muscle group. Pt should report smoking so dose can be regulated, take safety precautions w/CNS effects.

## cinacalcet hydrochloride (Sensipar)

**CLASS** Calcimimetic, calcium-lowering drug
**PREG/CONT** C/NA

**IND & DOSE** **Tx of hypercalcemia associated w/parathyroid carcinoma or severe hypercalcemia in pts w/ primary hyperparathyroidism.** *Adult:* Initially, 30 mg PO bid to maintain calcium within normal range; adjust dose q 2–4 wk in sequential doses of 60 mg bid, then 90 mg bid to max 90 mg tid–qid. **Tx of secondary hyperparathyroidism.** *Adult:* 30 mg/d PO. Monitor serum calcium and phosphorus within 1 wk; may increase dose 30 mg q 2–4 wk to max 180 mg/d. Target intact parathyroid hormone level, 150–300 pg/mL.

**ADV EFF** Dizziness, hallucinations, **hepatic impairment,** hypocalcemia, myalgia, n/v, **seizures**, upper GI bleeding
**INTERACTIONS** Amitriptyline, erythromycin, flecainide, ketoconazole, itraconazole, TCAs, thioridazine, vinblastine
**NC/PT** Monitor serum calcium before and regularly during tx. Hypocalcemia may lead to prolonged QT interval/arrhythmias, hypotension, and worsening HF. If pt on dialysis, also give vitamin D and phosphate binders. Give w/food. Not for use in breastfeeding. Pt should not cut/crush/chew tablets; should take safety measures w/CNS effects; report urine/stool color changes.

**ciprofloxacin** (Ciloxan, Cipro)
**CLASS** Antibacterial, fluoroquinolone
**PREG/CONT** C/NA

**BBW** Risk of tendinitis and tendon rupture; risk higher in pts >60 yr, those on steroids, and those w/kidney, heart, or lung transplant. Avoid use in pts w/hx of myasthenia gravis; drug may exacerbate weakness. Reserve use for pts w/no alternative tx options for exacerbation of chronic bronchitis, uncomplicated cystitis, acute sinusitis.
**IND & DOSE Tx of uncomplicated UTIs.** *Adult:* 250 mg PO q 12 hr for 3 d or 500 mg (ER tablets) PO daily for 3 d. **Tx of mild to moderate UTIs.** *Adult:* 250 mg PO q 12 hr for 7–14 d or 200 mg IV q 12 hr for 7–14 d. **Tx of complicated UTIs.** *Adult:* 500 mg PO q 12 hr for 7–14 d or 400 mg IV q 12 hr or 1,000 mg (ER tablets) PO daily q 7–14 d. **Tx of chronic bacterial prostatitis.** *Adult:* 500 mg PO q 12 hr for 28 d or 400 mg IV q 12 hr for 28 d. **Tx of infectious diarrhea.** *Adult:* 500 mg PO q 12 hr for 5–7 d. **Anthrax postexposure.** *Adult:* 500 mg PO q 12 hr for 60 d or 400 mg IV q 12 hr for 60 d. *Child:* 15 mg/kg/dose PO q 12 hr for 60 d or 10 mg/kg/dose IV q 12 hr for 60 d; max, 500 mg/dose PO or 400 mg/dose IV. **Tx of respiratory infections.** *Adult:* 500–750 mg PO q 12 hr or 400 mg IV q 8–12 hr for 7–14 d. **Tx of acute sinusitis.** *Adult:* 500 mg PO q 12 hr or 400 mg IV q 12 hr for 10 d. **Tx of acute uncomplicated pyelonephritis.** *Adult:* 1,000 mg (ER tablets) PO daily q 7–14 d. **Tx of bone, joint, skin infections.** 500–750 mg PO q 12 hr or 400 mg IV q 8–12 hr for 4–6 wk. **Tx of nosocomial pneumonia.** *Adult:* 400 mg IV q 8 hr for 10–14 d. **Tx of plaque.** *Adults:* 400 mg IV q 8–12 hr for 14 d. *Child:* 10 mg/kg IV (max, 400 mg/dose) q 8–12 hr for 10–21 d. **Tx of ophthal infections caused by susceptible organisms not responsive to other tx.** *Adult:* 1 or 2 drops q 2 hr in affected eye(s) while awake for 2 d or q 4 hr for 5 d; or ½-inch ribbon ointment into conjunctival sac tid on first 2 d, then ½-inch ribbon bid for next 5 d. **Tx of acute otitis externa.** *Adult:* 4 drops in infected ear tid–qid, or 1 single-use container (0.25 mL) in infected ear bid for 7 d.
**ADJUST DOSE** Renal impairment
**ADV EFF Aortic aneurysm/dissection**, **CDAD,** CNS effects, headache, **hepatotoxicity,** hypersensitivity reactions, n/v/d, **peripheral neuropathy**, **QT prolongation**, rash, **tendinitis, tendon rupture**
**INTERACTIONS** Antacids, antidiabetic agents, didanosine, foscarnet, methotrexate, phenytoin, QT-prolonging drugs, St. John's wort, sucralfate, theophylline, warfarin
**NC/PT** Culture before tx. Avoid use in pts w/hx of myasthenia gravis; may exacerbate weakness. Use cautiously w/child; increased incidence of joint/tissue injury. Discontinue if s&sx of acute adverse effects. Reserve use for serious infections. Give antacids at least 2 hr apart from dosing. Ensure hydration. Pt should not cut/crush/chew ER form; should report diarrhea, urine/stool color changes, sudden muscle pain.

DANGEROUS DRUG

**CISplatin** (CDDP) (generic)
**CLASS** Alkylating agent, antineoplastic, platinum agent
**PREG/CONT** D/NA

**BBW** Ensure adequate hydration, monitor renal function; severe toxicity related to dose possible. Can cause peripheral neuropathy. Premedicate w/antiemetics due to potential for severe n/v. Monitor blood counts for severe myelosuppression.
**IND & DOSE** **Tx of metastatic testicular tumors.** *Adult:* Remission induction: Cisplatin, 20 mg/m²/d IV for 5 consecutive d (days 1–5) q 3 wk for three courses; bleomycin, 30 units IV wkly (day 2 of each wk) for 12 consecutive doses; vinblastine, 0.15–0.2 mg/kg IV twice wkly (days 1 and 2) q 3 wk for four courses. Maint: Vinblastine, 0.3 mg/kg IV q 4 wk for 2 yr. **Tx of metastatic ovarian tumors.** *Adult:* 75–100 mg/m² IV once q 4 wk. For combo therapy, give sequentially: Cisplatin, 75–100 mg/m² IV once q 3–4 wk; cyclophosphamide, 600 mg/m² IV once q 4 wk. Single dose: 100 mg/m² IV once q 4 wk. **Tx of advanced bladder cancer.** *Adult:* 50–70 mg/m² IV once q 3–4 wk; in heavily pretreated (radiotherapy or chemo) pts, give initial dose of 50 mg/m² repeated q 4 wk. Do not give repeated courses until serum creatinine <1.5 mg/dL, BUN <25 mg/dL, or platelets >100,000/mm³ and WBCs >4,000/mm³. Do not give subsequent doses until audiometry indicates hearing within normal range.
**ADJUST DOSE** Renal impairment
**ADV EFF** **Anaphylaxis-like reactions,** anorexia, **bone marrow suppression, nephrotoxicity,** n/v/d, ocular toxicity, ototoxicity
**INTERACTIONS** Aminoglycosides, bumetanide, ethacrynic acid, furosemide, phenytoins
**NC/PT** Monitor renal function before and regularly during tx. Monitor hearing. Maintain hydration. Use antiemetics if needed. Monitor electrolytes regularly. Do not use needles containing aluminum. Use gloves when preparing IV. Not for use in preg/breastfeeding. Pt should report changes in hearing, difficulty breathing, unusual bleeding. Name confusion w/carboplatin; use extreme caution.

**citalopram hydrobromide** (CeleXA)
**CLASS** Antidepressant, SSRI
**PREG/CONT** C/NA

**BBW** Increased risk of suicidality in child, adolescent, young adult; monitor accordingly.
**IND & DOSE** **Tx of depression.** *Adult:* 20 mg/d PO as single daily dose. May increase to 40 mg/d; max, 40 mg/d.
**ADJUST DOSE** Elderly pts; renal/hepatic impairment
**ADV EFF** Dizziness, dry mouth, ejaculatory disorders, insomnia, nausea, **prolonged QT,** somnolence, **suicidality,** tremor
**INTERACTIONS** Azole antifungals, beta blockers, citalopram, erythromycin, linezolid, macrolide antibiotics, MAOIs, pimozide, QT-prolonging drugs, St. John's wort, TCAs, warfarin
**NC/PT** Avoid doses >40 mg; increased risk of prolonged QT interval. Limit drug to suicidal pts; monitor for suicidality. May take several wk to see effects. Not for use in preg/breastfeeding. Pt should avoid St. John's wort; report thoughts of suicide. Name confusion w/*Celexa* (citalopram), *Celebrex* (celecoxib), *Xanax* (alprazolam), and *Cerebyx* (fosphenytoin).

DANGEROUS DRUG

**cladribine** (Mavenclad)
**CLASS** Antimetabolite, antineoplastic, purine analog
**PREG/CONT** D/NA

**BBW** Monitor complete hematologic profile, LFTs, renal function tests

before and frequently during tx. Consult physician at first sign of toxicity; consider delaying dose or discontinuing if neurotoxicity or renal toxicity occurs (generic). Risk of malignancies and teratogenicity; contraindicated if current malignancy (*Mavenclad*).
**IND & DOSE** **Tx of active hairy cell leukemia.** *Adult:* Single course of 0.09–0.1 mg/kg/d by continuous IV infusion for 7 d. **Tx of relapsing forms of MS** (*Mavenclad*). *Adult:* 3.5 mg/kg PO in two treatment courses (1.75 mg/kg/treatment course) separated from other oral medications by at least 3 hr.
**ADV EFF** Abnormal breath sounds, anorexia, arthralgia, **bone marrow suppression,** chills, cough, fatigue, fever, headache, **hepatotoxicity,** injection-site reactions, **nephrotoxicity, neurotoxicity,** n/v/d
**NC/PT** Use gloves when handling drug. Must be given by continuous infusion for 7 d. Monitor renal function, LFTs, CBC before and regularly during tx. Not for use in preg (pt should use contraception during and for several wk [6 mo for *Mavenclad*] after tx ends)/breastfeeding. Pt should report numbness/tingling, pain at injection site, s&sx of infection, urine/stool color changes.

## clarithromycin (Biaxin XL)
**CLASS** Macrolide antibiotic
**PREG/CONT** C/NA

**IND & DOSE** **Tx of pharyngitis/tonsillitis, pneumonia, skin/skin-structure infections, lower respiratory infections caused by susceptible strains.** *Adult:* 250 mg PO q 12 hr for 7–14 d. *Child:* 15 mg/kg/d PO divided q 12 hr for 10 d. **Tx of acute maxillary sinusitis, acute otitis media, lower respiratory infections caused by susceptible strains.** *Adult:* 500 mg PO q 12 hr for 14 d or 1,000 mg (ER tablets) PO q 24 hr. **Tx of mycobacterial infections.** *Adult:* 500 mg PO bid. *Child:* 7.5 mg/kg PO bid; max, 500 mg PO bid. **Tx of duodenal ulcers.** *Adult:* 500 mg PO tid plus omeprazole 40 mg PO q a.m. for 14 d, then omeprazole 20 mg PO q a.m. for 14 d. **Tx of community-acquired pneumonia.** *Adult:* 250 mg PO q 12 hr for 7–14 d or 1,000 mg (ER tablets) PO q 24 hr for 7 d.
**ADJUST DOSE** Elderly pts, renal impairment
**ADV EFF** Abd pain, CDAD, diarrhea, prolonged QT, superinfections
**INTERACTIONS** Antidiabetics, carbamazepine, colchicine, grapefruit juice, lovastatin, phenytoin, QT-prolonging drugs, theophylline; serious reactions possible
**NC/PT** Culture before tx. Arrange for tx of superinfections. Do not refrigerate suspension. Not for use in preg/breastfeeding. Pt should take w/food if GI upset occurs; avoid grapefruit juice; not cut/crush/chew ER tablets; report persistent diarrhea.

## clemastine fumarate
(Dayhist-1, Tavist Allergy)
**CLASS** Antihistamine
**PREG/CONT** B/NA

**IND & DOSE** **Symptomatic relief of s&sx of allergic rhinitis.** *Adult:* 1.34 mg PO bid. Max, 8.04 mg/d (syrup), 2.68 mg/d (tablets). *Child 6–12 yr:* (syrup only) 0.67 mg PO bid; max, 4.02 mg/d. **Tx of mild, uncomplicated urticaria and angioedema.** *Adult:* 2.68 mg PO daily–tid; max, 8.04 mg/d. *Child 6–12 yr:* (syrup only) 1.34 mg PO bid; max, 4.02 mg/d.
**ADJUST DOSE** Elderly pts
**ADV EFF** **Anaphylactic shock,** bronchial secretion thickening, disturbed coordination, dizziness, drowsiness, epigastric distress, sedation
**INTERACTIONS** Alcohol, CNS depressants, MAOIs
**NC/PT** Use syrup if pt cannot swallow tablets. Give w/food if GI upset occurs. Pt should drink plenty of fluids; use humidifier; avoid alcohol; report difficulty breathing, irregular heartbeat.

## clevidipine butyrate
(Cleviprex)
**CLASS** Antihypertensive, calcium channel blocker
**PREG/CONT** C/NA

**IND & DOSE** **To reduce BP when oral tx not possible or desirable.** *Adult:* 1–2 mg/hr IV infusion; titrate quickly by doubling dose q 90 sec to achieve desired BP; maint, 4–6 mg/hr; max, 21 mg/hr/24 hr.
**ADV EFF** Headache, **HF,** n/v
**NC/PT** Continuously monitor BP, ECG during administration. Taper beta blockers before use. Handle drug w/ strict aseptic technique. Use within 4 hr of puncturing stopper. Rebound HTN possible within 8 hr of stopping drug; switch to oral antihypertensive as soon as possible.

## clindamycin hydrochloride (Cleocin), clindamycin palmitate hydrochloride (generic), clindamycin phosphate
(Cleocin T, Clindagel)
**CLASS** Lincosamide antibiotic
**PREG/CONT** Unkn (1st trimester); low risk (2nd, 3rd trimesters)/NA

**BBW** Serious to fatal colitis, including CDAD, possibly up to several wk after tx ends. Reserve use; monitor pt closely.
**IND & DOSE** **Serious infections caused by susceptible bacteria strains.** Reserve use for penicillin-allergic pts or when penicillin inappropriate. *Adult:* 150–300 mg PO q 6 hr (up to 300–450 mg PO q 6 hr in more severe infections) or 600–2,700 mg/d IV or IM in two–four equal doses (up to 4.8 g/d IV or IM for life-threatening situations). *Child:* Clindamycin hydrochloride, 8–16 mg/kg/d PO (serious infections) or 16–20 mg/kg/d PO (more serious infections in three or four equal doses). *Child <10 kg:* 37.5 mg PO tid as min dose. *Child >1 mo:* 20–40 mg/kg/d IV or IM in three or four equal doses or 350–450 mg/m²/d. *Neonates:* 15–20 mg/kg/d IV or IM in three or four equal doses. **Tx of bacterial vaginosis.** *Adult:* 1 applicator (100 mg clindamycin phosphate) intravaginally, preferably at bedtime for 7 consecutive d in preg women and 3 or 7 d in nonpreg women. **Tx of acne vulgaris.** *Adult:* Apply thin film to affected area bid.
**ADJUST DOSE** Renal impairment
**ADV EFF** Abd pain, **agranulocytosis, anaphylactic reactions,** anorexia, **cardiac arrest,** CDAD, contact dermatitis, esophagitis, n/v/d, pain after injection, **pseudomembranous colitis,** rash
**INTERACTIONS** Aluminum salts, kaolin, NMJ blockers
**NC/PT** Culture before tx. Consider changing to different drug if pt is preg (1st trimester) or breastfeeding. Give orally w/full glass of water or food. Do not give IM injection of more than 600 mg; inject deeply into muscle. Monitor LFTs, renal function. Pt should avoid eye contact w/topical sol; give intravaginally at bedtime; report severe or watery diarrhea, diarrhea w/ blood or mucus, difficulty breathing.

## cloBAZam (Onfi, Sympazan)
**CLASS** Antiepileptic, benzodiazepine
**PREG/CONT** C/C-IV

**IND & DOSE** **Adjunct tx of seizures associated w/Lennox-Gastaut syndrome.** *Adult, child ≥2 yr:* >30 kg, initially 5 mg PO bid; increase as tolerated up to 40 mg/d. ≤30 kg, initially 5 mg/d; titrate as tolerated up to 20 mg/d.
**ADJUST DOSE** Elderly pts, mild to moderate hepatic impairment, poor CYP2C19 metabolizers
**ADV EFF** Aggression, ataxia, constipation, drooling, dysarthria, fatigue, fever, insomnia, sedation, somnolence, **suicidality**
**INTERACTIONS** Alcohol, fluconazole, fluvoxamine, hormonal contraceptives, omeprazole, ticlopidine

**NC/PT** Taper drug after long-term use; dispense least amount feasible. Administer whole or crush and mix in applesauce. Dose adjustment needed for older pts, poor metabolizers of CYP2C19 drugs, hepatic impairment. Not for use in preg/breastfeeding. Dizziness, sleepiness possible; safety precautions advised. Pt should take bid if dose greater than 5 mg/d; swallow whole or crush and take in applesauce; avoid alcohol; report thoughts of suicide, increase in seizure activity.

## clofarabine (Clolar)

**CLASS** Antimetabolite, antineoplastic
**PREG/CONT** D/NA

**IND & DOSE** **Tx of pts w/ALL who relapsed after at least two other regimens.** *Child 1–21 yr:* 52 mg/m$^2$ IV over 2 hr daily for 5 consecutive d of 28-d cycle; repeat q 2–6 wk.
**ADV EFF** Anxiety, **bone marrow suppression, capillary leak syndrome,** fatigue, flushing, headache, **hemorrhage, hepatotoxicity, hyperuricemia, infections,** mucosal inflammation, n/v/d, pruritus, rash, **renal toxicity, skin reactions, TLS**
**NC/PT** Premedicate w/antiemetic. Monitor LFTs, renal function, CBC regularly; dose adjustment may be needed. Protect pt from infection, injury. Not for use in preg/breastfeeding. Pt should report bleeding, urine/stool color changes, s&sx of infection, rash.

## clomiPHENE citrate (generic)

**CLASS** Fertility drug, hormone
**PREG/CONT** X/NA

**IND & DOSE** **Tx of ovulatory failure in pts w/normal liver function, normal endogenous estrogen level.** *Adult:* 50 mg/d PO for 5 d started anytime there has been no recent uterine bleeding. If no ovulation occurs, 100 mg/d PO for 5 d as early as 30 d after first. May repeat if no response.
**ADV EFF** Abd discomfort/distention, bloating, breast tenderness, endometrial thickness, flushing, multiple births, n/v, ovarian enlargement, ovarian overstimulation, pancreatitis, visual disturbances
**NC/PT** Perform pelvic exam, obtain urine estrogen and estriol levels before tx. Discontinue if s&sx of ovarian overstimulation. Prepare calendar of tx days. Risk of multiple births. Failure after three courses indicates tx not effective and will be discontinued. Name confusion between *Serophene* (clomiphene) and *Sarafem* (fluoxetine).

## clomiPRAMINE hydrochloride (Anafranil)

**CLASS** Anxiolytic, TCA
**PREG/CONT** C/NA

**BBW** Increased risk of suicidality in child, adolescent, young adult; monitor pt carefully.
**IND & DOSE** **Tx of obsessions/compulsions in pts w/OCD.** *Adult:* Initially, 25 mg PO daily. Increase as tolerated to approx 100 mg during first 2 wk; max, 250 mg/d. Maint, adjust dose to maintain lowest effective dose; effectiveness after 10 wk not documented. *Child:* Initially, 25 mg PO daily. Increase as tolerated during first 2 wk; max, 3 mg/kg or 100 mg, whichever smaller. Maint, adjust dose to maintain lowest effective dosage; effectiveness after 10 wk not documented.
**ADV EFF** **Agranulocytosis,** anticholinergic effects, confusion, constipation, disturbed concentration, dry mouth, **MI,** nasal congestion, orthostatic hypotension, photosensitivity, rash w/systemic symptoms, sedation, **seizures,** serotonin syndrome, **stroke**
**INTERACTIONS** Anticholinergics, barbiturates, cimetidine, clonidine, disulfiram, ephedrine, epinephrine, fluoxetine, furazolidone, hormonal contraceptives, levodopa, MAOIs, methylphenidate, nicotine,

norepinephrine, phenothiazines, QT-prolonging drugs, St. John's wort, thyroid medication
**NC/PT** Restrict drug access in depressed, suicidal pts. Give major portion at bedtime. Obtain periodic CBC w/long-term therapy. In rare case of DRESS, discontinue medication. Pt should not mix w/other sleep-inducing drugs; avoid driving, etc, until drug's effects known; avoid St. John's wort, prolonged exposure to sun/sunlamps; report thoughts of suicide. Name confusion between clomipramine and chlorpromazine.

## clonazePAM (KlonoPIN)

**CLASS** Antiepileptic, benzodiazepine
**PREG/CONT** D/C-IV

**IND & DOSE** **Tx of Lennox-Gastaut syndrome (petit mal variant); akinetic and myoclonic seizures.** *Adult:* 1.5 mg/d PO divided into three doses; increase in increments of 0.5–1 mg PO q 3 d until seizures adequately controlled. Max, 20 mg/d. *Child at least 10 yr or 30 kg:* 0.01–0.03 mg/kg/d PO. Max, 0.05 mg/kg/d PO in two or three doses; maint, 0.1–0.2 mg/kg. **Tx of panic disorder w/ or w/o agoraphobia.** *Adult:* Initially, 0.25 mg PO bid; gradually increase to target dose of 1 mg/d.
**ADV EFF** **Agranulocytosis,** apathy, confusion, constipation, **CV collapse,** depression, diarrhea, disorientation, drowsiness, drug dependence w/ withdrawal, fatigue, incontinence, lethargy, light-headedness, restlessness, **suicidality,** urine retention
**INTERACTIONS** Alcohol, aminophylline, cimetidine, digoxin, disulfiram, dyphylline, hormonal contraceptives, omeprazole, theophylline
**NC/PT** Monitor suicidal and addiction-prone pts closely. Monitor LFTs. Monitor for therapeutic level (20–80 ng/mL). Taper gradually after long-term tx. Not for use in preg/breastfeeding. Pt should avoid alcohol, wear or carry medical alert notice, take safety precautions w/CNS effects. Name confusion between *Klonopin* (clonazepam) and clonidine.

## cloNIDine hydrochloride (Catapres, Duraclon, Kapvay)

**CLASS** Antihypertensive, central analgesic, sympatholytic
**PREG/CONT** C/NA

**BBW** Epidural route not recommended for obstetric, postpartum, or periop pain because of risk of hemodynamic instability.
**IND & DOSE** **Tx of HTN.** *Adult:* 0.1 mg bid PO. For maint, increase in increments of 0.1 or 0.2 mg to reach desired response; common range, 0.2–0.6 mg/d or 0.1-mg transdermal system (releases 0.1 mg/24 hr). If, after 1–2 wk desired BP reduction not achieved, add another 0.1-mg system or use larger system. More than two 0.3-mg systems does not improve efficacy. **Pain mgt.** *Adult:* 30 mcg/hr by epidural infusion. **Tx of ADHD.** *Child 6–17 yr:* 0.1 mg PO at bedtime; titrate at 0.1 mg/wk to total of 0.2 mg, w/0.1 mg in a.m. and 0.1 mg in p.m., then 0.1 mg in a.m. and 0.2 mg in p.m. Maint, 0.2 mg in a.m. and 0.2 mg in p.m. (*Kapvay* only).
**ADV EFF** Cardiac conduction abnormalities, constipation, dizziness, drowsiness, dry mouth, hypotension, local reactions to transdermal system, sedation, somnolence
**INTERACTIONS** Alcohol, antihypertensives, drugs affecting cardiac conduction, CNS depressants, propranolol, TCAs
**NC/PT** Taper when withdrawing to avoid rebound effects. *Kapvay* not interchangeable w/other form; baseline ECG before *Kapvay* use. Must remove old patch before applying new to clean, dry skin; rotate skin sites. Remove transdermal patch before defibrillation and MRI. Pt should swallow tablet whole and not cut/crush/chew; avoid alcohol; take safety precautions w/CNS effects. Name confusion

between clonidine and *Klonopin* (clonazepam).

## clopidogrel bisulfate
(Plavix)
**CLASS** ADP receptor antagonist, antiplatelet
**PREG/CONT** B/NA

**BBW** Slow metabolizers may experience less effects, as drug is activated in liver by CYP2C19. Genotype testing for poor metabolizers suggested before tx.
**IND & DOSE** **Tx of pts at risk for ischemic events (recent MI, stroke, established peripheral arterial disease).** *Adult:* 75 mg/d PO. **Tx of acute coronary syndrome.** *Adult:* 300 mg PO loading dose, then 75 mg/d PO w/aspirin, at dose from 75–325 mg once daily.
**ADV EFF** Bleeding risk, dizziness, **GI bleed**, headache, rash
**INTERACTIONS** NSAIDs, warfarin
**NC/PT** Genotype testing before tx. Monitor for bleeding. May give w/ meals. Pt should report unusual bleeding.

## clorazepate dipotassium bisulfate (Tranxene)
**CLASS** Antiepileptic, anxiolytic, benzodiazepine
**PREG/CONT** D/C-IV

**IND & DOSE** **Mgt of anxiety disorders.** *Adult:* 30 mg/d PO in divided doses tid. **Adjunct to antiepileptics.** *Adult:* Max initial dose, 7.5 mg PO tid. Increase dose by no more than 7.5 mg q wk; max, 90 mg/d. *Child 9–12 yr:* Max initial dose, 7.5 mg PO bid. Increase dose by no more than 7.5 mg q wk; max, 60 mg/d. **Acute alcohol withdrawal.** *Adult:* Day 1, 30 mg PO initially, then 30–60 mg in divided doses. Day 2, 45–90 mg PO in divided doses. Day 3, 22.5–45 mg PO in divided doses. Day 4, 15–30 mg PO in divided doses. Thereafter, gradually reduce dose to 7.5–15 mg/d PO; stop as soon as condition stable.
**ADJUST DOSE** Elderly pts, debilitating disease
**ADV EFF** **Agranulocytosis,** apathy, **CV collapse,** constipation, depression, diarrhea, disorientation, dizziness, drowsiness, dry mouth, lethargy, light-headedness, mild paradoxical excitatory reactions during first 2 wk
**INTERACTIONS** Alcohol, cimetidine, CNS depressants, digoxin, disulfiram, hormonal contraceptives, kava, omeprazole, theophylline
**NC/PT** Taper gradually after long-term use. Monitor for suicidality. Encourage use of medical alert tag. Not for use in preg. Pt should avoid alcohol, take safety precautions for CNS effects. Name confusion between clorazepate and clofibrate.

## clotrimazole (Cruex, Desenex, Gyne-Lotrimin, Lotrimin)
**CLASS** Antifungal
**PREG/CONT** B (topical/vaginal); C (oral)/NA

**IND & DOSE** **Tx of oropharyngeal candidiasis; px of oropharyngeal candidiasis in immunocompromised pts receiving radiation, chemo, steroid therapy** (troche). *Adult, child ≥2 yr:* Dissolve slowly in mouth 5 ×/d for 14 d. For prevention, tid for duration of chemo, radiation. **Local tx of vulvovaginal candidiasis.** *Adult, child ≥12 yr:* 100-mg suppository intravaginally at bedtime for 7 consecutive nights, or 200-mg suppository for 3 consecutive nights, or 1 applicator (5 g/d) vaginal cream, preferably at bedtime for 3–7 consecutive d. Topical tx of susceptible fungal infections. *Adult, child ≥2 yr:* Gently massage into affected area and surrounding skin bid in a.m. and p.m. for 14 d. Treat for 2–4 wk.
**ADV EFF** Abd cramps, abnormal LFTs, local reaction to topical forms, n/v, urinary frequency
**NC/PT** Culture before tx. Dissolve troche in mouth. Insert vaginal

suppository or cream high into vagina using applicator; apply even during menstrual period. Apply topically to clean, dry area. Pt should take full course of tx. Name confusion between clotrimazole and co-trimoxazole.

## cloZAPine (Clozaril, FazaClo)

**CLASS** Antipsychotic, dopaminergic blocker
**PREG/CONT** B/NA

**BBW** Use only when pt unresponsive to conventional antipsychotics. Risk of serious CV and respiratory effects, including myocarditis. Risk of severe neutropenia; monitor WBC count wkly during and for 4 wk after tx; dosage must be adjusted based on WBC count. Potentially fatal agranulocytosis has occurred. Elderly pts w/ dementia-related psychosis are at increased risk for death; drug not approved for these pts. Monitor for seizures; risk increases in pts w/hx of seizures and as dose increases. Available only through restricted access program.
**IND & DOSE** **Mgt of severely ill schizophrenics unresponsive to standard antipsychotics; to reduce risk of recurrent suicidal behavior in pts w/schizophrenia.** *Adult:* 12.5 mg PO daily or bid. Continue to 25 mg PO daily or bid, then gradually increase w/daily increments of 25–50 mg/d, if tolerated, to 300–450 mg/d by end of second wk; max, 900 mg/d. Maintain at lowest effective dose. Withdraw slowly over 2–4 wk when discontinuing.
**ADV EFF** **Agranulocytosis,** cognitive changes, constipation, dizziness, **DRESS,** drowsiness, dry mouth, fever, headache, hypotension, **myocarditis (potentially fatal),** n/v, NMS, PE, sedation, **seizures,** syncope
**INTERACTIONS** Anticholinergics, caffeine, cimetidine, CYP450 inducers/inhibitors, ethotoin, phenytoin
**NC/PT** Obtain through limited access program. Monitor WBC closely; ensure adequate neutrophil count before starting drug. Monitor temp; report fever. Monitor for seizures. Monitor cardiac status. Ensure hydration in elderly pts. Not for use in preg. Pt should empty bladder before taking, use sugarless lozenges for dry mouth, obtain wkly blood tests, take safety precautions w/CNS effects, report s&sx of infection, rash. Name confusion between *Clozaril* (clozapine) and *Colazal* (balsalazide); dangerous effects possible.

## coagulation factor VIIa (recombinant) (NovoSeven, NovoSeven RT)

**CLASS** Antihemophilic
**PREG/CONT** C/NA

**BBW** Serious thrombotic events associated w/off-label use. Use only for approved indication.
**IND & DOSE** **Tx of bleeding episodes, in hemophilia A or B pts w/ inhibitors to factor VIII or IX.** *Adult:* 90 mcg/kg as IV bolus q 2 hr until bleeding controlled. Continue dosing at 3- to 6-hr intervals after hemostasis in severe bleeds.
**ADV EFF** Arthralgia, edema, fever, headache, **hemorrhage,** HTN, **hypersensitivity reactions,** hypotension, injection-site reactions, n/v, rash, **thromboembolic events**
**INTERACTIONS** Do not mix in sol w/other drugs
**NC/PT** Use only for approved indication. Monitor for hypersensitivity reactions, thrombotic events; alert pt to warning signs of each.

## coagulation factor IX, recombinant (Ixinity, Rixubis)

**CLASS** Antihemophilic factor
**PREG/CONT** C/NA

**IND & DOSE** **Control/px of bleeding, periop mgt w/hemophilia B.** *Adult:* International units (IU) needed = body weight (kg) × desired factor IX increase

(% of normal) × reciprocal of observed recovery (IU/kg per IU/dL). **Routine px of hemophilia B.** *Adult:* 40–60 international units/kg IV twice wkly. *Child:* 60–80 international units/kg IV twice wkly.
**ADV EFF** Hypersensitivity reactions, nephrotic syndrome, neutralizing antibody development, thrombotic events
**NC/PT** Ensure proper dx. Do not use w/DIC; fibrinolysis; known hypersensitivity to hamster proteins; preg/breastfeeding. Pt should take safety measures to prevent injury, blood loss; report difficulty breathing, rash, chest pain, increased bleeding.

## coagulation factor IX (recombinant), albumin fusion protein (Idelvion), Fe fusion protein (Alprolix, Benefix)

**CLASS** Clotting factor
**PREG/CONT** High risk/NA

**IND & DOSE** **Control/px of bleeding episodes; periop mgt of pts w/ hemophilia B.** *Adult, child ≥12 yr:* Required dose = body wt (kg) × desired factor X rise (% of normal or international units (IU)/d) × reciprocal of recovery (IU/kg per IU/dL). **Routine px.** *Adult, child ≥12 yr:* 25–40 IU/kg IV q 7 d; may switch to q 14 d w/good control; *Alprolix,* 50 IU/kg IV q 7 d or 100 IU/kg IV q 10 d. *Child <12 yr:* 40–55 IU/kg IV q 7 d; *Alprolix,* 60 IU/kg IV q 7 d.
**ADV EFF** **Anaphylaxis,** headache, nephrotic syndrome, neutralizing antibody development, **thrombotic events**
**NC/PT** One IU is expected to increase circulation activity of factor X 1.3 IU/dL per IU/kg for adults and adolescents, 1 IU/dL per IU/kg for child <12 yr. Monitor blood work before use. Do not exceed rate of 10 mL/min IV. Pt should avoid preg/breastfeeding if possible; report difficulty breathing, unusual swelling, rash, chest pain, increased bleeding.

## coagulation factor IX (recombinant), glyco PEGylated (Rebinyn)

**CLASS** Coagulation factor
**PREG/CONT** Unkn/NA

**IND & DOSE** **Tx of hemophilia B; periop mgt of hemophilia B.** *Adult, child:* 40–80 international units/kg IV over 4–8 min.
**ADV EFF** Hypersensitivity/injection-site reactions, itching, **thrombotic complications**
**NC/PT** Monitor for anaphylaxis; provide immediate tx. Monitor for neutralizing antibodies if response is not as expected. Teach pt proper preparation/administration of drug for on-demand bleeding episodes, proper disposal of needles/syringes, and to report difficulty breathing (stop drug and call prescriber), leg pain, severe headache, unresponsive bleeding, hives, rash.

## coagulation factor X (human) (Coagadex)

**CLASS** Clotting factor
**PREG/CONT** Unkn/NA

**IND & DOSE** **Tx/control of bleeding episodes w/factor X deficiency.** *Adult, child ≥12 yr:* 25 international units (IU)/kg IV; *child <12 yr:* 30 IU/kg IV; *both:* repeated q 24 hr until bleeding stops. **Mgt of periop bleeding w/mild hereditary factor X deficiency.** *Adult, child:* Raise factor X levels to 70–90 IU/dL (preop) and maintain factor X levels 50 IU/dL or more (postop): required dose = body wt in kg × desired factor X rise in IU/dL × 0.5 (adult/child ≥12 yr) or × 0.6 (child <12 yr) infused IV. Postop: Repeat dose as necessary to maintain factor X level at minimum 50 IU/dL. **Px to reduce frequency of bleeding episodes.** *Adult, child ≥12 yr:* 25 IU/kg IV twice/wk. *Child <12 yr:* 40 IU/kg IV twice/wk. *Both:* monitor trough levels of factor X targeting 5 IU/dL or more and adjust dose; peak level, 120 IU/dL.

**ADV EFF** Back pain, factor X antibody production, fatigue, **hypersensitivity reactions,** injection-site reaction
**NC/PT** Drug is a blood product; explain disease risk to pt. Reconstitute w/Sterile Water for Injection, resulting in 100 international units/mL. Use caution in preg/breastfeeding. Pt should report difficulty breathing, chest pain, pain at injection site.

## coagulation factor Xa (recombinant) (Andexxa)
**CLASS** Antidote, reversal agent
**PREG/CONT** Unkn/NA

**IND & DOSE Reversal of anticoagulation from apixaban or rivaroxaban.** *Adult: Low dose*—400 mg IV bolus at 30 mg/min, followed 2 min later by 4 mg/min IV infusion for up to 120 min. *High dose*—800 mg IV bolus at 30 mg/min, followed 2 min later by 8 mg/min IV infusion up to 120 min. Choice of high vs low dose based on timing and anticoagulation dose.
**ADV EFF Acute respiratory failure,** infusion-site reaction, pneumonia, UTI; **thromboembolic events, including DVT, ischemic stroke, MI, PE, cardiogenic shock, worsening HF**
**NC/PT** Drug only administered IV. Risk of clot development that may cause tissue/organ ischemia. Pt should report bleeding; s&sx of allergy, UTI, MI/stroke; difficulty breathing.

▶NEW DRUG

## coagulation factor XIIIA-subunit (recombinant) (Tretten)
**CLASS** Blood product
**PREG/CONT** C/NA

**IND & DOSE Px of bleeding in congenital factor XIII A-subunit deficiency.** *Adult, child:* 35 IU/kg IV monthly to achieve a target level of factor XIII activity at or above 10% using validated assay. Do not exceed 1–2 mL/min.
**ADV EFF** D dimer increase, extremity pain, headache, **hypersensitivity,** injection-site pain, **thrombosis**
**NC/PT** Not for pts w/congenital factor XIII B-subunit deficiency. Discontinue if sx of allergy.

## cobimetinib (Cotellic)
**CLASS** Antineoplastic, kinase inhibitor
**PREG/CONT** High risk/NA

**IND & DOSE Tx of unresectable or metastatic melanoma w/BRAF V600E or V600K mutation, w/vemurafenib.** *Adult:* 60 mg/d PO for first 21 d of 28-d cycle until progression.
**ADV EFF Cardiomyopathy,** fever, **hemorrhage, hepatotoxicity,** n/v/d, **new malignancies, retinopathy/retinal vein occlusion, rhabdomyolysis, severe photosensitivity**
**INTERACTIONS** Strong CYP3A inducers/inhibitors; avoid combo
**NC/PT** Ensure proper dx. Perform LFTs before and periodically during use. Monitor liver function, vision. Evaluate skin for skin cancers q 2 mo. Not for use in preg (contraceptives advised)/breastfeeding during and for 2 wk after tx. Pt should avoid sun exposure, wear protective clothing; report difficulty breathing, swelling, shortness of breath, bleeding, skin/vision changes, muscle pain, urine/stool color changes.

DANGEROUS DRUG

## codeine sulfate (generic)
**CLASS** Antitussive, opioid agonist analgesic
**PREG/CONT** C (preg); D (labor)/C-II

**BBW** Risk of addiction/abuse/misuse; life-threatening respiratory depression; death related to ultrarapid metabolism of codeine to morphine in child after tonsillectomy/adenoidectomy (T&A); neonatal opioid withdrawal syndrome.

Interactions w/drugs affecting CYP450 isoenzymes and w/concomitant use of benzodiazepines or CNS depressants.
**IND & DOSE Relief of mild to moderate pain.** *Adult:* 15–60 mg PO, IM, IV, or subcut q 4–6 hr; max, 360 mg/24 hr. *Child ≥1 yr:* 0.5 mg/kg or 15 mg/m² IM or subcut q 4 hr. **Suppression of coughing induced by chemical or mechanical irritation.** *Adult:* 10–20 mg PO q 4–6 hr; max, 120 mg/24 hr. *Child 6–12 yr:* 5–10 mg PO q 4–6 hr; max, 60 mg/24 hr. *Child 2–6 yr:* 2.5–5 mg PO q 4–6 hr; max, 12–18 mg/d.
**ADJUST DOSE** Elderly pts, impaired adults
**ADV EFF Cardiac arrest,** clamminess, confusion, constipation, dizziness, floating feeling, lethargy, light-headedness, n/v, sedation, **shock**
**INTERACTIONS** Anticholinergics, barbiturate anesthetics, CNS depressants
**NC/PT** Do not give IV in child. Do not use to manage postop pain in child w/T&A. Ensure opioid antagonist available during parenteral administration. Ensure perfusion of subcut area before injecting. Monitor bowel function; use of laxatives advised. Use in preg only if benefit clearly outweighs fetal risk. Breastfeeding women should receive drug 4–6 hr before next feeding and should monitor infant closely for s&sx of sedation or difficulty breathing. Serious withdrawal sx possible if drug stopped abruptly in physically dependent pt. Pt should take safety precautions for CNS effects. Name confusion between codeine and *Cardene* (nicardipine).

**DANGEROUS DRUG**

## colchicine (Colcrys, Gloperba, Mitigare)
**CLASS** Antigout drug
**PREG/CONT** C/NA

**IND & DOSE Tx of acute gout flares.** *Adult:* 1.2 mg PO at first sign of gout flare, then 0.6 mg 1 hr later; max, 1.8 mg over 1-hr period. **Px of gout flares.** *Adult, child ≥16 yr:* 0.6 mg PO once or twice daily; max, 1.2 mg/d. **Tx of familial Mediterranean fever.** *Adult:* 1.2–2.4 mg/d PO in one or two divided doses; increase or decrease in 0.3-mg increments as needed. *Child >12 yr:* Use adult dosage. *Child 6–12 yr:* 0.9–1.8 mg/d PO. *Child 4–6 yr:* 0.3–1.8 mg/d PO.
**ADJUST DOSE** Hepatic/renal impairment
**ADV EFF** Abd pain, **bone marrow suppression,** n/v/d, rash, **rhabdomyolysis**
**INTERACTIONS** Amprenavir, aprepitant, atazanavir, atorvastatin, clarithromycin, cyclosporine, digoxin, diltiazem, erythromycin, fibrates, fluconazole, fluvastatin, fosamprenavir, gemfibrozil, grapefruit juice, indinavir, itraconazole, ketoconazole, nefazodone, nelfinavir, ranolazine, pravastatin, ritonavir, saquinavir, simvastatin, telithromycin, verapamil
**NC/PT** Obtain baseline and periodic CBC, LFTs, renal function tests. Check complete drug list; many drug interactions require dose adjustments. Monitor for pain relief. Fatal overdoses have occurred; keep out of reach of child. Pt should avoid grapefruit juice, report to all providers all drugs and herbs taken (many potentially serious drug interactions possible), ensure protection from infection and injury, obtain periodic medical exams.

## colesevelam hydrochloride (WelChol)
**CLASS** Antihyperlipidemic, bile acid sequestrant
**PREG/CONT** B/NA

**IND & DOSE Monotherapy for tx of hyperlipidemia.** *Adult:* 3 tablets PO bid w/meals or 6 tablets/d PO w/meal; max, 7 tablets/d. **To lower lipid levels, w/HMG-CoA inhibitor.** *Adult:* 3 tablets PO bid w/meals or 6 tablets PO once a day w/meal; max,

6 tablets/d. **To improve glycemic control in type 2 diabetes.** *Adult:* 6 tablets/d PO or 3 tablets PO bid. **Tx of familial hypercholesterolemia.** *Child 10–17 yr:* 1.8 g PO bid or 3.7 g/d PO oral suspension.
**ADV EFF** Constipation to fecal impaction, flatulence, **hypertriglyceridemia/pancreatitis,** increased bleeding tendencies
**INTERACTIONS** Fat-soluble vitamins, oral drugs, verapamil
**NC/PT** Used w/diet, exercise program. Give other oral drugs 1 hr before or 4–6 hr after drug. Monitor blood lipids before starting and during tx. Mix oral suspension in 4–8 oz water; do not use dry. Suspension contains phenylalanine; use caution w/phenylketonuria. Establish bowel program for constipation. Pt should report unusual bleeding, severe constipation.

## colestipol hydrochloride (Colestid)

**CLASS** Antihyperlipidemic, bile acid sequestrant
**PREG/CONT** C/NA

**IND & DOSE Adjunct tx for primary hypercholesterolemia.** *Adult:* 5–30 g/d PO suspension once a day or in divided doses bid–qid. Start w/5 g PO daily or bid; increase in 5-g/d increments at 1- to 2-mo intervals. For tablets, 2–16 g/d PO in one–two divided doses; initially, 2 g once or twice daily, increasing in 2-g increments at 1- to 2-mo intervals.
**ADV EFF** Constipation to fecal impaction, flatulence, headache, increased bleeding tendencies
**INTERACTIONS** Digoxin, fat-soluble vitamins, oral drugs, thiazide diuretics
**NC/PT** Used w/diet, exercise program. Give other oral drugs 1 hr before or 4–6 hr after drug. Give before meals. Monitor blood lipids. Mix in liquids, soups, cereal, carbonated beverages; do not give dry (inhalation and esophageal distress possible). Contains phenylalanine; use caution w/phenylketonuria. Establish bowel program for constipation. Pt should swallow tablets whole and not cut/crush/chew them; report unusual bleeding, severe constipation; use analgesic for headache.

## collagenase clostridium histolyticum (Xiaflex)

**CLASS** Proteinase enzyme
**PREG/CONT** Low risk/NA

**BBW** Risk of corporal rupture (penile fracture) or other serious penile injury when used in tx of Peyronie disease. Available for this use only through restricted access program.
**IND & DOSE Tx of pts w/Dupuytren contraction w/palpable cord.** *Adult:* 0.58 mg injected into palpable cord by health care provider, up to 2 cords/hand/tx session; may repeat up to 3 ×/cord at 4-wk intervals. **Tx of pts w/Peyronie disease w/penile curvature deformity of 30 degrees or more.** *Adult:* 2 injections into the collagen-containing structure followed by penile remodeling; may repeat max of eight times.
**ADV EFF Corporal rupture, hypersensitivity reactions,** injection-site reaction, pain, **severe allergic reaction, severe penile hematoma, tendon rupture,** swelling in involved hand
**INTERACTIONS** Anticoagulants, aspirin
**NC/PT** Be prepared for possible severe allergic reaction. Risk of bleeding if pt on anticoagulants. Tendon rupture, damage to nerves and tissue of hand possible. Monitor penile injection site closely for adverse reactions.

## copanlisib (Aliqopa)

**CLASS** Antineoplastic, kinase inhibitor
**PREG/CONT** High risk/NA

**IND & DOSE Tx of relapsed follicular lymphoma after two failed therapies.**

*Adult:* 60 mg IV over 1 hr on days 1, 8, and 15 of 28-day cycle.
**ADV EFF Bone marrow depression**, diarrhea, HTN, hyperglycemia, infections, **pneumonitis, severe skin reactions**
**INTERACTIONS** CYP3A inducers/ inhibitors
**NC/PT** Monitor blood counts, blood glucose, BP, respiratory status, skin reactions; dosage may need adjustment based on toxicity. Pt should avoid preg (contraceptives advised)/ breastfeeding; mark calendar w/ infusion days; report fever, rash, headache, difficulty breathing, s&sx of infection.

## corticotropin (H.P. Acthar Gel)

**CLASS** Anterior pituitary hormone, diagnostic agent
**PREG/CONT** C/NA

**IND & DOSE Tx of allergic states, glucocorticoid-sensitive disorders, nonsuppurative thyroiditis, tuberculous meningitis, trichinosis w/CNS and cardiac involvement; rheumatic disorders; palliative mgt of leukemias, lymphomas.** *Adult:* 40–80 units IM or subcut q 24–72 hr. **Tx of acute exacerbations of MS.** *Adult:* 80–120 units/d IM for 2–3 wk. **Tx of infantile spasms.** *Infant, child <2 yr:* 75 units/m$^2$ IM bid.
**ADV EFF** Acne, amenorrhea, **anaphylactoid reactions,** depression, ecchymoses, euphoria, fluid and electrolyte disturbances, fragile skin, HTN, immunosuppression, impaired wound healing, infections, muscle weakness, petechiae
**INTERACTIONS** Anticholinesterases, antidiabetics, barbiturates, live vaccines
**NC/PT** Verify adrenal responsiveness before tx. Give only IM or subcut. Taper dose when discontinuing after long-term use. Give rapidly acting corticosteroid in times of stress. Pt should avoid exposure to infections; monitor blood glucose periodically; avoid immunizations; report difficulty breathing, bruising.

## cosyntropin (Cortrosyn)

**CLASS** Diagnostic agent
**PREG/CONT** C/NA

**IND & DOSE Diagnostic tests of adrenal function.** *Adult:* 0.25–0.75 mg IV or IM or as IV infusion at 0.04 mg/hr.
**ADV EFF Anaphylactoid reactions,** bradycardia, edema, HTN, rash, **seizures,** tachycardia
**INTERACTIONS** Diuretics
**NC/PT** Plasma cortisol levels usually peak within 45–60 min of injection. Normally, expect doubling of baseline levels. Pt should report difficulty breathing.

## crizotinib (Xalkori)

**CLASS** Antineoplastic, kinase inhibitor
**PREG/CONT** High risk/NA

**IND & DOSE Tx of locally advanced or metastatic NSCLC that is anaplastic lymphoma kinase–positive as detected by Vysis ALK Break Apart FISH Probe Kit; tx of metastatic NSCLC that is ROS1-positive.** *Adult:* 250 mg PO bid w/o regard to food.
**ADJUST DOSE** Renal or hepatic impairment
**ADV EFF** Bradycardia, constipation, **hepatotoxicity,** n/v/d, **prolonged QT, serious to fatal pneumonitis,** vision changes including blurry vision to **severe vision loss**, light sensitivity, floaters, flashes of light
**INTERACTIONS** CYP3A inducers/ inhibitors, QT-prolonging drugs; avoid these combos
**NC/PT** Ensure pt has been tested for appropriate sensitivity. Monitor LFTs, pulmonary function, vision. Institute bowel program as needed; advise safety precautions w/vision changes. Pt should avoid preg (contraceptives advised)/breastfeeding; driving, operating

machinery w/vision changes. Pt should report difficulty breathing, urine/stool color changes, vision changes.

**crofelemer** (Fulyzaq)
**CLASS** Antidiarrheal, calcium channel stimulator
**PREG/CONT** C/NA

**IND & DOSE** **Relief of noninfectious diarrhea in adults w/HIV/AIDS on antiretroviral therapy.** *Adult:* 125 mg PO bid.
**ADV EFF** Bronchitis, cough, flatulence, possible URI
**NC/PT** Ensure cause of diarrhea is not infectious and pt also taking antiretroviral. Not for use in preg/breastfeeding. Monitor diarrhea. Pt should take as directed; swallow capsule whole and not cut/crush/chew it; report cough, increased diarrhea.

**cromolyn sodium** (Crolom)
**CLASS** Antiallergy drug
**PREG/CONT** C/NA

**IND & DOSE** **Px/tx of allergic rhinitis.** *Adult, child ≥2 yr:* 1 spray in each nostril 3–6 ×/d as needed. **Tx of allergic eye disorders.** *Adult:* 1 or 2 drops in each eye 4–6 ×/d as needed.
**ADV EFF** Allergic reaction, burning or stinging, shortness of breath, wheezing
**NC/PT** Eyedrops not for use w/soft contact lenses. May take several days to 2 wk for noticeable effects; pt should continue use. If preg or breastfeeding, consult provider.

**cyanocobalamin, intranasal** (Nascobal)
**CLASS** Synthetic vitamin
**PREG/CONT** C/NA

**IND & DOSE** **Maint of pts in hematologic remission after IM vitamin $B_{12}$ tx for pernicious anemia, inadequate secretion of intrinsic factor, dietary deficiency, malabsorption, competition by intestinal bacteria or parasites, inadequate utilization of vitamin $B_{12}$; maint of effective therapeutic vitamin $B_{12}$ levels in pts w/HIV infection, AIDS, MS, Crohn disease.** *Adult:* 1 spray (500 mcg) in one nostril once/wk
**ADV EFF** Headache, nasal congestion, rhinitis
**INTERACTIONS** Alcohol, antibiotics, colchicine, methotrexate, para-aminosalicylic acid
**NC/PT** Confirm dx before tx. Monitor serum vitamin $B_{12}$ before, at 1 mo, then q 3–6 mo during tx. Do not give w/nasal congestion, rhinitis, URI. Pt should take drug 1 hr before or after ingesting hot foods or liquids, which can cause nasal congestion.

**cyclobenzaprine hydrochloride** (Amrix)
**CLASS** Centrally acting skeletal muscle relaxant
**PREG/CONT** B/NA

**IND & DOSE** **Relief of discomfort associated w/acute, painful musculoskeletal conditions, as adjunct to rest/physical therapy.** *Adult:* 5 mg PO tid, up to 10 mg PO tid. Do not use for longer than 2–3 wk. For ER capsules, 15 mg once/d PO.
**ADJUST DOSE** Elderly pts, hepatic impairment
**ADV EFF** Dizziness, drowsiness, dry mouth, **MI**
**INTERACTIONS** Alcohol, barbiturates, CNS depressants, MAOIs, TCAs, tramadol
**NC/PT** Give analgesics for headache. Monitor elderly pts closely. Pt should swallow capsules whole and not cut/crush/chew them (may sprinkle capsule contents on applesauce and swallow immediately); take safety precautions for CNS effects; avoid alcohol.

DANGEROUS DRUG

## cyclophosphamide
(generic)
**CLASS** Alkylating agent, antineoplastic, nitrogen mustard
**PREG/CONT** D/NA

**IND & DOSE** **Tx of malignant lymphoma, multiple myeloma, leukemias, mycosis fungoides, neuroblastoma, adenocarcinoma of ovary, retinoblastoma, carcinoma of breast; used concurrently or sequentially w/other antineoplastics.** *Adult:* Induction, 40–50 mg/kg IV in divided doses over 2–5 d or 1–5 mg/kg/d PO for 2–5 d. Or, 1–5 mg/kg/d PO, 10–15 mg/kg IV q 7–10 d, or 3–5 mg/kg IV twice wkly. **Tx of minimal change nephrotic syndrome.** *Child:* 2.5–3 mg/d PO for 60–90 d.
**ADJUST DOSE** Renal/hepatic impairment
**ADV EFF** Alopecia, anorexia, **bone marrow suppression,** hematuria to **potentially fatal hemorrhagic cystitis, interstitial pulmonary fibrosis,** n/v/d, stomatitis
**INTERACTIONS** Allopurinol, anticoagulants, chloramphenicol, digoxin, doxorubicin, grapefruit juice, succinylcholine
**NC/PT** Monitor CBC, respiratory status; dose adjustment may be needed. Do not give full dose within 4 wk of radiation or chemo. Ensure pt well hydrated. Pt should use contraceptive measures (can cause fetal abnormalities); take oral drug on empty stomach; wear protective gloves when handling drug; avoid grapefruit juice; cover head at temp extremes (hair loss may occur); report difficulty breathing, bleeding, pain when emptying bladder.

## cycloSERINE (Seromycin Pulvules)
**CLASS** Antibiotic, antituberculotic
**PREG/CONT** C/NA

**IND & DOSE** **Tx of active pulmonary, extrapulmonary (including renal) TB unresponsive to first-line antituberculotics, w/other antituberculotics; UTIs caused by susceptible bacteria.** *Adult:* 250 mg PO bid at 12-hr intervals for first 2 wk. Max, 1 g/d; maint, 500 mg–1 g/d PO in divided doses.
**ADV EFF** Confusion, drowsiness, headache, **HF,** somnolence, tremor, vertigo
**INTERACTIONS** Alcohol, high-fat meals
**NC/PT** Culture before tx. Use only when other drugs have failed. Use w/ other anti-TB agents. Pt should avoid alcohol; take safety precautions for CNS effects; not take w/high-fat meal or discontinue drug w/o consulting prescriber. Name confusion w/ cycloserine, cyclosporine, and cyclophosphamide.

## cycloSPORINE (Gengraf, Neoral, Sandimmune)
**CLASS** Immunosuppressant
**PREG/CONT** C/NA

**BBW** Monitor pts for infections, malignancies; risks increase. Monitor LFTs, renal function before and during tx; marked decreases in function may require dose adjustment or discontinuation. Monitor BP. Heart transplant pts may need concomitant antihypertensive tx. Should be used only by physicians trained in tx w/immunosuppressants.
**IND & DOSE** **Px/tx of organ rejection in pts w/kidney, liver, heart transplants.** *Adult:* 15 mg/kg/d PO (*Sandimmune*) initially given 4–12 hr before transplantation; continue dose postop for 1–2 wk, then taper by 5% per wk to maint level of 5–10 mg/kg/d. Or by IV infusion (*Sandimmune*) at 1/3 oral dose (ie, 5–6 mg/kg/d 4–12 hr before transplantation as slow infusion over 2–6 hr); continue this daily dose postop. Switch to oral drug as soon as possible. **Tx of RA.** *Adult:* 2.5 mg/kg/d (*Gengraf, Neoral*) PO in divided doses bid; may increase up to 4 mg/kg/d. If no benefit after 16 wk,

discontinue. **Tx of recalcitrant plaque psoriasis.** *Adult:* 2.5 mg/kg/d (*Gengraf, Neoral*) PO divided bid for 4 wk, then may increase up to 4 mg/kg/d. If response unsatisfactory after 6 wk at 4 mg/kg/d, discontinue.
**ADV EFF** Acne, diarrhea, gum hyperplasia, hirsutism, HTN, hyperkalemia, hypomagnesemia, renal impairment, tremors
**INTERACTIONS** Amiodarone, androgens, azole antifungals, carbamazepine, colchicine, diltiazem, foscarnet, grapefruit juice, high-fat meal, HMG-CoA reductase inhibitors, hormonal contraceptives, hydantoins, macrolides, metoclopramide, nephrotoxic agents, nicardipine, orlistat, phenobarbital, rifampin, St. John's wort, SSRIs
**NC/PT** Mix oral sol w/milk, chocolate milk, orange juice at room temp; do not allow to stand before drinking. Do not refrigerate. Use parenteral route only if pt cannot take oral form. Monitor LFTs, renal function, CBC, BP carefully; toxicity possible. Not for use in preg (barrier contraceptives advised). Pt should avoid grapefruit juice, St. John's wort, exposure to infection; should not take w/high-fat meal or discontinue w/o consulting prescriber. Interacts w/many drugs; pt should inform all caregivers he is taking drug. Name confusion w/cyclosporine, cycloserine, and cyclophosphamide.

## cyproheptadine hydrochloride (generic)

**CLASS** Antihistamine
**PREG/CONT** B/NA

**IND & DOSE** **Relief of s&sx associated w/perennial, seasonal allergic rhinitis; other allergic reactions; tx of cold urticaria.** *Adult:* 4 mg PO tid. Maint, 4–20 mg/d in three divided doses; max, 0.5 mg/kg/d. *Child 7–14 yr:* 4 mg PO bid–tid. Max, 16 mg/d. *Child 2–6 yr:* 2 mg PO bid. Max, 12 mg/d.
**ADJUST DOSE** Elderly pts
**ADV EFF** **Agranulocytosis, anaphylactic shock,** bronchial secretion thickening, dizziness, drowsiness, epigastric distress, disturbed coordination, **pancytopenia**
**INTERACTIONS** Alcohol, anticholinergics, CNS depressants, fluoxetine, metyrapone, MAOIs
**NC/PT** Use syrup if pt cannot swallow tablets. Give w/food. Monitor response.

## cysteamine bitartrate (Procysbi)

**CLASS** Cystine-depleting agent
**PREG/CONT** High risk/NA

**IND & DOSE** **Tx of nephropathic cystinosis.** *Adult, child ≥2 yr:* Dosage is weight-based; see manufacturer's insert for details. Given orally q 12 hr. Maint dose titrated based on cysteine levels.
**ADV EFF** Alkaline phosphatase elevations, benign intracranial HTN, bone/skin lesions, CNS symptoms, fatigue, GI ulcers/bleeding, headache, leukopenia, n/v/d, **severe rash,** skin odor
**INTERACTIONS** Alcohol, antacids, bicarbonate, grapefruit juice
**NC/PT** Ensure proper dx. Not for use in preg/breastfeeding. Pt should swallow capsule whole and not cut/crush/chew it; not eat for 2 hr before and at least 30 min after taking capsule (if food is essential when taking capsule, pt should limit food to ½ cup 1 hr before or 1 hr after dose; may take w/juice [not grapefruit juice]); avoid high-fat foods near dosing time, alcohol, antacids; report rash, tarry stools.

**DANGEROUS DRUG**

## cytarabine (cytosine arabinoside) (generic)

**CLASS** Antimetabolite, antineoplastic
**PREG/CONT** D/NA

**BBW** Chemical arachnoiditis (n/v, headache, fever) can be fatal if untreated; concurrently treat w/dexamethasone.

**IND & DOSE AML, ALL induction, maint of remission.** *Adult:* For induction, 100 mg/m²/d by continuous IV infusion (days 1–7) or 100 mg/m² IV q 12 hr (days 1–7); same dose for maint. Longer rest period may be needed. *Child:* Dose based on body weight and surface area. **Tx of meningeal leukemia.** *Adult:* 5–75 mg/m² IV once daily for 4 d or once q 4 d. Most common dose, 30 mg/m² q 4 d until CSF normal, then one more tx. **Tx of lymphomatous meningitis.** *Adult:* 50 mg liposomal cytarabine intrathecal q 14 d for two doses, then q 14 d for three doses. Repeat q 28 d for four doses.

**ADV EFF** Alopecia, anorexia, **bone marrow depression,** fever, n/v/d, neurotoxicity, rash, stomatitis, thrombophlebitis

**INTERACTIONS** Digoxin

**NC/PT** Monitor CBC; dose adjustment based on bone marrow response. Monitor neuro function; reduce dose as needed. Premedicate w/antiemetics, dexamethasone. Do not come in contact w/liposomal forms. Provide mouth care, comfort measures. Not for use in preg. Pt should take safety measures w/CNS effects; avoid exposure to infection; cover head at temp extremes (hair loss possible); report s&sx of infection, chest pain.

## dabigatran etexilate mesylate hydrochloride

(Pradaxa)

**CLASS** Anticoagulant, direct thrombin inhibitor

**PREG/CONT** C/NA

**BBW** Increased risk of thrombotic events when discontinuing. Consider adding another anticoagulant if stopping drug for any reason other than pathological bleeding. Spinal/epidural hematoma in pts w/spinal puncture/anesthesia.

**IND & DOSE To reduce risk of stroke/systemic embolism in pts w/ nonvalvular atrial fibrillation.** *Adult:* 150 mg PO bid. Converting from warfarin: Stop warfarin and begin dabigatran when INR is <2. Converting from parenteral anticoagulant: Start dabigatran 0–2 hr before next dose of parenteral drug would have been given, or at discontinuation of continuous infusion of parenteral anticoagulant. If starting on parenteral anticoagulant, wait 12 hr (if CrCl 30 mL/min or more) or 24 hr (if CrCl <30 mL/min) after last dose of dabigatran before starting parenteral drug. **Tx of DVT/PE in pts treated w/parenteral anticoagulant for 5–10 d.** *Adult:* 150 mg PO bid after 5–10 d of parenteral anticoagulation. **Px of recurrent DVT/PE in previously treated pts.** *Adult:* 150 mg PO bid after previous tx. **Px of DVT/PE in pts undergoing hip replacement surgery.** *Adult:* 110 mg PO first day postop, then 220 mg PO once daily.

**ADJUST DOSE** Renal impairment

**ADV EFF Bleeding,** dyspepsia, **gastric hemorrhage,** gastritis, gastritis-like s&sx, **rebound increased risk of thrombotic events w/abrupt withdrawal, serious hypersensitivity reactions**

**INTERACTIONS** Aspirin, NSAIDs, platelet inhibitors, rifampin, warfarin

**NC/PT** Contraindicated in pts w/ artificial heart valves or active bleeding. Increased risk of bleeding; use caution. Consider using another anticoagulant if stopping drug. Reverse effects w/idarucizumab (*Praxbind*) for life-threatening bleeds, emergency surgery. Not for use in preg/breastfeeding. Pt should take at about same time each day; swallow capsule whole and not cut/crush/chew it; not double-up doses; not stop drug suddenly; ensure prescription does not run out (risk of thrombotic events); protect drug from moisture; keep in original container or blister pack; mark container and use within 4 mo; alert all health care providers he is taking drug; report chest pain, difficulty breathing, unusual bleeding, swelling, rash.

## dabrafenib (Tafinlar)

**CLASS** Antineoplastic, kinase inhibitor

**PREG/CONT** High risk/NA

**IND & DOSE** **Tx of unresectable or metastatic melanoma w/BRAF V600E or V600K mutations alone or w/ trametinib; tx of metastatic NSCLC w/ BRAF V600E mutation w/trametinib; tx of advanced or metastatic anaplastic thyroid cancer w/BRAF V600E mutation and no satisfactory locoregional tx options w/trametinib.** *Adult:* 150 mg PO bid at least 1 hr before or 2 hr after meal; if combo being used, add trametinib 2 mg/d PO.

**ADV EFF** Alopecia, arthralgia, **cardiomyopathy, DVT,** fever, headache, **hemolytic anemia, hemorrhage,** hyperglycemia, hyperkeratosis, **malignancies,** ocular toxicity, palmar-plantar erythrodysesthesia, **tumor promotion of wild-type BRAF melanoma,** uveitis/iritis

**INTERACTIONS** CYP3A4/CYP2C8 inhibitors/inducers

**NC/PT** Ensure proper dx and appropriate BRAF mutation. Not for use in wild-type BRAF melanoma. Assess for other malignancies; monitor temp, CBC, blood glucose; have pt schedule eye exams. Pt should avoid preg/breastfeeding; use analgesics for headache; monitor skin; report vision changes, rash or skin lesions, fever, chest pain, bleeding.

**DANGEROUS DRUG**

## dacarbazine hydrochloride (generic)

**CLASS** Alkylating agent, antineoplastic

**PREG/CONT** C/NA

**BBW** Arrange for lab tests (LFTs; WBC, RBC, platelet count) before and frequently during tx; serious bone marrow suppression, hepatotoxicity possible. Carcinogenic in animals; monitor accordingly.

**IND & DOSE** **Tx of metastatic malignant melanoma.** *Adult, child:* 2–4.5 mg/kg/d IV for 10 d, repeated at 4-wk intervals, or 250 mg/m²/d IV for 5 d, repeated q 3 wk. **Second line tx of Hodgkin disease.** *Adult, child:* 150 mg/m²/d IV for 5 d w/other drugs, repeated q 4 wk, or 375 mg/m² IV on day 1 w/other drugs, repeated q 15 d.

**ADV EFF** **Anaphylaxis,** anorexia, **bone marrow suppression, hepatic necrosis,** local tissue damage w/ extravasation, n/v/d, photosensitivity

**NC/PT** Monitor CBC, LFTs carefully; may limit dose. Give IV only; monitor site carefully. Extravasation can cause serious local damage; apply hot packs if this occurs. Restrict fluids and food for 4–6 hr before tx; may use antiemetics. Prepare calendar of tx days. Pt should avoid exposure to infection, sun; report difficulty breathing.

## daclatasvir (Daklinza)

**CLASS** Antiviral, HCV inhibitor

**PREG/CONT** Unkn/NA

**BBW** Risk of HBV reactivation in pts coinfected w/HCV and HBV.

**IND & DOSE** **Tx of HCV, genotype 1 or 3, w/sofosbuvir.** *Adult:* 60 mg/d PO for 12 wk.

**ADV EFF** **Bradycardia,** fatigue, headache, n/d

**INTERACTIONS** Amiodarone, carbamazepine, phenytoin, rifampin, St. John's wort, strong CYP3A inducers; warfarin (frequent INR monitoring needed)

**NC/PT** Test genotype; test for presence of virus if genotype 1a. Give w/ sofosbuvir; may be used w/ribavirin. Monitor cardiac function in pt w/ cardiac comorbidities. Carefully review drug regimen; many potentially serious interactions possible. Monitor lungs/HR regularly; adjust dose as needed. Use caution in preg/breastfeeding. Pt should take daily for 12 wk w/sofosbuvir; avoid St. John's wort; report all drugs being taken, dizziness, chest pain, severe fatigue.

## daclizumab (Zinbryta)
**CLASS** Interleukin blocker, monoclonal antibody, MS drug
**PREG/CONT** High risk/NA

**BBW** Risk of severe hepatotoxicity; monitor LFTs for up to 6 mo after use. Contraindicated in pts w/hepatic disease/impairment. Risk of severe immune-mediated disorders. Available only through limited access program.
**IND & DOSE Tx of relapsing MS in pts w/inadequate response to other tx.** *Adult:* 150 mg subcut monthly.
**ADJUST DOSE** Hepatic impairment
**ADV EFF Anaphylaxis,** bronchitis, depression, dermatitis, eczema, **hepatotoxicity, immune disorders,** infections, lymphadenopathy, nasopharyngitis, **suicidality,** URI
**INTERACTIONS** Hepatotoxic drugs
**NC/PT** Do not give w/severe hepatic impairment, hx of immune hepatic dx. Monitor LFTs before, periodically during tx. Teach pt proper subcutaneous administration, disposal of needles/ syringes. Pt should avoid preg (contraceptives advised)/breastfeeding; mark calendar w/injection days; report difficulty breathing, unusual swelling, urine/stool color changes, thoughts of suicide, fever, s&sx of infection.

## dacomitinib (Vizimpro)
**CLASS** Antineoplastic, epidermal growth factor receptor (EGFR) antagonist, kinase inhibitor
**PREG/CONT** High risk/NA

**IND & DOSE Tx of pts w/metastatic NSCLC w/EGFR exon 19 deletion or exon 21 L858R substitution mutations as detected by FDA-approved test.** *Adult:* 45 mg PO daily.
**ADV EFF** Alopecia, cough, decreased appetite/weight, diarrhea, dry skin, paronychia, pruritus, rash, stomatitis
**INTERACTIONS** CYP2D6 substrates, proton pump inhibitors
**NC/PT** Obtain preg test. Pt should use contraceptives/avoid breastfeeding during and for at least 17 d after tx. Pt should take w/ or w/o food; report respiratory s&sx, rash, severe diarrhea.

**DANGEROUS DRUG**

## dactinomycin (Cosmegen)
**CLASS** Antibiotic, antineoplastic
**PREG/CONT** D/NA

**BBW** Use strict handling procedures; extremely toxic to skin and eyes. If extravasation/burning/ stinging occur at injection site, stop infusion immediately, apply cold compresses to area, and restart in another vein. Tx local infiltration w/injectable corticosteroid and flushing w/saline; may lessen reaction.
**IND & DOSE Tx of Wilms' tumor.** *Adult, child:* 45 mcg/kg IV q 3–6 wk for up to 26 wk as combo chemo regimen. **Tx of rhabdomyosarcoma.** *Adult, child:* 15 mcg/kg IV q day for 5 d q 3–9 wk for up to 112 wk as combo chemo regimen. **Tx of Ewing sarcoma.** *Adult, child:* 1,250 mcg/m$^2$ IV q 3 wk for 51 wk as combo chemo regimen. **Tx of testicular cancer (metastatic nonseminomatous).** *Adult, child:* 1,000 mcg/m$^2$ IV q 3 wk as part of cisplatin-based multidrug chemo regimen. **Tx of gestational trophoblastic neoplasia.** *Adult, child:* 12 mcg/kg/d IV for 5 d when used as monotherapy; 500 mcg IV on days 1 and 2 q 2 wk for up to 8 wk in combo therapy. **Palliative tx or adjunct to tumor resection via isolation-perfusion technique for solid malignancies.** *Adult:* 50 mcg/kg for lower extremity or pelvis; 35 mcg/kg for upper extremity.
**ADV EFF Agranulocytosis,** alopecia, anemia, **aplastic anemia, bone marrow suppression,** cheilitis, dysphagia, esophagitis, fatigue, fever, **hepatotoxicity,** lethargy, myalgia, skin

eruptions, stomatitis, tissue necrosis w/extravasation
**NC/PT** Use strict handling procedures; toxic to skin and eyes. Monitor CBC, LFTs carefully; may limit dose. Give IV only. Monitor site carefully; extravasation can cause serious local damage. Monitor for adverse effects, which may worsen 1–2 wk after tx. Prepare calendar of tx days. Pt should cover head at temp extremes (hair loss possible); avoid infections; report urine/stool color changes. Name confusion between dactinomycin and daptomycin.

## dalbavancin (Dalvance)
**CLASS** Lipoglycopeptide antibiotic
**PREG/CONT** Moderate risk/NA

**IND & DOSE** **Tx of acute skin/skin-structure infections caused by susceptible strains of gram-positive bacteria.** *Adult:* 1,000 mg IV over 30 min, then 500 mg IV over 30 min 1 wk later, or 1,500 mg IV over 30 min as a single dose.
**ADJUST DOSE** Renal impairment
**ADV EFF** CDAD, headache, **hypersensitivity reactions,** LFT changes, n/v/d, skin reactions
**NC/PT** Perform culture before tx. Ensure appropriate use of drug. Monitor pt during infusion; reactions possible, especially if administered rapidly. Not for use in preg/breastfeeding. Pt should mark calendar for return date for second infusion; report difficulty breathing, severe diarrhea, diarrhea w/blood or mucus, rash.

## dalfampridine (Ampyra)
**CLASS** Potassium channel blocker, MS drug
**PREG/CONT** C/NA

**IND & DOSE** **To improve walking in pts w/MS.** *Adult:* 10 mg PO bid, 12 hr apart.
**ADJUST DOSE** Renal impairment, seizure disorder
**ADV EFF** **Anaphylaxis,** asthenia, back pain, balance disorder, constipation, dizziness, dyspepsia, headache, insomnia, MS relapse, nasopharyngitis, nausea, paresthesia, pharyngolaryngeal pain, **seizures,** UTIs
**INTERACTIONS** OCT2 inhibitors (may increase seizure risk)
**NC/PT** Do not use w/hx of seizure disorders, renal impairment. Not for use in preg/breastfeeding. Pt should swallow tablet whole and not cut/crush/chew it; use safety precautions w/CNS effects; report difficulty breathing, facial swelling.

**DANGEROUS DRUG**

## dalteparin sodium (Fragmin)
**CLASS** Anticoagulant, low-molecular-weight heparin
**PREG/CONT** Low risk/NA

**BBW** Carefully monitor pts w/spinal epidural anesthesia for neuro impairment. Risk of spinal hematoma and paralysis; provide urgent tx as necessary.
**IND & DOSE** **Tx of unstable angina.** *Adult:* 120 international units (IU)/kg subcut q 12 hr w/aspirin therapy for 5–8 d; max, 10,000 IU q 12 hr. **DVT px, abd surgery.** *Adult:* 2,500 IU subcut 1–2 hr before surgery, repeated once daily for 5–10 d after surgery. High-risk pts, 5,000 IU subcut starting evening before surgery, then daily for 5–10 d. **DVT px w/hip replacement surgery.** *Adult:* 5,000 IU subcut evening before surgery *or* 2,500 IU within 2 hr before surgery *or* 2,500 IU 4–8 hr after surgery. Then, 5,000 IU subcut each day for 5–10 d or up to 14 d *or* 2,500 IU subcut 4–8 hr after surgery, then 5,000 IU subcut once daily. **Px for DVT in pts w/restricted mobility.** *Adult:* 5,000 IU/d subcut. **Extended tx of VTE.** *Adult:* Mo 1, 200 IU/kg/d subcut; max, 18,000 IU/d. Mo 2–6, 150 IU/kg/d subcut; max,

18,000 IU/d. *Child 8–<17 yr:* 100 IU/kg subcut bid; *2–<8 yr:* 125 IU/kg subcut bid; *4 wk–<2 yr:* 150 IU/kg subcut bid.
**ADJUST DOSE** Thrombocytopenia, renal impairment
**ADV EFF** Bruising, chills, fever, **hemorrhage,** injection-site reaction
**INTERACTIONS** Antiplatelet drugs, chamomile, clopidogrel, garlic, ginger, ginkgo, ginseng, heparin, high-dose vitamin E, oral anticoagulants, salicylates, ticlopidine
**NC/PT** Do not give IM. Give subcut, alternating left and right abd wall. Cannot be interchanged w/other heparin product. Check dosing; timing varies per indication. Do not mix w/other injection or infusion. Have protamine sulfate on hand as antidote. Use caution in preg/breastfeeding. Teach proper administration/disposal of needles/syringes. Pt should avoid injury, report excessive bleeding.

## dantrolene sodium
(Dantrium, Ryanodex)
**CLASS** Direct acting skeletal muscle relaxant
**PREG/CONT** C/NA

**BBW** Monitor LFTs periodically. Arrange to discontinue at first sign of abnormality; early detection of liver abnormalities may permit reversion to normal function. Hepatotoxicity possible.
**IND & DOSE** **Control of clinical spasticity resulting from upper motor neuron disorders.** *Adult:* 25 mg PO daily. Increase to 25 mg PO tid for 7 d; then increase to 50 mg PO tid and to 100 mg PO tid if needed. *Child >5 yr:* 0.5 mg/kg PO once daily for 7 d, then 0.5 mg/kg PO tid for 7 d, then 1 mg/kg PO tid for 7 d, then 2 mg/kg PO tid if needed. Max, 100 mg PO qid. **Preop px of malignant hyperthermia.** *Adult, child:* 4–8 mg/kg/d PO in three–four divided doses for 1–2 d before surgery; give last dose about 3–4 hr before scheduled surgery. Or, for adult, child >5 yr, 2.5 mg/kg IV 1¼ hr before surgery infused over 1 hr. **Postcrisis follow-up.** 4–8 mg/kg/d PO in four divided doses for 1–3 d to prevent recurrence. **Tx of malignant hyperthermia.** *Adult, child >5 yr:* Discontinue all anesthetics as soon as problem recognized. Give dantrolene by continuous rapid IV push beginning at minimum of 1 mg/kg and continuing until sx subside or maximum cumulative dose of 10 mg/kg reached.
**ADV EFF** **Aplastic anemia,** diarrhea, dizziness, drowsiness, fatigue, **hepatitis, HF,** malaise, weakness
**INTERACTIONS** Alcohol, verapamil
**NC/PT** Monitor baseline and periodic LFTs. Monitor IV site to prevent extravasation. Use all appropriate support and tx for malignant hyperthermia, including mannitol. Establish tx goal w/oral drug; stop occasionally to assess spasticity. Discontinue if diarrhea is severe. Pt should take safety precautions, avoid alcohol.

## dapagliflozin (Farxiga)
**CLASS** Antidiabetic, sodium-glucose cotransporter 2 inhibitor
**PREG/CONT** C/NA

**IND & DOSE** **Adjunct to diet/exercise to improve glycemic control in type 2 diabetes.** *Adult:* 5 mg/d PO in a.m.; max, 10 mg/d. **To reduce risk of hospitalization for HF in pts w/ type 2 diabetes.** *Adult:* 10 mg/d PO.
**ADJUST DOSE** Renal impairment; severe renal impairment (not recommended)
**ADV EFF** **Bladder cancer,** dehydration, genital mycotic infections, hypoglycemia, hyponatremia, hypotension, increased LDLs, ketoacidosis, **necrotizing fasciitis of perineum, renal impairment,** UTI
**INTERACTIONS** Celery, coriander, dandelion root, digoxin, fenugreek, garlic, ginger, juniper berries, phenobarbital, phenytoin, rifampin
**NC/PT** Not for use w/type 1 diabetes, diabetic ketoacidosis. Monitor

blood glucose, $HbA_{1c}$, BP periodically. Not for use in preg/breastfeeding. Pt should continue diet/exercise program, other antidiabetics as ordered; take safety measures w/dehydration; watch for UTI, genital infections.

## dapsone (generic)

**CLASS** Leprostatic
**PREG/CONT** C/NA

**IND & DOSE** **Tx of leprosy.** *Adult, child:* 50–100 mg/d PO. Adults may need up to 300 mg/d; max in child, 100 mg/d PO. **Tx of dermatitis herpetiformis.** *Adult:* 50–300 mg/d PO. Smaller doses in child; max, 100 mg/d.
**ADV EFF** Blurred vision, headache, **hepatic impairment,** insomnia, n/v/d, photosensitivity, **severe allergic reactions,** tinnitus
**INTERACTIONS** Probenecid, rifampin, trimethoprim
**NC/PT** Obtain baseline, periodic LFTs. Not for use in preg/breastfeeding. Pt should complete full course of therapy; avoid sun exposure; take safety precautions w/vision changes; report difficulty breathing, urine/stool color changes.

## DAPTOmycin (Cubicin)

**CLASS** Cyclic-lipopeptide antibiotic
**PREG/CONT** Unkn/NA

**IND & DOSE** **Tx of complicated skin/skin-structure infections caused by susceptible strains of gram-positive bacteria.** *Adult:* 4 mg/kg IV over 30 min or as IV injection over 2 min in normal saline injection q 24 hr for 7–14 d. **Tx of *Staphylococcus aureus* bacteremia.** *Adult:* 6 mg/kg/d IV over 30 min or as IV injection over 2 min for 2–6 wk or longer.
**ADJUST DOSE** Renal impairment
**ADV EFF** **Anaphylaxis,** CNS and musculoskeletal system effects in child <12 mo, CDAD, constipation, dizziness, dyspnea, eosinophilic pneumonia, injection-site reactions, insomnia, myopathy, n/v/d, peripheral neuropathy, **pseudomembranous colitis,** superinfections
**INTERACTIONS** HMG-CoA inhibitors, oral anticoagulants, tobramycin
**NC/PT** Culture before tx. Ensure proper use. Do not use in child <12 mo. Use caution in preg/breastfeeding. Monitor CK for myopathy. Discontinue and give support for pseudomembranous colitis. Discontinue if s&sx of eosinophilic pneumonia. Treat superinfections. Pt should report persistent diarrhea, chest pain, difficulty breathing, numbness/tingling. Name confusion between dactinomycin and daptomycin.

## daratumumab (Darzalex)

**CLASS** Antineoplastic, monoclonal antibody
**PREG/CONT** Unkn/NA

**IND & DOSE** **Tx of multiple myeloma in pts who have had at least three prior lines of therapy; in pts who have received at least two prior therapies w/pomalidomide and dexamethasone; in pts who have received at least one prior therapy w/lenalidomide and dexamethasone or bortezomib and dexamethasone; in pts who are ineligible for autologous stem cell transplant w/bortezomib, melphalan, prednisone.** *Adult:* 16 mg/kg IV. Dose frequency depends on if combo therapy or monotherapy used.
**ADV EFF** Back pain, cough, fatigue, fever, infusion reactions, URI
**NC/PT** Ensure proper dx. Premedicate w/corticosteroids/antipyretics/antihistamines. Dilute and administer at initially 50 mL/hr; max, 200 mL/hr. Give corticosteroids on days 1 and 2 postinfusion. Monitor for infusion reactions; stop if life-threatening reactions occur. Use caution in preg/breastfeeding. Pt should mark calendar for tx days; report difficulty breathing, rash, fever.

## darbepoetin alfa (Aranesp)

**CLASS** Erythropoiesis-stimulating hormone
**PREG/CONT** C/NA

**BBW** Increased risk of death and serious CV events if Hgb target exceeds 11 g/dL. Use lowest level of drugs needed to increase Hgb to lowest level needed to avoid transfusion. Risk of DVT is higher in pts receiving erythropoietin-stimulating agents preop to decrease need for transfusion; note darbepoetin not approved for this use. Increased risk of death or tumor progression when drug used in cancer pts w/Hgb target range exceeding 11 g/dL; monitor Hgb closely in these pts.
**IND & DOSE** **Tx of anemia associated w/chronic renal failure, including during dialysis.** *Adult:* 0.45 mcg/kg IV or subcut once/wk. Target Hgb, 11 g/dL. **Tx of chemo-induced anemia in pts w/nonmyeloid malignancies.** 2.25 mcg/kg subcut once/wk; adjust to maintain acceptable Hgb levels. Or 500 mcg by subcut injection once q 3 wk; adjust to maintain Hgb level no higher than 11 g/dL.
**ADJUST DOSE** Chronic renal failure
**ADV EFF** Abd pain, arthralgia, asthenia, cough, **development of anti-erythropoietin antibodies w/subsequent pure red cell aplasia and extreme anemia,** diarrhea, dizziness, dyspnea, edema, fatigue, headache, HTN, hypotension, **MI,** myalgias, n/v/d, **rapid cancer growth, seizure, stroke,** thromboembolism, URI
**NC/PT** Ensure correct dx; not substitute for emergency transfusion. Monitor Hgb closely; max, 11 g/dL. Monitor preop pt for increased risk of DVTs. Discontinue if severe cutaneous reaction. Do not give in sol w/other drugs. Evaluate iron stores before and periodically during tx. Frequent blood tests will be needed. Teach pt proper administration/disposal of needles/syringes. Pt should take safety precautions for CNS effects; mark calendar for injection dates; report chest pain, extreme fatigue.

## darifenacin hydrobromide

(Darifenacin, Enablex)
**CLASS** Urinary antispasmodic, muscarinic receptor antagonist
**PREG/CONT** C/NA

**IND & DOSE** **Tx of overactive bladder.** *Adult:* 7.5 mg/d PO w/liquid and swallowed whole. May increase to 15 mg/d PO as early as wk 2.
**ADJUST DOSE** Gastric retention, hepatic impairment, somnolence, urine retention
**INTERACTIONS** Anticholinergics, clarithromycin, flecainide, itraconazole, ketoconazole, nefazodone, nelfinavir, ritonavir, thioridazine, TCAs
**NC/PT** Ensure correct dx; rule out underlying medical issues. Monitor IOP. Not for use in preg/breastfeeding. Pt should swallow tablet whole and not cut/crush/chew it; use sugarless lozenges for dry mouth; use safety precautions w/somnolence.

## darunavir (Prezista)

**CLASS** Antiviral/protease inhibitor
**PREG/CONT** C/NA

**IND & DOSE** **Tx of pts w/HIV infection that has progressed after standard tx.** *Adult:* 600 mg PO bid w/ritonavir 100 mg PO bid w/food (tx-experienced) 800 mg PO bid w/ritonavir 100 mg PO bid (tx-naïve). *Child 3–<18 yr, 10 kg or more:* Base dose on weight and surface area (see manufacturer's guidelines).
**ADJUST DOSE** Hepatic impairment
**ADV EFF** Abd pain, diabetes, headache, **hepatitis,** hyperglycemia, **increased bleeding w/hemophilia,** n/v/d, rash to **SJS,** redistribution of body fat
**INTERACTIONS** Alfuzosin, cisapride, dihydroergotamine, ergotamine,

lovastatin, methylergonovine, oral midazolam, pimozide, rifampin, St. John's wort, sildenafil, simvastatin, triazolam. Contraindicated w/drugs highly dependent on CYP3A for clearance
**NC/PT** Contraindicated for use w/ many other drugs; check complete drug list before tx. Monitor LFTs regularly; not for use w/severe hepatic impairment. Not for use in child <3; fatalities have occurred. Monitor blood glucose. Not for use in preg/breastfeeding. Pt should report rash, urine/stool color changes.

**DANGEROUS DRUG**

## dasatinib (Sprycel)

**CLASS** Antineoplastic, kinase inhibitor
**PREG/CONT** High risk/NA

**IND & DOSE** **Tx of adults w/all stages of CML; newly diagnosed or resistant Philadelphia chromosome–positive (Ph+) ALL.** *Adult:* Chronic CML, 100 mg/d PO. ALL/other phases of CML, 140 mg/d PO. **Tx of child w/ Ph+ CML in chronic phase or newly diagnosed w/combo chemo.** *Child:* Dose based on body weight.
**ADV EFF** **Bone marrow suppression, cardiac dysfx,** diarrhea, dyspnea, fatigue, fluid retention, hemorrhage, **HF,** nausea, **pulmonary artery HTN, prolonged QT,** rash to severe dermatologic reactions
**INTERACTIONS** Antacids; CYP3A4 inducers/inhibitors; grapefruit juice, proton pump inhibitors
**NC/PT** Obtain baseline and periodic ECG. Monitor CBC closely; dose adjustment may be needed. Not for use in preg/breastfeeding. Men should not father a child during tx. Pt should swallow tablet whole w/ or w/o a meal and not cut/crush/chew it; avoid grapefruit juice; avoid exposure to infection, injury; report severe swelling, bleeding, chest pain, difficulty breathing.

**DANGEROUS DRUG**

## DAUNOrubicin citrate

(generic)
**CLASS** Antineoplastic
**PREG/CONT** D/NA

**BBW** Cardiotoxicity possible; monitor ECG, enzymes (dose adjustment may be needed). Serious bone marrow depression possible; monitor CBC (dose adjustment may be needed).
**IND & DOSE** **Tx of advanced HIV-associated Kaposi sarcoma.** *Adult:* 400 mg/m² IV over 1 hr q 2 wk.
**ADJUST DOSE** Renal/hepatic impairment
**ADV EFF** Abd pain, anorexia, **bone marrow suppression, cancer, cardiotoxicity,** fatigue, fever, headache, **hepatotoxicity,** n/v/d
**INTERACTIONS** Cyclophosphamide, hepatotoxic drugs, myelosuppressants
**NC/PT** Obtain baseline and periodic ECG, enzymes. Monitor CBC closely; dose adjustment may be needed. Encourage cancer screening. Monitor injection site; extravasation can cause serious damage. Not for use in preg/breastfeeding.

**DANGEROUS DRUG**

## decitabine (Dacogen)

**CLASS** Antineoplastic antibiotic, nucleoside metabolic inhibitor
**PREG/CONT** High risk/NA

**IND & DOSE** **Tx of pts w/myelodysplastic syndromes.** *Adult:* 15 mg/m² IV over 3 hr q 8 hr for 3 d; repeat q 6 wk *or* 20 mg/m² IV over 1 hr daily for 5 d, repeated q 4 wk
**ADJUST DOSE** Renal/hepatic impairment
**ADV EFF** Anemia, constipation, cough, diarrhea, fatigue, hyperglycemia, nausea, neutropenia, petechiae, pyrexia, thrombocytopenia
**NC/PT** Monitor CBC closely; dose adjustment may be needed. Premedicate w/antiemetic. Not for use in preg

(contraceptive use during and for 1 mo after tx)/breastfeeding. Men should not father a child during and for 2 mo after tx. Pt should avoid exposure to infection, injury.

## deferasirox (Exjade, Jadenu)

**CLASS** Chelate
**PREG/CONT** High risk/NA

**BBW** May cause potentially fatal renal/hepatic reactions, gastric hemorrhage; monitor closely.
**IND & DOSE** **Tx of chronic iron overload from blood transfusions.** *Adult, child ≥2 yr:* 20 mg/kg/d PO; max, 30 mg/kg/d. Adjust dose based on serum ferritin. **Tx of iron overload related to thalassemia.** *Adult, child ≥10 yr:* 10 mg/kg/d PO. Adjust dose based on serum ferritin.
**ADJUST DOSE** Moderate hepatic impairment, renal impairment (contraindicated if GFR <40 mL/min/1.73 $m^2$).
**ADV EFF** Abd pain, **bone marrow suppression, GI hemorrhage, hepatic/renal impairment, hypersensitivity reaction,** n/v/d, rash to **SJS;** vision/hearing changes
**INTERACTIONS** Aluminum-containing drugs, bisphosphonates, iron chelating agents.
**NC/PT** Monitor LFTs, renal function before, wkly for 2 wk, then monthly during tx. Dose adjusted based on serum ferritin levels. Contraindicated in pts w/high-risk myelodysplastic syndromes, advanced malignancies, platelet count <50 × $10^9$/L. Not for use in preg/breastfeeding. Pt should not chew or swallow tablets whole but should disperse in water or apple or orange juice, resuspend any residue and swallow liquid. Pt should take on empty stomach at least 30 min before food; take safety precautions for CNS effects; report unusual bleeding, rash, urine/stool color changes, difficulty breathing.

## deferoxamine mesylate (Desferal)

**CLASS** Chelate
**PREG/CONT** C/NA

**IND & DOSE** **Tx of chronic iron overload.** *Adult, child ≥2 yr:* 0.5–1 g IM qid; 2 g IV w/each unit of blood, or 2,040 mg/kg/d as continuous subcut infusion over 8–24 hr. IM preferred. **Tx of acute iron toxicity.** *Adult, child:* 1 g IM or IV, then 0.5 g q 4 hr for two doses, then q 4–12 hr based on pt response. Max for child, 6 g/d.
**ADV EFF** Abd pain, hearing/vision changes, infections, injection-site reactions, n/v/d, **RDS,** rash, discolored urine
**NC/PT** Not for use in primary hemochromatosis. Monitor hearing, vision, lung function. Use caution in preg/breastfeeding. Urine may be discolored. Pt should take safety measures for CNS effects.

## defibrotide (Defitelio)

**CLASS** Plasmin enhancer
**PREG/CONT** High risk/NA

**IND & DOSE** **Tx of pts w/hepatic veno-occlusive dx w/renal or pulmonary dysfx.** *Adult, child:* 6.25 mg/kg IV q 6 hr for at least 21 d. May continue tx if no disease resolution.
**ADV EFF** Epistaxis, **hemorrhage,** hypotension, n/v/d, **severe hypersensitivity reactions**
**INTERACTIONS** Systemic anticoagulants, fibrinolytic therapy; contraindicated
**NC/PT** Do not give w/anticoagulants, fibrinolytic therapy; monitor closely for bleeding, hypersensitivity reactions. Pt should avoid preg/breastfeeding; report bleeding, difficulty breathing, unusual swelling.

## deflazacort (Emflaza)
**CLASS** Corticosteroid
**PREG/CONT** High risk/NA

**IND & DOSE** **Tx of Duchenne muscular dystrophy.** *Adult, child ≥2 yr:* 0.9 mg/kg/d PO.
**ADV EFF** **Cushing syndrome, GI perforation,** hyperglycemia, hypernatremia, hypertension, **hypokalemia, immune suppression,** loss of bone density, mood changes, **serious rash,** vision changes
**INTERACTIONS** Moderate to strong CYP34A inhibitors (give 1/3 recommended dose), moderate to strong CYP341 inducers (avoid use), live vaccines
**NC/PT** Do not use in child <2 yr (benzyl alcohol in sol). Pt may swallow tablet whole or crush and take immediately in applesauce. Must taper drug when discontinuing. Not for use in preg/breastfeeding. Monitor BP; serum potassium, sodium, and glucose; bone density (w/long-term use); growth in child. Pt should use safety measures w/vision changes; avoid infection; report mood changes, s&sx of infection, rash, swelling, acute abd pain.

## degarelix (Firmagon)
**CLASS** Antineoplastic
**PREG/CONT** X/NA

**IND & DOSE** **Tx of advanced prostate cancer.** *Adult:* 240 mg subcut as two 120-mg injections, then maint of 80 mg subcut q 28 d.
**ADV EFF** Hot flashes, **hypersensitivity reactions,** injection-site reaction, loss of libido, **prolonged QT,** weight gain
**INTERACTIONS** QT-prolonging drugs
**NC/PT** Obtain baseline and periodic ECG. Monitor injection sites for reaction. Not for use in preg/breastfeeding. Alert pt that flushing, hot flashes, changes in libido possible. Pt should report rash, difficulty breathing, facial swelling.

**DANGEROUS DRUG**

## delafloxacin (Baxdela)
**CLASS** Antibiotic, fluoroquinolone
**PREG/CONT** Unkn/NA

**BBW** Associated w/disabling and potentially irreversible serious adverse reactions, including tendinitis/tendon rupture, peripheral neuropathy, CNS effects. Discontinue immediately; avoid fluoroquinolones if any of these serious adverse reactions occur. Fluoroquinolones may exacerbate muscle weakness in pts w/myasthenia gravis; avoid in pts w/history of myasthenia gravis.
**IND & DOSE** **Tx of acute bacterial skin/skin structure infections caused by susceptible bacteria; tx of community-acquired bacterial pneumonia.** *Adult:* 300 mg IV over 60 min q 12 hr *or* 450 mg PO q 12 hr for 5–14 d; 200 mg q 12 hr if GFR is 15–29.
**ADV EFF** **CDAD, CNS effects,** diarrhea, headache, **hypersensitivity,** nausea, **peripheral neuropathy, tendinitis/tendon rupture,** vomiting
**NC/PT** May reduce dose if renal impairment. Contraindicated in ESRD. Not recommended in pts <18 yr or >65 yr (greater risk of tendon disorders). Pt should take w/ or w/o food at least 2 hr before or 6 hr after antacids containing magnesium, aluminum, sucralfate; metal cations such as iron, multivitamins/preparations containing zinc or iron, or w/didanosine buffered tablets for oral suspension or pediatric powder for oral sol.

## delavirdine mesylate (Rescriptor)
**CLASS** Antiviral, nonnucleoside reverse transcriptase inhibitor
**PREG/CONT** C/NA

**BBW** Give concurrently w/appropriate antiretrovirals; not for monotherapy.

**IND & DOSE Tx of HIV-1 infection, w/other appropriate antiretrovirals.** *Adult, child>16 yr:* 400 mg PO tid w/ appropriate antiretrovirals.
**ADV EFF** Diarrhea, flulike sx, headache, nausea, rash
**INTERACTIONS** Antacids, antiarrhythmics, benzodiazepines, calcium channel blockers, clarithromycin, dapsone, ergot derivatives, indinavir, quinidine, rifabutin, saquinavir, St. John's wort, warfarin
**NC/PT** Must give w/other antiretrovirals. Monitor T cells, LFTs. Monitor for opportunistic infections. Disperse 100-mg tablets in water before giving; let stand. Stir to form uniform dispersion. Have pt drink, rinse glass, and drink the rinse. Pt should use appropriate precautions (drug not a cure); consult all health care providers (drug interacts w/many drugs); avoid St. John's wort; report severe diarrhea.

## demeclocycline hydrochloride (generic)

**CLASS** Tetracycline
**PREG/CONT** D/NA

**IND & DOSE Tx of infections caused by susceptible bacteria strains; when penicillin contraindicated.** *Adult:* General guidelines, 150 mg PO qid or 300 mg PO bid. *Child≥8 yr:* 3–6 mg/lb/d (6.6–13.2 mg/kg/d) PO in two–four divided doses. **Tx of gonococcal infections.** *Adult:* 600 mg PO, then 300 mg q 12 hr for 4 d to total 3 g. **Tx of streptococcal infections.** *Adult:* 150 mg PO qid for 10 d.
**ADV EFF** **Anemia;** anorexia; discoloration, inadequate calcification of fetal primary teeth if used in preg; discoloration, inadequate calcification of permanent teeth if used during dental development; **eosinophilia;** glossitis; **hemolytic thrombocytopenia; leukocytosis; leukopenia; liver failure; neutropenia;** n/v/d; phototoxic reaction; rash
**INTERACTIONS** Antacids, dairy products, digoxin, hormonal contraceptives, iron, magnesium, penicillin
**NC/PT** Not for use in preg (barrier contraceptives advised)/breastfeeding. Pt should take on empty stomach w/full glass of water; not take w/iron or dairy products; avoid sun exposure; report urine/stool color changes.

## denileukin diftitox

(Ontak)
**CLASS** Biological protein
**PREG/CONT** D/NA

**BBW** Severe hypersensitivity reactions possible; have life support equipment on hand. Capillary leak syndrome possible; pt may lose visual acuity, color vision.
**IND & DOSE Tx of cutaneous T-cell lymphoma in pts who express CD25 component of IL-2 receptor.** *Adult:* 9 or 18 mcg/kg/d IV over 30–60 min for 5 consecutive days q 21 d for eight cycles
**ADV EFF** **Capillary leak syndrome,** cough, diarrhea, dyspnea, fatigue, headache, **infusion reaction,** n/v, peripheral edema, pruritus, pyrexia, rigors, vision changes
**NC/PT** Premedicate w/antihistamine and acetaminophen. Have emergency equipment available for hypersensitivity reactions. Warn pt of potential vision loss. Use caution in preg; not for use in breastfeeding. Pt should report sudden weight gain, rash, difficulty breathing, vision changes.

## denosumab (Prolia, Xgeva)

**CLASS** RANK ligand inhibitor
**PREG/CONT** High risk/NA

**IND & DOSE Tx of postmenopausal osteoporosis in women at high risk for fracture; tx of bone loss in breast cancer pts receiving aromatase inhibitors; tx of bone loss in prostate cancer pts receiving androgen deprivation therapy.** *Adult:* 60 mg by subcut injection in upper arm, thigh, or abdomen q 6 mo (*Prolia* only). **Tx of multiple myeloma skeletal-related events in pts w/bone metastases from solid tumors.** *Adult:* 120 mg by subcut injection q 4 wk (*Xgeva* only). **Tx of unresectable giant cell tumor of the bone** (*Xgeva*). *Adult, adolescent:* 120 mg subcut q 4 wk w/additional 120 mg subcut on days 8, 15 of first month, w/calcium, vitamin D. **Tx of hypercalcemia of malignancy refractory to bisphosphonates** (*Xgeva*). *Adult:* 120 mg subcut q 4 wk w/added 120-mg doses on days 8 and 15 of first mo.

**ADJUST DOSE** Renal impairment

**ADV EFF** Anemia, atypical femur fractures, back pain, **cancer, constipation,** cystitis, diarrhea, hypercholesterolemia, hypocalcemia, **infection (serious to life-threatening),** nausea, **osteonecrosis of jaw, serious skin infections**

**NC/PT** Obtain baseline serum calcium; repeat regularly. Give subcut into abdomen, upper thigh, or upper arm; rotate injection sites. Not for use in preg (contraceptives advised)/breastfeeding. Pt should take 1,000 mg/d calcium and 400 units/d vitamin D; have regular cancer screening; get regular dental care to prevent jaw problems; avoid exposure to infection; report s&sx of infection, rash, jaw pain.

## deoxycholic acid (Kybella)

**CLASS** Cytolytic agent
**PREG/CONT** Moderate risk/NA

**IND & DOSE To improve appearance of moderate to severe convexity in fullness associated w/submental fat "double chin" in adults.** *Adult:* 0.2 mL injected 1 cm apart at all sites in planned tx area; up to 50 injections/session, up to six sessions at intervals no less than 1 mo apart.

**ADV EFF** Dysphagia, local edema/swelling, local redness/pain, mandibular nerve injury, numbness, submental bruising

**NC/PT** Follow prescribed injection technique to avoid injury. Avoid injection if infection or alopecia in tx area. Use caution in preg/breastfeeding. Pt should mark calendar for possible tx days; report difficulty swallowing, continued pain/swelling/bruising at injection site.

## desipramine hydrochloride (Norpramin)

**CLASS** Antidepressant, TCA
**PREG/CONT** C/NA

**BBW** Risk of suicidality in child, adolescent, young adult. Monitor pt; inform caregivers.

**IND & DOSE Relief of depression sx.** *Adult:* 100–200 mg/d PO as single dose or in divided doses; max, 300 mg/d.

**ADJUST DOSE** Adolescents, elderly pts

**ADV EFF Agranulocytosis,** anticholinergic effects, confusion, constipation, disturbed concentration, dry mouth, **MI,** nasal congestion, orthostatic hypotension, photosensitivity, sedation, serotonin syndrome, **stroke,** urine retention, withdrawal sx after prolonged use

**INTERACTIONS** Anticholinergics, cimetidine, clonidine, fluoxetine, MAOIs, oral anticoagulants, quinolones, sympathomimetics

**NC/PT** Give major portion of dose at bedtime. Monitor elderly pts for increased adverse effects. Screen for bipolar disorder. Use caution in preg/breastfeeding. Obtain CBC if fever, s&sx of infection occur. Pt should avoid alcohol, sun exposure; use sugarless lozenges for dry mouth; take safety precautions w/CNS effects; report difficulty urinating, fever, thoughts of suicide.

**DANGEROUS DRUG**

## desirudin (Iprivask)

**CLASS** Anticoagulant, thrombin inhibitor
**PREG/CONT** C/NA

**BBW** Risk of epidural, spinal hematoma w/resultant long-term or permanent

paralysis. Weigh risks before using epidural or spinal anesthesia, spinal puncture.
**IND & DOSE Px of DVT in pts undergoing elective hip replacement.** *Adult:* 15 mg subcut q 12 hr given up to 5–15 min before surgery after induction of anesthesia.
**ADJUST DOSE** Renal impairment
**ADV EFF Hemorrhage,** injection-site reactions
**INTERACTIONS** Drugs/herbs that prolong bleeding
**NC/PT** Give by deep subcut injection; alternate sites. Monitor blood clotting tests carefully. Protect pt from injury. Pt should report difficulty breathing, numbness/tingling, unusual bleeding.

## desloratadine (Clarinex, Clarinex Reditabs)
**CLASS** Antihistamine
**PREG/CONT** C/NA

**IND & DOSE Relief of nasal and nonnasal sx of seasonal allergic rhinitis in pts ≥2 yr; tx of chronic idiopathic urticaria and perennial allergies caused by indoor and outdoor allergens in pts ≥6 mo.** *Adult, child ≥12 yr:* 5 mg/d PO or 2 tsp (5 mg/10 mL) syrup/d PO. *Child 6–11 yr:* 1 tsp syrup (2.5 mg/5 mL)/d PO, or 2.5-mg rapidly disintegrating tablet/d PO. *Child 12 mo–5 yr:* ½ tsp syrup/d (1.25 mg/2.5 mL) PO. *Child 6–11 mo:* 2 mL syrup/d (1 mg) PO.
**ADJUST DOSE** Renal/hepatic impairment
**ADV EFF** Dry mouth/throat, dizziness, hypersensitivity reactions
**NC/PT** Do not use *Clarinex Reditabs* w/phenylketonuria. Pt should use humidifier if dryness a problem, suck sugarless lozenges for dry mouth, take safety precautions if dizzy.

## desmopressin acetate
(DDAVP, Noctiva, Stimate)
**CLASS** Hormone
**PREG/CONT** B/NA

**BBW** Nasal spray (*Noctiva*) associated w/potentially life-threatening hyponatremia; contraindicated w/high risk of hyponatremia. Ensure normal sodium level; monitor sodium at 7 d and monthly, more frequently in elderly pts.
**IND & DOSE Tx of neurogenic diabetes insipidus.** *Adult:* 0.1–0.4 mL/d intranasally as single dose or divided into two–three doses, or 0.5–1 mL/d subcut or IV divided into two doses, or 0.05 mg PO bid; adjust according to water turnover pattern (*DDAVP* only). *Child 3 mo–12 yr:* 0.05–0.3 mL/d intranasally as single dose or divided into two doses, or 0.05 mg PO daily; adjust according to water turnover pattern (*DDAVP* only). **Tx of hemophilia A, von Willebrand disease (type I).** *Adult:* 0.3 mcg/kg diluted in 50 mL sterile physiologic saline; infuse IV slowly over 15–30 min 30 min preop; intranasal, 1 spray/nostril 2 hr preop for total dose of 300 mcg. *Child ≥11 mo:* 1 spray/nostril (150 mcg); total dose, 300 mcg. <50 kg, 150 mcg as single spray. **Tx of nocturia due to nocturnal polyuria in adults who awaken at least 2 ×/night to void.** *Adults ≥50 yr:* ≥65 yr or pts at risk for hyponatremia: 0.83 mcg (1 spray) in either nostril/night about 30 min before bed. <65 yr: 1.66 mcg (1 spray) in either nostril/night about 30 min before bed.
**ADV EFF** Fluid retention, nasal congestion/pain, sneezing w/nasal spray; local redness, swelling, burning at injection site; sodium retention, **water intoxication**
**INTERACTIONS** Carbamazepine, chlorpropamide, furosemide, glucocorticoids, lamotrigine, NSAIDs, opiates, SSRIs, TCAs
**NC/PT** Refrigerate some sol, injection (check label; some no longer

need refrigeration). Use rhinal tube to deposit deep into nasal cavity; use air-filled syringe or blow into tube. Monitor nasal passages. Nasal spray not for use w/uncontrolled BP, SIADH, impaired renal function, nasal lesions, HF, preg, or in child. Monitor water balance closely. Monitor for hyponatremia. Monitor pts w/CV disorders. Individualize dose to establish diurnal water turnover patterns to allow sleep. Teach proper administration. Pt using nasal spray will need regular blood tests. Pt should report nose drainage, severe stuffiness, diarrhea, loss of fluid, s&sx of infection.

## desvenlafaxine succinate (Pristiq)

**CLASS** Antidepressant, serotonin-norepinephrine reuptake inhibitor
**PREG/CONT** Moderate risk/NA

**BBW** High risk of suicidality in child, adolescent, young adult; monitor for suicidal ideation, especially when beginning tx or changing dose. Not approved for child.
**IND & DOSE** **Tx of major depressive disorders.** *Adult:* 50 mg/d PO w/ or w/o food; reduce dose gradually when stopping.
**ADJUST DOSE** Hepatic/renal impairment
**ADV EFF** Activation of mania, angle-closure glaucoma, bleeding, constipation, decreased appetite, dizziness, dry mouth, **eosinophilic pneumonia**, fatigue, glaucoma, headache, **HTN**, hyperhidrosis, **ILD**, n/v/d, **seizures**, **serotonin syndrome**, **suicidal ideation**
**INTERACTIONS** Alcohol, aspirin, CNS depressants, MAOIs, NSAIDs, SSRIs, St. John's wort, venlafaxine, warfarin
**NC/PT** Limit access in suicidal pts. Do not give within 14 d of MAOIs. Taper gradually when stopping. Monitor IOP periodically. Not for use in preg/breastfeeding. May take several wks to see effects. Tablet matrix may appear in stool. Pt should swallow tablet whole and not cut/crush/chew it; report thoughts of suicide, abnormal bleeding, difficulty breathing.

## deutetrabenazine (Austedo)

**CLASS** Vesicular monoamine transporter 2 inhibitor
**PREG/CONT** Unkn/NA

**BBW** Risk of depression and suicidality in pts w/Huntington disease; contraindicated in suicidal pts. Monitor pts carefully; inform pts/caregivers/families of risk.
**IND & DOSE** **Tx of chorea associated w/Huntington disease.** *Adult:* 6–48 mg/d PO. **Tx of tardive dyskinesia.** *Adult:* 12 mg/d PO; may increase to max of 48 mg/d.
**ADJUST DOSE** Hepatic impairment
**ADV EFF** Agitation, akathisia, diarrhea, dry mouth, hepatic impairment, **NMS**, parkinsonism, **QT prolongation**, sedation, somnolence, suicidality
**INTERACTIONS** Alcohol, CYP2D6 inhibitors, QT-prolonging drugs, sedating drugs
**NC/PT** Assess QT interval before use. Monitor LFTs; monitor and support depression. Pt should take drug w/food; swallow tablets whole and not cut, crush, or chew; take safety precautions w/CNS effects; report depression, thoughts of suicide, restlessness, urine/stool color changes.

## dexamethasone (generic), dexamethasone (Hemady), dexamethasone sodium phosphate (generic)

**CLASS** Glucocorticoid, hormone
**PREG/CONT** C/NA

**IND & DOSE** **Short-term tx of various inflammatory, allergic disorders.** *Adult:* 0.75–9 mg/d PO, or 0.5–9 mg/d IM or IV. *Child:* Base dose on formulas for child dosing using

age, body weight. **Tx of cerebral edema.** *Adult:* 10 mg IV, then 4 mg IM q 6 hr until cerebral edema sx subside. Change to oral therapy, 1–3 mg tid, as soon as possible; taper over 5–7 d. **Tx of unresponsive shock.** *Child:* 1–6 mg/kg as single IV injection (as much as 20 mg initially; repeated injections q 2–6 hr have been used). **Intra-articular or soft-tissue administration for tx of arthritis, psoriatic plaques.** *Adult:* 0.2–6 mg (depending on joint or soft-tissue injection site). **Control of bronchial asthma requiring corticosteroids.** *Adult:* 3 inhalations tid–qid; max, 12 inhalations/d. *Child:* 2 inhalations tid–qid; max, 8 inhalations/d. **Relief of seasonal or perennial rhinitis sx.** *Adult:* 2 sprays (168 mcg) into each nostril bid–tid; max, 12 sprays (1,008 mcg)/d. *Child:* 1 or 2 sprays (84–168 mcg) into each nostril bid, depending on age; max, 8 sprays (672 mcg)/d. **Tx of inflammation of eyelid, conjunctiva, cornea, globe.** *Adult, child:* Instill 1 or 2 drops into conjunctival sac q hr during day and q 2 hr during night; taper as 1 drop q 4 hr, then 1 drop tid–qid. For ointment, apply thin coating in lower conjunctival sac tid–qid; reduce dose to bid, then once daily. **Relief of inflammatory and pruritic manifestations of dermatoses.** *Adult, child:* Apply sparingly to affected area bid–qid. **Tx w/other anti-myeloma products for multiple myeloma** (*Hemady*). *Adult:* 20 or 40 mg PO daily.
**ADV EFF** Acne, amenorrhea, depression, euphoria, fluid/electrolyte disturbances, headache, HPA suppression, HTN, hyperglycemia, immunosuppression, impaired wound healing, infection, insomnia, irregular menses, local irritation, muscle weakness, secondary adrenal suppression, **seizures,** vertigo
**INTERACTIONS** Corticotropin, live vaccines, phenobarbital, phenytoin, rifampin, salicylates
**NC/PT** Give daily doses before 9 a.m. to mimic normal peak corticosteroid blood level. Taper dose w/high doses or long-term use. Monitor serum glucose. Protect pt from exposure to infection; do not give to pt w/active infection. Not for use in breastfeeding. Apply topical drug sparingly to intact skin. Pt should not overuse joints after intra-articular injection.

## dexchlorpheniramine maleate (Polmon)

**CLASS** Antihistamine
**PREG/CONT** B/NA

**IND & DOSE Relief of sx associated w/perennial, seasonal allergic rhinitis; vasomotor rhinitis; allergic conjunctivitis; mild/uncomplicated urticaria, angioedema; amelioration of allergic reactions to blood/plasma; dermatographism; adjunct tx in anaphylactic reactions.** *Adult, child >12 yr:* 4–6 mg PO at bedtime or q 8–10 hr during day. *Child 6–12 yr:* 4 mg PO once daily at bedtime.
**ADJUST DOSE** Elderly pts
**ADV EFF Agranulocytosis, anaphylactic shock,** disturbed coordination, dizziness, drowsiness, epigastric distress, **pancytopenia,** sedation, thickening of bronchial secretions, **thrombocytopenia**
**INTERACTIONS** Alcohol, CNS depressants
**NC/PT** Adjust dose to lowest possible to manage sx. Available in oral syrup only. Pt should avoid alcohol; take safety precautions for CNS effects; report difficulty breathing, s&sx of infection.

## dexlansoprazole (Dexilant)

**CLASS** Antisecretory, proton pump inhibitor
**PREG/CONT** Low risk/NA

**IND & DOSE Healing, maint of healing of erosive esophagitis.** *Adult, child ≥12 yr:* 60 mg/d PO for up to 8 wk, then 30 mg/d PO. **Tx of heartburn, GERD.** *Adult, child ≥12 yr:* 30 mg/d PO for up to 4 wk.

**ADJUST DOSE** Hepatic impairment
**ADV EFF** Acute interstitial nephritis, CDAD, **gastric cancer,** hypomagnesemia, n/v/d, possible loss of bone density and fracture, vitamin $B_{12}$ deficiency
**INTERACTIONS** Ampicillin, atazanavir, digoxin, iron salts, ketoconazole, methotrexate, tacrolimus, warfarin; contraindicated w/rilpivirine
**NC/PT** If pt able, should swallow capsule whole and not chew. If pt unable, may open capsule, sprinkle contents over 1 tbsp applesauce, and swallow immediately (pt should not chew granules). Not for use in breastfeeding. Pt should report severe diarrhea.

**DANGEROUS DRUG**

## dexmedetomidine hydrochloride (Precedex)

**CLASS** Sedative/hypnotic
**PREG/CONT** C/NA

**IND & DOSE** **ICU sedation of mechanically ventilated pts.** *Adult:* 1 mcg/kg IV over 10 min, then 0.2–0.7 mcg/kg/hr using IV infusion pump. **Sedation of nonintubated pts before and/or during surgery or procedures.** *Adult:* 1 mcg/kg IV over 10 min, then maint dose 0.6 mcg/kg/hr; range 0.2–1 mcg/kg/hr.
**ADJUST DOSE** Elderly pts, hepatic impairment
**ADV EFF** Agitation, bradycardia, dry mouth, hypotension, **respiratory failure**
**INTERACTIONS** Anesthetics, CNS depressants, opioids
**NC/PT** Not for use in preg/breastfeeding. Monitor pt continuously during tx. Do not use for longer than 24 hr.

## dexmethylphenidate hydrochloride (Focalin, Focalin XR)

**CLASS** CNS stimulant
**PREG/CONT** C/C-II

**BBW** Use caution w/hx of substance dependence or alcoholism. Dependence, severe depression, psychotic reactions possible w/withdrawal.
**IND & DOSE** **Tx of ADHD as part of total tx program.** *Adult, child ≥6 yr:* 2.5 mg PO bid; may increase as needed in 2.5- to 5-mg increments to max 10 mg PO bid. ER capsules: Initially 5 mg/d PO for child; increase in 5-mg increments to 30 mg/d. Start adults at 10 mg/d PO; increase in 10-mg increments to 20 mg/d. *Already on methylphenidate:* Start at one-half methylphenidate dose w/max of 10 mg PO bid.
**ADV EFF** Abd pain, anorexia, **CV events including mortality,** dizziness, growth suppression, insomnia, nausea, nervousness, **priapism,** tachycardia
**INTERACTIONS** Alcohol, antihypertensives, dopamine, epinephrine, MAOIs, phenobarbital, phenytoin, primidone, SSRIs, TCAs, warfarin
**NC/PT** Ensure proper dx before use; interrupt periodically to reevaluate. Baseline ECG recommended. Use as part of comprehensive tx program. Do not give within 14 d of MAOIs. Monitor growth in child. Controlled substance; secure storage. May sprinkle contents on applesauce; pt should take immediately. Pt should swallow ER capsules whole and not cut/crush/chew them; take early in day to avoid interrupting sleep; avoid alcohol and OTC products; report chest pain, insomnia.

## dexpanthenol (Panthoderm)

**CLASS** Emollient
**PREG/CONT** C/NA

**IND & DOSE** **Topical tx of mild eczema, dermatosis, bee stings, diaper rash, chafing.** *Adult, child:* Apply once or twice daily to affected areas.
**ADV EFF** Local irritation
**NC/PT** Promote hydration; remove old skin. Pt should avoid contact w/eyes; report application-site reaction.

## dexrazoxane (Totect, Zinecard)

**CLASS** Lyophilizate
**PREG/CONT** D/NA

**IND & DOSE** **Tx of extravasation of IV anthracycline chemo.** *Adult:* Days 1, 2: 1,000 mg/m² IV; max, 2,000 mg IV. Day 3: 500 mg/m² IV; max, 1,000 mg infused over 2 hr.
**ADJUST DOSE** Renal impairment
**ADV EFF** **Bone marrow suppression,** injection-site pain, n/v/d, pyrexia
**NC/PT** Available in emergency kit. Monitor bone marrow. Not for use in preg/breastfeeding. Use pain-relief measures for extravasation site.

## dextran, low-molecular-weight (Dextran 40, 10% LMD, Rheomacrodex)

**CLASS** Plasma volume expander
**PREG/CONT** C/NA

**IND & DOSE** **Adjunct tx of shock or impending shock when blood or blood products are not available.** *Adult, child:* Total dose of 20 mL/kg IV in first 24 hr; max, 10 mL/kg beyond 24 hr. Discontinue after 5 d. **Hemodiluent in extracorporeal circulation.** *Adult:* 10–20 mL/kg added to perfusion circuit; max, 20 mL/kg. **Px for DVT/PE in pts undergoing procedures w/high risk of thromboembolic events.** *Adult:* 500–1,000 mL IV on day of surgery. Continue at 500 mL/d IV for additional 2–3 d. Thereafter, may give 500 mL q second–third day for up to 2 wk.
**ADV EFF** Hypotension, hypervolemia, injection-site reactions, rash
**NC/PT** Give IV only. Use clear sols only. Monitor for hypervolemia. Monitor urine output. Pt should report difficulty breathing.

## dextroamphetamine sulfate (Dexedrine)

**CLASS** Amphetamine, CNS stimulant
**PREG/CONT** C/C-II

**BBW** High abuse potential. Avoid prolonged use; prescribe sparingly. Misuse may cause sudden death or serious CV events. Increased risk w/ heart problems or structural heart anomalies.
**IND & DOSE** **Tx of narcolepsy.** *Adult, child >12 yr:* 10 mg/d PO in divided doses. Increase in 10-mg/d increments at wkly intervals; range, 5–60 mg/d PO in divided doses. *Child 6–12 yr:* 5 mg/d PO. Increase in 5-mg increments at wkly intervals until optimal response obtained. **Adjunct tx for ADHD w/hyperactivity.** *Adult:* 5 mg PO once or twice daily; max, 40 mg/d. *Child ≥6 yr:* 5 mg PO daily–bid. Increase in 5-mg/d increments at wkly intervals; max, 40 mg/d. *Child 3–5 yr:* 2.5 mg/d PO. Increase in 2.5-mg/d increments at wkly intervals.
**ADV EFF** Alopecia, diarrhea, dizziness, dry mouth, HTN, insomnia, overstimulation, palpitations, restlessness, tachycardia, unpleasant taste
**INTERACTIONS** Acetazolamide, antihypertensives, furazolidone, MAOIs, sodium bicarbonate, urinary acidifiers
**NC/PT** Baseline ECG recommended. Ensure proper dx. Do not give within 14 d of MAOIs. Incorporate into comprehensive social and behavioral tx plan. Controlled substance; store securely. Give early in day. Provide periodic drug breaks. Monitor BP, growth in child. Not for use in preg. Pt/caregiver should report manic or aggressive behavior, numbness in fingers or toes, chest pain, shortness of breath.

**dextromethorphan hydrobromide** (Creo-Terpin, Delsym, DexAlone, Hold DM, etc)
**CLASS** Nonopioid antitussive
**PREG/CONT** C/NA

**IND & DOSE Control of nonproductive cough.** *Adult, child ≥12 yr:* Gelcaps, 30 mg PO q 6–8 hr; max, 120 mg/d. Lozenges, 5–15 mg PO q 1–4 hr; max, 120 mg/d. Liquid, syrup, strips, 10–20 mg PO q 4 hr or 30 mg q 6–8 hr; max, 120 mg/d. ER suspension, 60 mg PO q 12 hr; max, 120 mg/d. *Child 6–11 yr:* Lozenges, 5–10 mg PO q 1–4 hr; max, 60 mg/d. Liquid, syrup, strips, 15 mg PO q 6–8 hr; max, 60 mg/d. Freezer pops, 2 pops q 6–8 hr. *Child 2–6 yr:* Liquid, syrup, 7.5 mg PO q 6–8 hr; max, 30 mg/d. Freezer pops, 1 pop q 6–8 hr.
**ADV EFF Respiratory depression** (w/overdose)
**INTERACTIONS** MAOIs
**NC/PT** Ensure proper use and advisability of suppressing cough. Do not use within 14 d of MAOIs. Pt should avoid OTC products w/same ingredients, report persistent cough w/fever.

**diazePAM** (Diastat, Diastat AcuDial, Valium)
**CLASS** Antiepileptic, anxiolytic, benzodiazepine
**PREG/CONT** High risk/C-IV

**IND & DOSE Tx of anxiety disorders, skeletal muscle spasm, seizure disorders.** *Adult:* 2–10 mg PO bid–qid, or 0.2 mg/kg rectally. Treat no more than one episode q 5 d. May give second dose in 4–12 hr. *Child 6–11 yr:* 0.3 mg/kg rectally. *Child 2–5 yr:* 0.5 mg/kg rectally.
**ADJUST DOSE** Elderly pts, debilitating diseases
**ADV EFF** Apathy, bradycardia, confusion, constipation, **CV collapse,** depression, diarrhea, disorientation, fatigue, incontinence, lethargy, libido changes, light-headedness, paradoxical excitement, tachycardia, urine retention
**INTERACTIONS** Alcohol, cimetidine, disulfiram, hormonal contraceptives, omeprazole, ranitidine, theophylline
**NC/PT** Taper dose after long-term use. Suggest medical alert tag. Not for use in preg (barrier contraceptives advised). Pt should take safety precautions w/CNS effects.

**diazoxide** (Proglycem)
**CLASS** Glucose-elevating drug
**PREG/CONT** C/NA

**IND & DOSE Mgt of hypoglycemia due to hyperinsulinism in infant/child and to inoperable pancreatic islet cell malignancies.** *Adult, child:* 3–8 mg/kg/d PO in two–three divided doses q 8–12 hr. *Infant, newborn:* 8–15 mg/kg/d PO in two–three doses q 8–12 hr.
**ADJUST DOSE** Renal impairment
**ADV EFF** Anxiety, hirsutism, hyperglycemia, hypotension, **HF,** n/v, pulmonary HTN in newborns, **thrombocytopenia**
**INTERACTIONS** Chlorpropamide, glipizide, glyburide, hydantoins, tolazamide, tolbutamide, thiazides
**NC/PT** Check serum glucose, daily weight to monitor fluid retention. Protect suspension from light; have insulin on hand if hyperglycemia occurs. Pulmonary HTN in neonate reported when used during preg; advise against use in preg. Not for use in breastfeeding. Excessive hair growth will end when drug stopped. Pt should report weight gain of >3 lb/d.

**diclofenac** (Zorvolex), **diclofenac epolamine** (Flector, Voltaren), **diclofenac potassium** (Cambia, Cataflam, Zipsor), **diclofenac sodium** (Solaraze)

**CLASS** Analgesic

**PREG/CONT** Moderate risk (1st, 2nd trimesters); high risk (3rd trimester)/NA

**BBW** Possible increased risk of CV events, GI bleed, renal insufficiency; monitor accordingly. Not for use in CABG surgery.

**IND & DOSE Tx of pain, including dysmenorrhea.** *Adult:* 50 mg PO tid or 1 transdermal patch (*Flector*) applied to most painful area bid. **Tx of osteoarthritis.** *Adult:* 100–150 mg/d PO in divided doses (*Voltaren*), or 50 mg bid–tid PO (*Cataflam*). For upper extremities, apply 2 g gel to affected area qid; for lower extremities, apply 4 g gel to affected area qid (*Voltaren*). **Tx of RA.** *Adult:* 150–200 mg/d PO in divided doses (*Voltaren*), or 50 mg bid–tid PO (*Cataflam*). **Tx of ankylosing spondylitis.** *Adult:* 100–125 mg/d PO. Give as 25 mg qid, w/extra 25-mg dose at bedtime (*Voltaren*), or 25 mg qid PO w/additional 25 mg at bedtime if needed (*Cataflam*). **Tx of acute migraine.** 50-mg packet mixed in 30–60 mL water PO as single dose at onset of headache (*Cambia*). **Tx of mild to moderate pain.** *Adult:* 25 mg liquid-filled capsule PO qid (*Zipsor;* not interchangeable w/other forms of diclofenac). **Tx of actinic keratosis.** *Adult:* Cover lesion w/topical gel, smooth into skin; do not cover w/dressings or cosmetics (*Solaraze*). **Relief of postop inflammation from cataract extraction.** *Adult:* 1 drop to affected eye qid starting 24 hr after surgery for 2 wk. **Tx of osteoarthritis pain.** *Adult:* 35 mg PO tid (*Zorvolex*). **Tx of mild to moderate acute pain.** *Adult:* 18–35 mg PO tid (*Zorvolex*).

**ADV EFF Anaphylactoid reactions to fatal anaphylactic shock,** constipation, **CV events,** diarrhea, dizziness, dyspepsia, edema, GI pain, headache, HF, nausea, renal impairment

**INTERACTIONS** Anticoagulants, lithium

**NC/PT** Be aware forms are not interchangeable. Give w/meals if GI upset occurs. Add packets for oral suspension to 30–60 mL water. Remove old transdermal patch before applying new one to intact, dry skin. Institute emergency procedures if overdose occurs. Pt should swallow tablets whole and not cut/crush/chew them; avoid sun if using topical gel; take safety precautions for CNS effects; report difficulty breathing, chest pain.

**dicyclomine hydrochloride** (Bentyl)

**CLASS** Anticholinergic, antispasmodic, parasympatholytic

**PREG/CONT** B/NA

**IND & DOSE Tx of functional bowel or IBS.** *Adult:* 160 mg/d PO divided into four equal doses or 40–80 mg/d IM in four divided doses for no longer than 1–2 d; do not give IV.

**ADJUST DOSE** Elderly pts

**ADV EFF** Altered taste perception, blurred vision, decreased sweating, dry mouth, dysphagia, irritation at injection site, n/v/d, urinary hesitancy, urine retention

**INTERACTIONS** Amantadine, antacids, anticholinergics, antipsychotics, atenolol, digoxin, TCAs

**NC/PT** IM use is only temporary; switch to oral form as soon as possible. Ensure hydration, temp control. Pt should avoid hot environments, empty bladder before taking if urine retention occurs, perform mouth care for dry mouth.

## didanosine (ddI, dideoxyinosine)

(Videx, Videx EC)
**CLASS** Antiviral
**PREG/CONT** B/NA

**BBW** Monitor for pancreatitis (abd pain, elevated enzymes, n/v). Stop drug; resume only if pancreatitis ruled out. Monitor pts w/hepatic impairment; decrease may be needed if toxicity occurs. Fatal liver toxicity w/ lactic acidosis possible. Noncirrhotic portal HTN, sometimes fatal, has occurred.
**IND & DOSE Tx of pts w/HIV infection w/other antiretrovirals.** *Adult, child:* DR capsules: 60 kg or more, 400 mg/d PO; 25–60 kg, 250 mg/d PO; 20–25 kg, 200 mg/d PO. Oral sol: 60 kg or more, 200 mg PO bid or 400 mg/d PO; <60 kg, 125 mg PO bid or 250 mg/d PO. *Child >8 mo:* Pediatric powder, 120 mg/m² PO bid. *Child 2 wk–8 mo:* 100 mg/m² PO bid.
**ADJUST DOSE** Renal/hepatic impairment
**ADV EFF** Abd pain, headache, hematopoietic depression, **hepatotoxicity, lactic acidosis,** n/v, **pancreatitis**
**INTERACTIONS** Antifungals, allopurinol, fluoroquinolones, ganciclovir, methadone, tetracyclines
**NC/PT** Monitor CBC, pancreatic enzymes, LFTs. Give on empty stomach 1 hr before or 2 hr after meals. Pediatric sol can be made by pharmacists; refrigerate. Pt should not cut/crush/chew ER forms; report abd pain, urine/stool color changes.

## diflunisal (generic)

**CLASS** Analgesic, anti-inflammatory, antipyretic, NSAIDs
**PREG/CONT** C/NA

**BBW** Possible increased risk of CV events, GI bleeding; monitor accordingly. Do not use to treat periop pain after CABG surgery.
**IND & DOSE Tx of mild to moderate pain.** *Adult, child >12 yr:* 1,000 mg PO initially, then 500 mg q 8–12 hr PO. **Tx of osteoarthritis, RA.** *Adult, child >12 yr:* 500–1,000 mg/d PO in two divided doses; maint, no more than 1,500 mg/d.
**ADV EFF Anaphylactoid reactions to anaphylactic shock, CV event,** diarrhea, dizziness, dyspepsia, GI pain, headache, insomnia, nausea, rash
**INTERACTIONS** Acetaminophen, antacids, aspirin
**NC/PT** Give w/food if GI upset. Pt should swallow tablets whole and not cut/crush/chew them; take safety precautions for CNS effects; report unusual bleeding, difficulty breathing.

**DANGEROUS DRUG**

## digoxin (Lanoxin)

**CLASS** Cardiac glycoside
**PREG/CONT** C/NA

**IND & DOSE Tx of HF, atrial fibrillation.** *Adult:* Loading dose, 0.25 mg/d IV or PO for pts <70 yr w/good renal function; 0.125 mg/d PO or IV for pts >70 yr or w/impaired renal function; 0.0625 mg/d PO or IV w/marked renal impairment. Maint, 0.125–0.5 mg/d PO. *Child: Premature,* 20 mcg/kg PO or 15–25 mcg/kg IV; *neonate,* 30 mcg/kg PO or 20–30 mcg/kg IV; *1–24 mo,* 40–50 mcg/kg PO or 30–50 mcg/kg IV; *2–10 yr,* 30–40 mcg/kg PO or 25–35 mcg/kg IV; *>10 yr,* 10–15 mcg/kg PO or 8–12 mcg/kg IV as loading dose. Maint, 25%–35% of loading dose in divided doses; range, 0.125–0.5 mg/d PO.
**ADJUST DOSE** Elderly pts, impaired renal function
**ADV EFF** Arrhythmias, GI upset, headache, weakness, yellow vision
**INTERACTIONS** Amiodarone, bleomycin, charcoal, cholestyramine, colestipol, cyclophosphamide, cyclosporine, dobutamine in sol, erythromycin, ginseng, hawthorn, licorice, loop diuretics, metoclopramide, methotrexate, oral

aminoglycosides, penicillamine, psyllium, quinidine, St. John's wort, tetracyclines, thiazide diuretics, thyroid hormone, verapamil
**NC/PT** Monitor apical P; withhold if <60 in adult, <90 in child. Check dose carefully. Do not give IM. Give on empty stomach. Monitor for therapeutic drug levels: 0.5–2 ng/mL. Pt should learn to take P; weigh self daily; consult prescriber before taking OTC drugs or herbs; avoid St. John's wort; report slow or irregular P, yellow vision, weight change of 3 lb or more/d.

## digoxin immune fab
(DigiFab)
**CLASS** Antidote
**PREG/CONT** C/NA

**IND & DOSE** **Tx of potentially life-threatening digoxin toxicity (serum digoxin >10 ng/mL, serum potassium >5 mEq/L in setting of digoxin toxicity).** *Adult, child:* Dose determined by serum digoxin level or estimate of amount of digoxin ingested. If no estimate possible and serum digoxin level unavailable, use 800 mg IV (20 vials). See manufacturer's details; dose varies by digoxin level.
**ADV EFF** **Anaphylaxis, HF,** low cardiac output, hypokalemia
**NC/PT** Ensure no sheep allergies. Monitor serum digoxin before tx. Have life-support equipment on hand. Do not redigitalize until drug has cleared (several days–a wk). Serum digoxin level unreliable for up to 3 d after administration. Pt should report difficulty breathing.

## dihydroergotamine mesylate (D.H.E. 45, Migranal)
**CLASS** Antimigraine, ergot
**PREG/CONT** X/NA

**BBW** Serious to life-threatening ischemia if taken w/potent CYP3A4 inhibitors, including protease inhibitors, macrolide antibiotics; concurrent use contraindicated.
**IND & DOSE** **Tx of migraine w/ or w/o aura; acute tx of cluster headaches.** *Adult:* 1 mg IM, IV, or subcut at first sign of headache; may repeat at 1-hr intervals. Max, 3 mg, or 1 intranasal spray (0.5 mg) in each nostril followed in 15 min by another spray in each nostril (max, 3 mg).
**ADV EFF** **CV events,** nausea, numbness, rhinitis, tingling
**INTERACTIONS** CYP3A4 inhibitors (contraindicated), peripheral vasoconstrictors, sumatriptan
**NC/PT** Not for use in preg/breastfeeding. May give antiemetic if nausea severe. Monitor BP; look for s&sx of vasospasm. Pt should prime pump four times before use (nasal spray), limit total daily dose; report numbness/tingling, chest pain.

## dilTIAZem hydrochloride (Cardizem, Cardizem LA, Cartia XT, Diltzac, Taztia XT, Tiazac)
**CLASS** Antianginal, antihypertensive, calcium channel blocker
**PREG/CONT** C/NA

**IND & DOSE** **Tx of angina pectoris.** *Adult:* Initially, 30 mg PO qid before meals and at bedtime; gradually increase at 1- to 2-day intervals to 180–360 mg PO in three–four divided doses. Or, 120–360 mg/d (ER, SR forms) PO, depending on brand. **Tx of essential HTN.** *Adult:* 180–240 mg PO daily (*Cardizem CD, Cartia XT*). 120–540 mg PO daily (*Cardizem LA*). 180–240 mg PO daily. 120–240 mg PO daily (*Tiazac, Taztia XT*). **Tx of supraventricular tachycardia, atrial fibrillation, atrial flutter.** *Adult:* Direct IV bolus, 0.25 mg/kg over 2 min; second bolus of 0.35 mg/kg over 2 min after 15 min if response inadequate. Or, 5–10 mg/hr by continuous

IV infusion w/increases up to 15 mg/hr; may continue for up to 24 hr.
**ADV EFF** Asthenia, **asystole,** bradycardia, dizziness, edema, flushing, light-headedness, nausea
**INTERACTIONS** Beta blockers, cyclosporine, grapefruit juice
**NC/PT** Monitor closely while establishing dose. Pt should swallow ER/SR tablets whole and not cut/crush/chew them; avoid grapefruit juice; report irregular heartbeat, swelling.

## dimenhyDRINATE
(Dimetabs, Dramanate, Dymenate)
**CLASS** Anticholinergic, antihistamine, anti–motion sickness drug
**PREG/CONT** B/NA

**IND & DOSE** **Px/tx of n/v or vertigo of motion sickness.** *Adult:* 50–100 mg PO q 4–6 hr; for px, pt should take first dose 30 min before exposure to motion. Max, 400 mg/24 hr. Or, 50 mg IM as needed, or 50 mg in 10 mL sodium chloride injection IV over 2 min. *Child 6–12 yr:* 25–50 mg PO q 6–8 hr; max, 150 mg/d.
**ADJUST DOSE** Elderly pts
**ADV EFF** **Anaphylaxis,** confusion, dizziness, drowsiness, headache, heaviness/weakness of hands, lassitude, nervousness, restlessness, vertigo
**INTERACTIONS** Alcohol, CNS depressants
**NC/PT** Have epinephrine on hand during IV use. Pt should use 30 min before motion sickness–inducing event; avoid alcohol; take safety precautions w/CNS effects; report difficulty breathing.

## dimercaprol (BAL)
**CLASS** Antidote, chelate
**PREG/CONT** C/NA

**IND & DOSE** **Tx of arsenic/gold poisoning.** *Adult, child:* 25 mg/kg deep IM four × /d for 2 d, two ×/d on third day, then once daily for 10 d. **Tx of mercury poisoning.** *Adult, child:* 5 mg/kg IM, then 2.5 mg/kg once daily or bid for 10 d. **Tx of lead poisoning w/edetate calcium.** *Adult, child:* 4 mg/kg IM for first dose, then at 4-hr intervals w/edetate calcium for 2–7 d.
**ADJUST DOSE** Hepatic impairment
**ADV EFF** Abd pain, burning sensation in lips/mouth, constricted feeling in throat/chest, headache, nausea, sweating
**INTERACTIONS** Alcohol, CNS depressants
**NC/PT** Use extreme caution w/peanut allergy. Use deep IM injection. Pt should report constricted feeling in throat/chest, difficulty breathing.

## dimethyl fumarate
(Tecfidera)
**CLASS** MS drug, nicotinic receptor agonist
**PREG/CONT** Moderate risk/NA

**IND & DOSE** **Tx of relapsing MS.** *Adult:* 120 mg PO bid for 7 d; then 240 mg PO bid.
**ADV EFF** Abd pain, **anaphylaxis, angioedema,** dizziness, dyspepsia, flushing, herpes zoster/opportunistic infections, liver injury, lymphopenia, n/v/d, **progressive multifocal leukoencephalopathy,** rash
**NC/PT** Obtain baseline and periodic CBC, LFTs; withhold w/serious infection. Use caution in preg/breastfeeding. Pt should swallow capsule whole and not cut/crush/chew it (may open and sprinkle contents on food); avoid infections; dress in layers if flushing occurs; report continued n/v/d, severe rash, worsening of MS sx.

## dinoprostone (Cervidil, Prepidil, Prostin E2)
**CLASS** Abortifacient, prostaglandin
**PREG/CONT** Low risk/NA

**IND & DOSE** **Termination of preg 12–20 wk from first day of last**

**menstrual period; evacuation of uterus in mgt of missed abortion.** *Adult:* 1 suppository (20 mg) high into vagina; keep pt supine for 10 min after insertion. May give additional suppositories at 3- to 5-hr intervals, based on uterine response and tolerance, for up to 2 d. **Initiation of cervical ripening before labor induction.** *Adult:* 0.5 mg gel via provided cervical catheter w/pt in dorsal position and cervix visualized using speculum. May repeat dose if no response in 6 hr. Wait 6–12 hr before beginning oxytocin IV to initiate labor. For insert: Place 1 insert transversely in posterior fornix of vagina. Keep pt supine for 2 hr (1 insert delivers 0.3 mg/hr over 12 hr). Remove, using retrieval system, at onset of active labor or 12 hr after insertion.

**ADV EFF** Dizziness, headache, hypotension, n/v/d, **perforated uterus**

**NC/PT** Store suppositories in freezer; bring to room temp before insertion. Keep pt supine after vaginal insertion. Ensure abortion complete. Give antiemetics, antidiarrheals if needed. Monitor for uterine tone, bleeding. Give support, encouragement for procedure/progressing labor. Name confusion among *Prostin VR Pediatric* (alprostadil), *Prostin FZ* (dinoprost), *Prostin E2* (dinoprostone), *Prostin 15* (carboprost in Europe); use extreme caution.

## dinutuximab (Unituxin)

**CLASS** Antineoplastic, monoclonal antibody

**PREG/CONT** High risk/NA

**BBW** Risk of life-threatening infusion reactions; prehydrate, premedicate. Interrupt severe reaction and stop if anaphylaxis occurs. Risk of severe neuropathic pain: Give IV opioid before, during, and for 2 hr after infusion; stop w/severe unresponsive pain, severe sensory neuropathy, or moderate to severe motor neuropathy.

**IND & DOSE** **As part of chemo in tx of child w/high-risk neuroblastoma w/at least partial response to prior first-line regimens.** *Child:* 17.5 mg/m²/d IV over 10–20 hr for 4 consecutive days for 5 cycles: days 4, 5, 6, 7 for cycles 1, 3, and 5 (24-day cycles); days 8, 9, 10, and 11 for cycles 2 and 4 (32-day cycles).

**ADV EFF** **Bone marrow suppression, capillary leak syndrome,** fever, **hemolytic uremic syndrome, infusion reactions,** hypokalemia, hypotension, infection, n/v/d, **neuropathies**

**NC/PT** Prehydrate w/0.9% Sodium Chloride Injection 10 mL/kg over 1 hr before starting infusion. Premedicate w/IV morphine before and continuously during infusion; continue for 2 hr after infusion. Give antihistamine IV over 10–15 min starting 20 min before infusion and q 4–6 hr during infusion, and acetaminophen 10–15 mg/kg PO starting 20 min before and q 4–6 hr during infusion. Give ibuprofen 5–10 mg/kg PO q 4–6 hr for fever, pain control. Not for use in preg/breastfeeding. Alert pt/caregiver of risks, adverse effects to anticipate. Pt should take safety precautions w/CNS effects; report s&sx of infection, difficulty breathing, swelling, dizziness, severe pain, vision changes.

## diphenhydrAMINE hydrochloride (generic)

**CLASS** Antihistamine, anti–motion sickness, antiparkinsonian, sedative

**PREG/CONT** B/NA

**IND & DOSE** **Relief of sx of various allergic reactions, motion sickness.** *Adult:* 25–50 mg PO q 4–6 hr; max, 300 mg/24 hr. Or, 10–50 mg IV or deep IM or up to 100 mg if needed; max, 400 mg/d. *Child 6–12 yr:* 12.5–25 mg PO tid–qid, or 5 mg/kg/d PO, or 150 mg/m²/d PO; max, 150 mg/d. Or, 5 mg/kg/d or 150 mg/m²/d IV or deep IM injection. Max, 300 mg/d divided into four doses. **Nighttime**

**sleep aid.** *Adult:* 50 mg PO at bedtime. **Cough suppression.** *Adult:* 25 mg PO q 4 hr; max, 150 mg/d (syrup). *Child 6–12 yr:* 12.5 mg PO q 4 hr. Max, 75 mg/24 hr (syrup).
**ADJUST DOSE** Elderly pts
**ADV EFF** **Agranulocytosis, anaphylactic shock,** bronchial secretion thickening, disturbed coordination, dizziness, drowsiness, epigastric distress, **hemolytic anemia, hypoplastic anemia, leukopenia, pancytopenia, thrombocytopenia**
**INTERACTIONS** Alcohol, CNS depressants, MAOIs
**NC/PT** Monitor response; use smallest dose possible. Use syrup if swallowing tablets difficult. Pt should avoid alcohol; take safety precautions w/CNS effect; report difficulty breathing.

## dipyridamole (Persantine)
**CLASS** Antianginal, antiplatelet, diagnostic agent
**PREG/CONT** B/NA

**IND & DOSE** **Px of thromboembolism in pts w/artificial heart valves, w/warfarin.** *Adult:* 75–100 mg PO qid. **Diagnostic aid to assess CAD in pts unable to exercise.** *Adult:* 0.142 mg/kg/min IV over 4 min.
**ADV EFF** Abd distress, dizziness, headache
**INTERACTIONS** Adenosine
**NC/PT** Monitor continually w/IV use. Give oral drug at least 1 hr before meals. Pt should take safety precautions for light-headedness.

## disopyramide phosphate (Norpace, Norpace CR)
**CLASS** Antiarrhythmic
**PREG/CONT** C/NA

**BBW** Monitor for possible refractory arrhythmias that can be life-threatening; reserve use for life-threatening arrhythmias.

**IND & DOSE** **Tx of life-threatening ventricular arrhythmias.** *Adult, child:* 400–800 mg/d PO in divided doses q 6 hr, or q 12 hr if using CR forms. **Rapid control of ventricular arrhythmias.** *Adult:* 300 mg (immediate-release) PO. If no response within 6 hr, 200 mg PO q 6 hr; may increase to 250–300 mg q 6 hr if no response in 48 hr. For pts w/cardiomyopathy, no loading dose; 100 mg (immediate-release) PO q 6–8 hr.
**ADJUST DOSE** Renal/hepatic failure
**ADV EFF** Blurred vision, constipation, dry nose/eye/throat, **HF,** itching, malaise, muscle aches and pains, urinary hesitancy, urine retention
**INTERACTIONS** Antiarrhythmics, erythromycin, phenytoin, quinidine
**NC/PT** Monitor ECG carefully. Make pediatric suspension (1–10 mg/mL) by adding contents of immediate-release capsule to cherry syrup, if desired. Store in amber glass bottle; refrigerate up to 1 mo. Evaluate pt for safe, effective serum levels (2–8 mcg/mL). Pt should swallow CR forms whole and not cut/crush/chew them; not stop taking w/o consulting prescriber; maintain hydration; empty bladder before taking; take safety precautions w/CNS effects; report swelling.

## disulfiram (Antabuse)
**CLASS** Antialcoholic, enzyme inhibitor
**PREG/CONT** C/NA

**BBW** Never give to intoxicated pt or w/o pt's knowledge. Do not give until pt has abstained from alcohol for at least 12 hr.
**IND & DOSE** **Aid in mgt of selected chronic alcoholics who want to remain in state of enforced sobriety.** *Adult:* 500 mg/d PO in single dose for 1–2 wk. If sedative effect occurs, give at bedtime or decrease dose. Maint, 125–500 mg/d PO; max, 500 mg/d.
**ADV EFF** Dizziness, fatigue, headache, metal- or garlic-like aftertaste,

skin eruptions; if taken w/alcohol, **arrhythmias, CV collapse, death, HF, MI**
**INTERACTIONS** Alcohol, caffeine, chlordiazepoxide, diazepam, metronidazole, oral anticoagulants, theophyllines
**NC/PT** Do not give until pt has abstained from alcohol for at least 12 hr. Monitor LFTs, CBC before and q 6 mo of tx. May crush tablets and mix w/liquid beverages. Institute supportive measures if pt drinks alcohol during tx. Pt should abstain from all forms of alcohol (serious to fatal reactions possible if combined); wear/carry medical tag; take safety precautions for CNS effects; report chest pain, edema.

**DANGEROUS DRUG**

## DOBUTamine hydrochloride (generic)

**CLASS** Beta$_1$-selective adrenergic agonist, sympathomimetic
**PREG/CONT** B/NA

**IND & DOSE Short-term tx of cardiac decompensation.** *Adult:* Usual rate, 2–20 mcg/kg/min IV to increase cardiac output; rarely, rates up to 40 mcg/kg/min. *Child:* 0.5–1 mcg/kg/min as continuous IV infusion. Maint, 2–20 mcg/kg/min.
**ADV EFF** Headache, HTN, nausea, PVCs, tachycardia
**INTERACTIONS** Methyldopa, TCAs
**NC/PT** Monitor urine flow, cardiac output, pulmonary wedge pressure, ECG, BP closely during infusion; adjust dose, rate accordingly. Arrange to digitalize pt w/atrial fibrillation w/rapid ventricular rate before giving dobutamine (dobutamine facilitates AV conduction). Name confusion between dobutamine and dopamine.

**DANGEROUS DRUG**

## DOCEtaxel (Docefrez, Taxotere)

**CLASS** Antineoplastic
**PREG/CONT** High risk/NA

**BBW** Do not give unless blood counts are within acceptable range (neutrophils >1,500 cells/m$^2$). Do not give w/hepatic impairment; increased risk of toxicity and death. Monitor LFTs carefully. Monitor for hypersensitivity reactions, possibly severe. Do not give w/hx of hypersensitivity. Monitor carefully for fluid retention; treat accordingly.
**IND & DOSE Tx of breast cancer.** *Adult:* 60–100 mg/m$^2$ IV infused over 1 hr q 3 wk. **Tx of NSCLC.** *Adult:* 75 mg/m$^2$ IV over 1 hr q 3 wk. **First-line tx of NSCLC.** *Adult:* 75 mg/m$^2$ over 1 hr, then 75 mg/m$^2$ cisplatin IV over 30–60 min q 3 wk. **Tx of androgen-independent metastatic prostate cancer.** *Adult:* 75 mg/m$^2$ IV q 3 wk as 1-hr infusion w/5 mg prednisone PO bid constantly throughout tx. Reduce dose to 60 mg/m$^2$ if febrile neutropenia, severe or cumulative cutaneous reactions, moderate neurosensory s&sx, or neutrophil count <500/mm$^3$ occurs for longer than 1 wk. Stop tx if reactions continue w/reduced dose. **Tx of operable node-positive breast cancer.** *Adult:* 75 mg/m$^2$ IV 1 hr after doxorubicin 50 mg/m$^2$ and cyclophosphamide 500 mg/m$^2$ q 3 wk for 6 courses. **Induction for squamous cell cancer of head/neck before radiotherapy.** *Adult:* 75 mg/m$^2$ as 1-hr IV infusion, then cisplatin 75 mg/m$^2$ IV over 1 hr on day 1, then 5-FU 750 mg/m$^2$/d IV for 5 d. Repeat q 3 wk for four cycles before radiotherapy starts. **Induction for squamous cell cancer of head/neck before chemoradiotherapy.** *Adult:* 75 mg/m$^2$ as 1-hr IV infusion, then cisplatin 100 mg/m$^2$ as 30-min–3-hr infusion, then 5-FU 1,000 mg/m$^2$/d as continuous infusion on days 1–4. Give q 3 wk for three cycles before

chemoradiotherapy starts. **Tx of advanced gastric adenocarcinoma.** *Adult:* 75 mg/m² IV as 1-hr infusion, then cisplatin 75 mg/m² IV as 1–3-hr infusion (both on day 1), then 5-FU 750 mg/m²/d IV as 24-hr infusion for 5 d. Repeat cycle q 3 wk.
**ADJUST DOSE** Hepatic impairment
**ADV EFF** **Acute myeloid leukemia,** alopecia, arthralgia, asthenia, **bone marrow suppression, CNS impairment, cystoid macular edema, fluid retention,** hypersensitivity reactions, infection, myalgia, n/v/d, pain, **skin toxicity,** stomatitis
**INTERACTIONS** Cyclosporine, erythromycin, immunosuppressants, ketoconazole
**NC/PT** Handle drug carefully. Premedicate w/oral corticosteroids to reduce fluid retention. Monitor CBC before each dose; adjust dose as needed. Monitor LFTs; do not give w/ hepatic impairment. Monitor for fluid retention; treat accordingly. Protect from infection. Give antiemetics if needed. High alcohol level in *Taxotere* may impair pt. Pt should cover head at temp extremes (hair loss possible); mark calendar for tx days; take safety precautions for CNS effects; report rash, s&sx of infection/bleeding. Name confusion between *Taxotere* (docetaxel) and *Taxol* (paclitaxel); use extreme caution.

## dofetilide (Tikosyn)
**CLASS** Antiarrhythmic
**PREG/CONT** C/NA

**BBW** Monitor ECG before and periodically during administration. Monitor pt continually for at least 3 d. May adjust dose based on maint of sinus rhythm. Risk of induced arrhythmias.
**IND & DOSE** **Conversion of atrial fibrillation (AF) or flutter to normal sinus rhythm; maint of sinus rhythm after conversion from AF.** *Adult:* Dose based on ECG response and CrCl. CrCl >60 mL/min, 500 mcg PO bid; CrCl 40–60 mL/min, 250 mcg PO bid; CrCl 20–<40 mL/min, 125 mcg PO bid; CrCl <20 mL/min, use contraindicated.
**ADJUST DOSE** Renal impairment
**ADV EFF** Fatigue, dizziness, headache, **ventricular arrhythmias**
**INTERACTIONS** Antihistamines, cimetidine, ketoconazole, phenothiazines, TCAs, trimethoprim, verapamil; contraindicated w/amiodarone, disopyramide, procainamide, quinidine, sotalol
**NC/PT** Determine time of arrhythmia onset. Monitor ECG before and periodically during tx. Have pt in facility for continual monitoring and cardiac resuscitation for 3 d when beginning or reinitiating tx. Monitor serum creatinine before and q 3 mo during tx. Do not attempt cardioversion within 24 hr of starting tx. Not for use in breastfeeding. Pt should take bid at about same time each day; keep follow-up appointments; take safety precautions w/CNS effects.

## dolutegravir (Tivicay)
**CLASS** Antiviral, integrase inhibitor
**PREG/CONT** High risk/NA

**IND & DOSE** **Tx of HIV-1 infection, w/other antiretrovirals; tx in combo w/rilpivirine as complete regimen to replace current antiretroviral regimen in pts virologically suppressed (HIV-1 RNA <50 copies/mL) on a stable antiretroviral regimen for at least 6 mo w/no history of tx failure or known substitutions associated w/resistance to either antiretroviral.** *Adult, child at least 40 kg: Treatment-naïve,* 50 mg/d PO; *treatment-naïve or experienced w/efavirenz, fosamprenavir/ritonavir, tipranavir/ritonavir, rifampin, or suspected resistance,* 50 mg PO bid. *Child 30–<40 kg:* 35 mg/d PO.
**ADV EFF** Abd pain, diarrhea, headache, hepatotoxicity in pts w/HBV or

HCV, **hypersensitivity reactions,** insomnia, nausea
**INTERACTIONS** Antacids, buffered drugs, calcium supplements, efavirenz, fosamprenavir/ritonavir, iron supplements, laxatives, rifampin, sucralfate, tipranavir/ritonavir
**NC/PT** Obtain preg test and screen for HBV or HCV before tx. Must be given w/other antiretrovirals; give cation-containing drugs at least 2 hr before or 6 hr after dolutegravir. Pt should continue other HIV drugs; space antacids apart from dosing; avoid preg/breastfeeding during tx; take precautions to avoid spread; not run out of prescription; report s&sx of infection, difficulty breathing, urine/stool color changes, rash.

## donepezil hydrochloride

(Aricept, Aricept ODT)
**CLASS** Alzheimer drug, anticholinesterase inhibitor
**PREG/CONT** C/NA

**IND & DOSE Tx of Alzheimer-type dementia, including severe dementia.** *Adult:* 5 mg/d PO at bedtime; may increase to 10 mg daily after 4–6 wk; 10 mg PO daily for severe disease. For severe disease, may use 23 mg/d after 10 mg/d for at least 3 mo.
**ADV EFF** Abd pain, anorexia, bradycardia, dyspepsia, fatigue, GI bleed, **hepatotoxicity,** insomnia, muscle cramps, n/v/d, rash
**INTERACTIONS** Anticholinergics, cholinesterase inhibitors, NMJ blockers, NSAIDs, theophylline
**NC/PT** Monitor hepatic function. Give at bedtime. Pt should place disintegrating tablet on tongue, allow to dissolve, then drink water; take safety precautions; report severe n/v/d. Name confusion between *Aricept* (donepezil) and *Aciphex* (rabeprazole).

**DANGEROUS DRUG**

## DOPamine hydrochloride (generic)

**CLASS** Dopaminergic, sympathomimetic
**PREG/CONT** C/NA

**BBW** To prevent sloughing/necrosis after extravasation, infiltrate area w/10–15 mL saline containing 5–10 mg phentolamine as soon as possible after extravasation.
**IND & DOSE Correction of hemodynamic imbalance, low cardiac output, hypotension.** *Adult:* Pts likely to respond to modest increments of cardiac contractility and renal perfusion, 2–5 mcg/kg/min IV initially. More seriously ill pts, 5 mcg/kg/min IV initially. Increase in increments of 5–10 mcg/kg/min to rate of 20–50 mcg/kg/min.
**ADV EFF** Angina, dyspnea, ectopic beats, hypotension, n/v, palpitations, tachycardia
**INTERACTIONS** MAOIs, methyldopa, phenytoin, TCAs; do not mix in IV sol w/other drugs
**NC/PT** Use extreme caution in calculating doses. Base dosing on pt response. Give in large vein; avoid extravasation. Monitor urine output, cardiac output, BP during infusion. Name confusion between dopamine and dobutamine.

## doripenem (Doribax)

**CLASS** Carbapenem antibiotic
**PREG/CONT** B/NA

**IND & DOSE Tx of complicated intra-abd infections, UTIs caused by susceptible bacteria strains.** *Adult:* 500 mg IV over 1 hr q 8 hr for 5–14 d (intra-abd infection) or 10 d (UTI, pyelonephritis).
**ADJUST DOSE** Renal impairment
**ADV EFF** Diarrhea including CDAD, headache, **hypersensitivity reactions,** increased risk of death in ventilator-associated bacterial pneumonia, nausea, phlebitis, rash, **seizures**

**INTERACTIONS** Probenecid, valproic acid
**NC/PT** Culture, sensitivity before tx. Monitor injection site for phlebitis. Not for use in preg (barrier contraceptives advised)/breastfeeding. Monitor for CDAD. Provide supportive tx for up to 2 mo after tx ends. Pt should report difficulty breathing, severe diarrhea.

## dornase alfa (Pulmozyme)
**CLASS** Cystic fibrosis drug
**PREG/CONT** B/NA

**IND & DOSE** **Mgt of cystic fibrosis to improve pulmonary function, w/other drugs.** *Adult, child:* 2.5 mg inhaled through recommended nebulizer; bid use beneficial to some.
**ADV EFF** Chest pain, laryngitis, pharyngitis, rash, rhinitis
**NC/PT** Assess respiratory function regularly. Store in refrigerator; not stable after 24 hr at room temp. Do not mix in nebulizer w/other drugs; review proper use of nebulizer. Pt should continue other drugs for cystic fibrosis.

## doxapram hydrochloride (Dopram)
**CLASS** Analeptic, respiratory stimulant
**PREG/CONT** B/NA

**IND & DOSE** **Stimulation of respiration in pts w/drug-induced postanesthesia respiratory depression.** *Adult:* Single injection of 0.5–1 mg/kg IV; max, 1.5 mg/kg as total single injection or 2 mg/kg when given as multiple injections at 5-min intervals. **Tx of COPD-associated acute hypercapnia.** *Adult:* Mix 400 mg in 180 mL IV infusion; start infusion at 1–2 mg/min (0.5–1 mL/min); no longer than 2 hr. Max, 3 mg/min. **Mgt of drug-induced CNS depression.** 1–2 mg/kg IV; repeat in 5 min. Repeat q 1–2 hr until pt awakens. Or, priming dose of 1–2 mg/kg IV; if no response, infuse 250 mg in 250 mL dextrose or saline sol at rate of 1–3 mg/min, discontinue after 2 hr if pt awakens; repeat in 30 min–2 hr if relapse occurs. Max, 3 g/d.
**ADV EFF** **Bronchospasm,** cough, HTN, increased reflexes, **seizures**
**INTERACTIONS** Enflurane, halothane, MAOIs, muscle relaxants, sympathomimetics, theophylline
**NC/PT** Give IV only. Monitor for extravasation. Continuously monitor pt until fully awake. Discontinue if sudden hypotension, deterioration occur.

## doxazosin mesylate (Cardura, Cardura XL)
**CLASS** Antihypertensive, alpha-adrenergic blocker
**PREG/CONT** C/NA

**IND & DOSE** **Tx of mild to moderate HTN.** *Adult:* 1 mg PO daily; maint, 2, 4, 8, or 16 mg PO daily. May increase q 2 wk. Do not use ER tablets. **Tx of BPH.** *Adult:* 1 mg PO daily; maint, 2, 4, 8 mg daily. Or, ER tablets, 4 mg PO once daily at breakfast. Max, 8 mg/d PO.
**ADV EFF** Diarrhea, dizziness, dyspepsia, edema, fatigue, headache, lethargy, nausea, orthostatic hypotension, palpitations, priapism, sexual dysfx, tachycardia
**INTERACTIONS** Alcohol, antihypertensives, nitrates, sildenafil
**NC/PT** Monitor pt carefully w/first dose; chance of orthostatic hypotension, dizziness, syncope greatest w/first dose. Monitor for edema, BPH s&sx. Pt should swallow ER tablets whole and not cut/crush/chew them; take safety precautions.

## doxepin hydrochloride (Silenor, Zonalon)
**CLASS** Antidepressant, TCA
**PREG/CONT** C/NA

**BBW** Increased risk of suicidality in child, adolescent, young adult; monitor carefully.

**IND & DOSE** **Tx of mild to moderate anxiety, depression.** *Adult:* 25 mg PO tid. Individualize dose; range, 75–150 mg/d. **Tx of more severe anxiety, depression.** *Adult:* 50 mg PO tid; max, 300 mg/d. **Tx of mild sx or emotional sx accompanying organic disease.** *Adult:* 25–50 mg PO. **Tx of pruritus.** *Adult:* Apply cream 4 ×/d at least 3–4 hr apart for 8 d. Do not cover dressing. **Tx of insomnia w/difficulty in sleep maintenance** (*Silenor*). *Adult:* 3–6 mg PO 30 min before bed.
**ADV EFF** Anticholinergic effects, confusion, constipation, disturbed concentration, dry mouth, **MI,** orthostatic hypotension, photosensitivity, sedation, **stroke,** urine retention, withdrawal sx w/prolonged use
**INTERACTIONS** Alcohol, anticholinergics, barbiturates, cimetidine, clonidine, disulfiram, ephedrine, epinephrine, fluoxetine, furazolidone, hormonal contraceptives, levodopa, MAOIs, methylphenidate, nicotine, norepinephrine, phenothiazines, QT-prolonging drugs, thyroid medication
**NC/PT** Restrict drug access in depressed, suicidal pts. Give major portion at bedtime. Dilute oral concentrate w/approx 120 mL water, milk, fruit juice just before administration. Pt should be aware of sedative effects (avoid driving, etc); not mix w/other sleep-inducing drugs, alcohol; avoid prolonged exposure to sun, sunlamps; report thoughts of suicide. Name confusion between *Sinequan* and saquinavir.

## doxercalciferol (Hectorol)

**CLASS** Vitamin D analog
**PREG/CONT** B/NA

**IND & DOSE** **To reduce parathyroid hormone in mgt of secondary hyperparathyroidism in pts undergoing chronic renal dialysis; secondary hyperparathyroidism in pts w/stage 3, 4 chronic kidney disease w/o dialysis.** *Adult:* 10 mcg PO three ×/wk at dialysis; max, 20 mcg three ×/wk. W/o dialysis, 1 mcg/d PO; max, 3.5 mcg/d.
**ADV EFF** Dizziness, dyspnea, edema, headache, malaise, n/v
**INTERACTIONS** Cholestyramine, magnesium-containing antacids, mineral oil, phenothiazines, QT-prolonging drugs, thyroid medication
**NC/PT** Monitor for vitamin D toxicity. Give w/non-aluminum-containing phosphate binders. Monitor vitamin D level predialysis. Pt should take safety precautions w/CNS effects.

DANGEROUS DRUG

## DOXOrubicin hydrochloride (Doxil)

**CLASS** Antineoplastic
**PREG/CONT** High risk/NA

**BBW** Accidental substitution of liposomal form for conventional form has caused serious adverse reactions; check carefully before giving. Monitor for extravasation, burning, stinging. If these occur, discontinue; restart in another vein. For local subcut extravasation, local infiltration w/corticosteroid may be ordered. Flood area w/normal saline; apply cold compress. If ulceration, arrange consult w/plastic surgeon. Monitor pt's response often at start of tx: serum uric acid, cardiac output (listen for $S_3$). CBC changes may require dose decrease; consult physician. Acute to fatal infusion reactions have occurred. Risk of HF/myocardial damage, myelosuppression, liver damage. Record doses given to monitor total dosage; toxic effects often dose-related as total dose approaches 550 mg/m$^2$.
**IND & DOSE** **To produce regression in ALL, AML; Wilms' tumor; neuroblastoma; soft-tissue, bone sarcoma; breast, ovarian carcinoma; transitional cell bladder carcinoma; thyroid carcinoma; Hodgkin, non-Hodgkin lymphoma; bronchogenic carcinoma.** *Adult:* 60–75 mg/m$^2$ as single IV injection given at 21-day intervals. Alternate schedule: 30 mg/m$^2$ IV on

each of 3 successive d, repeated q 4 wk. **Tx of AIDS-related Kaposi sarcoma** (liposomal form). *Adult:* 20 mg/$m^2$ IV q 3 wk starting w/initial rate of 1 mg/min. **Tx of ovarian cancer that has progressed or recurred after platinum-based chemo** (liposomal form). *Adult:* 50 mg/$m^2$ IV at 1 mg/min; if no adverse effects, complete infusion in 1 hr. Repeat q 4 wk. **Tx of multiple myeloma** (liposomal form). *Adult:* 30 mg/$m^2$ IV on day 4 after bortezomib.

**ADJUST DOSE** Elevated bilirubin

**ADV EFF** **Anaphylaxis, cardiotoxicity,** complete but reversible alopecia, hand-foot syndrome, hypersensitivity reactions, infusion reactions, mucositis, **myelosuppression**, n/v, red urine

**INTERACTIONS** Digoxin

**NC/PT** Do not give IM or subcut. Monitor for extravasation. Ensure hydration. Not for use in preg (contraceptives advised)/breastfeeding. Pt should be aware that urine will be pink/red and hair loss is common; avoid infection; report difficulty breathing, chest pain. Name confusion between conventional doxorubicin and liposomal doxorubicin.

## doxycycline (Atridox, Doryx, Doxy 100, Oracea, Vibramycin)

**CLASS** Tetracycline

**PREG/CONT** Moderate risk/NA

**IND & DOSE** **Tx of infections caused by susceptible bacteria strains; tx of infections when penicillin contraindicated.** *Adult, child >8 yr, >45 kg:* 200 mg IV in one or two infusions (each over 1–4 hr) on first tx day, then 100–200 mg/d IV, depending on infection severity. Or, 200 mg PO on day 1, then 100 mg/d PO. *Child >8 yr, <45 kg:* 4.4 mg/kg IV in one or two infusions, then 2.2–4.4 mg/kg/d IV in one or two infusions. Or, 4.4 mg/kg PO in two divided doses on first tx day, then 2.2–4.4 mg/kg/d on subsequent days. **Tx of rosacea.** *Adult:* 40 mg/d PO in a.m. on empty stomach w/full glass of water for up to 9 mo. **Tx of primary or secondary syphilis.** *Adult, child >8 yr, >45 kg:* 100 mg PO bid for 14 d. **Tx of acute gonococcal infection.** *Adult, child >8 yr, >45 kg:* 100 mg PO, then 100 mg at bedtime, then 100 mg bid for 3 d. Or, 300 mg PO, then 300 mg in 1 hr. **Px of traveler's diarrhea.** *Adult, child >8 yr, >45 kg:* 100 mg/d PO. **Px of malaria.** *Adult, child >8 yr, >45 kg:* 100 mg PO daily. *Child >8 yr, <45 kg:* 2 mg/kg/d PO; max, 100 mg/d. **Px of anthrax.** *Adult, child >8 yr, >45 kg:* 100 mg PO bid for 60 d. *Child >8 yr, <45 kg:* 2.2 mg/kg PO bid for 60 d. **CDC recommendations for STDs.** *Adult, child >8 yr, >45 kg:* 100 mg PO bid for 7–28 d depending on disease. **Periodontal disease.** *Adult, child >8 yr, >45 kg:* 20 mg PO bid, after scaling, root planing. **Tx of Lyme disease.** *Child >8 yr, <45 kg:* 2.2 mg/kg PO bid for 60 d or 100 mg PO bid for 14–21 d.

**ADJUST DOSE** Elderly pts, renal impairment

**ADV EFF** Anorexia, **bone marrow suppression, CDAD,** discoloring of teeth/inadequate bone calcification (of fetus when used during preg, of child when used if <8yr), **exfoliative dermatitis,** glossitis, **hepatic failure,** HTN, n/v/d, phototoxic reactions, rash, superinfections

**INTERACTIONS** Alkali, antacids, barbiturates, carbamazepine, dairy foods, digoxin, iron, penicillins, phenytoins

**NC/PT** Culture before tx. Give w/food if GI upset severe, avoiding dairy products. Not for use in preg/breastfeeding. Pt should complete full course of therapy; avoid sun exposure; report severe diarrhea, urine/stool color changes.

**dronabinol (delta-9-tetrahydrocannabinol, delta-9-THC)** (Marinol, Syndros)
**CLASS** Antiemetic, appetite suppressant
**PREG/CONT** High risk/C-III

**IND & DOSE** **Tx of n/v associated w/cancer chemo.** *Adult, child:* 5 mg/$m^2$ PO 1–3 hr before chemo administration. Repeat q 2–4 hr after chemo, for total of four–six doses/d. If 5 mg/$m^2$ ineffective and no significant side effects, increase by 2.5-mg/$m^2$ increments to max, 15 mg/$m^2$/dose. Or, 4.2 mg/$m^2$ PO sol (*Syndros*) 1–3 hr before chemo, given on empty stomach at least 30 min before eating, then q 2–4 hr after therapy w/o regard to meals, for max four–six doses/d. **Tx of anorexia associated w/weight loss in pts w/AIDS.** *Adult, child:* 2.5 mg PO bid before lunch and dinner. May reduce to 2.5 mg/d as single evening or bedtime dose; max, 10 mg PO bid (max not recommended for child). Or, 2.1 mg sol (*Syndros*) PO bid, 1 hr before lunch and dinner.
**ADV EFF** Dependence w/use over 30 d, depression, dry mouth, dizziness, drowsiness, hallucinations, headache, heightened awareness, impaired coordination, irritability, sluggishness, unsteadiness, visual disturbances
**INTERACTIONS** Alcohol, anticholinergics, antihistamines, CNS depressants, dofetilide, metronidazole, ritonavir, TCAs
**NC/PT** Do not use w/hx of alcohol sensitivity, use of disulfiram, metronidazole in past 14 d. Store capsules in refrigerator. If using sol, always give dose w/provided calibrated syringe. Supervise pt during first use to evaluate CNS effects. Discontinue if psychotic reactions; warn pt about CNS effects. Not for use in preg/breastfeeding. Pt should avoid marijuana (drug contains same active ingredient); take safety precautions for CNS effects; avoid alcohol and OTC sleeping aids.

**dronedarone** (Multaq)
**CLASS** Antiarrhythmic
**PREG/CONT** X/NA

**BBW** Contraindicated in pts w/symptomatic HF or recent hospitalization for HF; doubles risk of death. Contraindicated in pts w/atrial fibrillation (AF) who cannot be cardioverted; doubles risk of death, stroke.
**IND & DOSE** **To reduce risk of CV hospitalization in pts w/paroxysmal or persistent AF or atrial flutter w/recent episode of either and associated CV risk factors who are in sinus rhythm or will be cardioverted.** *Adult:* 400 mg PO bid w/a.m. and p.m. meal.
**ADV EFF** Asthenia, **HF,** hypokalemia, n/v/d, prolonged QT, rash, renal impairment, **serious hepatotoxicity, serious pulmonary toxicity, stroke**
**INTERACTIONS** Antiarrhythmics, beta blockers, calcium channel blockers, CYP3A inhibitors/inducers, digoxin, grapefruit juice, sirolimus, statins, St. John's wort, tacrolimus, warfarin
**NC/PT** Obtain baseline, periodic ECG. Do not use in pt w/permanent AF or serious HF. Monitor LFTs, pulmonary function, serum potassium during tx. Not for use in preg/breastfeeding. Pt should avoid grapefruit juice, St. John's wort; keep complete list of all drugs and report use to all health care providers; comply w/frequent ECG monitoring; not make up missed doses; report difficulty breathing, rapid weight gain, extreme fatigue.

**droperidol** (Inapsine)
**CLASS** General anesthetic
**PREG/CONT** C/NA

**BBW** May prolong QT; reserve use for pts unresponsive to other tx. Monitor pt carefully.

**IND & DOSE To reduce n/v associated w/surgical procedures.** *Adult:* 2.5 mg IM or IV. May use additional 1.2 mg w/caution. *Child 2–12 yr:* 0.1 mg/kg IM or IV.
**ADJUST DOSE** Renal/hepatic impairment
**ADV EFF** Chills, drowsiness, hallucinations, hypotension, **prolonged QT w/potentially fatal arrhythmias,** tachycardia
**INTERACTIONS** CNS depressants, opioids, QT-prolonging drugs
**NC/PT** Reserve use. Monitor ECG continually during tx and recovery. Pt should take safety precautions for CNS effects.

## droxidopa (Northera)
**CLASS** Norepinephrine precursor
**PREG/CONT** Moderate risk/NA

**BBW** Risk of supine HTN. Raise head of bed to lessen effects; lower dose or discontinue drug if supine HTN cannot be managed.
**IND & DOSE Tx of orthostatic hypotension in adults w/neurogenic orthostatic hypotension caused by autonomic failure.** *Adult:* 100 mg PO tid; titrate in 100-mg-tid segments to max 600 mg PO tid. Effectiveness beyond 2 wk is unkn.
**ADJUST DOSE** Renal impairment
**ADV EFF** Confusion, dizziness, **exacerbation of ischemic heart disease,** fatigue, fever, headache, HTN, nausea, **supine HTN**
**INTERACTIONS** Carbidopa, levodopa
**NC/PT** Monitor BP carefully; raise head of bed to decrease supine HTN. Administer last dose at least 3 hr before bedtime. Pt should avoid breastfeeding; take safety precautions w/CNS changes; report severe headache, chest pain, palpitations, drugs used for tx of Parkinson disease.

## dulaglutide (Trulicity)
**CLASS** Antidiabetic, glucagon-like peptide-1 agonist
**PREG/CONT** C/NA

**BBW** Increased risk of thyroid C-cell cancer, medullary thyroid cancers. Contraindicated w/history of thyroid cancer or multiple endocrine neoplasia syndrome type 2.
**IND & DOSE Adjunct to diet/exercise to improve glycemic control in pts w/type 2 diabetes.** *Adult:* 0.75 mg subcut once/wk. May increase to 1.5 mg subcut once/wk if needed and tolerated.
**ADV EFF** Abd pain, hypoglycemia, hypersensitivity reactions (anaphylaxis and angioedema), microvascular events, n/v/d, **pancreatitis,** renal impairment, **thyroid C-cell tumors**
**INTERACTIONS** Oral medications (slow GI emptying; may impact absorption)
**NC/PT** Ensure safe use of drug; screen for thyroid cancers. Teach proper subcut administration/disposal of needles/syringes. Not for use in preg/breastfeeding. Monitor for hypoglycemia, dehydration. Pt should continue diet/exercise program; report serious diarrhea, difficulty breathing, lack of glycemic control.

## DULoxetine hydrochloride (Cymbalta)
**CLASS** Antidepressant, serotonin/norepinephrine reuptake inhibitor
**PREG/CONT** High risk/NA

**BBW** Monitor for increased depression (agitation, irritability, increased suicidality), especially at start of tx and dose change; most likely in child, adolescent, young adult. Provide appropriate interventions, protection. Drug not approved for child.
**IND & DOSE Tx of major depressive disorder.** *Adult:* 20 mg PO bid; max, 120 mg/d. Allow at least 14 d if

switching from MAOI, 5 d if switching to MAOI. **Tx of generalized anxiety disorder.** *Adult:* 60 mg/d PO; max, 120 mg/d. **Tx of diabetic neuropathic pain.** *Adult:* 60 mg/d PO as single dose. **Tx of fibromyalgia; chronic musculoskeletal pain.** *Adult:* 30 mg/d PO for 1 wk; then increase to 60 mg/d.
**ADV EFF** Constipation, diarrhea, dizziness, dry mouth, fatigue, **hepatotoxicity,** orthostatic hypotension, serotonin syndrome, sweating, urinary hesitancy
**INTERACTIONS** Alcohol, aspirin, flecainide, fluvoxamine, linezolid, lithium, MAOIs, NSAIDs, phenothiazines, propafenone, quinidine, SSRIs, St. John's wort, tramadol, TCAs, triptans, warfarin
**NC/PT** Not for use in preg/breastfeeding. Taper when discontinuing. Pt should swallow capsules whole and not cut/crush/chew them; avoid alcohol, St. John's wort; report thoughts of suicide; take safety precautions w/ dizziness.

## dupilumab (Dupixent)

**CLASS** Interleukin-4 receptor alpha antagonist
**PREG/CONT** Unkn/NA

**IND & DOSE** **Tx of pts w/moderate to severe atopic dermatitis whose disease is not adequately controlled w/topical prescription therapies or when those therapies are not advisable.** *Adult, adolescent ≥60 kg:* Initially, 600 mg subcut (two 300-mg injections at different sites) followed by 300 mg q other wk. *Adolescent <60 kg:* Initially, 400 mg subcut (two 200-mg injections at different sites); then 200 mg q other wk. **Tx of moderate to severe asthma as add-on maint if eosinophilic phenotype or oral corticosteroid–dependent asthma.** *Adult, child ≥12 yr:* Initially, 400 mg subcut (two 200-mg injections at different sites); then 200 mg q other wk. Or initially, 600 mg subcut (two 300-mg injections at different sites); than 300 mg q other wk.
**ADV EFF** Blepharitis, conjunctivitis/keratitis, dry eye, eye pruritus, herpes simplex, **hypersensitivity,** injection-site reactions, oral herpes
**INTERACTIONS** Live vaccines
**NC/PT** May give w/ or w/o topical corticosteroids. Teach pt/caregivers proper injection technique/sharps disposal. Not for relief of acute bronchospasm/status asthmaticus. Pt should stop drug and immediately report hypersensitivity; report new or worsening eye s&sx; continue asthma medication (pt w/asthma).

## durvalumab (Imfinzi)

**CLASS** Antineoplastic, monoclonal antibody
**PREG/CONT** High risk/NA

**IND & DOSE** **Tx of pts w/locally advanced or metastatic urothelial carcinoma who have disease progression during or after platinum-containing chemo or within 12 mo of neoadjuvant or adjuvant tx w/ platinum-containing chemo.** *Adult:* 10 mg/kg IV over 60 min q 2 wk.
**ADV EFF** **Colitis,** constipation, decreased appetite, diarrhea, **endocrinopathies,** fatigue, **hepatitis, infection, infusion-related reaction,** musculoskeletal pain, nausea, **nephritis,** peripheral edema, **pneumonitis,** UTI
**NC/PT** Dilute before infusion; do not infuse w/other drugs. Slow, withhold, or discontinue for pneumonitis, hepatitis, colitis, hyperthyroidism, adrenal insufficiency, nephritis, type 1 diabetes, rash, infection, infusion-related reactions. Pt should use effective contraception/avoid breastfeeding during tx and for at least 3 mo after tx.

**dutasteride** (Avodart)
**CLASS** Androgen hormone inhibitor, BPH drug
**PREG/CONT** X/NA

**IND & DOSE Tx of symptomatic BPH in men w/enlarged prostate gland.** *Adult:* 0.5 mg/d PO. W/ tamsulosin, 0.5 mg/d PO w/tamsulosin 0.4. mg/d PO.
**ADV EFF** Decreased libido, enlarged breasts, GI upset
**INTERACTIONS** Cimetidine, ciprofloxacin, diltiazem, ketoconazole, ritonavir, saw palmetto, verapamil
**NC/PT** Assess to ensure BPH dx. Monitor prostate periodically. Pt should not father child or donate blood during and for 6 mo after tx. Preg women should not handle capsule. Pt should swallow capsule whole and not cut/crush/chew it; avoid saw palmetto.

**DANGEROUS DRUG**

**duvelisib** (Copiktra)
**CLASS** Antineoplastic, phosphatidylinositol 3-kinase inhibitor
**PREG/CONT** High risk/NA

**BBW** May cause fatal and serious toxicities (infections, diarrhea/colitis, cutaneous reactions, pneumonitis).
**IND & DOSE Tx of relapsed or refractory chronic lymphocytic leukemia or small lymphocytic lymphoma after at least two prior therapies; relapsed or refractory follicular lymphoma after at least two prior systemic therapies.** *Adult:* 25 mg PO bid.
**ADV EFF** Anemia, colitis, cough, diarrhea, fatigue, **hepatotoxicity,** musculoskeletal pain, nausea, **neutropenia**, pneumonia, pyrexia, rash, URI
**NC/PT** Monitor for infection. Withhold for severe diarrhea/colitis, cutaneous reaction, pulmonary s&sx. Monitor LFTs/blood counts. Pt should use contraceptives/avoid breastfeeding during tx and for at least 1 mo after tx; take w/ or w/o food; swallow capsules whole; notify providers of all concomitant drugs.

**ecallantide** (Kalbitor)
**CLASS** Plasma kallikrein inhibitor
**PREG/CONT** C/NA

**BBW** Risk of severe anaphylaxis; have medical support on hand.
**IND & DOSE Tx of acute attacks of hereditary angioedema.** *Adult, child ≥12 yr:* 30 mg subcut as three 10-mg injections; may repeat once in 24 hr.
**ADV EFF Anaphylaxis,** fever, headache, injection-site reactions, nasopharyngitis, n/v/d
**NC/PT** Give only when able to provide medical support for anaphylaxis; not for self-administration. Not for use in preg/breastfeeding. Pt should report difficulty breathing.

**eculizumab** (Soliris)
**CLASS** Complement inhibitor, monoclonal antibody
**PREG/CONT** High risk/NA

**BBW** Pt must have received meningococcal vaccine at least 2 wk before tx. Drug increases risk of infection; serious to fatal meningococcal infections have occurred. Monitor closely for early s&sx of meningitis. Only available through restricted program.
**IND & DOSE Tx of pts w/paroxysmal nocturnal hemoglobinuria to reduce hemolysis.** *Adult:* 600 mg IV over 35 min q 7 days for first 4 wk, then 900 mg IV as fifth dose 7 days later, then 900 mg IV q 14 days. *Child <18 yr:* Base dose on body weight; see manufacturer's recommendations.
**Tx of atypical hemolytic uremic syndrome to inhibit complement-mediated thrombotic microangiopathy; tx of pts w/generalized myasthenia gravis who are anti-acetylcholine receptor antibody positive; tx of**

**neuromyelitis optica spectrum disorder in pts who are anti-aquaporin-4-antibody positive.** *Adult:* 900 mg IV over 35 min for first 4 wk, then 1,200 mg IV for fifth dose 1 wk later, then 1,200 mg IV q 2 wk. *Child <18 yr:* Base dose on body weight; see manufacturer's recommendations.
**ADV EFF** Back pain, headache, **hemolysis,** HTN, **meningococcal infections,** nasopharyngitis, n/v/d, UTI
**NC/PT** Monitor for s&sx of meningococcal infection. Stopping drug can cause serious hemolysis. Must monitor pt for 8 wk after stopping; inform pt of risk of meningococcal infections. Not for use in preg/breastfeeding. Pt should wear medical alert tag; report s&sx of infection.

## edaravone (Radicava)

**CLASS** ALS drug
**PREG/CONT** High risk/NA

**IND & DOSE Tx of ALS.** *Adult:* 60 mg IV daily over 60 min for 14 days, 14 days of rest; then daily for 10 of 14 days followed by 14 days of rest.
**ADV EFF** Confusion, gait disturbances, headache, hypersensitivity reactions
**NC/PT** Monitor response to drug. Pt. should mark calendar for tx days; avoid preg (contraceptives advised)/ breastfeeding; report difficulty breathing, facial swelling, rash.

## edetate calcium disodium (Calcium Disodium Versenate)

**CLASS** Antidote
**PREG/CONT** B/NA

**BBW** Reserve use for serious conditions requiring aggressive therapy; serious toxicity possible.
**IND & DOSE Tx of acute/chronic lead poisoning, lead encephalopathy.** *Adult, child:* For blood levels 20–70 mcg/dL, 1,000 mg/m$^2$/d IV or IM for 5 days. Interrupt tx for 2–4 days; follow w/another 5 days of tx if indicated. For blood levels higher than 70 mcg/dL, combine w/dimercaprol.
**ADV EFF** Electrolyte imbalance, headache, n/v/d, orthostatic hypotension
**INTERACTIONS** Zinc insulin
**NC/PT** Give IM or IV. Avoid excess fluids w/encephalopathy. Establish urine flow by IV infusion before tx. Monitor BUN, electrolytes. Keep pt supine for short period after tx to prevent orthostatic hypotension. Pt should prepare calendar of tx days.

**DANGEROUS DRUG**

## edoxaban (Savaysa)

**CLASS** Anticoagulant, direct thrombin inhibitor
**PREG/CONT** Unkn/NA

**BBW** Premature discontinuation increases risk of thrombotic events; consider coverage w/another anticoagulant if discontinued for reasons other than pathological bleeding. Risk of epidural/spinal hematomas if used in pts w/spinal puncture of anesthesia. Reduced efficacy w/CrCl >95 mL/min.
**IND & DOSE To reduce stroke/ embolism in pts w/nonvalvular atrial fibrillation; tx of DVT/PE after 5–10 days of parenteral anticoagulant.** *Adult w/CrCl >50–≤95 mL/min:* 60 mg/d PO. Reduce dose to 30 mg PO daily if CrCl 15–50 mL/min. Not recommended in hepatic impairment or if CrCl >95 mL/min.
**ADV EFF Bleeding, rebound thrombotic events w/discontinuation, severe hypersensitivity reactions**
**INTERACTIONS** Carbamazepine, clarithromycin, itraconazole, ketoconazole, other drugs that increase bleeding, phenytoin, rifampin, ritonavir, St. John's wort
**NC/PT** Not for use w/artificial heart valves. May crush tablets and mix w/2–3 oz water and immediately give by mouth or through gastric tube, or

may mix into applesauce and immediately administer orally. Monitor for bleeding. Breastfeeding not recommended. Pt should avoid OTC drugs that affect bleeding; not stop drug suddenly; take safety precautions to avoid injury; report increased bleeding, chest pain, headache, dizziness.

## efavirenz (Sustiva)

**CLASS** Antiviral, nonnucleoside reverse transcriptase inhibitor

**PREG/CONT** High risk/NA

**IND & DOSE Tx of HIV/AIDS, w/other antiretrovirals.** *Adult:* 600 mg/d PO w/ protease inhibitor or other nucleoside reverse transcriptase inhibitor. In combo w/voriconazole 400 mg PO q 12 hr: 300 mg/d efavirenz PO. *Child ≥3 mo:* ≥40 kg, 600 mg/d PO; 32.5–<40 kg, 400 mg/d PO; 25–<32.5 kg, 350 mg/d PO; 20–<25 kg, 300 mg/d PO; 15–<20 kg, 250 mg/d PO; 10–<15 kg, 200 m/d P; 5–<10 kg, 150 mg/d PO; 3.5–<5 kg, 100 mg/d PO.

**ADJUST DOSE** Hepatic impairment

**ADV EFF** Asthenia, body fat redistribution, CNS sx, dizziness, drowsiness, headache, hepatotoxicity, hyperlipidemia, n/v/d, **prolonged QT,** rash to **SJS**

**INTERACTIONS** Alcohol, cisapride, elbasvir, ergot derivatives, grazoprevir, hepatotoxic drugs, indinavir, methadone, midazolam, pimozide, QT-prolonging drugs, rifabutin, rifampin, ritonavir, saquinavir, St. John's wort, triazolam, voriconazole

**NC/PT** Not recommended in pts w/ moderate or severe hepatic impairment. Blood test needed q 2 wk. Ensure drug part of combo therapy. Monitor all drugs taken; many interactions possible. Give at bedtime for first 2–4 wk to minimize CNS effects. Monitor LFTs, lipids. Not for use in preg/breastfeeding. Not a cure; pt should use precautions. Pt should swallow forms whole and not cut/crush/chew them; avoid alcohol; report all drugs/herbs taken (including St. John's wort) to health care provider; seek regular medical care; report rash, urine/stool color changes.

## efinaconazole (Jublia)

**CLASS** Azole antifungal

**PREG/CONT** C/NA

**IND & DOSE Topical tx of toenail onychomycosis.** *Adult:* Apply to toenail once daily using flow-through brush applicator for 48 wk.

**ADV EFF** Application-site dermatitis/vesicles/pain, ingrown toenails

**NC/PT** For external use only. Pt should completely cover entire toenail, toenail folds, toenail bed, undersurface of toenail plate; apply to clean, dry nails; avoid nail polish; avoid using near heat or open flame (drug is flammable); report s&sx of infection.

## elapegademase-lvlr (Revcovi)

**CLASS** Enzyme

**PREG/CONT** Unkn/ NA

**IND & DOSE Tx of adenosine deaminase severe combined immune deficiency.** *Pt on Adagen:* 0.2 mg/kg IM wkly. *Pt Adagen-naïve:* 0.4 mg/kg IM wkly *or* 0.2 mg/kg twice a wk.

**ADV EFF** Cough, vomiting

**NC/PT** Use caution when giving to pt w/thrombocytopenia due to increased bleeding risk. Pt should follow recommended drug schedule.

## eletriptan hydrobromide (Relpax)

**CLASS** Antimigraine, triptan

**PREG/CONT** C/NA

**IND & DOSE Tx of acute migraine w/ or w/o aura.** *Adult:* 20–40 mg PO. If headache improves, then returns, may give second dose after at least 2 hr. Max, 80 mg/d.

**ADV EFF** HTN, hypertonia, hypoesthesia, **MI,** pharyngitis, **serotonin syndrome,** sweating, vertigo
**INTERACTIONS** Clarithromycin, ergots, itraconazole, ketoconazole, nefazodone, nelfinavir, ritonavir, SSRIs, other triptans
**NC/PT** Tx only; not for migraine px. No more than two doses in 24 hr. Closely monitor BP w/known CAD; stop if s&sx of angina, peripheral vascular obstruction. Not for use in preg. Pt should take safety precautions for CNS effects, maintain usual measures for migraine relief.

## eliglustat (Cerdelga)
**CLASS** Glucosylceramide synthase inhibitor
**PREG/CONT** C/NA

**IND & DOSE Long-term tx of pts w/ Gaucher disease type 1 who are extensive, intermediate, or poor CYP2D6 metabolizers.** *Adult:* 84 mg PO bid in extensive/intermediate metabolizers, 85 mg/d PO in poor metabolizers.
**ADJUST DOSE** Renal/hepatic impairment
**ADV EFF** Arrhythmias, back pain, fatigue, headache, n/v/d, pain, **prolonged QT**
**INTERACTIONS** CYP2D6 inhibitors/inducers, grapefruit juice, QT-prolonging drugs
**NC/PT** Monitor for cardiac disease before tx, then periodically. Test metabolizer status per FDA-cleared test. Check drug regimens; many interactions possible. Not for use in preg/breastfeeding. Pt should swallow capsule whole and not cut/crush/chew it; avoid grapefruit juice; report chest pain, palpitations, severe GI s&sx.

## elosulfase alfa (Vimizim)
**CLASS** Enzyme
**PREG/CONT** Moderate risk/NA

**BBW** Risk of life-threatening anaphylaxis, hypersensitivity reaction. Monitor pt closely; be prepared to deal w/anaphylaxis. Pts w/acute respiratory illness at risk for life-threatening pulmonary complications; delay use w/respiratory illness.
**IND & DOSE Tx of mucopolysaccharidosis type IVA (Morquio A syndrome).** *Adult, child ≥5 yr:* 2 mg/kg IV infused over 3.5–4.5 hr once a wk.
**ADV EFF** Abd pain, chills, fatigue, fever, headache, **hypersensitivity reaction,** respiratory complications, vomiting
**NC/PT** Pretreat w/antihistamines, antipyretic 30–60 min before infusion. Slow or stop infusion if sx of hypersensitivity reaction. Use cautiously in preg; not for use in breastfeeding. Pt should report difficulty breathing, cough, rash, chest pain.

## elotuzumab (Empliciti)
**CLASS** Immunostimulatory antibody
**PREG/CONT** High risk/NA

**IND & DOSE Tx of multiple myeloma in pts who have received one–three prior therapies.** *Adult:* 10 mg/kg IV q wk for two cycles, then q 2 wk until progression, given w/lenalidomide, dexamethasone. **Tx of multiple myeloma in pts who have received at least two prior therapies, including lenalidomide and a proteasome inhibitor.** *Adult:* 10 mg/kg IV q wk for two cycles, then 20 mg/kg q 4 wk until progression, given w/pomalidomide, dexamethasone.
**ADV EFF** Constipation, cough, diarrhea, fatigue, fever, **hepatotoxicity, infections, infusion reactions, malignancy**
**NC/PT** Ensure dx. Give w/lenalidomide, dexamethasone. Premedicate w/dexamethasone, diphenhydramine, ranitidine, acetaminophen. Monitor for infusion reactions; interrupt infusion or discontinue if severe. Monitor liver function. Assess for infection, other malignancies. Pt should avoid preg/breastfeeding (combo drugs

have high risk); report difficulty breathing, rash, fever, flulike sx, urine/stool color changes.

**eltrombopag** (Promacta)
**CLASS** Thrombopoietin receptor agonist
**PREG/CONT** C/NA

**BBW** Risk of severe to fatal hepatotoxicity w/interferon, ribavirin in pts w/chronic hepatitis C. Monitor LFTs closely; adjust dose or discontinue as needed.
**IND & DOSE** **Tx of chronic immune idiopathic thrombocytopenic purpura in pts unresponsive to usual tx.** *Adult, child ≥6 yr:* 50–75 mg/d PO. Start Eastern Asian pts at 25 mg/d. *Child 1–5 yr:* 25 mg/d PO. **Tx of HCV-associated thrombocytopenia.** *Adult:* 25 mg/d PO; max, 100 mg/d. **Tx of severe aplastic anemia after no response to immunosuppressants.** *Adult:* 50 mg/d PO; max, 150 mg. **First-line tx of severe aplastic anemia in combo w/standard immunosuppressive therapy.** *Adult, child ≥12 yr:* 150 mg PO daily. *Child 6–11 yr:* 75 mg PO daily. *Child 2–5 yr:* 2.5 mg/kg PO daily. Reduce initial dose for pts of Asian ancestry.
**ADJUST DOSE** Moderate hepatic failure, pts of East Asian ancestry
**ADV EFF** Back pain, **bone marrow fibrosis,** cataracts, headache, **hepatotoxicity,** n/v/d, pharyngitis, **thrombotic events,** URI, UTI
**INTERACTIONS** Antacids, dairy products, oral anticoagulants, statins
**NC/PT** Not indicated for tx of pts w/myelodysplastic syndrome. Safety/efficacy have not been established in combo w/direct-acting antivirals used w/o interferon for tx of chronic hepatitis C. Increased risk of death and progression of myelodysplastic syndromes to acute myeloid leukemia. Do not give within 4 hr of antacids/dairy products. Monitor CBC/LFTs regularly for safety, dose adjustment. Target platelets at $50 \times 10^9$/L or more. Not for use w/blood cancers; worsening possible. Monitor for cataracts/vision changes. Not for use in preg/breastfeeding. Pt should take on empty stomach 1 hr before or 2 hr after meals; report chest pain, bleeding, urine/stool color changes.

**eluxadoline** (Viberzi)
**CLASS** Antidiarrheal, mu-opioid receptor agonist
**PREG/CONT** Low risk/NA

**IND & DOSE** **Tx of IBS w/diarrhea.** *Adult:* 75–100 mg PO bid.
**ADJUST DOSE** Hepatic impairment
**ADV EFF** Abd pain, acute biliary pain, constipation, n/v, **pancreatitis,** sphincter of Oddi spasm
**NC/PT** Ensure proper use; not for use w/biliary obstruction, alcoholism, hx of pancreatitis, severe hepatic impairment, severe constipation, GI obstruction. Stop and notify provider if severe constipation for over 4 days occurs. Monitor pancreatic and liver enzymes. Pt should immediately stop drug and seek medical attention for hypersensitivity reaction, including anaphylaxis; report constipation, severe abd pain.

**emapalumab-izsg** (Gamifant)
**CLASS** Monoclonal antibody
**PREG/CONT** Unkn/NA

**IND & DOSE** **Tx of adult/child (newborn and older) w/primary hemophagocytic lymphohistiocytosis (HLH) w/refractory, recurrent, or progressive disease or intolerance to conventional HLH therapy.** *Adult, child:* 1 mg/kg IV over 1 hr twice a wk, w/dexamethasone.
**ADV EFF** HTN, infection, infusion-related reaction, pyrexia
**INTERACTIONS** Live vaccines
**NC/PT** Give drug w/dexamethasone. Monitor for s&sx of infection; treat promptly. Test for latent TB.

Administer px against herpes zoster, *Pneumocystis jiroveci* pneumonia, fungal infection. Do not give live or live attenuated vaccines during and for at least weeks after tx.

**DANGEROUS DRUG**

## emicizumab-kxwh
(Hemlibra)

**CLASS** Antihemophilic, monoclonal antibody
**PREG/CONT** Unkn/NA

**BBW** Thrombotic microangiopathy, thrombotic events were reported when on average a cumulative amount of >100 units/kg/24 hr of activated prothrombin complex concentrate (aPCC) was given for ≥24 hr.
**IND & DOSE To prevent or reduce frequency of bleeding episodes in adult/child w/hemophilia A (congenital factor VIII deficiency), w/factor VIII inhibitors.** *Adult, child:* 3 mg/kg subcut q wk for 4 wk; then 1.5 mg/kg once wkly.
**ADV EFF** Arthralgia, , headache, injection-site reaction, **thromboembolism**
**NC/PT** Lab coagulation tests interfering w/drug include ACT, aPTT, tests based on aPTT (including one-stage aPTT-based single-factor assays, aPTT-based activated protein C resistance, Bethesda assays [clotting-based] for factor VIII inhibitor titers). Pt should avoid preg (contraceptives advised).

## empagliflozin (Jardiance)

**CLASS** Antidiabetic, sodium-glucose cotransporter 2 inhibitor
**PREG/CONT** C/NA

**IND & DOSE Adjunct to diet/exercise to improve glycemic control in type 2 diabetes; to reduce risk of death in pts w/type 2 diabetes and CV disease.** *Adult:* 10 mg/d PO in a.m.; max, 25 mg/d.
**ADJUST DOSE** Severe renal impairment
**ADV EFF** Dehydration, **diabetic ketoacidosis**, genital mycotic infections, hypoglycemia, hyponatremia, hypotension, increased LDLs, **renal impairment**, urosepsis, UTI
**INTERACTIONS** Celery, coriander, dandelion root, digoxin, fenugreek, garlic, ginger, juniper berries, phenobarbital, phenytoin, rifampin
**NC/PT** Not for use w/type 1 diabetes or ketoacidosis. Monitor blood glucose, $HbA_{1c}$, BP periodically. Not for use in preg/breastfeeding. Discontinue promptly for hypersensitivity reaction or if estimated GFR <45 mL/min/1.73 $m^2$; monitor until s&sx resolve. Pt should continue diet/exercise program, other antidiabetics as ordered; monitor blood glucose; take safety measures w/ dehydration; monitor for UTI, genital infections.

## emtricitabine (Emtriva)

**CLASS** Antiviral, nucleoside reverse transcriptase inhibitor
**PREG/CONT** B/NA

**BBW** Use caution w/current/ suspected HBV; serious disease resurgence possible. Withdraw drug, monitor pt w/sx of lactic acidosis or hepatotoxicity, including hepatomegaly, steatosis.
**IND & DOSE Tx of HIV-1 infection, w/other antiretrovirals.** *Adult:* 200 mg/d PO or 240 mg (24 mL) oral sol/d PO. *Child 3 mo–17 yr:* 6 mg/ kg/d PO to max 240 mg (24 mL) oral sol. For child >33 kg able to swallow capsule, one 200-mg capsule/d PO. *Child <3 mo:* 3 mg/kg/d oral sol PO.
**ADJUST DOSE** Renal impairment
**ADV EFF** Abd pain, asthenia, cough, dizziness, headache, immune reconstitution syndrome, insomnia, **lactic acidosis,** n/v/d, rash, redistribution of body fat, rhinitis, **severe hepatomegaly w/steatosis**
**INTERACTIONS** *Atripla*, lamivudine, *Truvada;* contraindicated

**NC/PT** HIV antibody testing before tx. Monitor LFTs, renal function regularly. Ensure use w/other antiretrovirals. Not for use in preg/breastfeeding. Not a cure; pt should use precautions. Pt should try to maintain nutrition, hydration (GI effects will occur); report difficulty breathing, unusual muscle pain, dizziness, unusual heartbeat.

## enalapril maleate

(Epaned, Vasotec), enalaprilat (generic)

**CLASS** ACE inhibitor, antihypertensive

**PREG/CONT** High risk/NA

**BBW** Possible serious fetal injury or death if used in second, third trimesters; advise contraceptive use.

**IND & DOSE Tx of HTN.** *Adult:* Initially, 5 mg/d PO; range, 10–40 mg/d. Discontinue diuretics for 2–3 days before tx; if not possible, start w/2.5 mg/d PO or 1.25 mg IV q 6 hr; monitor pt response. If on diuretics, 0.625 mg IV over 5 min; repeat in 1 hr if needed, then 1.25 mg IV q 6 hr. *Child 2 mo–16 yr:* 0.08 mg/kg PO once daily; max, 5 mg. **Tx of HF.** *Adult:* 2.5 mg/d PO or bid w/diuretics, digitalis; max, 40 mg/d. **Tx of asymptomatic left ventricular dysfx.** *Adult:* 2.5 mg PO bid; target dose, 20 mg/d in two divided doses.

**ADJUST DOSE** Elderly pts, renal impairment, HF

**ADV EFF** **Anaphylaxis, angioedema,** cough; decreased Hct, Hgb; diarrhea; dizziness; fatigue; hyperkalemia, **renal failure**

**INTERACTIONS** ARBs, ACE inhibitors, indomethacin, lithium, NSAIDs, renin inhibitors, rifampin

**NC/PT** Adjust dose if pt also on diuretic. Peak effect may not occur for 4 hr. Monitor BP before giving second dose; monitor closely in situations that might lead to BP drop. Monitor potassium, renal function. Mark chart if surgery required; pt may need fluid support. Not for use in preg (contraceptives advised)/ breastfeeding. Pt should take safety precautions w/CNS effects; report difficulty breathing.

**DANGEROUS DRUG**

## enasidenib (Idhifa)

**CLASS** Antineoplastic, isocitrate dehydrogenase-2 inhibitor

**PREG/CONT** High risk/NA

**BBW** Risk of potentially fatal differentiation syndrome; if suspected, initiate corticosteroids and constant monitoring.

**IND & DOSE Tx of refractory AML w/an isocitrate dehydrogenase-2 mutation.** *Adult:* 100 mg/d PO.

**ADV EFF** Decreased appetite, elevated bilirubin, n/v/d

**NC/PT** Monitor for differentiation syndrome, dehydration. Pt should take once daily; avoid preg (contraceptives advised)/breastfeeding; report fever, weight gain, difficulty breathing.

## enfuvirtide (Fuzeon)

**CLASS** Anti-HIV drug, fusion inhibitor

**PREG/CONT** B/NA

**IND & DOSE Tx of HIV-1 infection in tx-experienced pts w/evidence of HIV-1 replication despite ongoing tx, w/other antiretrovirals.** *Adult:* 90 mg bid by subcut injection into upper arm, anterior thigh, or abdomen. *Child 6–16 yr:* 2 mg/kg bid by subcut injection; max, 90 mg/dose into upper arm, anterior thigh, or abdomen.

**ADV EFF** Dizziness, hypersensitivity reactions, injection-site reactions, n/v/d, **pneumonia**

**NC/PT** Ensure pt also on other antiretrovirals; rotate injection sites (upper arm, anterior thigh, abdomen).

Reconstitute only w/sol provided. Refrigerate reconstituted sol; use within 24 hr. Not for use in preg/breastfeeding; preg registry available. Not a cure; pt should use precautions. Teach pt proper administration/disposal of needles/syringes. Pt should report difficulty breathing, unusual breathing.

DANGEROUS DRUG

**enoxaparin** (Lovenox)
**CLASS** Low-molecular-weight heparin
**PREG/CONT** B/NA

**BBW** Increased risk of spinal hematoma, neuro damage if used w/spinal/epidural anesthesia. If must be used, monitor pt closely.
**IND & DOSE Px of DVT after hip/knee replacement surgery.** *Adult:* 30 mg subcut bid, w/initial dose 12–24 hr after surgery. Continue for 7–10 days; then may give 40 mg daily subcut for up to 3 wk. **Px of DVT after abd surgery.** *Adult:* 40 mg/d subcut begun within 2 hr before surgery, continued for 7–10 days. **Px of DVT in high-risk pts.** 40 mg/d subcut for 6–11 days; has been used up to 14 days. **Px of ischemic complications of unstable angina and non-Q-wave MI.** *Adult:* 1 mg/kg subcut q 12 hr for 2–8 days. **Tx of DVT.** *Adult:* 1 mg/kg subcut q 12 hr (for outpts); 1.5 mg/kg/d subcut or 1 mg/kg subcut q 12 hr (for inpts). **Tx of MI.** *Adult:* ≥75 yr, 0.75 mg/kg subcut q 12 hr (max, 75 mg for first two doses only). <75 yr, 30-mg IV bolus plus 1 mg/kg subcut followed by 1 mg/kg subcut q 12 hr w/aspirin (max, 100 mg for first two doses only).
**ADJUST DOSE** Renal impairment
**ADV EFF** Bruising, chills, fever, **hemorrhage,** injection-site reactions, thrombocytopenia
**INTERACTIONS** Aspirin, cephalosporins, chamomile, garlic, ginger, ginkgo, ginseng, high-dose vitamin E, NSAIDs, penicillins, oral anticoagulants, salicylates
**NC/PT** Contraindicated in pts w/hx of heparin-induced thrombocytopenia within past 100 days or in presence of circulating antibodies. Give as soon as possible after hip surgery, within 12 hr of knee surgery, and within 2 hr preop for abd surgery. Use deep subcut injection, not IM; alternate sites. Do not mix w/other injections or sols. Store at room temp. Have protamine sulfate on hand as antidote. Check for s&sx of bleeding; protect pt from injury. Teach pt proper administration/disposal of needles/syringes. Pt should report s&sx of bleeding.

**entacapone** (Comtan)
**CLASS** Antiparkinsonian, catechol-O-methyl transferase inhibitor
**PREG/CONT** C/NA

**IND & DOSE Adjunct w/levodopa/carbidopa in tx of s&sx of idiopathic Parkinson disease in pts experiencing "wearing off" of drug effects.** *Adult:* 200 mg PO concomitantly w/levodopa/carbidopa; max, 8 ×/d.
**ADV EFF** Confusion, disorientation, dizziness, dry mouth, dyskinesia, falling asleep during ADLs, **fever, hallucinations,** hyperkinesia, hypotension, loss of impulse control, n/v, orthostatic hypotension, renal impairment, **rhabdomyolysis,** somnolence
**INTERACTIONS** Ampicillin, apomorphine, chloramphenicol, cholestyramine, dobutamine, dopamine, epinephrine, erythromycin, isoetharine, isoproterenol, MAOIs, methyldopa, norepinephrine, rifampin
**NC/PT** Give only w/levodopa/carbidopa; do not give within 14 days of MAOIs. Not for use in preg (contraceptives advised)/breastfeeding. Pt should use sugarless lozenges for dry mouth, take safety precautions w/CNS effects.

**entecavir** (Baraclude)
**CLASS** Antiviral, nucleoside analog
**PREG/CONT** C/NA

**BBW** Withdraw drug, monitor pt if s&sx of lactic acidosis or hepatotoxicity, including hepatomegaly and steatosis. Do not use in pts w/HIV unless pt receiving highly active antiretroviral tx, because of high risk of HIV resistance. Offer HIV testing to all pts before starting entecavir. Severe, acute HBV exacerbations have occurred in pts who discontinue antihepatitis tx. Monitor pts for several mo after drug cessation; restarting antihepatitis tx may be warranted.
**IND & DOSE** **Tx of chronic HBV infection in pts w/evidence of active viral replication and active disease.** *Adult, child ≥16 yr w/no previous nucleoside tx:* 0.5 mg/d PO on empty stomach at least 2 hr after meal or 2 hr before next meal. *Adult, child ≥16 yr w/hx of viremia also receiving lamivudine or w/known resistance mutations:* 1 mg/d PO on empty stomach at least 2 hr after meal or 2 hr before next meal. *Child ≥2 yr, ≥10 kg:* Dosage based on weight.
**ADJUST DOSE** Hepatic/renal impairment
**ADV EFF** **Acute exacerbation of HBV when discontinuing, dizziness, fatigue, headache, lactic acidosis,** nausea, **severe hepatomegaly**
**INTERACTIONS** Nephrotoxic drugs
**NC/PT** Assess renal function regularly. Give on empty stomach at least 2 hr after meal or 2 hr before next meal. Not a cure; pt should take precautions. Not for use in preg/breastfeeding. Pt should not run out of or stop drug suddenly (severe hepatitis possible), should take safety precautions w/dizziness, report unusual muscle pain.

**▶ NEW DRUG**

**entrectinib** (Rozlytrek)
**CLASS** Kinase inhibitor
**PREG/CONT** High risk/NA

**IND & DOSE** **Tx of pts w/metastatic NSCLC whose tumors are ROS1-positive.** *Adult:* 600 mg PO daily. **Tx of pts w/NTRK gene fusion-positive solid tumors.** *Adult:* 600 mg PO daily. *Child ≥12 yr:* BSA >1.5 m$^2$, 600 mg PO daily; BSA 1.11–1.50 m$^2$, 500 mg PO daily; BSA 0.91–1.10 m$^2$, 400 mg PO daily.
**ADV EFF** Arthralgia, cognitive impairment, constipation, cough, diarrhea, dizziness, dysesthesia, dysgeusia, dyspnea, edema, fatigue, **hepatotoxicity, HF, hyperuricemia,** myalgia, n/v, **prolonged QT,** pyrexia, **skeletal fractures**, vision changes, weight increase
**INTERACTIONS** Moderate/strong CYP3A inducers/inhibitors
**NC/PT** Monitor for sx of heart/liver failure and CNS effects, including vision changes; dosage decrease/drug discontinuation may be needed. Pt should use contraception during and for at least 5 wk (women) or 3 mo (men) after tx.

**enzalutamide** (Xtandi)
**CLASS** Androgen receptor inhibitor, antineoplastic
**PREG/CONT** High risk/NA

**IND & DOSE** **Tx of castration-resistant or metastatic castration-sensitive prostate cancer.** *Adult:* 160 mg/d PO once daily, w/o regard to food.
**ADV EFF** Arthralgia, asthenia, anxiety, back pain, diarrhea, dizziness, edema, falls, flushing, fractures, headache, hematuria, HTN, hypersensitivity, **ischemic heart disease**, paresthesia, **RPLS, seizures,** weakness
**INTERACTIONS** Midazolam, omeprazole, pioglitazone, warfarin; avoid concurrent use. Gemfibrozil

**NC/PT** Give w/gonadotropin-releasing hormone analog or pt should have bilateral orchiectomy. Monitor for CNS and hypersensitivity reactions; provide safety precautions. Not for use in preg/breastfeeding. Pt should swallow capsule whole and not cut/crush/chew it; use caution w/CNS effects; report falls, severe headache, problems thinking clearly.

**DANGEROUS DRUG**

## ephedrine sulfate

(Akovaz, Corphedra)

**CLASS** Bronchodilator, sympathomimetic, vasopressor

**PREG/CONT** C/NA

**IND & DOSE** **Tx of hypotensive episodes, allergic disorders.** *Adult:* 25–50 mg IM (fast absorption) or subcut (slower absorption), or 5–25 mg IV slowly; may repeat in 5–10 min. *Child:* 0.5 mg/kg or 16.7 mg/m$^2$ IM or subcut q 4–6 hr. **Tx of clinically important hypotension during anesthesia.** *Adult:* 5–10 mg as IV bolus during anesthesia; max, 50 mg (*Akovaz, Corphedra*). **Tx of acute asthma, allergic disorders.** *Adult:* 12.5–25 mg PO q 4 hr.
**ADJUST DOSE** Elderly pts
**ADV EFF** Anxiety, **CV collapse w/ hypotension,** dizziness, dysuria, fear, **HTN resulting in intracranial hemorrhage,** pallor, **palpitations, precordial pain in pts w/ischemic heart disease,** restlessness, **tachycardia,** tenseness
**INTERACTIONS** Caffeine, cardiac glycosides, ephedra, guanethidine, guarana, ma huang, MAOIs, methyldopa, rocuronium, TCAs, theophylline, urinary acidifiers/alkalinizers
**NC/PT** Monitor newborn for acidosis if taken during preg. Not for use in breastfeeding. Protect sol from light. Give only if sol clear; discard unused portion. Monitor CV status, urine output. Avoid prolonged systemic use. Pt should avoid OTC products w/similar action; take safety precautions w/CNS effects; report chest pain, rapid HR.

**DANGEROUS DRUG**

## EPINEPHrine bitartrate, EPINEPHrine hydrochloride

(Adrenaclick, AsthmaNefrin, EpiPen)

**CLASS** Antiasthmatic, cardiac stimulant, sympathomimetic, vasopressor

**PREG/CONT** High risk/NA

**IND & DOSE** **Tx in cardiac arrest.** *Adult:* 0.5–1 mg (5–10 mL of 1:10,000 sol) IV during resuscitation, 0.5 mg q 5 min. Intracardiac injection into left ventricular chamber, 0.3–0.5 mg (3–5 mL of 1:10,000 sol). **Hypersensitivity, bronchospasm.** *Adult:* 0.1–0.25 mg (1–2.5 mL of 1:10,000 sol) injected slowly IV or 0.2–1 mL of 1:1,000 sol subcut or IM, or 0.1–0.3 mL (0.5–1.5 mg) of 1:200 sol subcut, or 0.3 mg IM or subcut w/autoinjector. *Child:* 1:1,000 sol, 0.01 mg/kg or 0.3 mL/m$^2$ (0.01 mg/kg or 0.3 mg/m$^2$) subcut. Repeat q 4 hr if needed; max, 0.5 mL (0.5 mg) in single dose. For neonates, 0.01 mg/kg subcut; for infants, 0.05 mg subcut as initial dose. Repeat q 20–30 min as needed. *Child ≤30 kg:* 1:10,000 sol, 0.15 mg or 0.01 mg/kg by autoinjector. **Temporary relief from acute attacks of bronchial asthma, COPD.** *Adult, child ≥4 yr:* 1 inhalation, wait 1 min, then may use once more. Do not repeat for at least 3 hr. Or, place not more than 10 drops into nebulizer reservoir, place nebulizer nozzle into partially opened mouth, have pt inhale deeply while bulb is squeezed one–three times (not more than q 3 hr).
**ADJUST DOSE** Elderly pts
**ADV EFF** Anxiety, **CV collapse w/ hypotension,** dizziness, dysuria, fear, **HTN resulting in intracranial hemorrhage,** pallor, **palpitations, precordial pain in pts w/ischemic heart disease,** restlessness, **tachycardia,** tenseness

**INTERACTIONS** Alpha blockers, beta blockers, cardiac glycosides, chlorpromazine, diuretics, ephedra, ergots, guarana, ma huang, methyldopa, propranolol, TCAs
**NC/PT** Use extreme caution when calculating doses; small margin of safety. Protect sol from light, heat. Rotate subcut injection sites. Have alpha-adrenergic blocker on hand for hypertensive crises/pulmonary edema, beta blocker on hand for cardiac arrhythmias. Do not exceed recommended dose of inhalants. Pt should take safety precautions w/CNS effects, seek medical help after emergency use.

**DANGEROUS DRUG**

## epiRUBicin hydrochloride (Ellence)

**CLASS** Antineoplastic antibiotic
**PREG/CONT** High risk/NA

**BBW** Cardiotoxicity possible; monitor ECG closely. Severe tissue necrosis w/extravasation. Secondary acute myelogenous leukemia possible. Reduce dose in hepatic impairment. Monitor for severe bone marrow suppression.
**IND & DOSE** **Adjunct tx in pts w/ evidence of axillary node tumor involvement after resection of primary breast cancer.** *Adult:* 100–120 mg/m² IV in repeated 3- to 4-wk cycles, all on day 1; given w/cyclophosphamide and 5-FU.
**ADJUST DOSE** Elderly pts; hepatic impairment, severe renal impairment
**ADV EFF** Alopecia, **bone marrow suppression, HF,** infection, **leukemia,** local injection-site toxicity/rash, n/v/d, **renal toxicity, thromboembolic events**
**INTERACTIONS** Cardiotoxic drugs, cimetidine, live vaccines
**NC/PT** Monitor baseline and periodic ECG to evaluate for toxicity. Premedicate w/antiemetic. Monitor injection site carefully. Monitor CBC regularly; dose adjustment may be needed. Not for use in preg/breastfeeding. Pt should mark calendar of tx dates; report swelling, s&sx of infection.

## eplerenone (Inspra)

**CLASS** Aldosterone receptor blocker, antihypertensive
**PREG/CONT** B/NA

**IND & DOSE** **Tx of HTN.** *Adult:* 50 mg/d PO as single dose; may increase to 50 mg PO bid after minimum 4-wk trial period. Max, 100 mg/d. **Tx of HF post MI.** *Adult:* Initially, 25 mg/d PO; titrate to 50 mg/d over 4 wk. If serum potassium lower than 5, increase dose; if 5–5.4, no adjustment needed; if 5.5–5.9, decrease dose; if 6 or higher, withhold dose.
**ADJUST DOSE** Hyperkalemia, renal impairment
**ADV EFF** Dizziness, gynecomastia, headache, **hyperkalemia, MI**
**INTERACTIONS** ACE inhibitors, amiloride, ARBs, NSAIDs, spironolactone, triamterene; serious reactions w/erythromycin, fluconazole, itraconazole, ketoconazole, lithium, renin inhibitors, saquinavir, verapamil
**NC/PT** Monitor potassium, renal function; suggest limiting potassium-rich foods. Not for use in preg/breastfeeding. Pt should avoid OTC drugs that might interact; weigh self daily, report changes of ≥3 lb/d, chest pain.

## epoetin alfa (EPO, erythropoietin) (Epogen, Procrit, Retacrit)

**CLASS** Recombinant human erythropoietin
**PREG/CONT** C/NA

**BBW** Increased risk of death, serious CV events if Hgb target is >11 g/dL. Use lowest levels of drug needed to increase Hgb to lowest level needed to avoid transfusion. Incidence of DVT higher in pts receiving erythropoietin-stimulating agents preop to reduce need for transfusion; consider antithrombotic px if used for this purpose.

Pts w/cancer at risk for more rapid tumor progression, shortened survival, death when Hgb target is >11 g/dL. Increased risk of death in cancer pts not receiving radiation or chemo.
**IND & DOSE Tx of anemia of chronic renal failure.** *Adult:* 50–100 units/kg 3 ×/wk IV for dialysis pts, IV or subcut for nondialysis pts. Maint, 75–100 units/kg 3 ×/wk. If on dialysis, median dose is 75 units/kg 3 ×/wk. Target Hgb range, 10–11 g/dL. *Child 1 mo–16 yr:* 50 units/kg IV or subcut 3 ×/wk. **Tx of anemia in HIV-infected pts on AZT therapy.** *Adult:* For pts receiving AZT dose of 4,200 mg/wk or less w/serum erythropoietin levels of 500 milliunits/mL or less, 100 units/kg IV or subcut 3 ×/wk for 8 wk. **Tx of anemia in cancer pts on chemo** (*Procrit* only). *Adult:* 150 units/kg subcut 3 ×/wk or 40,000 units subcut wkly. After 8 wk, can increase to 300 units/kg or 60,000 units subcut wkly. *Child 1 mo–16 yr:* 600 units/kg per wk IV; max, 60,000 units/dose in child ≥5 yr. **To reduce allogenic blood transfusions in surgery.** *Adult:* 300 units/kg/d subcut for 10 days before surgery, on day of surgery, and 4 days after surgery. Or, 600 units/kg/d subcut 21, 14, and 7 days before surgery and on day of surgery. **Tx of anemia of prematurity.** *Child:* 25–100 units/kg/dose IV 3 ×/wk.
**ADV EFF** Arthralgia, asthenia, chest pain, **development of anti-erythropoietin antibodies,** dizziness, edema, fatigue, headache, HTN, n/v/d, **seizures,** severe cutaneous reactions, **stroke, thrombotic events, tumor progression/shortened survival (w/cancers).**
**NC/PT** Confirm nature of anemia. Do not give in sol w/other drugs. Monitor access lines for clotting. Monitor Hgb (target range, 10–11 g/dL; max, 11 g/dL). Evaluate iron stores before and periodically during tx; supplemental iron may be needed. Monitor for sudden loss of response and severe anemia w/low reticulocyte count; withhold drug and check for anti-erythropoietin antibodies. Discontinue for severe cutaneous reactions or reactions due to benzyl alcohol preservative. Must give subcut 3 ×/wk. Pt should keep blood test appointments to monitor response to drug; report difficulty breathing, chest pain, severe headache.

## epoprostenol sodium
(Flolan, Veletri)
**CLASS** Prostaglandin
**PREG/CONT** B/NA

**IND & DOSE Tx of primary pulmonary HTN in pts unresponsive to standard tx.** *Adult:* 2 ng/kg/min IV w/increases of 1–2 ng/kg at least 15-min intervals as tolerated through infusion pump using central line; 20–40 ng/kg/min common range after 6 mo.
**ADV EFF** Anxiety, agitation, bleeding, chest pain, flushing, headache, hypotension, muscle aches, n/v/d, pain, pulmonary edema; **rebound pulmonary HTN** (w/sudden stopping)
**INTERACTIONS** Antihypertensives, diuretics, vasodilators
**NC/PT** Must deliver through continuous infusion pump. Use caution in preg; not for use in breastfeeding. Teach pt, significant other maint and use of pump. Do not stop suddenly; taper if discontinuing. Pt should use analgesics for headache, muscle aches; report chest pain, s&sx of infection.

## eprosartan mesylate
(generic)
**CLASS** Antihypertensive, ARB
**PREG/CONT** D/NA

**BBW** Rule out preg before starting tx. Suggest barrier birth control; fetal injury, deaths have occurred. If preg detected, discontinue as soon as possible.
**IND & DOSE Tx of HTN.** *Adult:* 600 mg PO daily. Can give in divided doses bid w/target dose of 400–800 mg/d.

**ADJUST DOSE** Renal impairment
**ADV EFF** Abd pain, diarrhea, dizziness, headache, hyperkalemia, hypotension, URI sx
**INTERACTIONS** ACE inhibitors, ARBs, lithium, NSAIDs, potassium-elevating drugs, renin inhibitors
**NC/PT** If BP not controlled, may add other antihypertensives, such as diuretics, calcium channel blocker. Monitor fluid intake, BP, potassium. Use caution if pt goes to surgery; volume depletion possible. Not for use in preg (barrier contraceptives advised)/breastfeeding. Pt should use care in situations that could lead to volume depletion.

DANGEROUS DRUG

**eptifibatide** (Integrelin)
**CLASS** Antiplatelet, glycoprotein IIb/IIIa receptor agonist
**PREG/CONT** B/NA

**IND & DOSE Tx of acute coronary syndrome.** *Adult:* 180 mcg/kg IV (max, 22.6 mg) over 1–2 min as soon as possible after dx, then 2 mcg/kg/min (max, 15 mg/hr) by continuous IV infusion for up to 72 hr. If pt is to undergo PCI, continue for 18–24 hr after procedure, up to 96 hr of tx. **Px of ischemia w/PCI.** 180 mcg/kg IV as bolus immediately before PCI, then 2 mcg/kg/min by continuous IV infusion for 18–24 hr. May give second bolus of 180 mcg/kg 10 min.
**ADJUST DOSE** Renal impairment
**ADV EFF** **Bleeding,** dizziness, headache, hypotension, rash
**INTERACTIONS** Anticoagulants, clopidogrel, dipyridamole, NSAIDs, thrombolytics, ticlopidine
**NC/PT** Used w/aspirin, heparin. Arrange for baseline and periodic CBC, PT, aPTT, active clotting time; maintain aPTT of 50–70 sec and active clotting time of 300–350 sec. Avoid invasive procedures. Ensure compression of sites. Pt should use analgesics for headache; take safety precautions for dizziness; report unusual bleeding.

▶NEW DRUG

**eravacycline** (Xerava)
**CLASS** Tetracycline
**PREG/CONT** High risk/NA

**IND & DOSE Tx of complicated intra-abd infections.** *Adult ≥18 yr:* 1 mg/kg IV q 12 hr for 4–14 days.
**ADV EFF** Bone growth inhibition, *Clostridium difficile* infection, **hypersensitivity,** infusion-site reactions, n/v, tooth discoloration/enamel hypoplasia
**INTERACTIONS** Anticoagulants, strong CYP3A inducers
**NC/PT** NOT indicated for UTIs. Give over 60 min. May decrease dose if hepatic impairment. May cause photosensitivity.

▶NEW DRUG

**erdafitinib** (Balversa)
**CLASS** Kinase inhibitor
**PREG/CONT** High risk/NA

**IND & DOSE Tx of pts w/locally advanced or metastatic urothelial carcinoma w/susceptible FGFR3 or FGFR2 genetic alterations that progressed after prior platinum-containing chemo.** *Adult:* 8 mg PO daily; may increase to 9 mg if criteria met.
**ADV EFF** Abd pain, alopecia, constipation, diarrhea, dry eye, dry mouth, dysgeusia, electrolyte/blood count changes, fatigue, hyperphosphatemia, musculoskeletal pain, nausea, ocular disorders, onycholysis, palmar-plantar erythrodysesthesia, stomatitis
**INTERACTIONS** CYP3A4 substrates, drugs that alter serum phosphate level, moderate/strong CYP3A inducers/inhibitors, OCT2/P-gp substrates
**NC/PT** Ophthal exam recommended monthly for 4 mo, then q 3 mo and when visual changes occur; dose

decrease/drug discontinuation may be needed for adverse effects. Pt should swallow whole w/ or w/o food. Pt should use contraception during and at least 1 mo after tx.

## erenumab-aooe (Aimovig)

**CLASS** Calcitonin gene-related peptide receptor antagonist; monoclonal antibody
**PREG/CONT** No data for human; no risk in animal studies/NA

**IND & DOSE Migraine px.** *Adult:* 70 or 140 mg subcut monthly.
**ADV EFF** Constipation (sometimes severe requiring surgery), hypersensitivity reactions rare but possible (rash, angioedema, anaphylaxis), injection-site reactions
**NC/PT** Needle/syringe components may cause latex-related allergic reactions. Give in abdomen/thigh/upper arm. If giving 140 mg, give two separate injections of 70 mg each.

## ergotamine tartrate

(Ergomar)
**CLASS** Antimigraine, ergot
**PREG/CONT** X/NA

**IND & DOSE Px, tx of vascular headaches.** *Adult:* 2 mg under tongue at first sign of headache. May repeat at 30-min intervals; max, 6 mg/d or 10 mg/wk.
**ADV EFF** Cyanosis, gangrene, headache, HTN, ischemia, itching, n/v, **pulmonary fibrosis,** tachycardia
**INTERACTIONS** Beta blockers, epinephrine, macrolide antibiotics, nicotine, protease inhibitors, sympathomimetics
**NC/PT** Not for use in preg/breastfeeding. Pt should take at first sign of headache; not take more than 3 tablets in 24 hr; report difficulty breathing, numbness/tingling, chest pain.

## eriBULin mesylate

(Halaven)
**CLASS** Antineoplastic, microtubular inhibitor
**PREG/CONT** High risk/NA

**IND & DOSE Tx of metastatic breast cancer in pts previously treated w/at least two chemo regimens; tx of unresectable or metastatic liposarcoma in pts who have received an anthracycline-containing regimen.** *Adult:* 1.4 mg/m$^2$ IV over 2–5 min on days 1 and 8 of 21-day cycle.
**ADJUST DOSE** Hepatic/renal impairment
**ADV EFF** Alopecia, asthenia, **bone marrow suppression,** constipation, nausea, **prolonged QT, peripheral neuropathy**
**INTERACTIONS** Dextrose-containing solutions, QT-prolonging drugs
**NC/PT** Obtain baseline ECG; monitor QT interval. Do not mix w/other drugs or dextrose-containing sol. Monitor for bone marrow suppression (adjust dose accordingly), peripheral neuropathy (dose adjustment may be needed). Not for use in preg/breastfeeding. Protect from infection. Pt should cover head at extremes of temp (hair loss possible); report fever, chills, cough, numbness/tingling in extremities.

## erlotinib (Tarceva)

**CLASS** Antineoplastic, kinase inhibitor
**PREG/CONT** High risk/NA

**IND & DOSE Tx of locally advanced or metastatic NSCLC w/EGFR exon 19 deletions or exon 21 L858R substitution mutations as first-line tx or after failure of other chemo.** *Adult:* 150 mg/d PO on empty stomach. **Tx of locally advanced, unresectable or metastatic pancreatic cancer, w/ gemcitabine.** *Adult:* 100 mg/d PO w/ IV gemcitabine.

**ADJUST DOSE** Hepatic/renal impairment, lung dysfx
**ADV EFF** Abd pain, anorexia, **bleeding, corneal ulcerations,** cough, dyspnea, **exfoliative skin disorders,** fatigue, **GI perforation, hepatic failure, hemolytic anemia, interstitial pulmonary disease, MI,** n/v/d, rash, **renal failure**
**INTERACTIONS** Antacids, cigarette smoking, CYP3A4 inducers/inhibitors, $H_2$ receptor antagonists (take 10 hr after *Tarceva*), midazolam; PPIs, avoid combo
**NC/PT** Monitor LFTs, renal function regularly. Monitor pulmonary status. Assess cornea before and periodically during tx. Provide skin care, including sunscreen, alcohol-free emollient cream. Not for use in preg/breastfeeding. Pt should report severe diarrhea, difficulty breathing, worsening rash, vision changes.

## ertapenem (INVanz)
**CLASS** Carbapenem antibiotic
**PREG/CONT** B/NA

**IND & DOSE Tx of community-acquired pneumonia; skin/skin-structure infections, including diabetic foot infections; complicated GU/intra-abd infections; acute pelvic infections caused by susceptible bacteria strains; px of surgical-site infection after colorectal surgery.** *Adult, child ≥13 yr:* 1 g IM or IV each day. Length of tx varies w/infection: intra-abd, 5–14 days; urinary tract, 10–14 days; skin/skin-structure, 7–14 days; community-acquired pneumonia, 10–14 days; acute pelvic, 3–10 days. *Child 3 mo–12 yr:* 15 mg/kg IV or IM bid for 3–14 days; max, 1 g/d.
**ADJUST DOSE** Renal impairment
**ADV EFF Anaphylaxis**, CDAD, headache, hypersensitivity reaction, local pain/phlebitis at injection site; n/v/d, **pseudomembranous colitis, seizures,** superinfections
**NC/PT** Culture before tx. Give by deep IM injection; have emergency equipment on hand for hypersensitivity reactions. Monitor injection site for reaction. Treat superinfections. Pt should report severe or bloody diarrhea, pain at injection site, difficulty breathing.

## ertugliflozin (Steglatro)
**CLASS** Antidiabetic, sodium-glucose cotransporter 2 inhibitor
**PREG/CONT** High risk/NA

**IND & DOSE Adjunct to diet/exercise to improve glycemic control in pts w/type 2 diabetes mellitus.** *Adult:* 5–15 mg PO daily.
**ADV EFF** Genital mycotic infection, hypoglycemia, **hypotension**, increased LDL-C, **ketoacidosis, kidney injury, pyelonephritis, urosepsis**
**INTERACTIONS** Insulin/insulin secretagogues
**NC/PT** May be contraindicated or decreased dosage needed in renal impairment. Monitor renal function/cholesterol/blood glucose; watch for ketoacidosis s&sx. Pt's urine will test positive for glucose during therapy. Monitor for infection/lower limb ulcer; discontinue drug if present. Potential for embryo-fetal toxicity, especially in 2nd and 3rd trimesters. Inform pt of increased risk of UTI/genital yeast infection.

## erythromycin salts (Eryc, Eryped, Ery-Tab, Erythrocin)
**CLASS** Macrolide antibiotic
**PREG/CONT** B/NA

**IND & DOSE Tx of infections caused by susceptible bacteria.** *Adult:* General guidelines, 15–20 mg/kg/d by continuous IV infusion or up to 4 g/d in divided doses q 6 hr; or 250 mg (400 mg ethylsuccinate) PO q 6 hr or 500 mg PO q 12 hr or 333 mg PO q 8 hr, up to 4 g/d, depending on infection severity. *Child:* General guidelines, 30–50 mg/kg/d PO in divided doses. Specific dose determined by infection severity, age, weight. **Tx of streptococcal infections.** *Adult:* 250 mg PO q 6 hr or 500 mg PO q 12 hr (for group A beta-hemolytic streptococcal infections, continue tx for at least 10 days). **Tx of Legionnaires' disease.** *Adult:* 1–4 g/d PO or IV in divided doses for 10–21 days. **Tx of dysenteric amebiasis.** *Adult:* 250 mg PO q 6 hr or 333 mg PO q 8 hr for 10–14 days. *Child:* 30–50 mg/kg/d PO in divided doses for 10–14 days. **Tx of acute PID** *(Neisseria gonorrhoeae). Adult:* 500 mg IV q 6 hr for 3 days, then 250 mg PO q 6 hr or 333 mg PO q 8 hr or 500 mg PO q 12 hr for 7 days. **Tx of chlamydial infections.** *Adult:* Urogenital infections during preg, 500 mg PO qid or 666 mg PO q 8 hr for at least 7 days; ½ this dose q 8 hr for at least 14 days if intolerant to first regimen. Urethritis in males, 800 mg ethylsuccinate PO tid for 7 days. *Child:* 50 mg/kg/d PO in divided doses, for at least 2 (conjunctivitis of newborn) or 3 (pneumonia of infancy) wk. **Tx of primary syphilis.** *Adult:* 30–40 g PO in divided doses over 10–15 days. **CDC recommendations for STDs.** *Adult:* 500 mg PO qid for 7–30 days, depending on infection. **Tx of pertussis.** *Child:* 40–50 mg/kg/d PO in divided doses for 14 days. **Tx of superficial ocular infections caused by susceptible strains.** *Adult, child:* ½-inch ribbon instilled into conjunctival sac of affected eye 2–6 ×/d, depending on infection severity. **Tx of acne** (dermatologic sol). *Adult, child:* Apply to affected areas a.m. and p.m. **Tx of skin infections caused by susceptible bacteria.** *Adult, child:* Apply flexible hydroactive dressings and granules; keep in place for 1–7 days.

**ADV EFF** Abd pain, **anaphylaxis,** anorexia, local irritation w/topical use; n/v/d, **pseudomembranous colitis,** superinfections

**INTERACTIONS** Calcium channel blockers, carbamazepine, corticosteroids, cyclosporine, digoxin, disopyramide, ergots, grapefruit juice, midazolam, oral anticoagulants, proton pump inhibitors, quinidine, statins, theophylline

**NC/PT** Culture before tx. Give oral drug on empty stomach round the clock for best results. Monitor LFTs w/long-term use. Apply topical form to clean, dry area. Pt should avoid grapefruit juice; report severe or bloody diarrhea, difficulty breathing.

## escitalopram oxalate

(Lexapro)

**CLASS** Antidepressant, SSRI

**PREG/CONT** C/NA

**BBW** Monitor for suicidality, especially when starting tx or altering dose. Increased risk in child, adolescent, young adult. Not approved for use in pt <12 yr.

**IND & DOSE** **Tx of major depressive disorder.** *Adult:* 10 mg/d PO as single dose; may increase to 20 mg/d after minimum of 1-wk trial period. Maint, 10–20 mg/d PO. *Child 12–17 yr:* 10 mg/d PO as single dose; max, 20 mg/d. **Tx of generalized anxiety disorder.** *Adult:* 10 mg/d PO; may increase to 20 mg/d after 1 wk if needed.

**ADJUST DOSE** Elderly pts, hepatic impairment

**ADV EFF** **Activation of mania/hypomania, anaphylaxis, angioedema,** angle-closure glaucoma, dizziness, ejaculatory disorders, nausea, **seizures, serotonin syndrome,** somnolence, suicidality

**INTERACTIONS** Alcohol, carbamazepine, citalopram, lithium, MAOIs, SSRIs, St. John's wort

**NC/PT** Limit supply in suicidal pts. Do not use within 14 days of MAOIs. Taper after long-term use. Not for use in preg/breastfeeding. Use safety precautions. May need 4 wk to see effects. Pt should not stop drug suddenly but should taper dose; avoid alcohol, St. John's wort; report thoughts of suicide. Name confusion between escitalopram and citalopram and *Lexapro* (escitalopram) and *Loxitane* (loxapine).

▶NEW DRUG

DANGEROUS DRUG

**esketamine** (Spravato)
**CLASS** Antidepressant, noncompetitive N-methyl-D-aspartate receptor antagonist
**PREG/CONT** High risk/C III

**BBW** Risk of sedation and dissociation. Available only through REMS program. Increased risk of suicidal thoughts/behaviors in child/young adult taking antidepressants. Closely monitor all antidepressant-treated pts for clinical worsening, emergence of suicidal thoughts/behaviors. Spravato is not approved for child.
**IND & DOSE Tx of tx-resistant depression, w/oral antidepressant.** *Adult:* 56 mg (4 sprays) intranasally w/health care provider supervision. May increase to 84 mg based on efficacy/tolerability.
**ADV EFF** Anxiety, cognitive impairment, dizziness, HTN, lethargy, n/v, vertigo
**NC/PT** Monitor for sedation for at least 2 hr after administration and for s&sx of abuse/misuse. Assess BP before and after administration. Give other intranasal drugs at least 1 hr before Spravato. Pt should avoid food for 2 hr and liquids for 30 min before administration.

**eslicarbazepine acetate** (Aptiom)
**CLASS** Antiepileptic, sodium channel blocker
**PREG/CONT** C/NA

**IND & DOSE Tx of partial-onset seizures, as monotherapy or w/other antiepileptics.** *Adult:* 400 mg/d PO; after 1 wk, increase to 800 mg/d PO. May increase by 400–600 mg/d wkly to max of 1,600 mg/d. *Child ≥4 yr:* Base dose on body weight and administer PO once daily. Increase dose in wkly intervals based on clinical response and tolerability, to recommended maintenance dose.
**ADJUST DOSE** Renal impairment
**ADV EFF Anaphylaxis,** dizziness, double vision, drowsiness, fatigue, headache, hyponatremia, **liver damage**, n/v, **suicidality**
**INTERACTIONS** Carbamazepine, hormonal contraceptives, phenobarbital, phenytoin, primidone
**NC/PT** Ensure proper dx. Taper dose when stopping to minimize seizure risk. Monitor LFTs, serum electrolytes; ensure safety precautions w/CNS effects. Pt should avoid preg/breastfeeding; take safety precautions w/CNS effects; report thoughts of suicide, difficulty breathing, urine/stool color changes.

DANGEROUS DRUG

**esmolol hydrochloride** (Brevibloc)
**CLASS** Antiarrhythmic, beta-selective adrenergic blocker
**PREG/CONT** C/NA

**IND & DOSE Tx of supraventricular tachycardia, noncompensatory tachycardia, intraop/postop tachycardia and HTN.** *Adult:* Initial loading dose, 500 mcg/kg/min IV for 1 min, then maint of 50 mcg/kg/min for 4 min. If response inadequate after 5 min, repeat loading dose and follow w/maint infusion of 100 mcg/kg/min. Repeat titration as needed, increasing rate of maint dose in 50-mcg/kg/min increments. As desired HR or safe endpoint is approached, omit loading infusion and decrease incremental dose in maint infusion to 25 mcg/kg/min (or less), or increase interval between titration steps from 5 to 10 min. Usual range, 50–200 mcg/kg/min. Up to 24-hr infusions have been used; up to 48 hr may be well tolerated. Individualize dose based on pt response; max, 300 mcg/kg/min.
**ADV EFF** Hypoglycemia, hypotension, injection-site inflammation,

light-headedness, midscapular pain, rigors, weakness
**INTERACTIONS** Anticholinergics, antihypertensives, calcium channel blockers, digoxin, ibuprofen, indomethacin, piroxicam, sympathomimetics
**NC/PT** Do not give undiluted. Do not mix in sol w/sodium bicarbonate, diazepam, furosemide, thiopental. Not for long-term use. Closely monitor BP, ECG. Pt should report difficulty breathing, chest pain.

## esomeprazole magnesium (Nexium)

**CLASS** Antisecretory, proton pump inhibitor
**PREG/CONT** B/NA

**IND & DOSE** **Healing of erosive esophagitis.** *Adult:* 20–40 mg PO daily for 4–8 wk. Maint, 20 mg PO daily. *Child 1–11 yr:* ≥20 kg, 10–20 mg/d PO for up to 8 wk; <20 kg, 10 mg/d PO for up to 8 wk. **Tx of symptomatic GERD.** *Adult:* 20 mg PO daily for 4 wk. Can use additional 4-wk course. *Child 12–17 yr:* 20–40 mg/d PO for up to 8 wk. *Child 1–11 yr:* 10 mg/d PO for up to 8 wk. **Tx of duodenal ulcer.** *Adult:* 40 mg/d PO for 10 days w/1,000 mg PO bid amoxicillin and 500 mg PO bid clarithromycin. **To reduce risk of gastric ulcers w/NSAID use.** *Adult:* 20–40 mg PO daily for 6 mo. **Short-term tx of GERD when oral therapy not possible.** *Adult, child 1 mo–17 yr:* 20–40 mg IV by injection over at least 3 min or IV infusion over 10–30 min.
**ADJUST DOSE** Severe hepatic impairment
**ADV EFF** Abd pain, acute interstitial nephritis, atrophic gastritis, **bone loss w/long-term use, CDAD,** dizziness, headache, hypomagnesemia, n/v/d, pneumonia, sinusitis, URI, vitamin $B_{12}$ deficiency
**INTERACTIONS** Atazanavir, benzodiazepines, cilostazol, clopidogrel, digoxin, iron salts, ketoconazole, rifampin, St. John's wort, tacrolimus
**NC/PT** Reevaluate use after 8 wk. Give at least 1 hr before meals; may give through NG tube. Monitor LFTs periodically. Limit IV use to max 10 days. Pt should swallow capsules whole and not cut/crush/chew them; take safety precautions w/CNS effects; report diarrhea, difficulty breathing. Name confusion between esomeprazole and omeprazole, *Nexium* (esomeprazole) and *Nexavar* (sorafenib).

## estazolam (generic)

**CLASS** Benzodiazepine, sedative-hypnotic
**PREG/CONT** X/C-IV

**IND & DOSE** **Tx of insomnia, recurring insomnia, acute or chronic medical conditions requiring restful sleep.** *Adult:* 1 mg PO before bedtime; may need up to 2 mg.
**ADJUST DOSE** Elderly pts, debilitating disease
**ADV EFF** **Anaphylaxis, angioedema,** apathy, bradycardia, constipation, **CV collapse,** depression, diarrhea, disorientation, drowsiness, drug dependence w/withdrawal syndrome, dyspepsia, lethargy, light-headedness, tachycardia, urine retention
**INTERACTIONS** Alcohol, aminophylline, barbiturates, opioids, phenothiazines, rifampin, TCAs, theophylline
**NC/PT** Monitor LFTs, renal function. Taper after long-term use. Pt should avoid alcohol; use only as needed (can be habit-forming); take safety precautions w/CNS effects; report difficulty breathing, swelling.

## estradiol, estradiol acetate, estradiol cypionate, estradiol hemihydrate, estradiol valerate (Delestrogen, Estrace, Estring, Estrogel, Evamist, Femring, Vagifem)

**CLASS** Estrogen
**PREG/CONT** X/NA

**BBW** Arrange for pretreatment and periodic (at least annual) hx and

physical; should include BP, breasts, abdomen, pelvic organs, Pap test. May increase risk of endometrial cancer. Do not use to prevent CV events, dementia; may increase risks, including thrombophlebitis, PE, stroke, MI. Caution pt of risks of estrogen use. Stress need for preg prevention during tx, frequent medical follow-up, periodic rests from tx.
**IND & DOSE** **Relief of moderate to severe vasomotor sx, atrophic vaginitis, kraurosis vulvae associated w/ menopause.** *Adult:* 1–2 mg/d PO. adjust dose to control sx. For gel, 0.25 g 0.1% gel applied to right or left upper thigh on alternating days; may increase to 0.5 or 1 g/d to control sx. For topical spray *(Evamist)*, 1 spray once daily to forearm; may increase to 2–3 sprays daily. Cyclic therapy (3 wk on/1 wk off) recommended, especially in women w/no hysterectomy. 1–5 mg estradiol cypionate in oil IM q 3–4 wk. 10–20 mg estradiol valerate in oil IM q 4 wk. 0.014- to 0.05-mg system applied to skin wkly or twice wkly. If oral estrogens have been used, start transdermal system 1 wk after withdrawal of oral form. Given on cyclic schedule (3 wk on/1 wk off). Attempt to taper or discontinue q 3–6 mo. Vaginal cream: 2–4 g intravaginally daily for 1–2 wk, then reduce to ½ dose for similar period followed by maint of 1 g 1–3 ×/wk thereafter. Discontinue or taper at 3- to 6-mo intervals. Vaginal ring: Insert one ring high into vagina. Replace q 90 days. Vaginal tablet: 1 tablet inserted vaginally daily for 2 wk, then twice wkly. Emulsion: Apply lotion to legs, thighs, or calves once daily. Apply gel to one arm once daily. **Tx of female hypogonadism, female castration, primary ovarian failure.** *Adult:* 1–2 mg/d PO. Adjust to control sx. Cyclic therapy (3 wk on/1 wk off) recommended. 1.5–2 mg estradiol cypionate in oil IM at monthly intervals. 10–20 mg estradiol valerate in oil IM q 4 wk. 0.05-mg system applied to skin twice wkly as above. **Tx of prostate cancer** (inoperable). *Adult:* 1–2 mg PO tid; give long-term. 30 mg or more estradiol valerate in oil IM q 1–2 wk. **Tx of breast cancer** (inoperable, progressing). *Adult:* 10 mg tid PO for at least 3 mo. **Px of postpartum breast engorgement.** *Adult:* 10–25 mg estradiol valerate in oil IM as single injection at end of first stage of labor. **Px of osteoporosis.** *Adult:* 0.5 mg/d PO cyclically (23 days on, 5 days rest) starting as soon after menopause as possible.
**ADV EFF** **Acute pancreatitis,** abd cramps, bloating, **cancer,** chloasma, **cholestatic jaundice, colitis,** dysmenorrhea, edema, **hepatic adenoma,** menstrual flow changes, n/v/d, pain at injection site, photosensitivity, premenstrual syndrome, **thrombotic events**
**INTERACTIONS** Barbiturates, carbamazepine, corticosteroids, phenytoins, rifampin
**NC/PT** Give cyclically for short-term use. Give w/progestin for women w/ intact uterus. Review proper administration for each drug type. Potentially serious adverse effects. Not for use in preg/breastfeeding. Pt should get regular pelvic exams, avoid sun exposure, report pain in calves/chest, lumps in breast, vision or speech changes.

## estrogens, conjugated
(Premarin)
**CLASS** Estrogen
**PREG/CONT** High risk/NA

**BBW** Arrange for pretreatment and periodic (at least annual) hx and physical; should include BP, breasts, abdomen, pelvic organs, Pap test. May increase risk of endometrial cancer. Do not use to prevent CV events, dementia; may increase risks, including thrombophlebitis, PE, stroke, MI. Caution pt of risks of estrogen use. Stress need for preg prevention during tx, frequent medical follow-up, periodic rests from tx.

**IND & DOSE Relief of moderate to severe vasomotor sx associated w/ menopause:** *Adult:* 0.3–0.625 mg/d PO. **Tx of atrophic vaginitis, kraurosis vulvae associated w/menopause.** *Adult:* 0.5–2 g vaginal cream daily intravaginally or topically, depending on severity. Taper or discontinue at 3- to 6-mo intervals. Or, 0.3 mg/d PO continually. **Tx of female hypogonadism.** *Adult:* 0.3–0.625 mg/d PO for 3 wk, then 1 wk rest. **Tx of female castration, primary ovarian failure.** *Adult:* 1.25 mg/d PO. **Tx of prostate cancer** (inoperable). *Adult:* 1.25–2.5 mg PO tid. **Tx of osteoporosis.** *Adult:* 0.3 mg/d PO continuously or cyclically (25 days on/5 days off). **Tx of breast cancer** (inoperable, progressing). *Adult:* 10 mg PO tid for at least 3 mo. **Tx of abnormal uterine bleeding due to hormonal imbalance.** 25 mg IV or IM. Repeat in 6–12 hr as needed. More rapid response w/IV route.

**ADJUST DOSE** Hepatic impairment

**ADV EFF Acute pancreatitis,** abd cramps, **anaphylaxis**, bloating, **cancer,** chloasma, **cholestatic jaundice, colitis**, dysmenorrhea, edema, gallbladder disease, headache, **hepatic adenoma,** hereditary angioedema exacerbations, menstrual flow changes, n/v/d, pain at injection site, photosensitivity, premenstrual syndrome, **thrombotic events**

**INTERACTIONS** Barbiturates, carbamazepine, corticosteroids, phenytoins, rifampin

**NC/PT** Give cyclically for short-term use. Give w/progestin for women w/ intact uterus. Do not give w/undiagnosed genital bleeding, active DVT, liver disease, hx of thrombotic events. Review proper administration for each drug type. Potentially serious adverse effects. Not for use in preg/breastfeeding. Pt should get regular pelvic exams; avoid sun exposure; report pain in calves/chest, lumps in breast, vision or speech changes.

## estrogens, esterified

(Menest)

**CLASS** Estrogen

**PREG/CONT** X/NA

**BBW** Arrange for pretreatment and periodic (at least annual) hx and physical; should include BP, breasts, abdomen, pelvic organs, Pap test. May increase risk of endometrial cancer. Do not use to prevent CV events or dementia; may increase risks, including thrombophlebitis, PE, stroke, MI. Caution pt of risks of estrogen use. Stress need for preg prevention during tx, frequent medical follow-up, periodic rests from drug tx. Give cyclically for short-term only when treating postmenopausal conditions because of endometrial neoplasm risk. Taper to lowest effective dose; provide drug-free wk each mo.

**IND & DOSE Relief of moderate to severe vasomotor sx, atrophic vaginitis, kraurosis vulvae associated w/ menopause.** *Adult:* 0.3–1.25 mg/d PO given cyclically (3 wk on/1 wk off). Use lowest possible dose. **Tx of female hypogonadism.** *Adult:* 2.5–7.5 mg/d PO in divided doses for 20 days on/10 days off. **Tx of female castration, primary ovarian failure.** *Adult:* 1.25 mg/d PO given cyclically. **Tx of prostate cancer** (inoperable). *Adult:* 1.25–2.5 mg PO tid. **Tx of inoperable, progressing breast cancer.** *Adult*: 10 mg PO tid for at least 3 mo.

**ADV EFF Acute pancreatitis,** abd cramps, bloating, **cancer,** chloasma, **cholestatic jaundice, colitis,** dysmenorrhea, edema, headache, **hepatic adenoma,** menstrual flow changes, n/v/d, pain at injection site, photosensitivity, premenstrual syndrome, **thrombotic events**

**INTERACTIONS** Barbiturates, carbamazepine, corticosteroids, phenytoins, rifampin

**NC/PT** Give cyclically for short-term use. Give w/progestin for women w/intact uterus. Review proper administration for each drug type. Potentially serious adverse effects. Not for use in preg/breastfeeding. Pt should get regular pelvic exams; avoid sun exposure; report pain in calves/chest, lumps in breast, vision or speech changes.

**estropipate** (generic)
**CLASS** Estrogen
**PREG/CONT** X/NA

**BBW** Arrange for pretreatment and periodic (at least annual) hx and physical; should include BP, breasts, abdomen, pelvic organs, Pap test. May increase risk of endometrial cancer. Do not use to prevent CV events or dementia; may increase risks, including thrombophlebitis, PE, stroke, MI. Caution pt of risks of estrogen use. Stress need for preg prevention during tx, frequent medical follow-up, periodic rests from drug tx. Give cyclically for short term only when treating postmenopausal conditions because of endometrial neoplasm risk. Taper to lowest effective dose; provide drug-free wk each mo.
**IND & DOSE** **Relief of moderate to severe vasomotor sx, atrophic vaginitis, kraurosis vulvae associated w/ menopause.** *Adult:* 0.75–6 mg/d PO given cyclically (3 wk on/1 wk off). Use lowest possible dose. **Tx of female hypogonadism, female castration, primary ovarian failure.** *Adult:* 1.5–9 mg/d PO for first 3 wk, then rest period of 8–10 days. Repeat if no bleeding at end of rest period. **Px of osteoporosis.** *Adult:* 0.75 mg/d PO for 25 days of 31-day cycle/mo.
**ADV EFF** **Acute pancreatitis,** abd cramps, bloating, **cancer,** chloasma, **cholestatic jaundice, colitis,** dysmenorrhea, edema, headache, **hepatic adenoma,** menstrual flow changes, n/v/d, pain at injection site, photosensitivity, premenstrual syndrome, **thrombotic events**
**INTERACTIONS** Barbiturates, carbamazepine, corticosteroids, phenytoins, rifampin
**NC/PT** Give cyclically for short-term use. Give w/progestin for women w/ intact uterus. Review proper administration for each drug type. Potentially serious adverse effects. Not for use in preg/breastfeeding. Pt should get regular pelvic exams; avoid sun exposure; report pain in calves/chest, lumps in breast, vision or speech changes.

**eszopiclone** (Lunesta)
**CLASS** Nonbenzodiazepine hypnotic, sedative-hypnotic
**PREG/CONT** C/C-IV

**BBW** Complex sleep behaviors (sleepwalking, sleep-driving) may occur while pt not fully awake, leading to serious injuries, including death.
**IND & DOSE** **Tx of insomnia.** *Adult:* 1 mg PO immediately before bedtime, w/7–8 hr remaining before planned awakening. May increase to 3 mg PO. Use lowest effective dose.
**ADJUST DOSE** CYP3A4 inhibitor use, elderly or debilitated pts, severe hepatic impairment
**ADV EFF** Abnormal thinking, **anaphylaxis, angioedema,** depression, dizziness, headache, impaired alertness/motor coordination, nervousness, somnolence, **suicidality**
**INTERACTIONS** Alcohol, clarithromycin, itraconazole, ketoconazole, nefazodone, nelfinavir, rifampin, ritonavir
**NC/PT** Not for use in preg/breastfeeding. Pt should swallow tablet whole and not cut/crush/chew it; take only if in bed and able to stay in bed for up to 8 hr; avoid alcohol; not take w/high-fat meal; avoid sudden withdrawal; use safety precautions w/CNS effects; report thoughts of suicide, difficulty breathing, swelling of face or neck.

**etanercept** (Enbrel), **etanercept-szzs** (Erelzi)
**CLASS** Antiarthritic, DMARD
**PREG/CONT** Moderate risk/NA

**BBW** Monitor for infection s&sx; discontinue if infection occurs. Risk

of serious infections (including TB), death. Increased risk of lymphoma, other cancers in child taking for juvenile RA, Crohn disease, other inflammatory conditions; monitor accordingly.
**IND & DOSE To reduce s&sx of ankylosing spondylitis, RA, psoriatic arthritis, juvenile idiopathic arthritis.** *Adult:* 50 mg/wk subcut. *Child 2–17 yr >63 kg:* 50 mg/wk subcut. **To reduce s&sx of plaque psoriasis.** *Adult:* 50 mg/dose subcut twice wkly 3 or 4 days apart for 3 mo; maint, 50 mg/wk subcut.
**ADV EFF Anaphylaxis, bone marrow suppression, demyelinating disorders (MS, myelitis, optic neuritis), cancers, increased risk of serious infections,** dizziness, headache, HF, injection-site irritation, URIs
**INTERACTIONS** Immunosuppressants, vaccines
**NC/PT** Obtain baseline and periodic CBC, neuro function tests. Monitor pt w/hx of HBV infection; reactivation possible. Rotate injection sites (abdomen, thigh, upper arm). Monitor for infection. Do regular cancer screening. Teach proper administration/disposal of needles/syringes. Pt should avoid exposure to infection; maintain other tx for rheumatoid disorder (drug not a cure); report s&sx of infection, difficulty breathing.

## etelcalcetide (Parsabiv)
**CLASS** Calcium-sensing receptor agonist
**PREG/CONT** Unkn/NA

**IND & DOSE Tx of secondary hyperparathyroidism in adults w/ chronic kidney disease on hemodialysis.** *Adult:* 5 mg by IV bolus 3 ×/wk at end of hemodialysis tx. Maint based on serum calcium response; range, 2.5–15 mg IV bolus 3 ×/wk.
**ADV EFF** Adynamic bone disease, headache, **hypocalcemia,** muscle spasms, n/v/d, paresthesia, **upper GI bleeding, worsening HF**
**NC/PT** Ensure serum calcium is within normal range. Use caution in preg; not for use in breastfeeding. Do not mix or dilute drug. Inject into venous end of dialysis line at end of hemodialysis tx during rinse back to give IV after rinse back. Measure parathyroid hormone level after 4 wk to adjust dosage. Pt should maintain regular serum calcium levels; report muscle spasms, coffee-ground vomiting, abd pain.

## eteplirsen (Exondys 51)
**CLASS** Antisense oligonucleotide
**PREG/CONT** Unkn/NA

**IND & DOSE Tx of Duchenne muscular dystrophy w/confirmed gene amenable to exon 51 skipping.** *Adult, child:* 30 mg/kg IV over 35–60 min once wkly.
**ADV EFF** Balance disorders, **hypersensitivity reactions,** nausea
**NC/PT** Ensure proper dx. Dilute before infusing. Monitor clinical effects. Pt should mark calendar w/tx days; be aware effects in preg/breastfeeding are unkn.

## ethacrynic acid (Edecrin)
**CLASS** Loop diuretic
**PREG/CONT** B/NA

**IND & DOSE To reduce edema associated w/systemic diseases.** *Adult:* 50–200 mg/d PO; may give IV as 50 mg slowly to max, 100 mg. *Child:* 25 mg/d PO; adjust in 25-mg/d increments if needed.
**ADV EFF** Abd pain, **agranulocytosis,** dehydration, dysphagia, fatigue, headache, hepatic impairment, hypokalemia, n/v/d, vertigo, weakness
**INTERACTIONS** Diuretics
**NC/PT** Switch to oral form as soon as possible. Give w/food if GI upset. Monitor potassium; supplement as needed. Not for use in breastfeeding.

Pt should weigh self daily; report changes of ≥3 lb/d.

**ethambutol hydrochloride** (Myambutol)
**CLASS** Antituberculotic
**PREG/CONT** C/NA

**IND & DOSE Tx of pulmonary TB, w/at least one other antituberculotic.** *Adult, child ≥13 yr:* 15 mg/kg/d PO as single oral dose. Continue until bacteriologic conversion permanent and max clinical improvement has occurred. Retreatment: 25 mg/kg/d as single oral dose. After 60 days, reduce to 15 mg/kg/d as single dose.
**ADV EFF** Anorexia, fever, headache, malaise, n/v/d, optic neuritis, **toxic epidermal necrolysis, thrombocytopenia**
**INTERACTIONS** Aluminum salts
**NC/PT** Ensure use w/other antituberculotics. Give w/food. Monitor CBC, LFTs, renal function, ophthal exam. Not for use in preg/breastfeeding. Pt should not stop suddenly; have regular medical checkups; report changes in vision, color perception; take safety precautions w/CNS effects.

**ethionamide** (Trecator)
**CLASS** Antituberculotic
**PREG/CONT** High risk/NA

**IND & DOSE Tx of pulmonary TB unresponsive to first-line tx, w/at least one other antituberculotic.** *Adult:* 15–20 mg/kg/d PO to max 1 g/d. *Child:* 10–20 mg/kg/d PO in two or three divided doses after meals (max, 1 g/d), or 15 mg/kg/24 hr as single dose.
**ADV EFF** Alopecia, asthenia, depression, drowsiness, **hepatitis,** metallic taste, n/v/d, orthostatic hypotension, peripheral neuritis
**NC/PT** Ensure use w/other antituberculotics. Concomitant use of pyridoxine recommended to prevent or minimize s&sx of peripheral neuritis. Give w/food. Monitor LFTs before tx and q 2–4 wk during tx. Not for use in preg. Pt should not stop suddenly; have regular medical checkups; take safety precautions w/CNS effects; report urine/stool color changes.

**ethosuximide** (Zarontin)
**CLASS** Antiepileptic, succinimide
**PREG/CONT** High risk/NA

**IND & DOSE Control of absence (petit mal) seizures.** *Adult, child ≥6 yr:* 500 mg/d PO. Increase by small increments to maint level; increase by 250 mg q 4–7 days until control achieved. *Child 3–6 yr:* 250 mg/d PO. Increase in small increments until optimal 20 mg/kg/d in one dose or two divided doses.
**ADV EFF** Abd pain, **agranulocytosis, aplastic anemia,** ataxia, blurred vision, constipation, cramps, dizziness, drowsiness, **eosinophilia, generalized tonic-clonic seizures, granulocytopenia,** irritability, **leukopenia, monocytosis,** nervousness, n/v/d, **pancytopenia, SJS, suicidality**
**INTERACTIONS** Alcohol, CNS depressants, primidone
**NC/PT** Reduce dose, discontinue, or substitute other antiepileptic gradually. Taper when discontinuing. Monitor CBC. Stop drug at signs of rash. Evaluate for therapeutic serum level (40–100 mcg/mL). Not for use in preg (contraceptives advised)/breastfeeding. Pt should avoid alcohol; wear medical alert tag; avoid exposure to infection; take safety precautions w/CNS effects; report s&sx of infection, thoughts of suicide.

**ethotoin** (Peganone)
**CLASS** Antiepileptic, hydantoin
**PREG/CONT** D/NA

**IND & DOSE Control of tonic-clonic, complex partial (psychomotor) seizures.** *Adult:* 1 g/d PO in four–six divided doses; increase gradually over several days. Usual maint dose, 2–3 g/d PO in four–six divided doses. *Child ≥1 yr:* 750 mg/d PO in four–six divided doses; maint range, 500 mg/d to 1 g/d PO in four–six divided doses.

**ADV EFF** Abd pain, **agranulocytosis, aplastic anemia,** ataxia, blurred vision, confusion, constipation, cramps, dizziness, drowsiness, **eosinophilia, epidermal necrolysis,** fatigue, **granulocytopenia,** gum dysplasia, **hepatotoxicity,** irritability, **leukopenia, lymphoma, monocytosis,** nervousness, n/v/d, nystagmus, **pancytopenia, pulmonary fibrosis, SJS, suicidality**

**INTERACTIONS** Acetaminophen, amiodarone, antineoplastics, carbamazepine, chloramphenicol, cimetidine, corticosteroids, cyclosporine, diazoxide, disopyramide, disulfiram, doxycycline, estrogens, fluconazole, folic acid, hormonal contraceptives, isoniazid, levodopa, methadone, metyrapone, mexiletine, phenacemide, phenylbutazone, primidone, rifampin, sulfonamides, theophyllines, trimethoprim, valproic acid

**NC/PT** May use w/other antiepileptics. Reduce dose, discontinue, or substitute other antiepileptic gradually. Taper when discontinuing. Monitor CBC. Stop drug at signs of rash. Monitor LFTs. Give w/food to enhance absorption. Evaluate for therapeutic serum levels (15–50 mcg/mL). Not for use in preg (contraceptives advised)/breastfeeding. Evaluate lymph node enlargement during tx. Frequent medical follow-up needed. Pt should avoid alcohol; wear medical alert tag; avoid exposure to infection; take safety precautions w/ CNS effects; use good dental care to limit gum hyperplasia; report s&sx of infection, thoughts of suicide.

---

## etodolac (generic)

**CLASS** Analgesic, NSAID

**PREG/CONT** C/NA

**BBW** Increased risk of CV events, GI bleeding; monitor accordingly.

**IND & DOSE Mgt of s&sx of osteoarthritis, RA.** *Adult:* 600–1,000 mg/d PO in divided doses. Maint range, 600–1,200 mg/d in divided doses; max, 1,200 mg/d (20 mg/kg for pts <60 kg). ER, 400–1,000 mg/d PO; max, 1,200 mg/d. **Mgt of s&sx of juvenile RA** (ER tablets). *Child 6–16 yr:* >60 kg, 1,000 mg/d PO as 500 mg PO bid; 46–60 kg, 800 mg/d PO as 400 mg PO bid; 31–45 kg, 600 mg/d PO; 20–30 kg, 400 mg/d PO. **Analgesia, acute pain.** *Adult:* 200–400 mg PO q 6–8 hr; max, 1,200 mg/d.

**ADV EFF Anaphylactoid reactions, bleeding,** blurred vision, constipation, **CV events,** diarrhea, dizziness, dyspepsia, GI pain, **hepatic failure, renal impairment**

**INTERACTIONS** Anticoagulants, antihypertensives, antiplatelets

**NC/PT** Pt should take w/meals; use safety precautions w/CNS effects; report bleeding, difficulty breathing, urine/stool color changes.

---

**DANGEROUS DRUG**

## etoposide (VP-16) (Etopophos)

**CLASS** Antineoplastic, mitotic inhibitor

**PREG/CONT** D/NA

**BBW** Obtain platelet count, Hgb, Hct, WBC count w/differential before tx and each dose. If severe response, discontinue; consult physician. Severe myelosuppression possible. Monitor for severe hypersensitivity reaction; arrange supportive care.

**IND & DOSE Tx of testicular cancer.** *Adult:* 50–100 mg/m²/d IV on days 1–5, or 100 mg/m²/d IV on days 1, 3, 5 q 3–4 wk w/other chemotherapeutics. **Tx of small-cell lung cancer.** *Adult:* 35 mg/m²/d IV for 4 days to 50 mg/m²/d for 5 days; repeat q 3–4 wk after recovery from toxicity or switch to oral form (two × IV dose rounded to nearest 50 mg).

**ADJUST DOSE** Renal impairment

**ADV EFF** Alopecia, **anaphylactoid reactions,** anorexia, fatigue, hypotension, **myelotoxicity**, n/v/d, somnolence
**INTERACTIONS** Anticoagulants, antihypertensives, antiplatelets
**NC/PT** Avoid skin contact; use rubber gloves. If contact occurs, immediately wash w/soap, water. Do not give IM, subcut. Monitor BP during infusion. Give antiemetic if nausea severe. Not for use in preg (contraceptives advised). Pt should cover head at temp extremes (hair loss possible); mark calendar of tx days; avoid exposure to infection; have blood tests regularly; report difficulty breathing, muscle pain.

## etravirine (Intelence)

**CLASS** Antiviral, nonnucleoside reverse transcriptase inhibitor
**PREG/CONT** B/NA

**IND & DOSE Tx of HIV-1 infection in tx-experienced pts w/evidence of viral replication and HIV-1 strains resistant to non-NRTIs and other antiretrovirals, w/other drugs.** *Adult, pregnant pt:* 200 mg PO bid after meal. *Child 2–<18 yr:* ≥30 kg, 200 mg PO bid; 25–<30 kg, 150 mg PO bid; 20–<25 mg, 125 mg PO bid; 16–<20 kg, 100 mg PO bid.
**ADV EFF** Altered fat distribution, diarrhea, fatigue, headache, **severe hypersensitivity reactions**
**INTERACTIONS** Antiarrhythmics, atazanavir, azole, carbamazepine, clarithromycin, clopidogrel, delavirdine, fosamprenavir, indinavir, maraviroc, nelfinavir, nevirapine, phenobarbital, phenytoin, rifabutin, rifampin, rifapentine, ritonavir, St. John's wort, tipranavir, warfarin
**NC/PT** Always give w/other antivirals. Stop at first sign of severe skin reaction. Pt should swallow tablets whole and not cut/crush/chew them. If pt cannot swallow, put tablets in glass of water, stir; when water is milky, have pt drink whole glass, rinse several times, and drink rinse each time to get full dose. Not for use in breastfeeding. Pt should avoid w/St. John's wort; take precautions to prevent transmission (drug not a cure); have blood tests regularly; report difficulty breathing.

## everolimus (Afinitor, Zortress)

**CLASS** Antineoplastic, kinase inhibitor
**PREG/CONT** High risk/NA

**BBW** *Zortress* only: Risk of serious infections, cancer development; risk of venous thrombosis, kidney loss; risk of nephrotoxicity w/cyclosporine. Increased mortality if used w/heart transplant; not approved for this use.
**IND & DOSE Tx of advanced renal carcinoma after failure w/sunitinib, sorafenib; tx of subependymal giant-cell astrocytoma in pts not candidates for surgery.** *Adult:* 5–10 mg/d PO w/food. **Tx of pts ≥1 yr w/tuberous sclerosis complex (TSC) who have developed brain tumor.** *Adult, child:* 4.5 mg/$m^2$ PO once/d w/food. **Tx of postmenopausal advanced hormone receptor–positive, HER2-negative breast cancer; advanced neuroendocrine pancreatic tumors; advanced renal cell carcinoma; renal angiomyolipoma w/TSC.** *Adult:* 10 mg/d PO at same time each day. **Px of organ rejection in adult at low to moderate risk receiving kidney transplant** (*Zortress*). *Adult:* 0.75 mg PO bid w/cyclosporine starting as soon as possible after transplant. **Adjunct for tx of TSC-associated partial-onset seizures** (*Afinitor*). *Adult, child ≥2 yr:* 5 mg/$m^2$ PO daily; adjust dose to attain trough of 5–15 ng/mL
**ADJUST DOSE** Hepatic impairment
**ADV EFF** Angioedema; elevated blood glucose, lipids, serum creatinine; myelosuppression, oral ulcerations, **pneumonitis, serious to fatal infections**, stomatitis

**INTERACTIONS** Live vaccines, strong CYP3A4 inducers (increase everolimus dose to 20 mg/d), CYP3A4 inhibitors
**NC/PT** Give w/food. Provide oral care. Monitor respiratory status; protect from infections. Not for use in preg (contraceptives advised)/breastfeeding. Mouth care may be needed. Pt should swallow tablet whole and not cut/crush/chew it; report difficulty breathing, fever.

## evolocumab (Repatha)
**CLASS** PCSK9 inhibitor antibody
**PREG/CONT** Moderate risk/NA

**IND & DOSE** **To reduce risk of MI, stroke, coronary revascularization in pts w/established CV disease; tx of pts w/primary hyperlipidemia (including heterozygous familial hypercholesterolemia) as adjunct to diet, alone or in combo w/other lipid-lowering therapies; adjunct to diet/exercise for tx of heterozygous familial hypercholesterolemia in pts w/maximum tolerated statin or other lipid-lowering therapy or clinical atherosclerotic CV disease.** *Adult:* 140 mg subcut once q 2 wk; or 420 mg subcut (three 140-mg injections given in 30 min) subcut once/mo.
**ADV EFF** Back pain, flulike sx, **hypersensitivity reactions,** injection-site reactions, nasopharyngitis
**NC/PT** Monitor LDL at baseline and periodically. Monitor for severe hypersensitivity reaction; stop drug, provide supportive care. Ensure use of diet/exercise program. Use caution in preg/breastfeeding. Teach proper administration/disposal of needles/syringes, not to reuse or share syringe or pen. Pt should rotate injection sites w/each use; mark calendar for injection days; review information w/each prescription; report difficulty breathing, rash, injection-site pain/inflammation.

## exemestane (Aromasin)
**CLASS** Antineoplastic
**PREG/CONT** High risk/NA

**IND & DOSE** **Tx of advanced breast cancer in postmenopausal women whose disease has progressed after tamoxifen; adjunct tx of postmenopausal women w/estrogen receptor–positive early breast cancer who have received 2–3 yr of tamoxifen; switch to exemestane to finish 5-yr course.** *Adult:* 25 mg/d PO w/meal.
**ADV EFF** Anxiety, decreased bone marrow density, depression, GI upset, headache, hot flashes, nausea, sweating
**INTERACTIONS** CYP3A4 inducers/inhibitors, estrogens, St. John's wort
**NC/PT** Monitor LFTs, renal function, bone density. Give supportive therapy for adverse effects. Not for use in preg/breastfeeding. Pt should not use St. John's wort.

## exenatide (Bydureon, Byetta)
**CLASS** Antidiabetic, incretin mimetic drug
**PREG/CONT** C/NA

**BBW** ER form increases risk of thyroid C-cell tumors; contraindicated w/personal, family hx of medullary thyroid cancer and in pts w/multiple endocrine neoplasia syndrome.
**IND & DOSE** **Adjunct to diet/exercise for tx of type 2 diabetes; to improve glycemic control in type 2 diabetes. Not a first-line therapy.** *Adult:* 5–10 mcg by subcut injection bid at any time within 60 min before a.m. and p.m. meals or two main meals of day, approx 6 hr apart. ER form, 2 mg by subcut injection once q 7 days.
**ADJUST DOSE** Renal impairment
**ADV EFF** **Anaphylaxis, angioedema,** dizziness, **hypoglycemia,** injection-site reaction, **hemorrhagic or necrotizing pancreatitis,** n/v/d, renal impairment, **thyroid C cell tumors**

**INTERACTIONS** Alcohol, antibiotics, oral contraceptives, warfarin
**NC/PT** Not for use in type 1 diabetes, ketoacidosis. Maintain diet/exercise, other drugs used to tx diabetes. Monitor serum glucose. Monitor for pancreatitis. Rotate injection sites (thigh, abdomen, upper arm). Give within 1 hr of meal; if pt not going to eat, do not give. Use caution in preg; not for use in breastfeeding. Review hypoglycemia s&sx. Pt should report difficulty breathing, swelling.

## ezetimibe (Zetia)

**CLASS** Cholesterol-absorption inhibitor, cholesterol-lowering drug
**PREG/CONT** C/NA

**IND & DOSE Adjunct to diet/exercise to lower cholesterol.** *Adult, child >10 yr:* 10 mg/d PO w/o regard to food. May give at same time as HMG-CoA reductase inhibitor, fenofibrate. If combined w/bile acid sequestrant, give at least 2 hr before or 4 hr after bile acid sequestrant.
**ADV EFF** Abd pain, diarrhea, dizziness, headache, URI
**INTERACTIONS** Cholestyramine, cyclosporine, fenofibrate, gemfibrozil
**NC/PT** Ensure use of diet/exercise program. Monitor serum lipid profile. Not for use in preg/breastfeeding. Frequent blood tests needed. Pt should use safety precautions w/CNS effects, continue other lipid-lowering drugs if prescribed.

## ezogabine (Potiga)

**CLASS** Antiepileptic, neuronal potassium channel opener
**PREG/CONT** C/NA

**BBW** Risk of suicidal ideation/suicidality; monitor accordingly. Risk of retinal abnormalities, vision loss. Obtain baseline and periodic ophthalmologic exams; if eye changes occur, stop drug unless no other tx possible.
**IND & DOSE Adjunct to tx of partial seizures when other measures have failed.** *Adult:* 100 mg PO tid for 1 wk; maint, 200–400 mg PO tid, w/other antiepileptics.
**ADV EFF** Abnormal coordination, aphasia, asthenia, blurred vision, confused state, dizziness, fatigue, **prolonged QT,** retinal abnormalities, skin discoloration, somnolence, tremor, urine retention, suicidal ideation, vertigo, **vision loss**
**INTERACTIONS** Alcohol, carbamazepine, digoxin, phenytoin
**NC/PT** Obtain baseline ECG; review QT interval periodically. Ensure baseline and periodic vision exam by ophthalmologist; discontinue w/pigmentary or vision changes. Taper slowly when withdrawing. Not for use in preg/breastfeeding. Pt should empty bladder before taking; continue other tx for seizures as prescribed; wear medical alert tag; avoid alcohol; use safety precautions for CNS effects; report thoughts of suicide, vision changes.

## factor XIII concentrate (human) (Corifact)

**CLASS** Clotting factor
**PREG/CONT** C/NA

**IND & DOSE Routine px of congenital factor XIII deficiency.** *Adult, child:* 40 units/kg IV over not less than 4 mL/min, then base dose on pt response. Repeat q 28 d, maintaining trough activity level of 5%–20%.
**ADV EFF Anaphylaxis,** arthralgia, **blood-transferred diseases,** chills, factor XIII antibody formation, fever, headache, hepatic impairment, **thrombotic events**
**NC/PT** Alert pt to risk of blood-related disease. Teach pt s&sx of thrombotic events, allergic reaction, immune reaction (break-through bleeding). Advise use of medical alert tag.

**famciclovir** (generic)
**CLASS** Antiviral
**PREG/CONT** B/NA

**IND & DOSE** **Mgt of herpes labialis.** *Adult:* 1,500 mg PO as single dose. **Tx of genital herpes, first episode in immunocompetent pts.** *Adult:* 1,000 mg PO bid for 1 day. **Suppression of recurrent genital herpes in immunocompetent pts.** *Adult:* 250 mg PO bid for up to 1 yr. **Tx of herpes zoster.** *Adult:* 500 mg PO q 8 hr for 7 d. **Tx of recurrent orolabial/genital herpes simplex infection in HIV-infected pts.** *Adult:* 500 mg PO bid for 7 d.
**ADJUST DOSE** Renal impairment
**ADV EFF** **Cancer,** diarrhea, fever, **granulocytopenia,** headache, nausea, rash, renal impairment, **thrombocytopenia**
**INTERACTIONS** Cimetidine, digoxin, probenecid
**NC/PT** Not for use in breastfeeding. Pt should continue precautions to prevent transmission (drug not a cure); avoid exposure to infection; take analgesics for headache; report bleeding.

**famotidine** (Pepcid)
**CLASS** Histamine-2 receptor antagonist
**PREG/CONT** B/NA

**IND & DOSE** **Acute tx of active duodenal ulcer.** *Adult:* 40 mg PO or IV at bedtime, or 20 mg PO or IV bid; discontinue after 6–8 wk. *Child 1–12 yr:* 0.5 mg/kg/d PO at bedtime or divided into two doses (up to 40 mg/d), or 0.25 mg/kg IV q 12 hr (up to 40 mg/d) if unable to take orally. **Maint tx of duodenal ulcer.** *Adult:* 20 mg PO at bedtime. **Benign gastric ulcer.** *Adult:* 40 mg PO daily at bedtime. **Tx of hypersecretory syndrome.** *Adult:* Initially, 20 mg PO q 6 hr. Taper; up to 160 mg PO q 6 hr has been used. Or, 20 mg IV q 12 hr in pts unable to take orally. *Child 1–12 yr:* 0.25 mg/kg IV q 12 hr (up to 40 mg/d) if unable to take orally. **Tx of GERD.** *Adult:* 20 mg PO bid for up to 6 wk. For GERD w/esophagitis, 20–40 mg PO bid for up to 12 wk. *Child 1–12 yr:* 1 mg/kg/d PO divided into two doses (up to 40 mg bid). *Child 3 mo–1 yr:* 0.5 mg/kg PO bid for up to 8 wk. *<3 mo:* 0.5 mg/kg/dose oral suspension once daily for up to 8 wk. **Px/relief of heartburn/acid indigestion.** *Adult:* 10–20 mg PO for relief; 10–20 mg PO 15–60 min before eating for prevention. Max, 20 mg/24 hr.
**ADJUST DOSE** Renal impairment
**ADV EFF** Arrhythmias, constipation, diarrhea, headache
**NC/PT** Reserve IV use for pts unable to take orally; switch to oral as soon as possible. Give at bedtime. May use concurrent antacid to relieve pain. Pt should place rapidly disintegrating tablet on tongue; swallow w/ or w/o water.

**▶NEW DRUG**

**fam-trastuzumab deruxtecan-nxki** (Enhertu)
**CLASS** Antibody/drug conjugate, antineoplastic
**PREG/CONT** High risk/NA

**BBW** Risk of ILD/pneumonitis, sometimes fatal. Risk of embryo-fetal harm.
**IND & DOSE** **Tx of unresectable or metastatic HER2-positive breast cancer after two or more anti-HER2-based regimens.** *Adult:* 5.4 mg/kg IV infusion q 21 d until disease progression or unacceptable toxicity.
**ADV EFF** Alopecia, **cardiomyopathy,** constipation, cough, diarrhea, dyspnea, fatigue, fever, **leukopenia, neutropenia, thrombocytopenia,** vomiting
**INTERACTIONS** Strong CYP3A inhibitors
**NC/PT** Do not substitute Enhertu for or w/trastuzumab or ado-trastuzumab emtansine. Give first infusion over

90 min, subsequent infusions over 30 min if prior infusions well tolerated. Slow/interrupt infusion rate if infusion-related sx develop. Dose reductions per label based on adverse reactions.

**fat emulsion, intravenous** (Intralipid)
**CLASS** Caloric drug, nutritional drug
**PREG/CONT** C/NA

**BBW** Give to preterm infants only if benefit clearly outweighs risk; deaths have occurred.
**IND & DOSE Parenteral nutrition.** *Adult:* Should not constitute more than 60% of total calorie intake. *10%:* Infuse IV at 1 mL/min for first 15–30 min; may increase to 2 mL/min. Infuse only 500 mL first day; increase following day. Max, 2.5 g/kg/d. *20%:* Infuse at 0.5 mL/min for first 15–30 min. Infuse only 250 mL *Intralipid* first day; increase following day. Max, 3 g/kg/d. *30%:* Infuse at 1 mL/min (0.1 g fat/min) for first 15–30 min; max, 2.5 g/kg/d. *Child:* Should not constitute more than 60% of total calorie intake. *10%:* Initial IV infusion rate, 0.1 mL/min for first 10–15 min. *20%:* Initial infusion rate, 0.05 mL/min for first 10–15 min. If no untoward reactions, increase rate to 1 g/kg in 4 hr; max, 3 g/kg/d. *30%:* Initial infusion rate, 0.1 mL/min (0.01 g fat/min) for first 10–15 min; max, 3 g/kg/d. **Tx of essential fatty acid deficiency.** Supply 8%–10% of caloric intake by IV fat emulsion.
**ADV EFF** Headache, **leukopenia,** nausea, **sepsis, thrombocytopenia,** thrombophlebitis
**NC/PT** Supplied in single-dose containers. Do not store partially used bottles or resterilize for later use. Do not use w/filters. Do not use bottle in which there appears to be separation from emulsion. Monitor pt closely for fluid, fat overload. Monitor lipid profile, nitrogen balance closely; monitor for thrombotic events, sepsis. Pt should report pain at injection site, s&sx of infection.

**febuxostat** (Uloric)
**CLASS** Antigout drug, xanthine oxidase inhibitor
**PREG/CONT** Unkn/NA

**BBW** Higher risk of CV death in gout pts w/established CV disease.
**IND & DOSE Long-term mgt of hyperuricemia in pts w/gout if inadequate control w/allopurinol.** *Adult:* 40 mg/d PO; if serum uric acid not <6 mg/dL in 2 wk, may increase to 80 mg/d PO.
**ADJUST DOSE** Hepatic/renal impairment
**ADV EFF** Gout flares, **MI,** nausea, **stroke**
**INTERACTIONS** Azathioprine, mercaptopurine theophyllines (use contraindicated)
**NC/PT** Not recommended for asymptomatic hyperuricemia. Obtain baseline, periodic uric acid level. May use w/antacids, other drugs to control gout. Store at room temp, protected from light. Use caution in preg/breastfeeding. Pt should report chest pain, numbness/tingling.

**▶NEW DRUG**

**fedratinib** (Inrebic)
**CLASS** Kinase inhibitor
**PREG/CONT** Unkn/NA

**BBW** Serious and fatal encephalopathy, including Wernicke's, has occurred. Assess thiamine level before/periodically during tx. Do not start if thiamine deficiency; replete thiamine before tx. If encephalopathy is suspected, immediately stop drug; initiate parenteral thiamine.
**IND & DOSE Tx of intermediate-2 or high risk primary or secondary (post-polycythemia vera or post-essential thrombocythemia) myelofibrosis.** *Adult:* 400 mg PO daily

w/ or w/o food if baseline platelet count ≥50 × $10^9$/L.
**ADV EFF** Amylase/lipase elevation, anemia, diarrhea, **hepatotoxicity,** n/v
**INTERACTIONS** Strong CYP3A4 inhibitors, strong/moderate CYP3A4 inducers
**NC/PT** Avoid if severe hepatic impairment; reduced dose may be needed if renal impairment. Risk to fetus unkn. Animal studies show embryo-fetal harm; no human studies exist. Pt should not breastfeed during tx and for at least 1 mo after tx.

## felodipine (generic)
**CLASS** Antihypertensive, calcium channel blocker
**PREG/CONT** C/NA

**IND & DOSE Tx of essential HTN.** *Adult:* 5 mg/d PO; range, 2.5–10 mg/d PO.
**ADJUST DOSE** Elderly pts, hepatic impairment
**ADV EFF** Dizziness, fatigue, flushing, headache, lethargy, light-headedness, nausea, peripheral edema
**INTERACTIONS** Antifungals, barbiturates, carbamazepine, cimetidine, grapefruit juice, hydantoins, ranitidine
**NC/PT** Monitor cardiac rhythm, BP carefully during dose adjustment. Pt should swallow tablet whole and not cut/crush/chew it; avoid grapefruit juice; take safety precautions w/CNS effects; report swelling in hands, feet.

## fenofibrate (Antara, Fenoglide, Lipofen, Lofibra, TriCor, Triglide, Trilipix)
**CLASS** Antihyperlipidemic
**PREG/CONT** C/NA

**IND & DOSE Adjunct to diet/exercise for tx of hypertriglyceridemia.** *Adult:* 48–145 mg (*TriCor*) PO, or 67–200 mg (*Lofibra*) PO w/meal, or 50–160 mg/d (*Triglide*) PO daily, or 43–130 mg/d PO (*Antara*), or 50–150 mg/d PO (*Lipofen*), or 40–120 mg/d PO (*Fenoglide*), or 45–135 mg/d PO (*Trilipix*). **Adjunct to diet/exercise for tx of primary hypercholesterolemia, mixed dyslipidemia.** *Adult:* 145 mg/d PO (*TriCor*), or 200 mg/d (*Lofibra*) PO w/meal, or 160 mg/d (*Triglide*), or 130 mg/d PO (*Antara*), or 150 mg/d PO (*Lipofen*), or 120 mg/d PO (*Fenoglide*), or 135 mg/d PO (*Trilipix*).
**ADJUST DOSE** Elderly pts, renal impairment
**ADV EFF** Decreased libido, ED, flu-like sx, hepatic impairment, myalgia, nausea, **pancreatitis,** rash
**INTERACTIONS** Anticoagulants, bile acid sequestrants, immunosuppressants, nephrotoxic drugs, statins, warfarin
**NC/PT** Obtain baseline, periodic lipid profile, LFTs, CBC w/long-term therapy. Differentiate between brand names; doses vary. Balance timing of administration if used w/other lipid-lowering drugs. Use caution in preg; not for use in breastfeeding. Pt should swallow DR capsules whole and not cut/crush/chew them; continue diet/exercise programs; report muscle weakness, aches.

## fenoprofen calcium (Nalfon)
**CLASS** Analgesic, NSAID
**PREG/CONT** Moderate risk (1st, 2nd trimesters); high risk (3rd trimester)/NA

**BBW** Increased risk of CV events, GI bleeding; monitor accordingly. Not for use in the setting of CABG surgery.
**IND & DOSE Tx of RA/osteoarthritis.** *Adult:* 400–600 mg PO tid or qid. May need 2–3 wk before improvement seen. **Tx of mild to moderate pain.** *Adult:* 200 mg PO q 4–6 hr as needed.
**ADJUST DOSE** Renal impairment
**ADV EFF Agranulocytosis, anaphylactoid reactions to fatal anaphylactic shock, aplastic anemia,** dizziness, dyspepsia, **eosinophilia,** GI pain, **granulocytopenia,** headache,

HF, impaired vision, insomnia, **leukopenia**, *nausea*, **neutropenia, pancytopenia**, rash, somnolence, **thrombotic events, thrombocytopenia**
**INTERACTIONS** ACE inhibitors, anticoagulants, antiplatelets, aspirin, phenobarbital
**NC/PT** Not for use in preg (contraceptives advised)/breastfeeding. Pt should take w/meals; use safety precautions w/CNS effects; report bleeding, tarry stools, vision changes.

**DANGEROUS DRUG**

**fentaNYL** (Actiq, Duragesic, Fentora, Lazanda, SUBSYS)
**CLASS** Opioid agonist analgesic
**PREG/CONT** C/C-II

**BBW** Ensure appropriate use because drug potentially dangerous (life-threatening respiratory depression). Have opioid antagonist, facilities for assisted or controlled respiration on hand during parenteral administration. Use caution when switching between forms; doses vary. Transdermal, nasal forms not for use in opioid–nontolerant pts. Not for acute or postop pain. Do not substitute for other fentanyl product. Keep out of child's reach; can be fatal. Potentiation of effects possible when given w/macrolide antibiotics, ketoconazole, itraconazole, protease inhibitors; potentially fatal respiratory depression possible.
**IND & DOSE Analgesic adjunct for anesthesia.** *Adult:* Premedication, 50–100 mcg IM 30–60 min before surgery. Adjunct to general anesthesia, initially, 2–20 mcg/kg; maint, 2–50 mcg IV or IM. 25–100 mcg IV or IM when vital sign changes indicate surgical stress, lightening of analgesia. W/oxygen for anesthesia, total high dose, 50–100 mcg/kg IV. Adjunct to regional anesthesia, 50–100 mcg IM or slowly IV over 1–2 min. *Child 2–12 yr:* 2–3 mcg/kg IV as vital signs indicate. **Control of postop pain, tachypnea, emergence delirium.** *Adult:* 50–100 mcg IM; repeat in 1–2 hr if needed. **Mgt of chronic pain in pts requiring continuous opioid analgesia over extended period.** *Adult:* 25 mcg/hr transdermal system; may need replacement in 72 hr if pain has not subsided. Do not use torn, damaged systems; serious overdose possible. *Child 2–12 yr:* 25 mcg/hr transdermal system; pts should be opioid-tolerant and receiving at least 60 mg oral morphine equivalents/d. **Tx of breakthrough pain in cancer pts treated w/and tolerant to opioids.** *Adult:* Place unit (*Actiq*) in mouth between cheek, lower gum. Start w/200 mcg; may start redosing 15 min after previous lozenge completed. No more than two lozenges/breakthrough pain episode. For buccal tablets, initially 100-mcg tablet between cheek, gum for 14–25 min; may repeat in 30 min. For buccal soluble film, remove film, place inside cheek; will dissolve within 5–30 min. For SL tablets (*Astral*), initially 100 mcg SL; wait at least 2 hr between doses. For nasal spray, 100 mcg as single spray in one nostril. Max, 800 mcg as single spray in one nostril or single spray in each nostril/episode. Wait at least 2 hr before treating new episode. No more than four doses in 24 hr.
**ADV EFF Apnea, cardiac arrest,** clamminess, confusion, constipation, dizziness, floating feeling, headache, lethargy, light-headedness, local irritation, n/v, **respiratory depression,** sedation, **shock,** sweating, vertigo
**INTERACTIONS** Alcohol, barbiturates, CNS depressants, grapefruit juice, itraconazole, ketoconazole, macrolide antibiotics, MAOIs, protease inhibitors
**NC/PT** Adjust dose as needed, tolerated for pain relief. Apply transdermal system to nonirritated, nonirradiated skin on flat surface of upper torso. Clip, do not shave, hair. May need 12 hr for full effect. Do not use torn, damaged transdermal systems;

serious overdose possible. Give to breastfeeding women 4–6 hr before next scheduled feeding. Buccal soluble film, nasal spray only available through restricted access program. Titrate carefully w/COPD. Pt should avoid grapefruit juice; remove old transdermal patch before applying new one; take safety precautions w/ CNS effects; report difficulty breathing. Name confusion between fentanyl and sufentanil; use extreme caution.

## ferrous salts: ferrous aspartate, ferrous fumarate, ferrous gluconate, ferrous sulfate, ferrous sulfate exsiccated (Femiron, Feosol, Slow Release Iron)

**CLASS** Iron preparation
**PREG/CONT** A/NA

**BBW** Warn pt to keep out of reach of child; leading cause of fatal poisoning in child <6 yr.
**IND & DOSE** **Dietary iron supplement.** *Adult:* Men, 8–11 mg/d PO; women, 8–18 mg/d PO. *Preg/breastfeeding women:* 9–27 mg/d PO. *Child:* 7–11 mg/d PO. **Px/tx of iron deficiency anemia.** *Adult:* 150–300 mg/d (6 mg/kg/d) PO for approx 6–10 mo. *Child:* 3–6 mg/kg/d PO.
**ADV EFF** Anorexia; **coma, death w/ overdose;** constipation; GI upset; n/v
**INTERACTIONS** Antacids, chloramphenicol, cimetidine, ciprofloxacin, coffee, eggs, levodopa, levothyroxine, milk, ofloxacin, tea, tetracycline
**NC/PT** Establish correct diagnosis. Regularly monitor Hct, Hgb. Use straw for liquid forms (may stain teeth). Give w/food if GI upset severe. Stool may be green to black; tx may take several mo. Laxative may be needed. Pt should avoid eggs, milk, coffee, tea; keep out of reach of child (serious to fatal toxicity possible).

## ferumoxytol (Feraheme)

**CLASS** Iron preparation
**PREG/CONT** C/NA

**BBW** Risk of serious hypersensitivity/ anaphylactic reactions; monitor pt closely during and for 30 min after infusion. Administer only when emergency support is available.
**IND & DOSE** **Tx of iron deficiency anemia in pts w/chronic renal failure or pts who have intolerance/unsatisfactory response to oral iron.** *Adult:* 510 mg IV then 510 mg IV in 3–8 d. Infuse in 50–200 mL 0.9% NSS or 5% dextrose injection over at least 15 min.
**ADV EFF** Constipation, diarrhea, dizziness, **hypersensitivity reactions, hypotension, iron overload,** nausea, peripheral edema
**NC/PT** Alters MRI results for up to 3 mo after use; will not alter CT scans or X-rays. Do not give if iron overload. Monitor for hypersensitivity reaction up to 30 min after infusion; have life support available; risk of anaphylaxis greatest w/hx of multiple drug allergies. Monitor BP during and for 30 min after administration. Use caution in preg; not for use in breastfeeding. Pt should take safety precautions w/CNS effects; report difficulty breathing, itching, swelling.

## fesoterodine fumarate (Toviaz)

**CLASS** Antimuscarinic
**PREG/CONT** Unkn/NA

**IND & DOSE** **Tx of overactive bladder.** *Adult:* 4 mg/d PO; may increase to max 8 mg/d.
**ADJUST DOSE** Renal impairment; hepatic impairment (not recommended)
**ADV EFF** Blurred vision, constipation, decreased sweating, dry eyes, dry mouth, increased IOP, urine retention
**INTERACTIONS** Alcohol, anticholinergics, clarithromycin, itraconazole, ketoconazole

**NC/PT** Monitor IOP before, periodically during tx. Pt should swallow tablet whole and not cut/crush/chew it; empty bladder before dose; use sugarless lozenges, mouth care for dry mouth; take safety precautions for vision changes; stay hydrated in heat conditions (decreased ability to sweat); avoid alcohol.

---

## fexofenadine hydrochloride (Allegra Allergy)

**CLASS** Antihistamine
**PREG/CONT** C/NA

**IND & DOSE Symptomatic relief of sx associated w/seasonal allergic rhinitis.** *Adult, child ≥12 yr:* 60 mg PO bid or 180 mg PO once daily; or 10 mL suspension PO bid. *Child 6–12 yr:* 30 mg orally disintegrating tablet (ODT) PO bid, or 5 mL suspension PO bid. *Child 2–12 yr:* 5 mL suspension PO bid. **Chronic idiopathic urticaria.** *Adult, child ≥12 yr:* 60 mg PO bid or 180 mg PO once daily. *Child 6–12 yr:* 30 mg ODT PO bid, or 5 mL suspension PO bid. *Child 2–12 yr:* 5 mL suspension PO bid.
**ADJUST DOSE** Elderly pts, renal impairment
**ADV EFF** Drowsiness, fatigue, nausea
**INTERACTIONS** Antacids, erythromycin, itraconazole ketoconazole
**NC/PT** Arrange for humidifier if nasal dryness, thickened secretions a problem; encourage hydration. Pt should use in a.m. before exposure to allergens; take safety precautions w/ CNS effects.

---

## fibrinogen concentrate, human (Fibryna, RiaSTAP)

**CLASS** Coagulation factor
**PREG/CONT** C/NA

**IND & DOSE Tx of acute bleeding episodes in pts w/congenital fibrinogen deficiency.** *Adult, child:* 70 mg/kg by slow IV injection not over 5 mL/min; adjust dose to target fibrinogen level of 100 mg/dL.
**ADJUST DOSE** Elderly pts, renal impairment
**ADV EFF Anaphylactic reactions, arterial thrombosis, blood-transmitted diseases,** chills, **DVT,** fever, **MI,** n/v, **PE,** rash
**NC/PT** Made from human blood; risk of blood-transmitted diseases. Risk of thromboembolic events, severe hypersensitivity reactions. Pt should report chest/leg pain, chest tightness, difficulty breathing, continued fever.

---

## fidaxomicin (Dificid)

**CLASS** Macrolide antibiotic
**PREG/CONT** B/NA

**IND & DOSE Tx of CDAD.** *Adult:* 200 mg PO bid for 10 d.
**ADV EFF** Abd pain, dyspepsia, **gastric hemorrhage, hypersensitivity,** n/v
**NC/PT** Culture stool before tx. Not for systemic infections; specific to *C. difficile* diarrhea. Pt should complete full course of tx; report severe vomiting, bloody diarrhea.

---

## filgrastim (Neupogen, Nivestym, Zarxio)

**CLASS** Colony-stimulating factor
**PREG/CONT** C/NA

**IND & DOSE To decrease incidence of infection in pts w/nonmyeloid malignancies receiving myelosuppressive anticancer drugs; to reduce time to neutrophil recovery, duration of fever after induction or consolidation chemo tx of acute myeloid leukemia.** *Adult:* 5 mcg/kg/d subcut or IV as single daily injection. May increase in increments of 5 mcg/kg for each chemo cycle; range, 4–8 mcg/kg/d. **To reduce duration of neutropenia after bone marrow transplant.** *Adult:* 10 mcg/kg/d IV or continuous subcut infusion. **Tx of severe chronic neutropenia.** *Adult:* 6 mcg/kg subcut bid (congenital neutropenia); 5 mcg/kg/d subcut as single injection (idiopathic, cyclic neutropenia). **To mobilize hematopoietic progenitor cells into blood for leukapheresis collection.** *Adult:* 10 mcg/kg/d subcut at least 4 d before first leukapheresis; continue to last leukapheresis. **To reduce incidence/duration of severe neutropenia in pts w/congenital, cyclic, or idiopathic neutropenia.** *Adult:* 6 mcg/kg subcut bid (congenital), or 5 mcg/kg/d subcut (cyclic, idiopathic). **To increase survival in pts exposed to myelosuppressive doses of radiation therapy.** *Adult:* 10 mcg/kg/d subcut

**ADV EFF** **Acute respiratory distress syndrome, alopecia, anaphylaxis,** bone pain, **fatal sickle cell crisis, fatal splenic rupture, glomerulonephritis,** n/v/d

**NC/PT** Obtain CBC, platelet count before and twice wkly during tx. Monitor renal function. Do not give within 24 hr of chemo. Give daily for up to 2 wk or neutrophils are 10,000/mm$^3$. Store in refrigerator. Do not shake vial; do not reuse vial, needles, syringes. Not for use in preg/breastfeeding. Teach pt proper administration/disposal of needles/syringes. Pt should avoid exposure to infection; cover head at temp extremes (hair loss possible); report difficulty breathing, severe abd or left shoulder pain.

## finafloxacin (Xtoro)

**CLASS** Antibiotic, quinolone
**PREG/CONT** Moderate risk/NA

**IND & DOSE** **Topical tx of acute otitis externa (swimmer's ear).** *Adult, child >1 yr:* 4 drops in affected ear(s) bid for 7 d. If using otowick, initial dose is 8 drops, then 4 drops bid for 7 d.

**ADV EFF** Allergic reaction, superinfection

**NC/PT** Warm bottle in hands before use; ensure full course of therapy. Pt/caregiver should report rash, worsening of condition.

## finasteride (Propecia, Proscar)

**CLASS** Androgen hormone inhibitor
**PREG/CONT** X/NA

**IND & DOSE** **Tx of symptomatic BPH.** *Adult:* 5 mg daily PO w/ or w/o meal; may take 6–12 mo for response (*Proscar*). **Px of male-pattern baldness.** *Adult:* 1 mg/d PO for 3 mo or more before benefit seen (*Propecia*).

**ADV EFF** Decreased libido, ED, gynecomastia

**INTERACTIONS** Saw palmetto

**NC/PT** Confirm dx of BPH. Protect from light. Preg women should not touch tablet. Pt may not donate blood and should not father a child during and for 6 mo after tx. Pt should monitor urine flow for improvement; may experience loss of libido.

## fingolimod (Gilenya)

**CLASS** MS drug
**PREG/CONT** High risk/NA

**IND & DOSE** **Tx of relapsing forms of MS.** *Adult, child ≥10 yr (>40 kg):* 0.5 mg/d PO w/ or w/o food. *≤40 kg:* 0.25 mg/d PO w/ or w/o food.

**ADV EFF** Back pain, bradycardia, cough, cutaneous malignancies, decreased lung capacity, depression, diarrhea, dyspnea, headache, increased liver enzymes, infections, macular edema, **PML, RPLS**

**INTERACTIONS** Ketoconazole, live vaccines, QT-prolonging drugs

**NC/PT** Contraindicated w/recent MI, stroke, angina, HF, heart block, long QT interval. Obtain CBC before start of tx; ECG before tx and at end of observation period. Monitor for infection during tx and for 2 mo after tx ends; do not start in pt w/active infections. Withhold at first s&sx suggesting

PML. Obtain baseline, periodic ophthal evaluation because of macular edema risk. Monitor for bradycardia for at least 6 hr after first dose; monitor P and BP hrly. Monitor symptomatic bradycardia w/ECG until resolved if hr <45 bpm in adults, <55 bpm in pts ≥12 yr, <60 bpm in pts 10 or 11 yr or if AV block. Obtain spirometry studies if dyspnea occurs. High probability of fetal risk; not for use in preg (contraceptives advised during and for 2 mo after tx)/breastfeeding. Pt should avoid exposure to infection; take safety precautions w/CNS effects; report difficulty breathing, chest pain, vision changes, s&sx of infection.

## flavoxate hydrochloride
(generic)

**CLASS** Parasympathetic blocker, urinary antispasmodic

**PREG/CONT** B/NA

**IND & DOSE** **Symptomatic relief of dysuria, urgency, nocturia, suprapubic pain, frequency/incontinence due to cystitis, prostatitis, urethritis, urethrocystitis, urethrotrigonitis.** *Adult, child ≥12 yr:* 100–200 mg PO tid or qid. Reduce dose when sx improve. Use max 1,200 mg/d in severe urinary urgency after pelvic radiotherapy.
**ADV EFF** Blurred vision, drowsiness, dry mouth, **eosinophilia**, headache, **leukopenia**, nervousness, n/v, vertigo
**INTERACTIONS** Anticholinergics, cholinergics
**NC/PT** Treat for underlying problem leading to s&sx. Obtain eye exam before, during tx. Pt should use sugarless lozenges for dry mouth; empty bladder before dose; use safety precautions w/CNS effects; report blurred vision.

## flecainide acetate
(Tambocor)

**CLASS** Antiarrhythmic

**PREG/CONT** C/NA

**BBW** Increased risk of nonfatal cardiac arrest, death in pts w/recent MI, chronic atrial fibrillation. Monitor cardiac rhythm carefully; risk of potentially fatal proarrhythmias.
**IND & DOSE** **Px/tx of life-threatening ventricular arrhythmias.** *Adult:* 100 mg PO q 12 hr. Increase in 50-mg increments bid q fourth day until efficacy achieved; max, 400 mg/d. **Px of paroxysmal atrial fibrillation/flutter, paroxysmal supraventricular tachycardias.** *Adult:* 50 mg PO q 12 hr; may increase in 50-mg increments bid q 4 d until efficacy achieved; max, 300 mg/d. **Transfer to flecainide.** Allow at least 2–4 plasma half-lives to elapse after other antiarrhythmics discontinued before starting flecainide.
**ADJUST DOSE** Elderly pts; renal/hepatic impairment
**ADV EFF** Abd pain, **arrhythmias**, chest pain, constipation, dizziness, drowsiness, dyspnea, fatigue, headache, **leukopenia**, n/v, visual changes
**INTERACTIONS** Amiodarone, cimetidine, disopyramide (avoid marked drop in cardiac output), propranolol
**NC/PT** Check serum potassium before starting tx; evaluate for therapeutic serum levels (0.2–1 mcg/mL). Monitor response closely; have life-support equipment on hand. Pt should take q 12 hr (arrange timing to avoid interrupting sleep); use safety precautions w/CNS effects; report chest pain, palpitations.

## flibanserin (Addyi)

**CLASS** Serotonin/dopamine agonist/antagonist

**PREG/CONT** Unkn/NA

**BBW** Risk of severe hypotension/syncope if combined w/alcohol; pt

must abstain. Contraindicated w/ CYP3A4 inhibitors or hepatic impairment.
**IND & DOSE** **Tx of premenopausal women w/acquired, generalized hypoactive sexual desire disorder.** *Adult:* 100 mg/d PO at bedtime; stop after 8 wk if no improvement.
**ADJUST DOSE** Hepatic impairment
**ADV EFF** Dizziness, dry mouth, fatigue, hypotension, insomnia, nausea, sedation, somnolence
**INTERACTIONS** Alcohol, CYP3A4 inducers/inhibitors, CYP2C19 inhibitors, digoxin, oral contraceptives
**NC/PT** Ensure appropriate use; not for postmenopausal women; does not enhance sexual performance. Not for use in preg/breastfeeding. Give at bedtime to decrease hypotension risks. May react w/many drugs; monitor regimen. Pt should not combine w/ alcohol; should take at bedtime; avoid tasks that require alertness for at least 6 hr after each dose; take safety precautions for CNS changes; use cautiously if low BP possible; monitor response and report after 8 wk; report fainting, continued sedation.

## floxuridine (generic)

**CLASS** Antimetabolite, antineoplastic
**PREG/CONT** D/NA

**IND & DOSE** **Palliative mgt of GI adenocarcinoma metastatic to liver.** *Adult:* 0.1–0.6 mg/kg/d via intra-arterial infusion.
**ADV EFF** **Bone marrow suppression, infections, gastric ulceration,** glossitis, **hepatic impairment,** n/v/d, **renal impairment,** stomatitis
**INTERACTIONS** Immunosuppressants, live vaccines
**NC/PT** Obtain baseline, periodic CBC. Check for mouth ulcerations, dental infections; mouth care essential. Protect from exposure to infections. Not for use in preg/breastfeeding. Pt should report severe GI pain, bloody diarrhea, s&sx of infection.

## fluconazole (Diflucan)

**CLASS** Antifungal
**PREG/CONT** D/NA

**IND & DOSE** **Tx of oropharyngeal candidiasis:** *Adult:* 200 mg PO or IV on first day, then 100 mg/d for at least 2 wk. *Child:* 6 mg/kg PO or IV on first day, then 3 mg/kg once daily for at least 2 wk. **Tx of esophageal candidiasis.** *Adult:* 200 mg PO or IV on first day, then 100 mg/d, up to 400 mg/d for minimum of 3 wk, at least 2 wk after resolution. *Child:* 6 mg/kg PO or IV on first day, then 3 mg/kg/d for 3 wk, at least 2 wk after resolution. **Tx of vaginal candidiasis.** *Adult:* 150 mg PO as single dose. **Tx of systemic candidiasis.** *Adult:* 400 mg PO or IV daily. *Child:* 6–12 mg/kg/d PO or IV. **Tx of candidal UTI/peritonitis.** *Adult:* 50–200 mg/d PO. **Tx of cryptococcal meningitis.** *Adult:* 400 mg PO or IV on first day, then 200 mg/d up to 400 mg/d for 10–12 wk after cultures of CSF become negative. *Child:* 12 mg/kg PO or IV on first day, then 6 mg/kg/d for 10–12 wk after cultures of CSF become negative. **Suppression of cryptococcal meningitis in AIDS pts.** *Adult:* 200 mg PO or IV daily. *Child:* 6 mg/kg PO or IV daily. **Px of candidiasis in bone marrow transplants.** *Adult:* 400 mg PO daily for several days before onset of neutropenia and for 7 d after neutrophil count above 1,000/mm$^3$.
**ADJUST DOSE** Hepatic/renal impairment
**ADV EFF** Abd pain, **anaphylaxis, exfoliative skin disorders,** headache, **hepatotoxicity,** n/v/d, **prolonged QT, renal toxicity**
**INTERACTIONS** Benzodiazepines, cimetidine, cyclosporine, oral hypoglycemics, phenytoin, pimozide, quinidine, QT-prolonging drugs, rifampin, warfarin anticoagulants, zidovudine
**NC/PT** Culture before tx. For IV, oral use only. Do not use oral form for tx of vaginal yeast infections during preg;

not for use in breastfeeding. Monitor renal/hepatic function wkly. Frequent medical follow-up needed. Pt should take hygiene measures to prevent infection spread; use analgesics for headache; report rash, difficulty breathing, urine/stool color changes.

## flucytosine (Ancobon)

**CLASS** Antifungal
**PREG/CONT** Moderate risk/NA

**BBW** Monitor serum flucytosine in pts w/renal impairment (levels >100 mcg/mL associated w/toxicity).
**IND & DOSE Tx of serious infections caused by susceptible *Candida, Cryptococcus* strains.** *Adult:* 50–150 mg/kg/d PO at 6-hr intervals.
**ADJUST DOSE** Renal impairment
**ADV EFF** Anemia, **cardiac arrest,** confusion, dizziness, **leukopenia,** n/v/d, **rash, respiratory arrest, thrombocytopenia**
**NC/PT** Give capsules few at a time over 15 min to decrease GI upset, diarrhea. Monitor LFTs, renal/hematologic function periodically during tx. Pt should take safety precautions w/CNS effects; report fever, difficulty breathing.

DANGEROUS DRUG

## fludarabine phosphate (generic)

**CLASS** Antimetabolite, antineoplastic
**PREG/CONT** D/NA

**BBW** Stop tx if s&sx of toxicity (CNS complaints, stomatitis, esophagopharyngitis, rapidly falling WBC count, intractable vomiting, diarrhea, GI ulceration/bleeding, thrombocytopenia, hemorrhage, hemolytic anemia); serious to life-threatening infections possible. Consult physician.
**IND & DOSE Chronic lymphocytic leukemia (CLL); unresponsive B-cell CLL.** *Adult:* 40 mg/m$^2$ PO or 25 mg/m$^2$ IV over 30 min for 5 consecutive d. Begin each 5-day course q 28 d.
**ADJUST DOSE** Renal impairment
**ADV EFF** Anorexia, **autoimmune hemolytic anemia,** bone marrow toxicity, chills, **CNS toxicity (including blindness, coma, death),** cough, dyspnea, edema, fatigue, fever, headache, infection, n/v/d, pneumonia, pruritus, **pulmonary toxicity,** stomatitis, **TLS,** visual disturbances, weakness
**INTERACTIONS** Pentostatin
**NC/PT** Obtain CBC before tx, each dose. Monitor pulmonary function regularly. Not for use in preg (contraceptives advised)/breastfeeding. Pt should not crush tablets; should avoid contact w/skin, mucous membranes; mark calendar of tx days; take safety precautions for CNS effects; avoid exposure to infections; report bruising, excess bleeding, black stools, difficulty breathing.

## fludrocortisone acetate (generic)

**CLASS** Corticosteroid
**PREG/CONT** C/NA

**IND & DOSE Partial replacement tx in adrenocortical insufficiency.** *Adult:* 0.05–0.1 mg/d PO. **Tx of salt-losing adrenogenital syndrome.** *Adult:* 0.1–0.2 mg/d PO.
**ADJUST DOSE** Elderly pts; hepatic/renal impairment
**ADV EFF** Anxiety, cardiac enlargement, depression, edema, HF, HTN, hypokalemic acidosis, infection, weakness
**INTERACTIONS** Amphotericin B, anabolic steroids, antidiabetics, aspirin, barbiturates, digitalis, diuretics, hormonal contraceptives, phenytoin, rifampin, warfarin
**NC/PT** Monitor BP, serum electrolytes, blood glucose before, periodically during tx. Protect from infection. Frequent medical follow-up, blood tests needed. Use caution in preg/breastfeeding. Pt should wear medical

alert tag, report all drugs used to health care provider (many drug interactions possible).

**flumazenil** (generic)
**CLASS** Antidote, benzodiazepine receptor antagonist
**PREG/CONT** C/NA

**BBW** Possible increased risk of seizures, especially in pts on long-term benzodiazepine tx and pts w/serious cyclic antidepressant overdose; take appropriate precautions.
**IND & DOSE** **Reversal of conscious sedation or in general anesthesia.** *Adult:* 0.2 mg (2 mL) IV over 15 sec, wait 45 sec; if ineffectual, repeat at 60-sec intervals. Max cumulative dose, 1 mg (10 mL). *Child >1 yr:* 0.01 mg/kg (up to 0.2 mg) IV over 15 sec; wait 45 sec. Repeat at 60-sec intervals. Max cumulative dose, 0.05 mg/kg or 1 mg, whichever lowest. **Mgt of suspected benzodiazepine overdose.** *Adult:* 0.2 mg IV over 30 sec; repeat w/0.3 mg IV q 30 sec. May give further doses of 0.5 mg over 30 sec at 1-min intervals. Max cumulative dose, 3 mg.
**ADV EFF** Amnesia, dizziness, increased sweating, n/v, pain at injection site, **seizures,** vertigo
**INTERACTIONS** Alcohol, CNS depressants, food
**NC/PT** IV use only, into running IV in large vein. Have emergency equipment on hand; continually monitor response. Provide safety measures for CNS effects for at least 18–24 hr after use. Give pt written information (amnesia may be prolonged). Pt should avoid alcohol for 18–24 hr after administration.

**flunisolide** (generic)
**CLASS** Corticosteroid
**PREG/CONT** C/NA

**IND & DOSE** **Intranasal relief/mgt of nasal sx of seasonal, perennial allergic rhinitis.** *Adult:* 2 sprays (50 mcg) in each nostril bid; may increase to 2 sprays in each nostril tid (total dose, 300 mcg/d). Max, 400 mcg/d. *Child 6–14 yr:* 1 spray in each nostril tid or 2 sprays in each nostril bid (total dose, 150–200 mcg/d). Max, 200 mcg/d. **Inhalation maint tx of asthma as px therapy.** *Adult, child ≥12 yr:* 160 mcg bid, not to exceed 320 mcg bid. *Child 6–11 yr:* 80 mcg bid, not to exceed 160 mcg bid. Should be taken w/adult supervision.
**ADV EFF** Epistaxis, fungal infection, headache, nasal irritation, rebound congestion
**NC/PT** May use decongestant drops to facilitate penetration if needed. Not for acute asthma attack. Pt should not stop suddenly; should shake well before each inhalation, rinse mouth after each inhaler use.

**DANGEROUS DRUG**

**fluorouracil** (Carac, Efudex, Fluoroplex, Tolak)
**CLASS** Antimetabolite, antineoplastic
**PREG/CONT** D/NA

**BBW** Stop tx at s&sx of toxicity (stomatitis, esophagopharyngitis, rapidly falling WBC count, intractable vomiting, diarrhea, GI ulceration/bleeding, thrombocytopenia, hemorrhage); serious to life-threatening reactions have occurred. Consult physician.
**IND & DOSE** **Palliative mgt of carcinoma of colon, rectum, breast, stomach, pancreas in selected pts considered incurable by surgery or other means.** *Adult:* 12 mg/kg/d IV for 4 successive d, infused slowly over 24 hr; max, 800 mg/d. If no toxicity, 6 mg/kg IV on days 6, 8, 10, 12, w/no drug tx on days 5, 7, 9, 11. Stop tx at end of day 12. If no toxicity, repeat q 30 d. If toxicity, 10–15 mg/kg/wk IV as single dose after s&sx of toxicity subside; max, 1 g/wk. Adjust dose based on response; tx may be

prolonged (12–60 mo). **Tx of actinic or solar keratoses.** *Adult:* Apply bid to cover lesions. 0.5% and 1% used on head, neck, chest; 2% and 5% used on hands. Continue until inflammatory response reaches erosion, necrosis, and ulceration stage, then stop. Usual tx course, 2–4 wk. Complete healing may not occur for 1–2 mo after tx stops. **Tx of superficial basal cell carcinoma.** *Adult:* 5% strength bid in amount sufficient to cover lesions, for at least 3–6 wk. Tx may be needed for 10–12 wk.
**ADJUST DOSE** Poor risk, undernourished pts
**ADV EFF** Alopecia, anorexia, cramps, dermatitis, duodenal ulcer, duodenitis, enteritis, gastritis, glossitis, lethargy, **leukopenia,** local irritation w/topical use, malaise, n/v/d, photosensitivity, rash, stomatitis, **thrombocytopenia**
**NC/PT** Obtain CBC before and regularly during tx. Ensure dx of topical lesions. Thoroughly wash hands after applying topical form; avoid occlusive dressings w/topical form. Stop tx at s&sx of toxicity. Frequent medical follow-up needed. Pt should mark calendar for tx days; cover head at temp extremes (hair loss possible); avoid exposure to sun, infections; report black tarry stools, unusual bleeding or bruising.

## FLUoxetine hydrochloride (Prozac, Sarafem, Selfemra)

**CLASS** Antidepressant, SSRI
**PREG/CONT** C/NA

**BBW** Establish suicide precautions for severely depressed pts. Limit quantity dispensed; high risk of suicidality in child, adolescent, young adult.
**IND & DOSE Tx of depression.** *Adult:* 20 mg/d PO in a.m.; max, 80 mg/d. Once stabilized, may switch to 90-mg DR capsules PO once/wk. *Child 8–18 yr:* 10 mg/d PO; may increase to 20 mg/d after 1 wk or after several wk for low-weight child. **Tx of depressive episodes of bipolar 1 disorder.** *Adult:* 20 mg/d PO w/5 mg olanzapine. **Tx of tx-resistant depression.** *Adult:* 20–50 mg/d PO w/5–20 mg olanzapine. **Tx of OCD.** *Adult:* 20 mg/d PO; range, 20–60 mg/d PO. May need up to 5 wk for effectiveness. Max, 80 mg/d. *Adolescent, higher-weight child:* 10 mg/d PO; range, 20–60 mg/d PO. Adolescent, lower-weight child: 10 mg/d PO; range, 20–30 mg/d. **Tx of bulimia.** *Adult:* 60 mg/d PO in a.m. **Tx of panic disorder.** *Adult:* 10 mg/d PO for first wk; max, 60 mg/d. **Tx of PMDD** *(Sarafem). Adult:* 20 mg/d PO. Or 20 mg/d PO starting 14 d before anticipated beginning of menses, continuing through first full day of menses; then no drug until 14 d before next menses. Max, 80 mg/d.
**ADJUST DOSE** Elderly pts, hepatic impairment
**ADV EFF Angle-closure glaucoma,** anorexia, anxiety, asthenia, constipation, dizziness, drowsiness, dry mouth, dyspepsia, fever, headache, insomnia, light-headedness, nervousness, n/v/d, painful menstruation, pharyngitis, pruritus, rash, **seizures,** serotonin syndrome, sexual dysfx, sweating, URI, urinary frequency, weight changes
**INTERACTIONS** Alcohol, benzodiazepines, ED drugs, linezolid, lithium, MAOIs, NSAIDs, opioids, pimozide, serotonergic drugs, St. John's wort, TCAs, thioridazine
**NC/PT** Do not use within 14 d of MAOIs, within 5 wk of thioridazine. Do not combine w/pimozide. Give in a.m. Full antidepressant effect may not occur for up to 4–6 wk. Taper when stopping. Not for use in preg. Pt should avoid alcohol, St. John's wort, NSAIDs; take safety precautions w/ CNS effects; report thoughts of suicide. Name confusion between *Sarafem* (fluoxetine) and *Serophene* (clomiphene).

## flurazepam hydrochloride (generic)

**CLASS** Benzodiazepine, sedative-hypnotic
**PREG/CONT** X/C-IV

**IND & DOSE Tx of insomnia.** *Adult:* 15–30 mg PO at bedtime.
**ADJUST DOSE** Elderly pts, debilitating disease
**ADV EFF Anaphylaxis, angioedema,** apathy, bradycardia, confusion, constipation, **CV collapse,** depression, diarrhea, disorientation, drowsiness, drug dependence w/withdrawal, fatigue, gynecomastia, lethargy, lightheadedness, restlessness, tachycardia, urine retention
**INTERACTIONS** Alcohol, aminophylline, barbiturates, cimetidine, disulfiram, hormonal contraceptives, opioids, phenothiazines, rifampin, SSRIs, theophylline, TCAs
**NC/PT** Monitor LFTs, renal function. Taper gradually after long-term use. Not for use in preg (barrier contraceptives advised)/breastfeeding. Pt should take safety precautions w/CNS effects; report worsening depression, difficulty breathing, edema.

## flurbiprofen (Ocufen)

**CLASS** Analgesic, NSAID
**PREG/CONT** B (oral); C (ophthal)/NA

**BBW** Increased risk of CV events, GI bleeding; monitor accordingly. Contraindicated for tx of periop CABG pain.
**IND & DOSE Acute or long-term tx of s&sx of RA/osteoarthritis; relief of moderate to mild pain.** *Adult:* 200–300 mg PO in divided doses bid, tid, or qid. Max, 100 mg/dose. **To inhibit intraop miosis.** *Adult:* 1 drop ophthal sol approx q 30 min, starting 2 hr before surgery (total, 4 drops).
**ADV EFF Agranulocytosis, aplastic anemia, bleeding, bone marrow depression, bronchospasm,** dizziness, dyspepsia, **eosinophilia, fatal anaphylactic shock,** fatigue, **gastric ulcer,** GI pain, **granulocytopenia,** headache, insomnia, **leukopenia,** nausea, **neutropenia, pancytopenia, renal impairment,** somnolence, **thrombocytopenia,** transient local stinging/burning w/ophthal sol
**NC/PT** Give w/food if GI upset severe. Not for use in preg (barrier contraceptives advised). Pt should take safety precautions w/CNS effects; report fever, rash, black stools, swelling in ankles/fingers.

**DANGEROUS DRUG**

## flutamide (generic)

**CLASS** Antiandrogen, antineoplastic
**PREG/CONT** D/NA

**BBW** Arrange for periodic monitoring of LFTs during long-term tx; severe hepatotoxicity possible.
**IND & DOSE Tx of locally advanced, metastatic prostatic carcinoma.** *Adult:* 250 mg PO tid. Begin tx at same time as initiation of LHRH analog.
**ADV EFF** Anemia, dizziness, drowsiness, ED, GI disturbances, gynecomastia, **hepatic necrosis, hepatitis,** hot flashes, leukopenia, loss of libido, n/v/d, photosensitivity, rash
**NC/PT** Give w/other drugs used for medical castration. Monitor LFTs regularly. Periodic blood tests will be needed. Pt should take safety precautions w/CNS effects; avoid exposure to sunlight; report urine/stool color changes.

## fluticasone furoate (Annuity Ellipta)

**CLASS** Asthma drug, corticosteroid
**PREG/CONT** Moderate risk/NA

**IND & DOSE Maint tx of asthma.** *Adult, child ≥12 yr:* 100–200 mcg/d by inhalation, 1 inhalation/d. *Child 5–11 yr:* 50 mcg/d, 1 inhalation/d.

**ADJUST DOSE** Hepatic impairment
**ADV EFF** Asthma episodes, **bronchospasm**, decreased bone density, headache, local infections, nasopharyngitis, slowed growth in adolescents, URI, worsening of glaucoma/cataracts
**INTERACTIONS** CYP3A4 inhibitors
**NC/PT** Not for use in acute bronchospasm, w/hypersensitivity to milk proteins. Monitor growth in adolescents. Review proper use and care of inhaler; pt should rinse mouth w/water w/o swallowing after each use. Not for use in breastfeeding. Pt should continue other regimen for asthma; not stop use w/o consulting provider; not use more than 1 inhalation/d; report difficulty breathing, worsening of asthma, vision changes.

## fluvastatin sodium

(Lescol XL)
**CLASS** Antihyperlipidemic, statin
**PREG/CONT** X/NA

**IND & DOSE** **Adjunct to diet/exercise to lower cholesterol/LDL; to slow progression of CAD, reduce risk of need for revascularization w/ CAD.** *Adult:* 40 mg/d PO. Maint, 20–80 mg/d PO; give 80 mg/d as two 40-mg doses, or use 80-mg ER form. **Tx of heterozygous familial hypercholesterolemia.** *Child 9–16 yr:* 20 mg/d PO. Adjust q 6 wk to max 40 mg bid or 80 mg ER form PO once/d.
**ADV EFF** Abd pain, blurred vision, cataracts, constipation, cramps, flatulence, headache, **rhabdomyolysis**
**INTERACTIONS** Azole antifungals, cyclosporine, erythromycin, gemfibrozil, grapefruit juice, niacin, other statins, phenytoin, warfarin
**NC/PT** Give in evening. Periodic ophthal exam will be needed. Not for use in preg (barrier contraceptives advised)/breastfeeding. Pt should swallow ER form whole and not cut/crush/chew it; continue diet/exercise program; avoid grapefruit juice; report muscle pain w/ fever, changes in vision.

## fluvoxaMINE maleate

(Luvox)
**CLASS** Antidepressant, SSRI
**PREG/CONT** Low risk/NA

**BBW** Establish suicide precautions for severely depressed pts. Limit quantity dispensed. Increased risk of suicidal ideation, behavior in child, adolescent, young adult.
**IND & DOSE** **Tx of OCD, social anxiety disorders.** *Adult:* 50 mg PO at bedtime; range, 100–300 mg/d. Or, 100–300 mg/d CR capsules PO. *Child 8–17 yr:* 25 mg PO at bedtime. Divide doses >50 mg/d; give larger dose at bedtime. Max for child up to 11 yr, 200 mg/d.
**ADJUST DOSE** Elderly pts, hepatic impairment
**ADV EFF** Anorexia, anxiety, asthenia, constipation, dizziness, drowsiness, dry mouth, dyspepsia, fever, headache, insomnia, light-headedness, nervousness, n/v/d, painful menstruation, pharyngitis, pruritus, rash, **seizures**, sexual dysfx, serotonin syndrome, sweating, URI, urinary frequency, weight changes
**INTERACTIONS** Alprazolam, beta blockers, carbamazepine, cigarette smoking, clozapine, diltiazem, MAOIs, methadone, quetiapine, serotonergic drugs, statins, St. John's wort, TCAs, theophylline, triazolam, warfarin
**NC/PT** Give in evening. Monitor for serotonin syndrome. Taper when stopping. Pt should swallow CR capsule whole and not cut/crush/chew it; take safety precautions w/CNS effects; report thoughts of suicide.

## folic acid (generic)

**CLASS** Folic acid, vitamin supplement
**PREG/CONT** A/NA

**IND & DOSE** **Tx of megaloblastic anemias due to sprue, nutritional**

**deficiency, preg; anemias of infancy, childhood.** *Adult:* 1 mg/d PO, IM, IV, subcut; maint, 0.4 mg/d. In preg/ breastfeeding, 0.8 mg/d PO. *Child (maint):* >4 yr, 0.4 mg/d PO; <4 yr, up to 0.3 mg/d PO; infants, 0.1 mg/d.
**ADV EFF** Pain, discomfort at injection site
**INTERACTIONS** Aminosalicylic acid, phenytoin, sulfasalazine
**NC/PT** Ensure correct anemia dx. Give orally if possible. Monitor for hypersensitivity reactions. Pt should report pain at injection site, difficulty breathing.

## follitropin alfa (Gonal-F, Gonal-F RFF, Gonal-F RFF Redi-Ject)

**CLASS** Fertility drug
**PREG/CONT** X/NA

**IND & DOSE To induce ovulation.** *Adult:* 75 international units (IU)/d subcut. Increase by 37.5 IU/d after 14 d; may increase again after 7 d. Do not use for longer than 35 d. **Stimulation of multiple follicles for in vitro fertilization.** *Adult*: 150 IU/d subcut on days 2, 3 of cycle; continue for 10 d. Adjust based on response. Max, 450 IU subcut; then 5,000–10,000 IU HCG. **To promote spermatogenesis.** *Adult:* 150–300 IU subcut 2–3 ×/wk w/HCG. May use for up to 18 mo.
**ADV EFF** Multiple births, nausea, ovarian cyst, **ovarian hyperstimulation, pulmonary/vascular complications,** URI
**NC/PT** Ensure uterine health. Monitor regularly; monitor for thrombotic events. Alert pt to risk of multiple births. Teach proper administration/ disposal of needles/syringes. Pt should report difficulty breathing, chest pain.

## follitropin beta (Follistim AQ)

**CLASS** Fertility drug
**PREG/CONT** X/NA

**IND & DOSE To induce ovulation.** *Adult:* 75 international units/d subcut. Increase by 37.5 international units/d after 14 d; may increase again after 7 d. Do not use for longer than 35 d. **Stimulation of multiple follicles for in vitro fertilization.** *Adult*: 150–225 international units/d subcut or IM for at least 4 d; adjust based on response. Follow w/HCG.
**ADV EFF** Multiple births, nausea, ovarian cyst, **ovarian hyperstimulation, pulmonary/vascular complications,** URI
**NC/PT** Ensure uterine health. Give subcut in navel or abdomen. Monitor regularly; monitor for thrombotic events. Alert pt to risk of multiple births. Teach proper administration/ disposal of needles/syringes. Pt should report difficulty breathing, chest pain.

## fomepizole (Antizol)

**CLASS** Antidote
**PREG/CONT** C/NA

**IND & DOSE Antidote for antifreeze, methanol poisoning.** *Adult:* 15 mg/kg loading dose IV, then 10 mg/kg IV q 12 hr for 12 doses by slow IV infusion over 30 min.
**ADV EFF** Acidosis, bradycardia, dizziness, electrolyte disturbances, headache, hypotension, injection-site reaction, lymphangitis, **multiorgan failure,** nausea, nystagmus, phlebitis, **seizures, shock**
**INTERACTIONS** Alcohol
**NC/PT** Monitor ECG, electrolytes, renal function, LFTs, BP. Monitor injection site. May be used w/hemodialysis if needed to clear toxins. Give q 4 hr during dialysis. Pt should take safety precautions w/CNS effects.

DANGEROUS DRUG

**fondaparinux** (Arixtra)
**CLASS** Antithrombotic, low-molecular-weight heparin
**PREG/CONT** Low risk/NA

**BBW** Carefully monitor pts receiving spinal/epidural anesthesia; risk of spinal hematoma, neuro damage.
**IND & DOSE Px of venous thrombotic events in pts undergoing surgery for hip fracture, hip or knee replacement; in pts undergoing abd surgery; extended px of DVT that may lead to PE after hip surgery.** *Adult:* 2.5 mg/d subcut starting 6–8 hr after surgical closure and continuing for 5–9 d. May add 24 d after initial course for pts undergoing hip fracture surgery. **Tx of DVT, acute PE, w/warfarin.** *Adult:* >100 kg, 10 mg/d subcut for 5–9 d; begin warfarin within 72 hr. 50–100 kg, 7.5 mg/d subcut for 5–9 d. <50 kg, 5 mg/d subcut for 5–9 d.
**ADJUST DOSE** Elderly pts, renal impairment
**ADV EFF** Anemia, **anaphylaxis,** bruising, fever, **hemorrhage,** hepatic impairment, local reaction at injection site, nausea
**INTERACTIONS** Cephalosporins, garlic, ginkgo, NSAIDs, oral anticoagulants, penicillins, platelet inhibitors, salicylates, vitamin E
**NC/PT** Give drug 6–8 hr after surgical closure. Give by deep subcut injections; do not give IM. Store at room temp. Do not mix w/other sols or massage injection site. Rotate injection sites. Monitor for spinal/epidural hematomas; may result in long-term or permanent paralysis. Bleeding risk is increased in renal impairment and in pt w/low body weight (<50 kg). Provide safety measures to prevent bleeding. Teach proper technique for injection, disposal of needles/syringes. Needle guard contains dry natural rubber; may cause allergic reactions w/latex sensibility. Pt should avoid NSAIDs; report bleeding, difficulty breathing, black tarry stools, severe headache.

**formoterol fumarate**
(Foradil Aerolizer, Perforomist)
**CLASS** Antiasthmatic, beta agonist
**PREG/CONT** Unkn/NA

**IND & DOSE Maint tx of COPD.** *Adult:* Oral inhalation of contents of 1 capsule (12 mcg) using *Aerolizer* inhaler q 12 hr; max, 24 mcg daily. Or, one 20-mcg/2 mL vial by oral inhalation using jet nebulizer connected to air compressor bid (a.m. and p.m.); max, 40 mcg/d. **Px of exercise-induced bronchospasm.** *Adult, child ≥12 yr:* Oral inhalation of contents of 1 capsule (12 mcg) using *Aerolizer* inhaler 15 min before exercise. Not indicated to treat deteriorations of COPD or to treat asthma.
**ADV EFF** Headache, nervousness, **prolonged QT,** throat/mouth irritation, tremors, viral infections
**INTERACTIONS** Beta blockers, QT-prolonging drugs
**NC/PT** Teach proper use of inhaler, nebulizer; periodically monitor use. Provide safety precautions for tremors, analgesics for headache. Ensure continued use of other drugs for COPD, bronchospasm.

**fosamprenavir** (Lexiva)
**CLASS** Antiviral, protease inhibitor
**PREG/CONT** Unkn/NA

**IND & DOSE Tx of HIV infection, w/other antiretrovirals.** *Adult:* 1,400 mg PO bid. W/ritonavir: 1,400 mg/d PO plus ritonavir 100 mg/d PO, or 1,400 mg/d PO plus ritonavir 200 mg/d PO, or 700 mg PO bid w/ritonavir 100 mg PO bid. In protease-experienced pts: 700 mg PO bid w/ritonavir 100 mg PO bid. *Child ≥6 yr (tx-naïve):* 30 mg/kg oral suspension PO bid; max, 1,400 mg bid. Or,

18 mg/kg oral suspension PO w/ ritonavir 3 mg/kg PO bid; max, 700 mg fosamprenavir plus 100 mg ritonavir bid. *Child ≥6 yr (tx-experienced):* 18 mg/kg oral suspension w/3 mg/kg ritonavir PO bid; max, 700 mg fosamprenavir w/100 mg ritonavir bid. *Child 2–5 yr (tx-naive):* 30 mg/kg oral suspension PO bid; max, 1,400 mg bid.
**ADJUST DOSE** Hepatic impairment
**ADV EFF** Depression, headache, hyperglycemia, **MI**, n/v/d, redistribution and/or increase of body fat, **SJS**
**INTERACTIONS** CYP3A4 inducers (may decrease efficacy); CYP3A4 inhibitors (may increase concentrations)
**NC/PT** Carefully check other drugs being used; interacts w/many drugs; potentially serious interactions possible. Give w/other antiretrovirals. Monitor LFTs, blood glucose. Monitor for rash. Not for use in preg (barrier contraceptives advised)/breastfeeding. Pt should monitor glucose carefully if diabetic; avoid St. John's wort; tell all health care providers about all drugs, herbs being taken; report rash, chest pain.

## fosfomycin tromethamine (Monurol)
**CLASS** Antibacterial, urinary tract anti-infective
**PREG/CONT** B/NA

**IND & DOSE** **Tx of uncomplicated UTIs in women caused by susceptible strains.** *Adult, child ≥12 yr:* 1 packet dissolved in water PO as single dose.
**ADV EFF** Dizziness, headache, nausea, rash
**INTERACTIONS** Metoclopramide
**NC/PT** Culture before tx. Do not give dry. Mix in 90–120 mL water (not hot); stir to dissolve. Pt should contact prescriber if no improvement, take safety precautions if dizziness occurs.

## fosinopril sodium (generic)
**CLASS** ACE inhibitor, antihypertensive
**PREG/CONT** D/NA

**BBW** Pt should avoid preg (suggest contraceptive); fetal damage possible if used in second, third trimesters. Switch to different drug if preg occurs.
**IND & DOSE** **Tx of HTN.** *Adult:* 10 mg/d PO. Range, 20–40 mg/d PO; max, 80 mg. **Adjunct tx of HF.** *Adult:* 10 mg/d PO; observe for 2 hr for hypotension. For pt w/moderate to severe renal failure, 5 mg/d PO; max, 40 mg/d.
**ADV EFF** **Angioedema,** cough, hyperkalemia, nausea, orthostatic hypotension, rash
**INTERACTIONS** ACE inhibitors, antacids, ARBs, indomethacin, lithium, NSAIDs, potassium-sparing diuretics, renin inhibitors
**NC/PT** Alert surgeon about use; postop fluid replacement may be needed. Not for use in preg (barrier contraceptives advised)/breastfeeding. Pt should use care in situations that might lead to BP drop, change positions slowly if light-headedness occurs. Name confusion between fosinopril and lisinopril.

## fosphenytoin sodium (Cerebyx)
**CLASS** Antiepileptic, hydantoin
**PREG/CONT** High risk/NA

**BBW** Pt should avoid preg; fetal damage possible. Suggest contraceptive. Risk of serious CV toxicity w/rapid infusion; monitor CV status continuously during infusion.
**IND & DOSE** **Short-term control of status epilepticus.** *Adult:* Loading dose, 15–20 mg PE/kg at 100–150 mg PE/min IV. **Px/tx of seizures during or after neurosurgery.** *Adult:* Loading dose, 10–20 mg PE/kg IM or IV; maint, 4–6 mg PE/kg/d. **Substitution**

**for oral phenytoin therapy.** *Adult:* Substitute IM or IV at same total daily dose as phenytoin; for short-term use only.
**ADJUST DOSE** Hepatic/renal impairment
**ADV EFF** **Angioedema,** ataxia, CV toxicity, dizziness, **DRESS**, drowsiness, hypotension, nausea, pruritus, rash to **SJS**, twitching
**INTERACTIONS** Acetaminophen, amiodarone, antineoplastics, carbamazepine, chloramphenicol, cimetidine, corticosteroids, cyclosporine, diazoxide, disopyramide, disulfiram, doxycycline, estrogens, fluconazole, folic acid, hormonal contraceptives, isoniazid, levodopa, methadone, metyrapone, mexiletine, phenacemide, phenylbutazone, primidone, rifampin, sulfonamides, theophyllines, trimethoprim, valproic acid
**NC/PT** Give IV slowly to prevent severe hypotension. Monitor infusion site carefully; sols are very alkaline, irritating. For short-term use only (up to 5 d); switch to oral phenytoin as soon as possible. Not for use in preg (contraceptives advised)/breastfeeding. Pt should take safety precautions w/CNS effects. Name confusion w/ *Cerebyx* (fosphenytoin), *Celebrex* (celecoxib), *Celexa* (citalopram), and *Xanax* (alprazolam).

## fostamatinib disodium
(Tavalisse)
**CLASS** Spleen tyrosine kinase inhibitor, tyrosine kinase inhibitor
**PREG/CONT** High risk/NA

**IND & DOSE** **Tx of chronic immune thrombocytopenia in pts w/insufficient response to a previous tx.** *Adult:* 100 mg PO bid. After 4 wk, increase to 150 mg bid, if needed, to achieve platelet count of at least $50 \times 10^9$/L as necessary to reduce bleeding risk.
**ADV EFF** Abd pain, chest pain, diarrhea, dizziness, fatigue, **hepatotoxicity,** HTN, nausea, **neutropenia,** respiratory infection, rash
**INTERACTIONS** Strong CYP3A4 inducers/inhibitors
**NC/PT** Monitor LFTs, CBC (including platelets) monthly until stable platelet count (at least $50 \times 10^9$/L). Monitor BP q 2 wk until stable dose achieved, then monthly. Contraceptives advised during tx and for at least 1 mo after tx. Pt should take w/ or w/o food, stay hydrated.

## fremanezumab-vfrm
(Ajovy)
**CLASS** Calcitonin gene-related peptide receptor antagonist; monoclonal antibody
**PREG/CONT** No data for humans; no risk in animal studies/NA

**IND & DOSE** **Px of migraine.** *Adult:* 225 mg subcut monthly or 675 mg subcut q 3 mo.
**ADV EFF** **Hypersensitivity,** injection-site reaction
**NC/PT** Give in abdomen/thigh/upper arm. Give 675 mg in three separate injections of 225 mg each. Monitor for hypersensitivity, including rash, itching, hives.

## frovatriptan succinate
(Frova)
**CLASS** Antimigraine, triptan
**PREG/CONT** C/NA

**IND & DOSE** **Tx of acute migraine w/ or w/o aura.** *Adult:* 2.5 mg PO as single dose at first sign of migraine; may repeat after 2 hr. Max, three doses/24 hr.
**ADV EFF** **Cerebrovascular events,** dizziness, headache, **MI,** n/v, tingling, **ventricular arrhythmias**
**INTERACTIONS** Ergots, SSRIs
**NC/PT** Ensure proper dx. For tx, not px. Ensure no ergots taken within 24 hr. Ensure 2 hr between doses, no more than three doses/d. Monitor BP.

Not for use in preg. Pt should take safety precautions w/CNS effects; report chest pain/pressure.

**DANGEROUS DRUG**

## fulvestrant (Faslodex)

**CLASS** Antineoplastic, estrogen receptor antagonist
**PREG/CONT** High risk/NA

**IND & DOSE** **Tx of HR-positive, HER2-negative breast cancer in postmenopausal women; tx of HR-positive, HER2-negative advanced or metastatic breast cancer w/ribociclib as initial tx or if disease progression after endocrine tx; tx of HR-positive, HER2-negative advanced or metastatic breast cancer w/palbociclib or abemaciclib w/disease progression after endocrine tx.** *Adult:* 500 mg IM on days 1, 15, 29, then monthly as two concomitant 5-mL injections over 1–2 min, one in each buttock.
**ADJUST DOSE** Hepatic impairment
**ADV EFF** Abd pain, anemia, arthritis, asthenia, back pain, bleeding, bone pain, dizziness, dyspnea, hot flashes, increased cough/sweating, injection-site reaction, n/v/d, pelvic pain
**INTERACTIONS** Oral anticoagulants
**NC/PT** Rule out preg; suggest contraceptives. Not for use in breastfeeding. Handle cautiously. Give by slow IM injection over 1–2 min. Hot flashes possible. Teach proper administration/disposal of needles/syringes. Pt should mark calendar of tx days, take safety precautions w/CNS effects.

## furosemide (Lasix)

**CLASS** Loop diuretic
**PREG/CONT** C/NA

**BBW** Profound diuresis w/water, electrolyte depletion possible; careful medical supervision needed.
**IND & DOSE** **Edema associated w/ systemic disease.** *Adult:* 20–80 mg/d PO as single dose; max, 600 mg/d. Or, 20–40 mg IM or IV (slow IV injection over 1–2 min); max, 4 mg/min. *Child:* 2 mg/kg/d PO; max, 6 mg/kg/d (1 mg/kg/d in preterm infants). **Tx of acute pulmonary edema.** *Adult:* 40 mg IV over 1–2 min. May increase to 80 mg IV over 1–2 min if response unsatisfactory after 1 hr. *Child:* 1 mg/kg IV or IM. May increase by 1 mg/kg in 2 hr until desired effect achieved. Max, 6 mg/kg. **Tx of HTN.** *Adult:* 40 mg bid PO.
**ADJUST DOSE** Renal impairment
**ADV EFF** Anemia, anorexia, dizziness, hyperglycemia, hypokalemia, leukopenia, muscle cramps, n/v, orthostatic hypotension, paresthesia, photosensitivity, pruritus, thrombocytopenia, urticaria, xanthopsia
**INTERACTIONS** Aminoglycosides, charcoal, cisplatin, digitalis, ibuprofen, indomethacin, NSAIDs, oral antidiabetics, phenytoin
**NC/PT** Give early in day so diuresis will not affect sleep. Do not expose to light. Record weight daily. Monitor potassium level; arrange for potassium replacement or potassium-rich diet. Use caution in preg/breastfeeding. Pt should avoid sun exposure; take safety precautions w/CNS effects; report loss or gain of more than 3 lb/d. Name confusion between furosemide and torsemide.

## gabapentin (Gralise, Horizant, Neurontin)

**CLASS** Antiepileptic
**PREG/CONT** C/NA

**IND & DOSE** **Adjunct tx of partial seizures.** *Adult:* 300 mg PO tid. Maint, 900–1,800 mg/d PO tid in divided doses; max of 2,400–3,600 mg/d has been used. Max interval between doses, 12 hr. *Child 3–12 yr:* 10–15 mg/kg/d PO in three divided doses. Range, 25–35 mg/kg/d in three divided doses (child ≥5 yr) and up to 40 mg/kg/d in three divided doses (child 3–4 yr). **Tx of postherpetic neuralgia.** *Adult:*

300 mg/d PO; 300 mg PO bid on day 2; 300 mg PO tid on day 3. Or, 1,800 mg/d PO w/evening meal (*Gralise*). **Tx of moderate to severe restless legs syndrome.** *Adult:* 600–800 mg/d PO w/food around 5 p.m.; max, 2,400 mg/d (*Horizant*).
**ADJUST DOSE** Elderly pts, renal impairment
**ADV EFF** **Anaphylaxis, angioedema.** ataxia, dizziness, insomnia, multiorgan hypersensitivity, neuropsychiatric reactions in child, **seizures**, somnolence, suicidal ideation, tremor, weight gain
**INTERACTIONS** Antacids
**NC/PT** *Gralise* not interchangeable w/other forms of gabapentin. Taper ER forms after long-term use. Monitor for anaphylaxis, angioedema; stop immediately. Pt may be at increased risk for suicidality; monitor. Not for use in preg; use caution in breastfeeding. Suggest medical alert tag. Pt should not cut/crush/chew ER forms; take safety precautions for CNS effects; report rash, difficulty breathing, swelling.

## gadobutrol (Gadavist)
**CLASS** Contrast agent
**PREG/CONT** Moderate risk/NA

**BBW** Risk of nephrogenic systemic fibrosis, more common w/higher-than-normal dosing or repeated dosing; monitor total dose. Screen for kidney injury before use.
**IND & DOSE** **Detection, visualization of areas w/disrupted blood-brain barrier and/or abnormal CNS vascularity; to assess malignant breast disease; to evaluate known or suspected supra-aortic or renal artery disease; to assess myocardial perfusion in adult w/known or suspected CAD.** *Adult, child (including neonates):* Dosage based on body weight: 0.1 mL/kg, given as IV bolus at 2 mL/sec; flush line w/NSS after injection.
**ADV EFF** Dysgeusia, feeling hot, headache, **hypersensitivity reaction**, injection-site reaction, nausea, **nephrogenic systemic fibrosis**
**NC/PT** Evaluate GFR before starting tx. Monitor total dose exposure; monitor for nephrogenic systemic fibrosis. Not for use in preg. Pt should report all exposure to contrast agents, itching, swelling or tightening, red or dark patches on skin, joint stiffness, muscle weakness, bone pain.

## galantamine hydrobromide (Razadyne)
**CLASS** Alzheimer drug, cholinesterase inhibitor
**PREG/CONT** B/NA

**IND & DOSE** **Tx of mild to moderate dementia of Alzheimer type.** *Adult:* 4 mg PO bid; after 4 wk, increase to 8 mg PO bid; after 4 more wk, increase to 12 mg PO bid. Range, 16–32 mg/d in two divided doses. ER capsules, 8 mg/d PO; titrate to 16–24 mg/d PO.
**ADJUST DOSE** Hepatic/renal impairment
**ADV EFF** Abd pain, anorexia, bladder outflow obstruction, bradycardia, diarrhea, dizziness, dyspepsia, n/v/d, insomnia, **serious skin reactions**, weight loss
**INTERACTIONS** Anticholinergics, bethanechol, cimetidine, erythromycin, ketoconazole, paroxetine, potent CYP2D6/CYP3A4 inhibitors, succinylcholine
**NC/PT** Does not cure disease; may slow degeneration. Establish baseline functional profile. Mix sol w/water, fruit juice, or soda. Do not cut/crush/allow pt to chew ER form; have pt swallow whole. Antiemetics may be helpful for GI upset. Pt should take safety measures for CNS effects; report rash, inability to empty bladder. Because of name confusion, manufacturer has changed name from *Reminyl* to *Razadyne*.

## galcanezumab-gnlm
(Emgality)
**CLASS** Calcitonin gene-related peptide receptor antagonist, monoclonal antibody
**PREG/CONT** Moderate risk/NA

**IND & DOSE** **Px of migraine.** *Adult:* 240 mg subcut loading dose (2 injections of 120 mg); then monthly doses of 120 mg subcut. **Tx of episodic cluster headache.** *Adult:* 300 mg subcut loading dose (3 injections of 100 mg); then monthly until end of cluster period.
**ADV EFF** **Hypersensitivity,** injection-site reaction
**INTERACTIONS** **Belimumab**
**NC/PT** Provide self-administration instructions. Pt should seek immediate medical attention for hypersensitivity s&sx.

## galsulfase (Naglazyme)
**CLASS** Enzyme
**PREG/CONT** B/NA

**IND & DOSE** **Tx of pts w/mucopolysaccharidosis VI to improve walking and stair climbing capacity.** *Adult:* 1 mg/kg/wk by IV infusion, diluted and infused over 4 hr.
**ADJUST DOSE** Hepatic/renal impairment
**ADV EFF** Abd pain, **anaphylaxis and allergic reactions, cardiorespiratory failure,** chills, dyspnea, fever, headache, **immune reactions, infusion reactions**, n/v, pruritus, rash, urticaria
**NC/PT** Establish baseline activity. Pretreat w/antihistamines and antipyretics; consider adding corticosteroids. Monitor continually during infusion; consider lowering dose or discontinuing w/severe reactions. Clinical surveillance program available if used in preg/breastfeeding.

## ganciclovir sodium
(Cytovene, Zirgan)
**CLASS** Antiviral
**PREG/CONT** High risk/NA

**BBW** Obtain CBC before tx, q 2 d during daily dosing, and at least wkly thereafter. Consult physician and arrange for reduced dose if WBC or platelet count falls. IV therapy is *only* for tx of CMV retinitis in immunocompromised pts and for px of CMV disease in transplant pts at risk for CMV. Potential for hematologic toxicity, impairment of fertility, fetal toxicity, mutagenesis, and carcinogenesis.
**IND & DOSE** **Tx of CMV retinitis.** *Adult:* 5 mg/kg IV at constant rate over 1 hr q 12 hr for 14–21 d; maint, 5 mg/kg by IV infusion over 1 hr once daily 7 d/wk *or* 6 mg/kg once daily 5 d/wk. *Child ≥2 yr:* Ophthal gel, 1 drop in affected eye(s) 5 ×/d (approx q 3 hr while awake) until ulcer heals. Maint, 1 drop 3 ×/d for 7 d. **Px of CMV disease in transplant recipients.** *Adult:* 5 mg/kg IV over 1 hr q 12 hr for 7–14 d; then 5 mg/kg/d IV once daily for 7 d/wk, *or* 6 mg/kg/d once daily for 5 d/wk.
**ADJUST DOSE** Renal impairment
**ADV EFF** Anemia, **bone marrow suppression, cancer,** fever, granulocytopenia, hepatic changes, inflammation at injection site, pain, rash, thrombocytopenia
**INTERACTIONS** Bone marrow suppressants, imipenem-cilastatin, probenecid, zidovudine
**NC/PT** Avoid contact w/sol; proper disposal necessary. Do not give IM or subcut. Monitor CBC before and periodically during tx. Not for use in preg (contraceptives for men/women advised). Frequent blood tests needed. Pt should have cancer screening; report rash, difficulty breathing.

## ganirelix acetate
(generic)
**CLASS** Fertility drug
**PREG/CONT** X/NA

**IND & DOSE To inhibit premature LH surges in women in fertility programs.** *Adult:* 250 mcg/d subcut starting on day 2 or 3 of cycle.
**ADV EFF** Abd pain, headache, injection-site reaction, n/v, **ovarian hyperstimulation,** vaginal bleeding
**NC/PT** Drug part of comprehensive fertility program. Show pt proper administration/disposal of needles/syringes. Pt should report swelling, shortness of breath, severe n/v, low urine output.

**DANGEROUS DRUG**

## gemcitabine hydrochloride (Gemzar, Infugem)
**CLASS** Antimetabolite, antineoplastic
**PREG/CONT** High risk/NA

**IND & DOSE Tx of pancreatic cancer.** *Adult:* 1,000 mg/m² IV over 30 min once wkly for up to 7 wk. Subsequent cycles of once wkly for 3 out of 4 consecutive wk can be given after 1-wk rest from tx. **First-line tx of inoperable, locally advanced, or metastatic NSCLC, w/cisplatin.** *Adult:* 1,000 mg/m² IV over 30 min, days 1, 8, and 15 of each 28-day cycle, w/100 mg/m² cisplatin on day 1 after gemcitabine infusion, *or* 1,250 mg/m² IV over 30 min, days 1 and 8 of each 21-day cycle, w/100 mg/m² cisplatin on day 1 after gemcitabine infusion. **First-line tx for metastatic breast cancer after failure of other adjuvant chemo, w/paclitaxel.** *Adult:* 1,250 mg/m² IV over 30 min, days 1 and 8 of each 21-day cycle, w/175 mg/m² paclitaxel IV as 3-hr infusion before gemcitabine on day 1 of cycle. **Tx of advanced ovarian cancer that has relapsed at least 6 mo after completion of platinum-based therapy.** *Adult:* 1,000 mg/m² IV over 30 min, days 1 and 8 of each 21-day cycle. Carboplatin given on day 1 after gemcitabine.
**ADV EFF** Alopecia, **bone marrow depression,** capillary leak syndrome, edema, fever, flulike sx, hemolytic-uremic syndrome, hepatotoxicity, **interstitial pneumonitis,** n/v, pain, rash, **RPLS**
**NC/PT** Monitor CBC/renal function/LFTS carefully; dose adjustment may be needed. Infuse over 30 min; longer infusions cause increased half-life/greater toxicity. Premedicate for n/v. Not for use in preg/breastfeeding. Pt should avoid exposure to infection; protect head in temp extremes (hair loss possible); report edema, difficulty breathing, urine/stool changes.

## gemfibrozil (Lopid)
**CLASS** Antihyperlipidemic
**PREG/CONT** High risk/NA

**IND & DOSE Adjunct to diet/exercise for tx of hypertriglyceridemia in pts w/very high triglycerides; reduction of CAD in pts unresponsive to traditional therapies.** *Adult:* 1,200 mg/d PO in two divided doses 30 min before morning and evening meals.
**ADJUST DOSE** Hepatic/renal impairment
**ADV EFF** Abd pain, blurred vision, cataract development, dizziness, dyspepsia, eczema, epigastric pain, **eosinophilia,** fatigue, gallstone development, headache, **hepatotoxicity, leukopenia,** n/v/d, **rhabdomyolysis**
**INTERACTIONS** Anticoagulants, enzalutamide, repaglinide, statins, sulfonylureas,
**NC/PT** Use only if strongly indicated and lipid studies show definite response; hepatic tumorigenicity occurs in lab animals. Not for use in preg/breastfeeding. Pt should take w/meals; continue diet/exercise program; take safety precautions w/CNS effects;

report muscle pain w/fever, upper abd pain, urine/stool color changes.

## gemifloxacin mesylate
(Factive)
**CLASS** Fluoroquinolone antibiotic
**PREG/CONT** High risk/NA

**BBW** Risk of disabling, potentially irreversible reactions that have occurred together, including tendinitis/tendon rupture, peripheral neuropathy, CNS effects. Risk of exacerbation of muscle weakness and potential crisis in pts w/myasthenia gravis; contraindicated for use in pts w/hx of myasthenia gravis. Reserve use for pts w/no other tx option for acute bacterial exacerbation of chronic bronchitis.
**IND & DOSE Tx of acute bacterial exacerbations of chronic bronchitis caused by susceptible strains.** *Adult:* 320 mg/d PO for 5 d. **Tx of community-acquired pneumonia caused by susceptible strains.** *Adult:* 320 mg/d PO for 5 d; 7 d for resistant strains.
**ADJUST DOSE** Renal impairment
**ADV EFF** Abd pain, **aortic aneurysm/dissection**, blood glucose changes, blurred vision, CDAD, dizziness, **hypersensitivity,** n/v/d, peripheral neuropathies, photosensitivity, **prolonged QT, rash to SJS, ulcerative colitis**
**INTERACTIONS** Aluminum- or potassium-containing antacids, amiodarone, antidepressants, antipsychotics, calcium, didanosine, erythromycin, iron, procainamide, quinidine, QT-prolonging drugs, sotalol, sucralfate, sulfonylureas
**NC/PT** Culture before tx. Ensure need for drug. Not for use in preg/breastfeeding. Pt should take 3 hr before or 2 hr after antacids; swallow tablet whole and not cut/crush/chew it; drink plenty of fluids; avoid sun exposure; report acute pain or tenderness in muscle or tendon, bloody diarrhea, palpitations, fainting, numbness/tingling, rash.

## gentamicin sulfate
(Gentak)
**CLASS** Aminoglycoside antibiotic
**PREG/CONT** High risk (systemic); unkn (ophthal)/NA

**BBW** Monitor hearing w/long-term tx; ototoxicity possible. Monitor renal function/CBC/serum drug levels during long-term tx; carefully monitor pt if combined w/other neurotoxic or nephrotoxic drugs.
**IND & DOSE Tx of community-acquired pneumonia caused by susceptible strains.** *Adult:* 3 mg/kg/d IM or IV in three equal doses q 8 hr. Up to 5 mg/kg/d in three–four equal doses in severe infections, usually for 7–10 d. For IV use, may infuse loading dose of 1–2 mg/kg over 30–60 min. *Child:* 2–2.5 mg/kg IM or IV q 8 hr. *Infants, neonates:* 2.5 mg/kg IM or IV q 8 hr. *Preterm, full-term neonates ≤1 wk:* 2.5 mg/kg IM or IV q 12 hr. *Preterm neonates <32 wk gestational age:* 2.5 mg/kg IM or IV q 18 hr or 3 mg/kg q 24 hr. **Tx of PID.** *Adult:* 2 mg/kg IV, then 1.5 mg/kg IV tid plus clindamycin 600 mg IV qid. Continue for at least 4 d and at least 48 hr after pt improves, then continue clindamycin 450 mg PO qid for 10–14 d total tx. **Tx of superficial ocular infections due to susceptible microorganism strains.** *Adult, child:* 1–2 drops in affected eye(s) q 4 hr; use up to 2 drops hrly in severe infections or apply about ½″ ointment to affected eye bid–tid. **Infection px in minor skin abrasions; tx of superficial skin infections.** *Adult, child:* Apply tid–qid. May cover w/sterile bandage.
**ADJUST DOSE** Elderly pts, renal failure
**ADV EFF** Anorexia, **apnea,** arachnoiditis at IM injection sites, **bone marrow suppression,** dizziness, local irritation, n/v/d, **nephrotoxicity, neuromuscular blockade,** ototoxicity, pain, purpura, rash, **seizures,** superinfections, tinnitus

**INTERACTIONS** Aminoglycosides, anesthetics, beta-lactam–type antibiotics, carbenicillin, cephalosporins, citrate-anticoagulated blood, diuretics (potent), enflurane, methoxyflurane, nondepolarizing NMJ blockers, penicillins, succinylcholine, ticarcillin, vancomycin
**NC/PT** Culture before tx. Systemic form not for use in preg/breastfeeding. Give by deep IM injection if possible. Avoid long-term use. Monitor serum levels. Max peak levels, 12 mcg/mL (6–8 mcg/mL usually adequate for most infections); max trough levels, 2 mcg/mL. Monitor CBC, renal function, hearing. Teach proper administration of ophthal and topical preparations. Pt should take safety precautions w/CNS effects; avoid exposure to infection; report severe headache, loss of hearing, difficult breathing.

▶NEW DRUG

## gilteritinib (Xospata)

**CLASS** Antineoplastic, kinase inhibitor, orphan
**PREG/CONT** High risk/NA

**IND & DOSE Tx of relapsed/refractory acute myeloid leukemia w/an FLT3 mutation.** *Adult:* 120 mg PO daily w/ or w/o food.
**ADV EFF** Cough, dizziness, fatigue, fever, headache, **hypersensitivity**, hypotension, malaise, myalgia/arthralgia, n/v, **pancreatitis**, pneumonia, **PRES**, **QT prolongation**, rash, stomatitis
**INTERACTIONS** Combined P-gp/strong CYP3A inducers, strong CYP3A inhibitors
**NC/PT** May need to adjust dose based on QT interval. Do not break/crush tablets. Obtain preg test before tx. Pt should avoid preg; contraception during and for at least 6 mo (4 mo for men) after tx advised.

DANGEROUS DRUG

## glasdegib (Daurismo)

**CLASS** Antineoplastic, hedgehog pathway inhibitor
**PREG/CONT** High risk/NA

**BBW** Can cause embryo-fetal death/severe birth defects when used in preg; conduct preg testing before start of tx. Advise males of potential for exposure through semen and to use condoms w/preg partner or partners of reproductive potential during tx and for at least 30 d after tx.
**IND & DOSE Tx of pts ≥75 yr w/contraindication to intensive induction chemo w/newly diagnosed acute myeloid leukemia.** *Adult:* 100 mg PO once a d.
**ADV EFF** Anemia, constipation, decreased appetite, dysgeusia, dyspnea, edema, fatigue, febrile neutropenia, hemorrhage, infertility, mucositis, musculoskeletal pain, nausea, **QT prolongation**, rash, thrombocytopenia
**NC/PT** Advise pts (male and female) to use effective contraception during tx and for at least 30 d after tx. Pts should not donate blood or blood products during tx and for at least 30 d after tx.

## glatiramer acetate (Copaxone, Glatopa)

**CLASS** MS drug
**PREG/CONT** B/NA

**IND & DOSE To reduce frequency of relapses in pts w/relapsing-remitting MS, including pts who have experienced a first clinical episode and have MRI features consistent w/MS.** *Adult:* 20 mg/d subcut. Or, 40 mg/d subcut 3 ×/wk.
**ADV EFF** Anxiety, asthenia, back pain, chest pain, infections, injection-site reactions (including lipoatrophy, skin necrosis), nausea, postinjection reaction, rash

**NC/PT** Rotate injection sites; do not use same site within a wk. Teach proper administration/disposal of needles/syringes. Use caution in breastfeeding. Monitor for infections. Pt should report severe injection-site reactions, chest pain w/sweating, trouble breathing.

DANGEROUS DRUG

## glimepiride (Amaryl)

**CLASS** Antidiabetic, sulfonylurea
**PREG/CONT** C/NA

**IND & DOSE** **Adjunct to diet to lower blood glucose in type 2 diabetes mellitus.** *Adult:* 1–2 mg PO once daily w/breakfast or first meal of day. Range, 1–4 mg PO once daily; max, 8 mg/d. **W/metformin or insulin to better control glucose as adjunct to diet/exercise in type 2 diabetes mellitus.** *Adult:* 8 mg PO daily w/first meal of day w/low-dose insulin or metformin.
**ADJUST DOSE** Adrenal or pituitary insufficiency; debilitated, elderly, malnourished pts; hepatic/renal impairment
**ADV EFF** Allergic skin reactions, anorexia, **CV mortality,** diarrhea, epigastric distress, **eosinophilia, hypoglycemia**
**INTERACTIONS** Alcohol, androgens, anticoagulants, azole antifungals, beta blockers, calcium channel blockers, celery, cholestyramine, chloramphenicol, clofibrate, coriander, corticosteroids, dandelion root, diazoxide, estrogens, fenugreek, fluconazole, garlic, gemfibrozil, ginseng, histamine-2 blockers, hormonal contraceptives, hydantoins, isoniazid, juniper berries, magnesium salts, MAOIs, methyldopa, nicotinic acid, phenothiazines, probenecid, rifampin, salicylates, sulfinpyrazone, sulfonamides, sympathomimetics, TCAs, thiazides, thyroid drugs, urinary acidifiers/alkalinizers
**NC/PT** Monitor blood glucose. Transfer to insulin temporarily in times of stress. Ensure diet/exercise program. Arrange for complete diabetic teaching program. Not for use in preg. Pt should avoid alcohol; report chest pain, uncontrolled glucose levels.

DANGEROUS DRUG

## glipiZIDE (Glucotrol)

**CLASS** Antidiabetic, sulfonylurea
**PREG/CONT** C/NA

**IND & DOSE** **Adjunct to diet/exercise to lower blood glucose in type 2 diabetes mellitus.** *Adult:* 5 mg PO before breakfast. Adjust dose in increments of 2.5–5 mg as determined by blood glucose response; max, 15 mg/dose. ER tablets, 5 mg/d PO; may increase to 10 mg/d after 3 mo.
**ADJUST DOSE** Elderly pts
**ADV EFF** Allergic skin reactions, anorexia, **bone marrow suppression, CV mortality,** diarrhea, epigastric distress, **eosinophilia, hypoglycemia**
**INTERACTIONS** Alcohol, beta blockers, chloramphenicol, clofibrate, coriander, dandelion root, diazoxide, fenugreek, garlic, gemfibrozil, ginseng, juniper berries, phenothiazines, rifampin, salicylates, sulfonamides
**NC/PT** Monitor blood glucose. Transfer to insulin temporarily in times of stress. Give 30 min before breakfast. Ensure diet/exercise program. Arrange for complete diabetic teaching program. Not for use in preg/breastfeeding. Pt should swallow ER tablets whole and not cut/crush/chew them; avoid alcohol; report chest pain, uncontrolled glucose levels.

## glucagon (Baqsimi, GlucaGen, Glucagon Emergency Kit, Gvoke)

**CLASS** Diagnostic agent, glucose-elevating drug
**PREG/CONT** B/NA

**IND & DOSE** **Tx of hypoglycemia.** *Adult, child >20 kg:* 0.5–1 mg IV, IM,

or subcut; severe hypoglycemia, 1 mL IV, IM, or subcut. Use IV if possible. *Child <20 kg:* 0.5 mg IM, IV, or subcut, or dose equivalent to 20–30 mcg/kg. *Adult, child ≥12 yr, child ≥2 yr >45 kg:* 1 mg subcut (*Gvoke*). *Child 2–12 yr <45 kg:* 0.5 mg subcut (*Gvoke*). *Adult, child ≥4 yr:* 3 mg intranasal into one nostril (*Baqsimi*). **Diagnostic aid in radiologic examination of stomach, duodenum, small bowel, colon.** *Adult, child >20 kg:* Usual dose, 0.25–2 mg IV or 1–2 mg IM.
**ADV EFF** Hypokalemia, hypotension, n/v, **respiratory distress**
**INTERACTIONS** Oral anticoagulants
**NC/PT** Arouse pt as soon as possible. Provide supplemental carbohydrates. Evaluate insulin dose in pts w/insulin overdose. Teach pt and significant other proper administration/disposal of needles/syringes.

## glucarpidase (Voraxaze)

**CLASS** Carboxypeptidase enzyme
**PREG/CONT** C/NA

**IND & DOSE Tx of pts w/toxic plasma methotrexate concentrations w/delayed methotrexate clearance due to impaired renal function.** *Adult, child:* 50 units/kg as single IV injection.
**ADV EFF** Flushing, headache, hypotension, n/v, paresthesia, **serious allergic reactions**
**INTERACTIONS** Folate, folate antimetabolites, leucovorin
**NC/PT** Continue hydration, alkalinization of urine. Do not administer within 2 hr of leucovorin. Monitor closely for allergic reaction during and directly after injection. Tell pt blood levels will be monitored repeatedly during tx. Pt should report fever, chills, rash, difficulty breathing, numbness/tingling, headache.

**DANGEROUS DRUG**

## glyBURIDE (DiaBeta, Glynase)

**CLASS** Antidiabetic, sulfonylurea
**PREG/CONT** B (Glynase); C (DiaBeta)/NA

**IND & DOSE Adjunct to diet/exercise to lower blood glucose in type 2 diabetes mellitus.** *Adult:* 2.5–5 mg PO w/breakfast (*DiaBeta*); 1.5–3 mg/d PO (*Glynase*); maint, 1.25–20 mg/d PO.
**ADJUST DOSE** Debilitated, elderly, malnourished pts
**ADV EFF** Allergic skin reactions, anorexia, blurred vision, **bone marrow suppression, CV mortality,** diarrhea, epigastric distress, **hypoglycemia**
**INTERACTIONS** Alcohol, beta blockers, bosentan, chloramphenicol, clofibrate, coriander, dandelion root, diazoxide, fenugreek, garlic, gemfibrozil, ginseng, juniper berries, phenothiazines, rifampin, salicylates, sulfonamides
**NC/PT** Note dosage difference between two forms; use w/care. Monitor blood glucose. Transfer to insulin temporarily in times of stress. Give before breakfast. Ensure diet/exercise program. Arrange for complete diabetic teaching program. Not for use in preg. Pt should avoid alcohol. Name confusion between *DiaBeta* (glyburide) and *Zebeta* (bisoprolol).

## glycerol phenylbutyrate (Ravicti)

**CLASS** Nitrogen-binding agent
**PREG/CONT** Unkn/NA

**IND & DOSE Long-term mgt of urea cycle disorders not managed by diet/amino acid supplementation.** *Adult, child ≥2 mo:* 4.5–11.2 mL/m²/d PO divided into three equal doses, rounded to nearest 0.5 mL, w/food; max, 17.5 mL/d.
**ADJUST DOSE** Hepatic impairment

**ADV EFF** Diarrhea, flatulence, headache, **neurotoxicity**
**INTERACTIONS** Corticosteroids, haloperidol, probenecid, valproic acid
**NC/PT** Must give w/protein-restricted diet; monitor ammonia levels; adjust dose as needed. Not for use in preg/breastfeeding. Pt should take w/food; report disorientation, confusion, impaired memory.

## **glycopyrrolate** (Cuvposa, Glyrx-PF, Lonhala Magnair, Seebri Neohaler)

**CLASS** Anticholinergic, antispasmodic, bronchodilator, parasympatholytic
**PREG/CONT** B/NA

**IND & DOSE** **Adjunct tx for peptic ulcer.** *Adult:* 1 mg PO tid or 2 mg bid–tid. Maint, 1 mg bid; max, 8 mg/d. **Tx of chronic, severe drooling caused by neuro disorders.** *Child: 3–16 yr:* 0.02 mg/kg PO tid; titrate in 0.02-mg increments q 5–7 d. Max, 0.1 mg/kg PO tid; do not exceed 1.5–3 mg/dose. **Tx of peptic ulcer.** *Adult:* 0.1–0.2 mg IM or IV tid–qid. **Preanesthetic medication.** *Adult:* 0.004 mg/kg IM 30–60 min before anesthesia. *Child 2 yr–<12 yr:* 0.004 mg/kg IM 30 min–1 hr before anesthesia. *Child 1 mo–2 yr:* Up to 0.009 mg/kg IM may be needed. **Intraop to decrease vagal traction reflexes.** *Adult:* 0.1 mg IV; repeat as needed at 2- to 3-min intervals. *Child >1 mo:* 0.004 mg/kg IV, not to exceed 0.1 mg in single dose. May repeat at 2- to 3-min intervals. **Reversal of neuromuscular blockade.** *Adult, child >1 mo:* W/neostigmine, pyridostigmine, 0.2 mg IV for each 1 mg neostigmine or 5 mg pyridostigmine; give IV simultaneously. **Long-term maint tx of airflow obstruction in COPD.** *Adult:* 15.6 mcg (one oral inhalation) bid w/*Neohaler* or *Lonhala* device.
**ADV EFF** Altered taste perception, blurred vision, decreased sweating, dry mouth, dysphagia, irritation at injection site, n/v, **paradoxical bronchospasm w/oral inhalation,** photosensitivity, urinary hesitancy, urine retention
**INTERACTIONS** Amantadine, anticholinergics, digitalis, haloperidol, phenothiazines
**NC/PT** Check dose carefully. Ensure adequate hydration. Oral inhalation is not for use in deteriorating COPD, acute bronchospasm. Teach proper use of *Neohaler* device for oral inhalation. Not for use in breastfeeding. Pt should empty bladder before each dose; avoid hot environments (may be subject to heat stroke) and sun exposure; suck sugarless lozenges; perform mouth care for dry mouth; not chew capsule if using *Seebri Neohaler* (only for use in *Neohaler* device); report sudden shortness of breath, vision problems, difficult/painful urination.

## **golimumab** (Simponi)

**CLASS** Monoclonal antibody, TNF inhibitor
**PREG/CONT** Unkn/NA

**BBW** Serious infections possible, including TB, sepsis, invasive fungal infections. Discontinue if infection or sepsis develops. Perform TB test before tx. If TB present, start TB tx and monitor pt carefully throughout tx. Increased risk of lymphoma and other cancers in child, adolescent; monitor accordingly.
**IND & DOSE** **Tx of active RA, active psoriatic arthritis, ankylosing spondylitis.** *Adult:* 50 mg/mo subcut or 2 mg/kg IV over 30 min wk 0, 4, then q 8 wk. **Tx of moderate to severe ulcerative colitis.** *Adult:* 200 mg subcut wk 0, then 100 mg subcut wk 2, then 100 mg subcut q 4 wk.
**ADV EFF** Dizziness, HF, increased risk of demyelinating disorders, infections, injection-site reactions, **invasive fungal infections, malignancies,** nasopharyngitis
**INTERACTIONS** Abatacept, anakinra, adalimumab, certolizumab, etanercept, infliximab, live vaccines, rituximab

**NC/PT** TB test before tx. Store in refrigerator; bring to room temp before use. Rotate injection sites. For IV, use inline filter; do not infuse w/other drugs. Monitor for CNS changes, infection. Not for use in breastfeeding. Teach proper administration/disposal of needles/syringes. Pt should avoid live vaccines; take safety precautions for dizziness; have regular medical follow-up; report fever, numbness/tingling, worsening of arthritis, s&sx of infection, difficulty breathing.

**DANGEROUS DRUG**

## goserelin acetate
(Zoladex)
**CLASS** Antineoplastic, hormone
**PREG/CONT** X; D (w/breast cancer)/NA

**IND & DOSE** **Palliative tx of advanced prostate or breast cancer.** *Adult:* 3.6 mg q 28 d subcut (long-term use). **Mgt of endometriosis.** *Adult:* 3.6 mg subcut q 28 d for 6 mo. **Endometrial thinning before ablation.** *Adult:* 1–2 3.6-mg subcut depots 4 wk apart; surgery should be done 4 wk after first dose (within 2–4 wk after second depot if two are used). **Tx of stage $B_{2-C}$ prostate cancer, w/flutamide.** *Adult:* Start tx 8 wk before start of radiation therapy and continue during radiation therapy; 3.6-mg depot 8 wk before radiation, then one 10.8-mg depot 28 d later. Or, four injections of 3.6-mg depot at 28-d intervals, two depots preceding and two during radiotherapy.
**ADV EFF** **Cancer,** decreased erections, dizziness, dysmenorrhea, edema, gynecomastia, hot flashes, injection-site infections, lower urinary tract sx, prolonged QT, sexual dysfx, vaginitis
**NC/PT** Implant in upper abdomen q 28 d or q 3 mo (q 6 mo for endometriosis). Mark calendar for injection dates. Not for use in preg (contraceptives advised)/breastfeeding. Pt should report pain at injection site, discuss sexual dysfx w/health care provider.

## granisetron hydrochloride (generic)
**CLASS** Antiemetic, 5-$HT_3$ receptor antagonist
**PREG/CONT** Low risk/NA

**IND & DOSE** **Px of chemo-induced n/v.** *Adult, child >2 yr:* 10 mcg/kg IV over 5 min starting within 30 min of chemo, only on days of chemo. Or, 2 mg/d PO 1 hr before chemo or 1 mg PO bid, given up to 1 hr before chemo, w/next dose 12 hr later. Or, for adults, apply 1 patch to clean, dry skin on upper, outer arm 24–48 hr before chemo. Keep patch in place minimum of 24 hr after completion of chemo, then remove; may be left in place for up to 7 d. Or, for adults, 10 mg subcut ER injection (*Sustol*) at least 30 min before chemo on day 1; do not administer more than once/7 d. **Px of radiation-induced n/v.** *Adult, child >2 yr:* 2 mg/d PO 1 hr before radiation.
**ADJUST DOSE** Renal impairment
**ADV EFF** Asthenia, chills, constipation, decreased appetite, fever, headache, injection-site reactions, serotonin syndrome
**NC/PT** Use only as directed. Apply transdermal patch to clean, dry skin; leave in place up to 7 d. Inject ER form over 20–30 sec, subcut in back of upper arm or in abdomen at least 1 inch from umbilicus; do not use more often than q 7 d. Pt should perform mouth care; use sugarless lozenges to help relieve nausea; report severe constipation, headache, injection-site reactions.

## grass pollen allergy extract (Oralair)
**CLASS** Allergen extract
**PREG/CONT** C/NA

**BBW** Risk of severe life-threatening allergic reactions; not for use in uncontrolled asthma. Observe pt for 30 min after initial dose; have emergency equipment available. Prescribe epinephrine auto-injector; train pt in

use. May not be suitable for pts who may not be responsive to epinephrine or inhaled bronchodilators (eg, pts taking beta blockers).
**IND & DOSE** **Tx of grass pollen–induced allergic rhinitis w/ or w/o conjunctivitis confirmed by skin test or in vitro for pollen-specific IgE antibodies for any grass species in pts 5–65 yr.** *Adult 18–65 yr:* 300 IR (index of reactivity) SL during grass season. *Child 5–17 yr:* 100 IR SL on day 1, 100 IR SL bid on day 2,300 IR SL on day 3 onward.
**ADV EFF** Cough, ear pruritus, eosinophilic esophagitis, mouth edema, oropharyngeal pain/pruritus, throat/tongue pruritus
**NC/PT** Ensure skin test confirms dx. Not for use w/uncontrolled asthma, hx of severe reactions, eosinophilic esophagitis. Begin 4 mo before expected grass season; continue through season. Monitor for at least 30 min after first dose; ensure pt has access to and can use emergency epinephrine auto-injector. Stop tx for oral wounds/inflammation; allow to heal completely before restarting. Pt should place tablet under tongue for at least 1 minute, until complete dissolution, then swallow; report difficulty breathing/swallowing.

## guaifenesin (Mucinex)

**CLASS** Expectorant
**PREG/CONT** C/NA

**IND & DOSE** **Symptomatic relief of respiratory conditions characterized by dry, nonproductive cough; mucus in respiratory tract.** *Adult, child >12 yr:* 200–400 mg PO q 4 hr; max, 2.4 g/d. Or 1–2 tablets PO (600-mg ER tablets) q 12 hr; max, 2.4 g/d. *Child 6–12 yr:* 100–200 mg PO q 4 hr; max, 1.2 g/d or 600 mg (ER) PO q 12 hr. *Child 2–6 yr:* 50–100 mg PO q 4 hr; max, 600 mg/d.
**ADV EFF** Dizziness, headache, n/v
**NC/PT** Pt should swallow ER tablet whole and not cut/crush/chew it; use for no longer than 1 wk; consult prescriber if cough persists; take safety precautions for dizziness.

## guanfacine hydrochloride (Intuniv)

**CLASS** Antihypertensive, sympatholytic
**PREG/CONT** Moderate risk/NA

**IND & DOSE** **Mgt of HTN.** *Adult, child >12 yr:* 1 mg/d PO at bedtime. **Tx of ADHD.** *Adult, child ≥6 yr:* 1 mg/d PO; titrate at increments of 1 mg/wk to range of 1–7 mg/d (0.05–0.12 mg/kg) (*Intuniv*).
**ADJUST DOSE** Elderly pts; hepatic/renal impairment
**ADV EFF** Constipation, dizziness, dry mouth, ED, sedation, weakness
**NC/PT** Taper when stopping; decrease by no more than 1 mg q 3–7 d. Pt should swallow ER form whole and not cut/crush/or chew it, take immediate-release form at bedtime; avoid high-fat meals around dosing time; continue tx program for ADHD; take safety precautions for CNS effects; use sugarless lozenges for dry mouth.

## guselkumab (Tremfya)

**CLASS** Antipsoriatic; interleukin-23 inhibitor
**PREG/CONT** Unkn/NA

**IND & DOSE** **Tx of pts w/moderate to severe plaque psoriasis who are candidates for systemic therapy or phototherapy.** *Adult:* 100 mg subcut at week 0, 4, and q 8 wk thereafter.
**ADV EFF** Arthralgia, diarrhea, gastroenteritis, headache, herpes simplex, injection-site reaction, respiratory infection, tinea infection
**INTERACTIONS** Live vaccines
**NC/PT** Evaluate for TB before start of tx. Teach proper administration/sharps disposal; monitor first self-administered dose. Advise pt about increased infection risk.

**haloperidol, haloperidol decanoate, haloperidol lactate** (Haldol)
**CLASS** Antipsychotic, dopaminergic blocker
**PREG/CONT** High risk/NA

**BBW** Increased risk of death in elderly pts w/dementia-related psychosis; drug not approved for this use.
**IND & DOSE Tx of psychiatric disorders, Tourette syndrome.** *Adult:* 0.5–2 mg PO bid–tid w/moderate sx; 3–5 mg PO bid–tid for more resistant pts. Or IM dose 10–15 × daily oral dose in elderly pts stabilized on 10 mg/d or less; 20 × daily oral dose in pts stabilized on high doses and tolerant to oral haloperidol. Max, 3 mL/injection site; repeat at 4-wk intervals. **Prompt control of acutely agitated pts w/severe sx.** *Adult:* 2–5 mg (up to 10–30 mg) q 60 min or q 4–8 hr IM as necessary. **Tx of psychiatric disorders.** *Child 3–12 yr or 15–40 kg:* 0.5 mg/d (25–50 mcg/kg/d) PO; may increase in increments of 0.5 mg q 5–7 d as needed in general, then 0.05–0.15 mcg/kg/d PO bid–tid. **Nonpsychotic and Tourette syndromes, behavioral disorders, hyperactivity.** *Child 3–12 yr or 15–40 kg:* 0.05–0.075 mg/kg/d PO bid–tid.
**ADJUST DOSE** Elderly pts
**ADV EFF** Akathisia, anemia, **aplastic anemia, autonomic disturbances, bronchospasm, cardiac arrest,** dry mouth, dystonia, **eosinophilia, hemolytic anemia,** hyperthermia, **hypoglycemia, laryngospasm,** leukocytosis, **leukopenia, NMS,** photosensitivity, pseudoparkinsonism, **refractory arrhythmias, seizures, sudden death related to asphyxia,** tardive dyskinesia, **thrombocytopenic or nonthrombocytopenic purpura**
**INTERACTIONS** Anticholinergics, carbamazepine, ginkgo, lithium
**NC/PT** Do not use in elderly pts w/dementia-related psychosis. Do not use IM in child. Do not give IV. Gradually withdraw after maint tx. Monitor for renal toxicity. Not for use in preg/breastfeeding. Urine may be pink to brown. Pt should take safety precautions for CNS effects, avoid sun exposure, maintain fluid intake, use sugarless lozenges for dry mouth, report difficulty breathing.

**DANGEROUS DRUG**

**heparin sodium** (generic)
**CLASS** Anticoagulant
**PREG/CONT** Low risk/NA

**IND & DOSE Px/tx of venous thrombotic events.** *Adult:* IV loading dose, 5,000 units; then 10,000–20,000 units subcut followed by 8,000–10,000 units subcut q 8 hr or 15,000–20,000 units q 12 hr. Or initial dose, 10,000 units IV, then 5,000–10,000 units IV q 4–6 hr. Or loading dose, 5,000 units IV, then 20,000–40,000 units/d by IV infusion. *Child:* IV bolus of 50 units/kg, then 100 units/kg IV q 4 hr, or 20,000 units/$m^2$/24 hr by continuous IV infusion. **Px of postop thromboembolism.** *Adult:* 5,000 units by deep subcut injection 2 hr before surgery and q 8–12 hr thereafter for 7 d or until pt fully ambulatory. **Surgery of heart and blood vessels for pts undergoing total body perfusion.** *Adult:* Not less than 150 units/kg IV. IV often-used guideline: 300 units/kg for procedures less than 60 min, 400 units/kg for longer procedures. Add 400–600 units to 100 mL whole blood. **Clot prevention in blood samples.** *Adult:* 70–150 units/10–20 mL whole blood.
**ADV EFF** Bleeding, bruising, chills, fever, **hemorrhage,** injection-site reactions, hair loss, liver enzyme changes, **white clot syndrome**
**INTERACTIONS** Aspirin, cephalosporins, chamomile, garlic, ginger, ginkgo, ginseng, high-dose vitamin E, NSAIDs, penicillins, oral anticoagulants, salicylates

**NC/PT** Adjust dose based on coagulation tests; target aPTT, 1.5–2.5 × control. Incompatible in sol w/many drugs; check before combining. Give by deep subcut injection; do not give IM. Apply pressure to all injection sites; check for s&sx of bleeding. Have protamine sulfate on hand as antidote. Use preservative-free formulation in preg pts, if possible. Pt should protect from injury, report bleeding gums, black or tarry stools, severe headache.

## hetastarch (Hespan, Hextend, Voluven)

**CLASS** Plasma expander
**PREG/CONT** Moderate risk/NA

**BBW** Increased risk of death, need for renal replacement in critically ill pts, including sepsis pts. Not for use in these pts.
**IND & DOSE** **Adjunct tx for plasma volume expansion in shock due to hemorrhage, burns, surgery, sepsis, trauma.** *Adult:* 500–1,000 mL IV; max, 1,500 mL/d. In acute hemorrhagic shock, rates approaching 20 mL/kg/hr IV often needed (*Hespan*); up to 50 mL/kg/d IV injection. *Child 2–12 yr:* 25–47 mL/kg/d IV (*Voluven*). *Newborn to <2 yr:* 13–25 mL/kg/d IV. **Adjunct tx in leukapheresis to improve harvesting, increase yield of granulocytes.** *Adult:* 250–700 mL infused at constant fixed ratio of 1:8 to 1:13 to venous whole blood. Safety of up to two procedures/wk and total of seven to ten procedures using hetastarch have been established.
**ADJUST DOSE** Critically ill pts, pts w/clotting disorders, renal impairment, severe liver impairment
**ADV EFF** **Bleeding,** chills, circulatory overload, coagulopathy, headache, hypersensitivity reactions, itching, mild flulike sx, submaxillary and parotid gland enlargement, n/v
**INTERACTIONS** Drugs affecting coagulation
**NC/PT** Do not use w/cardiac bypass pumps, severe liver disease, bleeding disorders. Monitor renal function; stop at first sign of renal injury. Do not mix in sol w/other drugs. Have emergency support on hand. Pt should report difficulty breathing, severe headache.

## histrelin implant (Vantas)

**CLASS** Antineoplastic, GNRH
**PREG/CONT** X/NA

**IND & DOSE** **Palliative tx of advanced prostate cancer.** *Adult:* 1 implant inserted subcut and left for 12 mo. May be removed after 12 mo and new implant inserted.
**ADV EFF** Diabetes, fatigue, hot flashes, hyperglycemia, injection-site reactions, **MI, renal impairment, spinal cord compression, stroke,** testicular atrophy
**NC/PT** Monitor serum glucose, renal function, injection site, CV status. Not for use in preg/breastfeeding. Pt should report chest pain, numbness/tingling, injection-site reactions.

## house dust mite allergen extract (Odactra)

**CLASS** Allergen extract
**PREG/CONT** B/NA

**BBW** Risk of severe, life-threatening allergic reactions. Not for use in uncontrolled asthma. Observe pt for 30 min after first dose; have emergency equipment on hand. Prescribe autoinjectable epinephrine; teach use.
**IND & DOSE** **Immunotherapy for tx of house dust mite–induced allergic rhinitis w/ or w/o conjunctivitis confirmed by skin test in pts 18–65 yr.** *Adult:* 1 tablet/d SL year round.
**ADV EFF** Ear pruritus, mouth/lip/tongue edema, nausea, oropharyngeal pain/pruritus, throat/tongue pruritus

**NC/PT** Ensure skin testing confirms allergy. Not for use in uncontrolled asthma, hx of severe reactions, eosinophilic esophagitis. First dose should be given under medical supervision; observe pt for at least 30 min and have emergency equipment on hand. Place tablet under tongue, allow to stay until completely dissolved; pt should not swallow for 1 min. Pt should also be prescribed auto-injectable epinephrine, taught its proper use, and instructed to seek medical help after using it. Stop tx if oral wounds/inflammation; allow to heal completely before restarting. Pt should report difficulty breathing/ swallowing.

## hyaluronic acid derivatives (Euflexxa, Hyalgan, Synvisc)

**CLASS** Glucosamine polysaccharide
**PREG/CONT** C/NA

**IND & DOSE Tx of pain in osteoarthritis of knee in pts unresponsive to traditional therapy.** *Adult:* 2 mL/wk by intra-articular injection in knee for total of three to five injections.
**ADV EFF** Headache, joint swelling, pain at injection site
**NC/PT** Headache may occur. Pt should avoid strenuous exercise and prolonged weight bearing for 48 hr after injection; report severe joint swelling, loss of movement.

## hyaluronidase (Amphadase, Hylenex, Vitrase)

**CLASS** Enzyme
**PREG/CONT** C/NA

**IND & DOSE To increase absorption of injected drugs.** *Adult, child:* Add 150 units to injection sol. **Hypodermoclysis.** *Adult:* 150 units injected under skin close to clysis. *Child <3 yr:* Limit total dose to 200 mL/clysis. *Premature infants:* Max, 25 mL/kg at rate of no more than 2 mL/min. **Adjunct to subcut urography.** *Adult:* 75 units subcut over each scapula followed by injection of contrast media at same sites.
**ADV EFF** Chills, dizziness, edema, hypotension, injection-site reactions, n/v
**INTERACTIONS** Benzodiazepines, furosemide, phenytoin
**NC/PT** Do not use w/dopamine or alpha-adrenergic drugs or in inflamed or infected areas. Do not apply to cornea or use for insect bites or stings; monitor injection site.

## hydrALAZINE hydrochloride (generic)

**CLASS** Antihypertensive, vasodilator
**PREG/CONT** C/NA

**IND & DOSE Tx of essential HTN.** *Adult:* 10 mg PO qid for first 2–4 d; increase to 25 mg PO qid for first wk. Second and subsequent wks: 50 mg PO qid. Or 20–40 mg IM or IV, repeated as necessary if unable to take orally. *Child:* 0.75 mg/kg/d PO in divided doses q 6 hr (max, 7.5 mg/kg/d PO in four divided doses, or 200 mg/d PO). Or 1.7–3.5 mg/kg IM or IV divided into four–six doses if unable to take orally. **Tx of eclampsia.** *Adult:* 5–10 mg q 20 min by IV bolus. If no response after 20 mg, try another drug.
**ADV EFF** Angina, anorexia, **blood dyscrasias,** dizziness, headache, n/v/d, orthostatic hypotension, palpitations, peripheral neuritis, rash, tachycardia
**INTERACTIONS** Adrenergic blockers
**NC/PT** Use parenteral drug immediately after opening ampule. Withdraw drug gradually, especially in pts who have experienced marked BP reduction. Pt should take safety precautions w/orthostatic hypotension, CNS effects; take w/food; report chest pain, numbness/ tingling, fever.

## hydroCHLOROthiazide
(Microzide Capsules)
**CLASS** Thiazide diuretic
**PREG/CONT** B/NA

**IND & DOSE** **Adjunct tx of edema from systemic disease.** *Adult:* 25–100 mg PO daily until dry weight attained. Then, 25–100 mg/d PO or intermittently, up to 200 mg/d. *Child:* 1–2 mg/kg/d PO in one or two doses. Max, 100 mg/d in two doses (2–12 yr), 37.5 mg/d in two doses (6 mo–2 yr), up to 3 mg/kg/d in two doses (under 6 mo). **Tx of HTN.** *Adult:* 12.5–50 mg PO; max, 50 mg/d.
**ADJUST DOSE** Elderly pts
**ADV EFF** Anorexia, dizziness, drowsiness, dry mouth, muscle cramps, nocturia, n/v, photosensitivity, polyuria, vertigo
**INTERACTIONS** Amphotericin B, antidiabetics, cholestyramine, colestipol, corticosteroids, lithium, loop diuretics, NMJ blockers
**NC/PT** Monitor BP; reduced dose of other antihypertensives may be needed. Give w/food. Mark calendar for intermittent therapy. Pt should measure weight daily, take early in day so sleep not interrupted, use safety precautions for CNS effects, avoid sun exposure, report weight changes of 3 lb/d.

**DANGEROUS DRUG**

## HYDROcodone bitartrate (Hysingla ER, Zohydro ER)
**CLASS** Opioid agonist analgesic
**PREG/CONT** High risk/C-II

**BBW** Risks of addiction, severe to fatal respiratory depression, death w/ accidental consumption by child, life-threatening neonatal withdrawal if used in preg, fatal plasma levels if combined w/alcohol. Initiating CYP3A4 inhibitors or stopping CYP3A4 inducers can cause fatal hydrocodone overdose; avoid this combo. FDA REMS in place.

**IND & DOSE** **Mgt of pain requiring continuous analgesic for prolonged period.** *Adult:* Initially, 10 mg PO q 12 hr for opioid-naïve or opioid-nontolerant pts; increase as needed in 10-mg increments q 12 hr q 3–7 d.
**ADJUST DOSE** Elderly, impaired pts; severe renal/hepatic impairment
**ADV EFF** Abd pain, back pain, confusion, constipation, dizziness, dry mouth, fatigue, headache, hypotension, n/v/d, pruritus, **respiratory depression**
**INTERACTIONS** Alcohol, anticholinergics, barbiturate anesthetics, CNS depressants, CYP3A4 inducers/ inhibitors, MAOIs, other opioids, protease inhibitors
**NC/PT** Monitor pt carefully. Ensure appropriate use of drug; abuse-resistant forms decrease risk of addiction, abuse. Ensure opioid antagonist and emergency equipment readily available. Safety issues w/ CNS changes. Taper when discontinuing. Pt should swallow capsule whole, not cut/crush/chew it; discontinue slowly; avoid preg/breastfeeding, alcohol; take safety precautions for CNS changes; report difficulty breathing, severe constipation, pain unrelieved by drug.

## hydrocortisone salts
(Colocort, Cortef, Cortenema, Pandel, Solu-Cortef)
**CLASS** Corticosteroid
**PREG/CONT** High risk/NA

**IND & DOSE** **Replacement tx in adrenal cortical insufficiency, allergic states, inflammatory disorders, hematologic disorders, trichinosis, ulcerative colitis, MS.** *Adult, child:* 5–200 mg/d PO based on severity and pt response, or 100–500 mg IM or IV q 2, 4, or 6 hr. **Retention enema for tx of ulcerative colitis/proctitis.** *Adult, child:* 100 mg nightly for 21 d. **Anorectal cream, suppositories to relieve discomfort of hemorrhoids/ perianal itching or irritation.** *Adult,*

*child:* 1 applicator daily or bid for 2 or 3 wk and q second day thereafter. **Dermatologic preparations to relieve inflammatory and pruritic manifestations of dermatoses.** *Adult, child:* Apply sparingly to affected area bid–qid. **Tx of acute/chronic ophthal inflammatory conditions.** *Adult, child:* 1–2 drops per eye one to two ×/d.
**ADV EFF Anaphylactoid reactions,** amenorrhea, ecchymoses, fluid retention, headache, **HF,** hypokalemia, hypotension, immunosuppression, infection, irregular menses, local pain or irritation at application site, muscle weakness, pancreatitis, peptic ulcer, **serious neuro reactions w/epidural use,** striae, vertigo
**INTERACTIONS** Anticoagulants, anticholinesterases, cholestyramine, estrogen, hormonal contraceptives, ketoconazole, live vaccines, phenobarbital, phenytoin, rifampin, salicylates
**NC/PT** Give daily before 9 a.m. to mimic normal peak diurnal corticosteroid levels and minimize HPA suppression. Rotate IM injection sites. IV, IM not for use in neonates; contains benzyl alcohol. Use minimal doses for minimal duration to minimize adverse effects. Taper doses when discontinuing high-dose or long-term tx; arrange for increased dose when pt is subject to unusual stress. W/topical use, use caution w/ occlusive dressings; tight or plastic diapers over affected area can increase systemic absorption. Suggest medical ID. Pt should protect from infection; report swelling, difficulty breathing.

**DANGEROUS DRUG**

## HYDROmorphone hydrochloride (Dilaudid)

**CLASS** Opioid agonist analgesic
**PREG/CONT** High risk/C-II

**BBW** Monitor dose and intended use; vary w/form. Serious effects, addiction, abuse, misuse possible. Extended-release form for opioid-tolerant pts only; fatal respiratory depression possible. Extended-release form not for use w/acute or postop pain or as an as-needed drug. Pt must swallow extended-release tablets whole; broken/chewed/crushed tablets allow rapid release of drug and could cause fatal overdose. Prolonged use in preg can lead to potentially fatal neonatal opioid withdrawal syndrome. Accidental ingestion by child can be fatal; secure drug out of reach of child. FDA requires a REMS to ensure that benefits of opioid analgesics outweigh risks of addiction/abuse/ misuse.
**IND & DOSE Relief of moderate to severe pain; acute/chronic pain.** *Adult:* 2–4 mg PO q 4–6 hr. Liquid, 2.5–10 mg PO q 3–6 hr. ER tablets, 8–64 mg/d PO. Or 1–2 mg IM or subcut q 4–6 hr as needed, or by slow IV injection over 2–3 min, or 3 mg rectally q 6–8 hr.
**ADJUST DOSE** Elderly or debilitated pts; hepatic/renal impairment
**ADV EFF Apnea, cardiac arrest, circulatory depression,** constipation, dizziness, flushing, light-headedness, n/v, **respiratory arrest, respiratory depression,** sedation, **shock,** sweating, visual disturbances
**INTERACTIONS** Alcohol, anticholinergics, antihistamines, barbiturate anesthetics, CNS depressants, MAOIs, opioid agonist/antagonists
**NC/PT** Ensure opioid antagonist and facilities for assisted or controlled respiration are readily available during parenteral administration. Monitor pt w/head injury carefully. Not for use in preg/labor. Breastfeeding pt should take 4–6 hr before scheduled feeding. Refrigerate rectal suppositories. Pt should swallow ER tablet whole, and not cut/crush/chew it; avoid alcohol, antihistamines; take laxative for constipation; use safety precautions for CNS effects; keep out of reach of child; report chest pain, difficulty breathing.

## hydroxocobalamin
(Cyanokit)
**CLASS** Antidote
**PREG/CONT** C/NA

**IND & DOSE Tx of known or suspected cyanide poisoning.** *Adult:* 5 g by IV infusion over 15 min; may give second dose over 15–120 min by IV infusion.
**ADV EFF Anaphylaxis,** chest tightness, dyspnea, edema, **HTN,** injection-site reactions, nausea, photosensitivity, rash, red skin and mucous membranes (up to 2 wk), red urine (up to 5 wk), renal injury
**NC/PT** Support pt during acute poisoning. Run in separate IV line; do not mix w/other drugs. Monitor BP. Monitor renal function for 7 d post tx. Not for use in preg/breastfeeding. Tell pt urine may be red for up to 5 wk, skin and mucous membranes may be red for 2 wk. Pt should avoid exposure to sunlight during that period, report difficulty breathing.

## hydroxyprogesterone caproate (Makena)
**CLASS** Progestin
**PREG/CONT** Low risk/NA

**IND & DOSE To reduce risk of preterm birth in women w/singleton preg and hx of singleton spontaneous preterm birth.** *Adult:* 250 mg IM (single and multidose vials) or subcut (auto-injector) once wkly, beginning between 16 wk, 0 days' and 20 wk, 6 days' gestation. Continue wkly injections until wk 37 of gestation, or until delivery, whichever comes first.
**ADV EFF** Depression, fluid retention, glucose intolerance, injection-site reactions, nausea, pruritus, **thromboembolic events,** urticaria
**NC/PT** IM injection into upper outer area of buttocks once/wk; injection must be given by health care professional. Vial stable for 5 wk at room temp; protect from light. Monitor injection sites; periodically check serum glucose. Mark calendar for injection days. Pt should report leg, chest pain.

**DANGEROUS DRUG**

## hydroxyurea (Droxia, Hydrea, Siklos)
**CLASS** Antineoplastic
**PREG/CONT** High risk/NA

**BBW** Risk of myelosuppression, infections, and malignancies; monitor pt closely.
**IND & DOSE Concomitant tx w/ radiation for primary squamous cell carcinoma of head/neck** *Adult:* 80 mg/kg PO as single daily dose q third day. Begin 7 d before irradiation; continue during and for a prolonged period after radiation therapy (*Hydrea*). **Tx of resistant chronic myelocytic leukemia.** *Adult:* 20–30 mg/kg PO as single daily dose (*Hydrea*). **To reduce sickle cell anemia crises** (*Droxia, Siklos*). *Adult:* 15 mg/kg/d PO (*Droxia*) or 20 mg/kg/d PO (*Siklos*) as single dose; may increase by 5 mg/kg/d q 12 wk until max of 35 mg/kg/d reached. If blood levels become toxic, stop drug and resume at 2.5 mg/kg/d less than dose that resulted in toxicity when blood levels return to normal; increase q 12 wk in 2.5-mg/kg/d intervals if blood levels remain acceptable.
**ADJUST DOSE** Renal impairment
**ADV EFF** Anorexia, **bone marrow depression, cancer,** dizziness, headache, n/v, pulmonary toxicity, stomatitis
**INTERACTIONS** Antiviral drugs, uricosuric agents
**NC/PT** Handle w/extreme care; may cause cancer. Use gloves when handling capsule. Monitor CBC before and q 2 wk during tx. Capsule should not be cut/crushed/chewed; have pt swallow whole. If pt unable to swallow capsule, may empty contents into glass of water; pt should swallow immediately. Not for use in preg (barrier contraceptives advised)/breastfeeding. Pt should drink 10–12 glasses of

fluid each day, take safety precautions for CNS effects, protect from exposure to infections, report unusual bleeding, s&sx of infection.

## hydrOXYzine hydrochloride (generic)

**CLASS** Antiemetic, antihistamine, anxiolytic
**PREG/CONT** C/NA

**IND & DOSE Relief of anxiety sx.** *Adult, child >6 yr:* 50–100 mg PO qid. *Child <6 yr:* 50 mg/d PO in divided doses. **Mgt of pruritus.** *Adult:* 25 mg PO tid–qid. **Sedation, antiemetic (preop/postop).** *Adult:* 50–100 mg PO. *Child:* 0.6 mg/kg PO.
**ADV EFF** Constipation, dizziness, drowsiness, dry mouth, fixed drug eruptions, hypersensitivity reactions, **prolonged QT,** sedation, tremors, urine retention
**INTERACTIONS** Alcohol, barbiturates, CNS depressants, opioids, QT-prolonging drugs
**NC/PT** Not for use in breastfeeding. Pt should use safety precautions for CNS effects; use sugarless lozenges for dry mouth; avoid alcohol; report rash, difficulty breathing.

## ibalizumab-uiyk (Trogarzo)

**CLASS** Anti-CD4 monoclonal antibody, antiretroviral
**PREG/CONT** Unkn/NA

**IND & DOSE Tx of pts w/HIV-1 infection who have been heavily treated and have multidrug-resistant HIV-1 infection and are failing their current antiretroviral regimen.** *Adult:* 2,000 mg IV loading dose, followed by 800 mg IV q 2 wk.
**ADV EFF** Diarrhea, dizziness, **immune reconstitution inflammatory syndrome,** nausea, rash
**INTERACTIONS** Belimumab; may enhance toxic effects
**NC/PT** Give initial infusion over at least 30 min; observe pt for 1 hr after completion. If no adverse reactions, may give subsequent infusions over 15 min and reduce observation to 15 min. Advise pt about antiretroviral preg registry (monitors fetal outcomes). Pt should not breastfeed, report s&sx of infection.

## ibandronate sodium (Boniva)

**CLASS** Bisphosphonate, calcium regulator
**PREG/CONT** C/NA

**IND & DOSE Tx/px of osteoporosis in postmenopausal women.** *Adult:* 150-mg tablet PO once/mo, or 3 mg IV over 15–30 sec q 3 mo.
**ADJUST DOSE** Renal impairment
**ADV EFF** Abd/back pain, **anaphylaxis,** atypical femur fractures, bronchitis, diarrhea, dizziness, dyspepsia, headache, HTN, hypocalcemia, **jaw osteonecrosis,** myalgia, pneumonia, **renal toxicity**
**INTERACTIONS** Aluminum, iron, magnesium antacids; food, milk
**NC/PT** Monitor serum calcium. Ensure adequate intake of vitamin D/calcium. Use caution in preg; not for use in breastfeeding. Obtain periodic bone density exams. Safety for use longer than 3–5 yr not established. Pt should take in a.m. w/full glass of water at least 60 min before first beverage, food, or medication of day; stay upright for 60 min after taking to avoid potentially serious esophageal erosion; mark calendar for once/mo or q-3-mo tx; report difficulty breathing/swallowing, pain/burning in esophagus.

**DANGEROUS DRUG**

## ibritumomab (Zevalin)

**CLASS** Antineoplastic, monoclonal antibody
**PREG/CONT** D/NA

**BBW** Risk of serious to fatal infusion reactions, prolonged bone marrow

suppression, cutaneous/mucocutaneous reactions; monitor, support pt accordingly. Max, 32 mCi total dose.
**IND & DOSE Tx of relapsed/refractory low-grade follicular transformed B-cell non-Hodgkin lymphoma; previously treated follicular non-Hodgkin lymphoma w/ relapse after first-line tx.** *Adult:* 250 mg/m$^2$ IV rituximab, then 5 mCi/kg as 10-min IV push. Repeat in 7–9 d.
**ADV EFF** Abd pain, asthenia, cough, fatigue, fever, **infusion reactions, leukemia**, nasopharyngitis, n/v/d, **prolonged bone marrow suppression, severe cutaneous/mucocutaneous reactions**
**INTERACTIONS** Live vaccines, platelet inhibitors
**NC/PT** Premedicate w/acetaminophen, diphenhydramine before each infusion. Monitor for extravasation; move to other limb if this occurs. Not for use in preg (barrier contraceptives advised)/breastfeeding. Pt should avoid exposure to infection; report bleeding, fever or s&sx of infection, rash, mouth sores.

## ibrutinib (Imbruvica)
**CLASS** Antineoplastic, kinase inhibitor
**PREG/CONT** High risk/NA

**IND & DOSE Tx of mantle cell lymphoma, marginal zone lymphoma when at least one other tx has been tried.** *Adult:* 560 mg PO once daily. **Tx of chronic lymphocytic leukemia (CLL); tx of CLL w/17p depletion; tx of Waldenström macroglobulinemia; chronic GVHD after failure of one or more lines of systemic therapy.** *Adult:* 420 mg PO once a day.
**ADJUST DOSE** Mild/moderate hepatic impairment (contraindicated w/severe impairment)
**ADV EFF** Abd pain, atrial fibrillation, anemia, **bone marrow suppression**, bruising, constipation, diarrhea, dyspnea, edema, fatigue, fever, **hemorrhage**, HTN, infections, musculoskeletal pain/spasms, n/v/d, rash, renal toxicity, **secondary malignancies**, TLS, URI
**INTERACTIONS** CYP3A inducers/inhibitors
**NC/PT** Ensure proper dx. Monitor renal function; check CBC monthly; screen for secondary malignancies. Not for use in preg (contraceptives advised)/breastfeeding. Pt must swallow capsule whole (not cut/crush/chew it) w/full glass of water. Pt should avoid exposure to infection; report urine/stool color changes, severe diarrhea, fever, bleeding, sx of infection.

## ibuprofen (Advil, Caldolor, Motrin)
**CLASS** Analgesic, NSAID
**PREG/CONT** Unkn (1st, 2nd trimesters); high risk (3rd trimester)/NA

**BBW** Increased risk of CV events, GI bleeding (especially in elderly pts, hx of GI ulcer or bleeds); monitor accordingly. Contraindicated for tx of periop pain after CABG.
**IND & DOSE Tx of mild to moderate pain, fever, migraine headache, primary dysmenorrhea.** *Adult, child ≥12 yr:* 400 mg PO q 4–6 hr; max, 3,200/d. Or, 400–800 mg IV over 30 min q 6 hr for pain. Or, 400 mg IV over 30 min for fever; may follow w/400 mg IV q 4–6 hr or 100–200 mg IV q 4 hr to control fever. *Child 6 mo–11 yr:* Base dose on weight, given q 6–8 hr. 32–42 kg, 300 mg PO; 27–31 kg, 250 mg PO; 22–26 kg, 200 mg PO; 16–21 kg, 150 mg PO; 11–15 kg, 100 mg PO; 8–10 kg, 75 mg PO; 5–7 kg, 50 mg PO. Oral drops: 9–11 kg or 12–23 mo, 1.875 mL (75 mg) PO; 5–8 kg or 6–11 mo, 1.25 mL (50 mg). Or 10 mg/kg IV over 10 min up to max dose of 400 mg q 4–6 hr as needed. **Tx of osteoarthritis, RA.** *Adult:* 1,200–3,200 mg/d PO (300 mg qid or 400, 600, 800 mg tid

or qid; individualize dose). **Tx of juvenile arthritis.** *Child 6 mo–11 yr:* 30–50 mg/kg/d PO in three–four divided doses; 20 mg/kg/d for milder disease.
**ADV EFF** **Agranulocytosis, anaphylactoid reactions to anaphylactic shock, bronchospasm,** dizziness, dyspepsia, edema, eye changes, headache, **GI bleeding,** GI pain, **HF,** hepatic impairment, insomnia, nausea, pancytopenia, rash, renal injury, **SJS,** somnolence, stomatitis, **thrombotic events**
**INTERACTIONS** ACE inhibitors, anticoagulants, beta blockers, bisphosphonates, bumetanide, ethacrynic acid, furosemide, ginkgo, lithium
**NC/PT** Ensure hydration w/IV use. Avoid use in 3rd trimester. Stop if eye changes, renal or hepatic impairment. Give w/food if GI upset. Pt should avoid OTC products that may contain ibuprofen; take safety precautions for CNS effects; report ankle swelling, black tarry stool, vision changes.

DANGEROUS DRUG

## ibutilide fumarate
(Corvert)
**CLASS** Antiarrhythmic
**PREG/CONT** C/NA

**BBW** Have emergency equipment on hand during and for at least 4 hr after administration; can cause potentially life-threatening arrhythmias. Use caution when selecting pts for tx.
**IND & DOSE** **Rapid conversion of atrial fibrillation (AF)/flutter of recent onset to sinus rhythm.** *Adult:* ≥60 kg, 1 vial (1 mg) IV over 10 min; may repeat after 10 min if arrhythmia not terminated; <60 kg, 0.1 mL/kg (0.01 mg/kg) IV over 10 min; may repeat after 10 min if arrhythmia not terminated.
**ADV EFF** Dizziness, headache, nausea, numbness/tingling in arms, **ventricular arrhythmias**
**INTERACTIONS** Amiodarone, antihistamines, digoxin, disopyramide, quinidine, phenothiazines, procainamide, sotalol, TCAs
**NC/PT** Determine time of arrhythmia onset; most effective if <90 d. Ensure pt anticoagulated for at least 2 wk if AF lasts >2 d. Have emergency equipment on hand. Provide follow-up for medical evaluation. Pt should report chest pain, difficulty breathing.

## icatibant (Firazyr)
**CLASS** Bradykinin receptor antagonist
**PREG/CONT** C/NA

**IND & DOSE** **Tx of acute attacks of hereditary angioedema.** *Adult:* 30 mg subcut in abdomen; may repeat after at least 6 hr. Max, 3 injections/d.
**ADV EFF** Dizziness, drowsiness, fever, injection-site reaction, rash
**INTERACTIONS** ACE inhibitors
**NC/PT** Teach proper administration/disposal of needles/syringes. Rotate injection sites in abdomen; do not inject into scars, inflamed/infected areas. Use caution in preg/breastfeeding. Pt should take safety precautions for CNS effects, go to emergency department after injecting if laryngeal attack occurs.

## icosapent ethyl (Vascepa)
**CLASS** Antithypertriglyceridemic, ethyl ester
**PREG/CONT** C/NA

**IND & DOSE** **Adjunct to diet to reduce triglycerides in adult w/severe (≥500 mg/dL) hypertriglyceridemia; adjunct to max tolerated statin tx to reduce risk of MI, stroke, coronary revascularization, unstable angina in adult w/elevated triglycerides (≥150 mg/dL) if CV disease or diabetes mellitus type 2/other risk factors for CV disease.** *Adult:* 2 g PO bid w/food.
**ADV EFF** Arthralgia, atrial fibrillation/flutter, bleeding, **hepatic impairment,** hypersensitivity reaction

**INTERACTIONS** Anticoagulants, platelet inhibitors
**NC/PT** Monitor LFTs carefully; use caution w/known fish/shellfish allergy. Pt should swallow capsule whole and not cut/crush/chew it; continue diet/exercise program.

**DANGEROUS DRUG**

## IDArubicin hydrochloride (Idamycin PFS)

**CLASS** Antineoplastic antibiotic
**PREG/CONT** High risk/NA

**BBW** Do not give IM/subcut because of severe local reaction, tissue necrosis; give slowly IV only. Risk of myocardial toxicity; monitor accordingly. Monitor response to tx frequently at start of tx. Monitor serum uric acid, CBC, cardiac output (listen for S3), LFTs. Changes in uric acid level may need dose decrease; consult physician.
**IND & DOSE** **Tx of AML w/other drugs.** *Adult:* 12 mg/m²/d for 3 d by slow IV injection (10–15 min) w/ cytarabine. May give cytarabine as 100 mg/m²/d by continuous IV infusion for 7 d or as 25-mg/m² IV bolus, then 200 mg/m²/d IV for 5 d by continuous infusion. May give second course when toxicity has subsided, if needed, at 25% dose reduction.
**ADJUST DOSE** Hepatic/renal impairment
**ADV EFF** Alopecia, **anaphylaxis,** anorexia, **cancer, cardiac toxicity,** headache, **HF,** injection-site reactions, **myelosuppression, mucositis,** n/v
**NC/PT** Monitor injection site for extravasation. Monitor CBC, LFTs, renal function, cardiac output frequently during tx. Ensure adequate hydration. Not for use in preg (barrier contraceptives advised)/breastfeeding. Pt should cover head at temp extremes (hair loss possible); get regular medical follow-up; report swelling, chest pain, difficulty breathing.

## idaruCIZUmab (Praxbind)

**CLASS** Monoclonal antibody, reversal agent
**PREG/CONT** Unkn/NA

**IND & DOSE** **To reverse anticoagulant effects of dabigatran in life-threatening or uncontrolled bleeding, need for emergency surgery/procedures.** *Adult:* 5 g IV as two consecutive infusions of 2.5 g/50 mL; consecutive bolus injections of 2.5 g each could be used.
**ADJUST DOSE** Conduction defects
**ADV EFF** Constipation, delirium, fever, headache, hypokalemia, hypersensitivity reactions, pneumonia, **thromboembolism**
**NC/PT** Risk of serious reaction w/hereditary fructose intolerance; monitor pt. Do not mix in sol w/other drugs; use aseptic handling when preparing infusion. Ensure consecutive infusions/injections. Risk of thromboembolism when pt off anticoagulant; restart anticoagulant when pt stable. Can restart dabigatran within 24 hr; other anticoagulants are not affected. Pt should report difficulty breathing, chest/leg pain, abnormal bleeding.

## idelalisib (Zydelig)

**CLASS** Antineoplastic, kinase inhibitor
**PREG/CONT** High risk/NA

**BBW** Risk of severe to fatal hepatotoxicity; serious to fatal diarrhea, colitis; serious to fatal pneumonitis; serious to fatal infections; GI perforation.
**IND & DOSE** **Tx of relapsed chronic lymphocytic leukemia w/rituximab, relapsed follicular B-cell non-Hodgkin lymphoma after at least two other tx, relapsed small lymphocytic lymphoma after at least two other tx.** *Adult:* 150 mg PO bid.
**ADV EFF** Abd pain, **anaphylaxis,** chills, **colitis,** cough, fatigue, **GI**

**perforation, hepatotoxicity,** hyperglycemia, neutropenia, **pneumonitis, severe cutaneous reactions**
**INTERACTIONS** CYP3A inducers/substrates
**NC/PT** Ensure dx. Monitor hepatic/respiratory function, CBC. Watch for diarrhea, s&sx of intestinal perforation. Not for use in preg (contraceptives advised)/breastfeeding. Frequent blood tests will be needed. Pt should take twice a day, report difficulty breathing, rash/skin sores, diarrhea w/blood or mucus, severe abd pain, urine/stool color changes, s&sx of infection.

## idursulfase (Elaprase)

**CLASS** Enzyme
**PREG/CONT** C/NA

**BBW** Risk of severe to life-threatening anaphylactic reactions during infusion; have emergency equipment on hand. Monitor closely.
**IND & DOSE Tx of Hunter syndrome.** *Adult, child >5 yr:* 0.5 mg/kg IV infused over 1–3 hr q wk.
**ADV EFF Anaphylaxis,** fever, HTN, rash, respiratory impairment
**NC/PT** Start first infusion slowly to monitor for infusion reaction (8 mL/min for first 15 min, then increase by 8 mL/min at 15-min intervals; max, 100 mL/hr). Do not infuse w/other products in same line. Use caution in preg/breastfeeding. Pt should report difficulty breathing, rash.

**DANGEROUS DRUG**

## ifosfamide (Ifex)

**CLASS** Alkylating agent, antineoplastic, nitrogen mustard
**PREG/CONT** D/NA

**BBW** Myelosuppression can be severe and lead to fatal infections. Arrange for blood tests to evaluate hematopoietic function before starting tx and wkly during tx; serious hemorrhagic toxicities have occurred. Provide extensive hydration consisting of at least 2 L oral or IV fluid/d to prevent bladder toxicity. Arrange to give protector such as mesna to prevent hemorrhagic cystitis, which can be severe. CNS toxicity can be severe to fatal. Nephrotoxicity can be severe and result in renal failure.
**IND & DOSE Third-line chemo of germ-cell testicular cancer w/other drugs.** *Adult:* 1.2 g/m²/d IV over at least 30 min for 5 consecutive d; repeat q 3 wk, or after recovery from hematologic toxicity. For px of bladder toxicity, give >2 L fluid/d IV or PO. Use mesna IV to prevent hemorrhagic cystitis.
**ADJUST DOSE** Elderly pts, renal impairment
**ADV EFF** Alopecia, **anaphylaxis,** anorexia, **cardiotoxicity,** confusion, hallucinations, immunosuppression, leukopenia, **neurotoxicity,** n/v, **potentially fatal hemorrhagic cystitis, pulmonary toxicity, secondary malignancies,** somnolence
**INTERACTIONS** CYP3A4 inducers/inhibitors, grapefruit juice
**NC/PT** For px of bladder toxicity, give >2 L fluid/d IV or PO. Use mesna IV to prevent hemorrhagic cystitis. Maintain hydration (at least 10–12 glasses fluid/d). Can cause fetal harm; contraceptives advised (for men/women) during and for few wks after tx. Not for use in breastfeeding. Pt should avoid grapefruit juice; cover head at temp extremes (hair loss possible); report painful urination, blood in urine, chest pain, difficulty breathing.

## iloperidone (Fanapt)

**CLASS** Atypical antipsychotic
**PREG/CONT** High risk/NA

**BBW** Increased risk of death if used in elderly pts w/dementia-related psychosis. Do not use for these pts; not approved for this use.
**IND & DOSE Tx of schizophrenia.** *Adult:* Range, 12–24 mg/d PO; titrate

based on orthostatic hypotension tolerance. Initially, 1 mg PO bid; then 2, 4, 6, 8, 10, 12 mg PO bid on days 2, 3, 4, 5, 6, 7, respectively, to reach 12–24 mg/d goal.
**ADJUST DOSE** Hepatic impairment, poor CYP2D6 metabolizers
**ADV EFF** Bone marrow suppression, cognitive/motor impairment, dizziness, fatigue, hyperglycemia, nausea, **NMS**, orthostatic hypotension, priapism, **prolonged QT, seizures,** suicidality, weight gain
**INTERACTIONS** Alcohol, antihypertensives, CNS depressants, fluoxetine, itraconazole, ketoconazole, other QT-prolonging drugs, paroxetine, St. John's wort
**NC/PT** Obtain baseline ECG; periodically monitor QT interval. Titrate over first wk to decrease orthostatic hypotension. Monitor serum glucose. Avoid use in preg; not for use in breastfeeding. Pt should take safety measures for CNS effects; avoid alcohol/St. John's wort; change positions carefully; report fever, thoughts of suicide, fainting.

## iloprost (Ventavis)

**CLASS** Vasodilator
**PREG/CONT** Low risk/NA

**IND & DOSE** **Tx of pulmonary artery HTN in pts w/NY Heart Association Class II–IV sx.** *Adult:* 2.5–5 mcg inhaled 6–9 ×/d while awake; max, 45 mcg/d.
**ADV EFF** Back pain, **bronchospasm,** cough, dizziness, headache, **hypotension,** insomnia, lightheadedness, muscle cramps, n/v, palpitations, **pulmonary hypotension,** syncope
**INTERACTIONS** Anticoagulants, antihypertensives, vasodilators
**NC/PT** Review proper use of inhaler. Use caution in preg; not for use in breastfeeding. Pt should take safety measures for CNS effects, report difficulty breathing, fainting.

DANGEROUS DRUG

## imatinib mesylate

(Gleevec)
**CLASS** Antineoplastic, protein tyrosine kinase inhibitor
**PREG/CONT** High risk/NA

**IND & DOSE** **Tx of chronic phase CML.** *Adult:* 400 mg/d PO as once-a-day dose; may consider 600 mg/d. *Child >2 yr:* 260 mg/m²/d PO as one dose, or divided a.m. and p.m. **Tx of accelerated phase or blast crisis CML.** *Adult:* 600 mg/d PO as single dose; may consider 400 mg PO bid. **Tx of newly diagnosed CML.** *Child >2 yr:* 340 mg/m² PO; max, 600 mg/d. **Tx of ALL.** *Adult:* 600 mg/d PO. **Tx of aggressive systemic mastocytosis (ASM), hypereosinophilic syndrome/chronic eosinophilic leukemia, myelodysplastic/myeloproliferative diseases, metastatic malignant GI stromal tumors; adjunct tx after surgical resection of Kit-positive GI stromal tumors.** *Adult:* 400 mg/d PO. **Tx of ASM w/eosinophilia.** *Adult:* 100 mg/d PO. **Tx of unresectable, recurrent, or metastatic dermatofibrosarcoma protuberans.** *Adult:* 800 mg/d PO.
**ADJUST DOSE** Hepatic/renal impairment
**ADV EFF** **Bone marrow suppression,** fluid retention, GI perforations, headache, hemorrhage, hepatic impairment, **left ventricular dysfx,** n/v/d, **rash to SJS,** renal toxicity, **severe HF,** TLS
**INTERACTIONS** Azithromycin, carbamazepine, clarithromycin, cyclosporine, dexamethasone, grapefruit juice, itraconazole, ketoconazole, levothyroxine, pimozide, phenobarbital, phenytoin, rifampin, simvastatin, St. John's wort, warfarin
**NC/PT** Monitor CBC. Not for use in preg (barrier contraceptives advised)/breastfeeding (avoid during and for 1 mo after tx). Monitor child for growth retardation. Give w/meals. May disperse in glass of water or

apple juice; give immediately using 50 mL for 10-mg tablet, 200 mL for 400-mg tablet. Pt should not cut or crush tablet, should take analgesics for headache, avoid grapefruit juice/ St. John's wort, report sudden fluid retention, unusual bleeding, rash, severe abd pain.

## imipramine hydrochloride, imipramine pamoate

(Tofranil)

**CLASS** Antidepressant, TCA

**PREG/CONT** C/NA

**BBW** Limit drug access for depressed, potentially suicidal pts. Increased risk of suicidality, especially in children, adolescents, young adults; monitor accordingly.

**IND & DOSE Tx of depression.** *Adult:* Hospitalized pts, 100–150 mg/d PO in divided doses; may increase to 200 mg/d. After 2 wk, may increase to 250–300 mg/d. Outpts, 75 mg/d PO, increasing to 150 mg/d. Max, 200 mg/d; range, 50–150 mg/d. *Adolescent:* 30–40 mg/d PO. **Tx of childhood enuresis.** *Child ≥6 yr:* 25 mg/d PO 1 hr before bedtime. May increase to 75 mg PO nightly in child >12 yr, 50 mg PO nightly in child <12 yr. Max, 2.5 mg/kg/d.

**ADJUST DOSE** Elderly pts

**ADV EFF** Anticholinergic effects, arrhythmias, **bone marrow depression**, confusion, constipation, disturbed concentration, dry mouth, **MI**, nervousness, orthostatic hypotension, photosensitivity, sedation, **stroke**, urine retention, withdrawal sx after prolonged use

**INTERACTIONS** Anticholinergics, clonidine, MAOIs, oral anticoagulants, St. John's wort, sympathomimetics

**NC/PT** Screen for bipolar disorder, angle-closure glaucoma. Give major portion at bedtime. Consider dose change w/adverse effects. Not for use in preg/breastfeeding. Pt should avoid sun exposure; take safety measures for CNS effects; report thoughts of suicide, excessive sedation.

## incobotulinumtoxinA

(Xeomin)

**CLASS** Neurotoxin

**PREG/CONT** Moderate risk/NA

**BBW** Drug not for tx of muscle spasticity; toxin may spread from injection area and cause s&sx of botulism (CNS alterations, trouble speaking and swallowing, loss of bladder control). Use only for approved indications.

**IND & DOSE Improvement of glabellar lines.** *Adult:* Total of 20 units (0.5 mL sol) injected as divided doses of 0.1 mL into each of five sites—two in each corrugator muscle, one in procerus muscle. Repetition usually needed q 3–4 mo to maintain effect. **Cervical dystonia.** *Adult:* 120 units/tx IM as four separate injections. **Blepharospasm in previously treated pts.** *Adult:* 25 units per eye. **Upper limb spasticity.** *Adult:* Up to 400 units/tx IM as several separate injections; repeat no sooner than q 12 wk. **Tx of chronic sialorrhea.** *Adult:* Total of 100 units injected, divided as 30 units per parotid gland and 20 units per submandibular gland no sooner than q 16 wk.

**ADV EFF Anaphylactic reactions,** dizziness, headache, local reactions, **MI, spread of toxin that can lead to death**

**INTERACTIONS** Aminoglycosides, anticholinesterases, lincosamides, magnesium sulfate, NMJ blockers, polymyxin, quinidine, succinylcholine

**NC/PT** Store in refrigerator. Have epinephrine available in case of anaphylactic reactions. Effects may not appear for 1–2 d; will persist for 3–4 mo. Not for use in preg. Pt should report difficulty breathing, chest pain.

## indacaterol (Arcapta Neohaler)

**CLASS** Bronchodilator, long-acting beta agonist
**PREG/CONT** C/NA

**IND & DOSE Long-term maint bronchodilator tx for pts w/COPD:** *Adult:* 75 mcg/d inhaled w/*Arcapta Neohaler.*
**ADV EFF Arrhythmias, asthma-related deaths, bronchospasm,** cough, headache, **HTN,** nausea, nasopharyngitis, pharyngeal pain, **seizures**
**INTERACTIONS** Adrenergic drugs, beta blockers, corticosteroids, diuretics, MAOIs, QT-prolonging drugs, TCAs, xanthines
**NC/PT** Not for asthma or acute or deteriorating situations. Do not exceed recommended dose. Should be used w/inhaled corticosteroid. Review proper use of inhaler. Pt should report worsening of condition, chest pain, severe difficulty breathing.

## indapamide (generic)

**CLASS** Thiazide-like diuretic
**PREG/CONT** B/NA

**IND & DOSE Tx of edema associated w/HF.** *Adult:* 2.5–5 mg/d PO. **Tx of HTN.** *Adult:* 1.25–2.5 mg/d PO. Consider adding another drug if control not achieved.
**ADV EFF Agranulocytosis,** anorexia, **aplastic anemia,** dizziness, dry mouth, hypotension, n/v, photosensitivity, vertigo
**INTERACTIONS** Antidiabetics, cholestyramine, colestipol, lithium, thiazide diuretics
**NC/PT** Give w/food if GI upset occurs. Give early in a.m. Pt should weigh self daily and record, report weight change of 3 lb/d, take safety precautions for CNS effects, use sugarless lozenges for dry mouth, avoid sun exposure.

## indinavir sulfate (Crixivan)

**CLASS** Antiviral, protease inhibitor
**PREG/CONT** C/NA

**IND & DOSE Tx of HIV infection w/ other drugs.** *Adult, child ≥12 yr:* 800 mg PO q 8 hr. W/delavirdine, 600 mg PO q 8 hr; w/delavirdine, 400 mg PO tid; w/didanosine, give more than 1 hr apart on empty stomach; w/itraconazole, 600 mg PO q 8 hr; w/itraconazole, 200 mg PO bid; w/ketoconazole, 600 mg PO q 8 hr; w/ rifabutin, 1,000 mg PO q 8 hr (reduce rifabutin by 50%).
**ADJUST DOSE** Hepatic impairment
**ADV EFF** Dry skin, flulike sx, headache, hyperbilirubinemia, n/v/d, nephrolithiasis/urolithiasis
**INTERACTIONS** Ergots, midazolam, pimozide, triazolam; do not use w/preceding drugs. Antidiabetic agents, atazanavir, azole antifungals, benzodiazepines, carbamazepine, delavirdine, efavirenz, fentanyl, grapefruit juice, interleukins, nelfinavir, nevirapine, phenobarbital, phenytoin, rifabutin, rifampin, rifamycin, ritonavir, sildenafil, St. John's wort, venlafaxine
**NC/PT** Protect capsules from moisture; store in container provided and keep desiccant in bottle. Give drug q 8 hr around clock. Maintain hydration. Check all drugs pt taking; many interactions possible. Not a cure for disease; advise pt to use precautions to prevent spread. Not for use in breastfeeding. Pt should avoid grapefruit juice/St. John's wort; continue other HIV drugs; drink at least 1.5 L of water/d; report severe diarrhea, flank pain.

**indomethacin, indomethacin sodium trihydrate** (Indocin, Tivorbex)
**CLASS** NSAID
**PREG/CONT** Unkn (1st, 2nd trimesters); high risk (3rd trimester)/NA

**BBW** Increased risk of CV events, GI bleeding; monitor accordingly. Adverse reactions dose-related; use lowest effective dose. Not for use for periop pain w/CABG surgery.
**IND & DOSE** **Relief of s&sx of osteoarthritis, RA, ankylosing spondylitis.** *Adult:* 25 mg PO bid or tid; may use total daily dose of 150–200 mg/d PO. **Tx of acute painful shoulder.** *Adult:* 75–150 mg/d PO in three or four divided doses for 7–14 d. **Tx of acute gouty arthritis.** *Adult:* 50 mg PO tid until pain tolerable; then decrease until not needed (within 3–5 d). Do not use SR form. **Closure of hemodynamically significant patent ductus arteriosus in preterm infants 500–1,750 g.** *Infant:* Three IV doses at 12- to 24-hr intervals. *2–7 d old:* 0.2 mg/kg IV for all three doses. *Under 48 hr old:* 0.2 mg/kg IV, then 0.1 mg/kg, then 0.1 mg/kg. **Tx of mild to moderate acute pain.** *Adult:* 20 mg PO tid or 40 mg PO two–three ×/d (*Tivorbex*).
**ADV EFF** **Anaphylactoid reactions to anaphylactic shock**, **aplastic anemia, apnea w/IV use, bleeding ulcer, bone marrow suppression**, depression, dizziness, drowsiness, edema, eye changes, headache, hepatic impairment, HF, HTN, insomnia, **MI**, n/v, **pulmonary hemorrhage w/IV use**, rash, thrombotic events
**INTERACTIONS** ACE inhibitors, adrenergic blockers, anticoagulants, ARBs, bisphosphonates, lithium, loop diuretics, platelet inhibitors, potassium-sparing diuretics
**NC/PT** Do not use SR form for gouty arthritic. Give w/food. Monitor eyes w/long-term therapy. Monitor LFTs, renal function. Pt should avoid OTC drugs w/o first checking w/prescriber. Pt should take safety precautions for CNS effects; report black/tarry stools, bleeding, difficulty breathing, chest pain.

**inFLIXimab** (Remicade), **inFLIXimab-abda** (Renflexis), **inFLIXimab-axxq** (Avsola), **inFLIXimab-dyyb** (Inflectra), **inFLIXimab-qbtx** (Ixifi)
**CLASS** Monoclonal antibody, TNF blocker
**PREG/CONT** Low risk/NA

**BBW** Risk of serious to life-threatening infections, activation of TB, malignancies, including fatal hepatosplenic T-cell lymphoma, especially in young males w/Crohn disease or ulcerative colitis. Monitor pt; reserve for approved uses.
**IND & DOSE** **Tx of Crohn disease, ulcerative colitis, ankylosing spondylitis, psoriatic arthritis, plaque psoriasis.** *Adult, child:* 5 mg/kg IV at 0, 2, 6 wk; maint, 5 mg/kg IV q 8 wk (q 6 wk for ankylosing spondylitis). **Tx of RA.** *Adult:* 3 mg/kg IV at 0, 2, 6 wk; maint, 3 mg/kg IV q 8 wk w/methotrexate.
**ADV EFF** Abd pain, **bone marrow suppression, cancer, demyelinating diseases, HBV reactivation**, headache, **hepatotoxicity, HF**, infusion reactions, **serious to fatal infections**
**INTERACTIONS** TNF blockers, tocilizumab, methotrexate, immunosuppressants, live vaccines
**NC/PT** Obtain TB test before starting tx. Administer IV over not less than 2 hr. Monitor CBC before each dose; adjustment may be needed. Monitor LFTs. Assess for s&sx of infection. Pt should get routine cancer screening; mark calendar for tx days; report edema, chest pain, fever, s&sx of infection, numbness/tingling.

DANGEROUS DRUG

## inotersen (Tegsedi)

**CLASS** Antisense oligonucleotide
**PREG/CONT** High risk/NA

**BBW** Reduced platelet count may result in sudden, unpredictable thrombocytopenia, which can be life-threatening; monitor platelet count before and q 8 wk during tx. Can cause glomerulonephritis that may require immunosuppressants; may result in dialysis-dependent renal failure. Available only through Tegsedi REMS Program.
**IND & DOSE** **Tx of polyneuropathy of hereditary transthyretin-mediated amyloidosis.** *Adult:* 284 mg subcut wkly.
**ADV EFF** **Cervicocephalic arterial dissection,** fatigue, fever, headache, **hepatic impairment, hypersensitivity reactions,** injection-site reactions, nausea, **ocular changes due to vitamin A deficiency, stroke,** thrombocytopenia
**NC/PT** Pt must enroll in Tegsedi REMS Program, comply w/ongoing monitoring requirements. Monitor platelet level, renal/hepatic function. Pt should immediately report prolonged bleeding, neck stiffness, atypical severe headache, stroke s&sx, ocular changes.

DANGEROUS DRUG

## inotuzumab ozogamicin (Besponsa)

**CLASS** Antineoplastic, CD22-directed antibody drug conjugate
**PREG/CONT** High risk/NA

**BBW** Risk of hepatotoxicity, hepatic veno-occlusive disease, post-hematopoietic stem cell transplant non-relapse mortality.
**IND & DOSE** **Tx of relapsed/refractory B-cell precursor ALL.** *Adult:* Cycle 1: 0.8 mg/m² IV on day 1, 0.5 mg/m² on days 8 and 15 of a 21-day cycle. For pt achieving a complete remission: 0.5 mg/m² IV on days 1, 8, and 15 of a 28-day cycle; w/out complete remission: repeat Cycle 1 dosing as a 28-day cycle.
**ADV EFF** Abd pain, **bone marrow suppression**, infusion reaction, **liver toxicity, QT prolongation**
**INTERACTIONS** QT-prolonging drugs
**NC/PT** Ensure proper use of drug. Monitor LFTs throughout tx; obtain baseline and periodic ECG to monitor QT interval. Premedicate w/corticosteroid, antipyretic, antihistamine before each infusion. Pt should avoid preg (contraceptives advised)/breastfeeding; mark calendar for infusion dates; report fever, difficulty breathing, urine/stool color changes, bleeding, extreme fatigue.

## insoluble Prussian blue (Radiogardase)

**CLASS** Ferric hexacyanoferrate
**PREG/CONT** C/NA

**IND & DOSE** **Tx of pts w/known or suspected internal contamination w/radioactive cesium and/or radioactive or nonradioactive thallium.** *Adult:* 3 g PO tid. *Child 2–12 yr:* 1 g PO tid.
**ADV EFF** Constipation
**NC/PT** Monitor radioactivity levels. Take appropriate precautions to avoid exposure. Begin as soon as possible after exposure. Treat for constipation if indicated. Stool, oral mucus, teeth may turn blue. Excreted in urine/feces; pt should flush toilet several times, clean up spilled urine/feces.

**DANGEROUS DRUG**

**insulin** (Novolin-R), **insulin inhaled** (Afrezza), **insulin lispro** (Admelog, Humalog), **insulin aspart** (Fiasp, Novolog), **insulin degludec** (Tresiba), **insulin detemir** (Levemir), **insulin glargine** (Basaglar, Lantus, Toujeo), **insulin glulisine** (Apidra), **insulin human** (Myxredlin), **isophane insulin** (Novolin N)
**CLASS** Hormone
**PREG/CONT** Low risk/NA

**BBW** Risk of acute bronchospasm w/inhaled insulin. Not for use w/ asthma or COPD. Baseline spirometry in all pts before use.
**IND & DOSE Tx of type 1 diabetes, severe ketoacidosis, diabetic coma; short-course tx when glucose control needed.** *Adult, child:* 0.5–1 unit/kg/d subcut. Base adjustment on serum glucose, pt response. Can give regular and glulisine IV. For inhaled insulin: 1 inhalation at start of each meal. **Tx of type 2 diabetes when glucose control cannot be maintained.** *Adult:* 10 mg/d subcut; range, 2–100 units/d (*Lantus, Tresiba*) or 0.1–0.2 units/kg subcut or 10 units/d or bid subcut (*Levemir*). See *Insulin pharmacokinetics.*
**ADV EFF Acute bronchospasm** (inhaled), **anaphylaxis, angioedema,** HF, hypoglycemia, injection-site reactions, ketoacidosis, **lung cancer** (inhaled), **pulmonary function decline** (inhaled), rash, renal impairment
**INTERACTIONS** Alcohol, atypical antipsychotics, beta blockers, celery, coriander, corticosteroids, dandelion root, diuretics, fenugreek, garlic, ginseng, juniper berries, MAOIs, salicylates, thiazolidinediones (inhaled)
**NC/PT** Spirometry evaluation before use of inhaled insulin. Double-check doses for child. Note *Lantus* and *Toujeo* are not interchangeable. Use caution when mixing two types of insulin; always draw regular insulin into syringe first. Change insulin reservoir at least q 6 d if using pump. If mixing w/lispro, draw lispro first. Use mixtures of regular and NPH or regular and lente within 5–15 min of combining. Do not mix *Lantus, Toujeo* (glargine), *Levemir* (detemir) in sol w/other drugs, including other insulins. Usage based on onset, peak, duration; varies among insulins. Do not freeze; protect from heat. Adjust dosage based on pt

**INSULIN PHARMACOKINETICS**

| Type | Onset | Peak | Duration |
|---|---|---|---|
| Regular | 30–60 min | 2–3 hr | 6–12 hr |
| NPH | 1–1.5 hr | 4–12 hr | 24 hr |
| Inhaled | <15 min | 50 min | 2–3 hr |
| Lispro | <15 min | 30–90 min | 2–5 hr |
| Aspart | 10–20 min | 1–3 hr | 3–5 hr |
| Degludec | 1 hr | 9 hr | 25 hr |
| Detemir | Slow | 3–6 hr | 6–23 hr |
| Glargine (Lantus, Basaglar) | 60 min | None | 24 hr |
| Glargine (Toujeo) | 1 hr | 12–16 hr | 24–36 hr |
| Glulisine | 2–5 min | 30–90 min | 1–2 hr |
| Combo insulins | 30–60 min, then 1–2 hr | 2–4 hr, then 6–12 hr | 6–8 hr, then 18–24 hr |

response. Monitor, rotate injections sites. Ensure total diabetic teaching, including diet/exercise, hygiene measures, recognition of hypo-, hyperglycemia. Teach proper use of inhaler, proper injection, disposal of needles/syringes and to never reuse or share pens/needles. Pt should avoid alcohol; if using herbs, check w/prescriber for insulin dose adjustment; wear medical ID; always eat when using insulin; report uncontrolled serum glucose.

**DANGEROUS DRUG**

## interferon alfa-2b

(Intron-A)
**CLASS** Antineoplastic
**PREG/CONT** High risk/NA

**BBW** Risk of serious to life-threatening reactions. Monitor for severe reactions (including hypersensitivity reactions), neuropsychiatric, autoimmune, ischemic, infectious disorders. Notify physician immediately if these occur; dose reduction/discontinuation may be needed.
**IND & DOSE** **Tx of hairy cell leukemia.** *Adult:* 2 million international units/m² subcut or IM three ×/wk for up to 6 mo. **Tx of condylomata acuminata.** *Adult:* 1 million international units/lesion intralesionally three ×/wk for 3 wk; can treat up to five lesions at one time. May repeat in 12–16 wk. **Tx of chronic HCV.** *Adult:* 3 million international units subcut or IM three ×/wk for 18–24 mo. **Tx of AIDS-related Kaposi sarcoma.** *Adult:* 30 million international units/m² subcut or IM three ×/wk. **Tx of chronic HBV.** *Adult:* 30–35 million international units/wk subcut or IM either as 5 million international units daily or 10 million international units three ×/wk for 16 wk. *Child:* 3 million international units/m² subcut three ×/wk for first wk, then 6 million international units/m² subcut three ×/wk for total of 16–24 wk (max, 10 million international units three ×/wk). **Tx of follicular lymphoma.** *Adult:* 5 million international units subcut three ×/wk for 18 mo w/other chemo. **Tx of malignant melanoma.** *Adult:* 20 million international units/m² IV over 20 min on 5 consecutive d/wk for 4 wk; maint, 10 million international units/m² IV three ×/wk for 48 wk.
**ADV EFF** Anorexia, **bone marrow suppression,** confusion, dizziness, flulike sx, n/v, pericarditis, rash
**NC/PT** Obtain baseline, periodic CBC, LFTs. Do not give IV. Pt should mark calendar of tx days, get blood tests regularly, take safety precautions for CNS effects, report bleeding, s&sx of infection.

## interferon beta-1a

(Avonex, Rebif)
**CLASS** Immunomodulator, MS drug
**PREG/CONT** C/NA

**IND & DOSE** **Tx of relapsing forms of MS.** *Adult:* 30 mcg IM once/wk (*Avonex*). Or, 22–44 mcg subcut three ×/wk (*Rebif*); start w/8.8 mcg three ×/wk; titrate up over 5 wk to full dose of 22–44 mcg.
**ADV EFF** **Anaphylaxis,** anorexia, **bone marrow suppression,** confusion, depression, dizziness, flulike sx, hepatotoxicity, nausea, photosensitivity, **seizures,** suicidality
**NC/PT** Obtain baseline, periodic CBC, LFTs. Rotate injection sites. Teach proper administration/disposal of needles/syringes. Maintain hydration. Pt should mark calendar of tx days; avoid exposure to infections, sun; report infection, unusual bleeding, thoughts of suicide, difficulty breathing.

## interferon beta-1b

(Betaseron, Extavia)
**CLASS** Immunomodulator, MS drug
**PREG/CONT** Low risk/NA

**IND & DOSE** **Tx of relapsing forms of MS.** *Adult:* 0.25 mg subcut q other day (target); discontinue if disease unremitting for >6 mo. Initially,

0.0625 mg subcut q other day, wks 1–2; then 0.125 mg subcut q other day, wks 3–4; then 0.1875 mg subcut q other day, wks 5–6; target 0.25 mg subcut q other day by wk 7.
**ADV EFF** **Anaphylaxis,** anorexia, **bone marrow suppression,** confusion, depression, dizziness, drug-induced SLE, flulike sx, hepatotoxicity, nausea, photosensitivity
**NC/PT** Obtain baseline, periodic CBC, LFTs. Rotate injection sites. Not for use in preg (barrier contraceptives advised)/breastfeeding. Maintain hydration. Teach proper administration/disposal of needles/syringes. Pt should mark calendar of tx day; avoid exposure to infection, sun; report infection, unusual bleeding, thoughts of suicide, difficulty breathing.

## interferon gamma-1b
(Actimmune)
**CLASS** Immunomodulator
**PREG/CONT** High risk/NA

**IND & DOSE** **To reduce frequency/severity of serious infections associated w/chronic granulomatous disease; to delay time to disease progression in pts w/severe, malignant osteopetrosis.** *Adult:* 50 mcg/m² (1 million international units/m²) subcut three ×/wk in pts w/body surface area (BSA) >0.5 m²; 1.5 mcg/kg/dose in pts w/BSA of 0.5 m² or less subcut three ×/wk. For severe reactions, withhold or reduce dose by 50%.
**ADV EFF** Anorexia, confusion, depression, dizziness, flulike sx, nausea, suicidality
**NC/PT** Obtain baseline, periodic CBC, LFTs. Store in refrigerator. Give at night if flulike sx a problem. Rotate injection sites. Teach proper administration/disposal of needles/syringes. Not for use in preg (barrier contraceptives advised)/breastfeeding. Maintain hydration. Pt should mark calendar of tx day; avoid exposure to infection, sun; report infection, unusual bleeding, thoughts of suicide.

## iodine thyroid products
(Iosat, Lugol's Solution, Pima, SSKI, Strong Iodine Solution, ThyroSafe, ThyroShield)
**CLASS** Thyroid suppressant
**PREG/CONT** D/NA

**IND & DOSE** **Tx of hyperthyroidism in preparation for surgery; thyrotoxic crisis.** *Adult, child >1 yr:* RDA, 150 mcg/d PO. Tx, 0.3 mL PO tid (*Strong Iodine Solution, Lugol's Solution*); range, 0.1–0.9 mL/d PO. **Thyroid blocking in radiation emergency.** *Adult, child >12 yr, ≥68 kg:* 130 mg PO q 24 hr (*Iosat, ThyroSafe, ThyroShield*). *Child 3–18 yr, <68 kg:* 65 mg/d PO. *Child 1 mo–3 yr:* 32.5 mg/d PO. *Child birth–1 mo:* 16.25 mg/d PO.
**ADV EFF** Iodism, rash, swelling of salivary glands
**INTERACTIONS** Lithium
**NC/PT** Dilute strong iodine sol w/fruit juice/water to improve taste. Crush tablets for small child. Discontinue if iodine toxicity.

## ipilimumab (Yervoy)
**CLASS** Cytotoxic T-cell antigen 4–blocking antibody
**PREG/CONT** High risk/NA

**BBW** Severe to fatal immune-mediated reactions involving many organs possible; may occur during tx or wks to mos after tx ends. Permanently stop drug, treat w/high-dose systemic corticosteroids if s&sx of immune reactions appear.
**IND & DOSE** **Tx of unresectable or metastatic melanoma.** *Adult:* 3 mg/kg IV over 90 min q 3 wk; total, four doses. **Tx of pts w/cutaneous melanoma w/regional lymph node involvement who have undergone complete resection.** *Adult:* 10 mg/kg IV over 90 min q 3 wk for four doses, then 10 mg/kg q 12 wk for up to 3 yr or progression, given w/nivolumab. **Tx of pts w/intermediate or poor risk, previously untreated advanced renal**

**cell carcinoma, w/nivolumab.** *Adults:* 1 mg/kg IV over 30 min after and on same d as nivolumab 3 mg/kg q 3 wks for four doses initially; then frequency varies. **Tx of microsatellite instability-high or mismatch repair deficient metastatic colorectal cancer that has progressed despite tx w/ nivolumab.** *Adult, child ≥12 yr:* 1 mg/kg IV after nivolumab 3 mg/kg q 3 wks for four doses.
**ADV EFF** Colitis, diarrhea, encephalitis, **endocrinopathies,** fatigue, **hepatitis, infusion reactions, nephritis,** pneumonitis, pruritus, rash, renal dysfx
**NC/PT** Establish baseline LFTs, thyroid/endocrine/GI/renal function, skin condition; assess regularly for changes. Not for use in preg/breastfeeding (stop during and for 3 mo after tx). Pt should mark calendar for tx days; report severe diarrhea, urine/stool color changes, increased thirst, unusual fatigue.

## ipratropium bromide (Atrovent HFA)

**CLASS** Anticholinergic, bronchodilator
**PREG/CONT** B/NA

**IND & DOSE Maint tx of bronchospasm associated w/COPD** (sol, aerosol), **chronic bronchitis, emphysema.** *Adult, child ≥12 yr:* 500 mcg tid–qid via nebulizer, w/doses 6–8 hr apart. **Sx relief of rhinorrhea associated w/common cold.** *Adult, child ≥12 yr:* 2 sprays 0.06%/nostril tid–qid. *Child 5–11 yr:* 2 sprays 0.06%/nostril tid. **Sx relief of rhinitis.** *Adult, child ≥6 yr:* 2 sprays 0.03%/nostril bid–tid. **Relief of rhinorrhea in seasonal allergic rhinitis.** *Adult, child >5 yr:* 2 sprays 0.06%/nostril qid for 3 wk.
**ADV EFF** Cough, dizziness, dry mouth, headache, nervousness, nausea, urine retention
**NC/PT** Do not use w/peanut, soy allergies. Protect sol from light. May mix in nebulizer w/albuterol for up to 1 hr. Review proper use of nebulizer. Ensure hydration. Pt should empty bladder before using; take safety precautions for CNS effects; report vision changes, rash.

## irbesartan (Avapro)

**CLASS** Antihypertensive, ARB
**PREG/CONT** D/NA

**BBW** Rule out preg before beginning tx. Suggest barrier contraceptives during tx; fetal injury, deaths have occurred.
**IND & DOSE Tx of HTN.** *Adult, child 13–16 yr:* 150 mg/d PO; max, 300 mg/d. *Child 6–12 y:* 75 mg/d PO; max, 150 mg/d. **To slow progression of nephropathy in pts w/HTN, type 2 diabetes.** *Adult:* 300 mg/d PO.
**ADJUST DOSE** Volume or salt depletion
**ADV EFF** Abd pain, **angioedema,** cough, dizziness, fatigue, headache, n/v/d, URI
**INTERACTIONS** ACE inhibitors, ARBs, CYP2C9-metabolized drugs, renin blockers
**NC/PT** Use caution w/surgery; volume expansion may be needed. Monitor closely when decreased BP secondary to fluid volume loss possible. May give w/meals. Not for use in preg (barrier contraceptives advised)/ breastfeeding. Pt should take safety precautions for CNS effects; report fever, chills, edema.

## irinotecan hydrochloride (Camptosar, Onivyde)

**CLASS** Antineoplastic, DNA topoisomerase inhibitor
**PREG/CONT** High risk/NA

**BBW** Obtain CBC before each infusion. Do not give when baseline neutrophil count <1,500/mm$^2$. Severe bone marrow depression possible; consult physician for dose reduction or withholding if bone marrow depression evident. Monitor for diarrhea; assess hydration. Arrange to

reduce dose if 4–6 stools/d; omit dose if 7–9 stools/d. If ≥10 stools/d, consult physician. May prevent or ameliorate early diarrhea w/atropine 0.25–1 mg IV or subcut. Treat late diarrhea lasting >24 hr w/loperamide; late diarrhea can be severe to life-threatening.
**IND & DOSE First-line tx w/5-FU and leucovorin for pts w/metastatic colon, rectal carcinomas.** *Adult:* 125 mg/m² IV over 90 min days 1, 8, 15, 22 w/leucovorin 20 mg/m² IV bolus days 1, 8, 15, 22 and 5-FU 500 mg/m² IV days 1, 8, 15, 22. Restart cycle on day 43. Or, 180 mg/m² IV over 90 min days 1, 15, 29 w/leucovorin 200 mg/m² IV over 2 hr days 1, 2, 15, 16, 29, 30 and 5-FU 400 mg/m² as IV bolus days 1, 2, 15, 16, 29, 30 followed by 5-FU 600 mg/m² IV infusion over 22 hr on days 1, 2, 15, 16, 29, 30. Restart cycle on day 43. **Tx of pts w/metastatic colon/rectal cancer whose disease has recurred or progressed after 5-FU therapy.** *Adult:* 125 mg/m² IV over 90 min once wkly for 4 wk, then 2-wk rest; repeat 6-wk regimen, or 350 mg/m² IV over 90 min once q 3 wk. **W/5-FU and leucovorin for tx of pts w/metastatic adenocarcinoma of pancreas after gemcitabine therapy.** 70 mg/m² IV over 90 min q 2 wk (*Onivyde*); 50 mg/m² IV q 2 wk (*Onivyde*) for pts homozygous w/ UGT1A1*28.
**ADV EFF** Alopecia, anorexia, **bone marrow suppression,** dizziness, dyspnea, fatigue, hypersensitivity reactions, interstitial pneumonitis, mucositis, n/v/d
**INTERACTIONS** CYP3A4 inducers/inhibitors, diuretics, ketoconazole, other antineoplastics, St. John's wort
**NC/PT** Check drug regimen; many interactions possible. Monitor CBC; dose adjustment based on bone marrow response. Premedicate w/ corticosteroid and antiemetic 30 min before IV *Onivyde.* Monitor IV site for extravasation. Not for use in preg (barrier contraceptives advised). Pt should mark calendar for tx days, cover head at temp extremes (hair loss possible), avoid exposure to infections, report pain at injection site, s&sx of infection, severe/bloody diarrhea.

## iron dextran (INFeD)
**CLASS** Iron preparation
**PREG/CONT** C/NA

**BBW** Monitor for hypersensitivity reactions; test dose highly recommended. Have epinephrine on hand for severe hypersensitivity reaction.
**IND & DOSE Tx of iron deficiency anemia only when PO route not possible.** *Adult, child:* 0.5 mL IM or IV test dose before tx; base dose on hematologic response w/frequent Hgb determinations. >25 kg: Dose (mL) = [0.0442 (desired Hgb – observed Hgb) × LBW] + (0.26 × LBW), where Hgb = Hgb in g/dL and LBW = lean body weight, IV or IM. Child >4 mo, 5–15 kg: Dose (mL) = 0.0442 (desired Hgb – observed Hgb) × W + (0.26 × W), where W = actual weight in kg, IV or IM. Iron replacement for blood loss. Adult, child: Replacement iron (in mg) = blood loss (in mL) × Hct.
**ADV EFF Anaphylaxis,** arthritic reactivation, **cardiac arrest,** discoloration/pain at injection site, local phlebitis, lymphadenopathy, n/v
**INTERACTIONS** Chloramphenicol
**NC/PT** Ensure actual iron deficiency. Perform test dose at least 5 min before tx. Inject IM only into upper outer quadrant of buttocks using Z-track technique. Monitor serum ferritin. Pt should avoid oral iron or vitamins w/ iron added, report pain at injection site, difficulty breathing.

## iron sucrose (Venofer)
**CLASS** Iron preparation
**PREG/CONT** B/NA

**IND & DOSE Tx of iron deficiency anemia in chronic kidney disease.** *Adult:* On dialysis, 100 mg IV injection over 2–5 min or 100 mg diluted IV infusion over at least 15 min. Not on dialysis, 200 mg IV injection over

2–5 min. Peritoneal dialysis, 300 mg over 1.5 hr on two occasions 14 d apart, then single infusion of 400 mg over 2.5 hr. *Child ≥2 yr:* 0.5 mg/kg slow IV injection or infusion.
**ADV EFF** **Anaphylaxis,** arthralgia, chest pain, dizziness, headache, **hypotension,** injection-site reactions, **iron overload,** muscle cramps, n/v/d
**NC/PT** Ensure actual iron deficiency. Pt should avoid oral iron or vitamins w/iron added, take safety precautions for CNS effects, report pain at injection site, difficulty breathing.

## isavuconazonium
(Cresemba)
**CLASS** Antifungal, azole
**PREG/CONT** High risk/NA

**IND & DOSE** **Tx of invasive aspergillosis, invasive mucormycosis.** *Adult:* Loading dose, 372 mg PO or IV q 8 hr for six doses; maintenance, 372 mg/d PO or IV starting 12–24 hr after last loading dose.
**ADV EFF** Back pain, constipation, cough, dyspnea, edema, **hepatotoxicity,** hypokalemia, **infusion reactions, serious hypersensitivity reactions**
**INTERACTIONS** CYP3A4 inhibitors/inducers (contraindicated), digoxin, immune suppressants
**NC/PT** Culture before tx. Review drug regimen; many interactions possible. Loading dose for 48 hours; then maintenance. Monitor LFTs. Administer IV through online filter. Monitor for infusion reactions; stop drug if these occur. Not for use in preg/breastfeeding. Pt should mark calendar for dose changes; report difficulty breathing, rash, urine/stool color changes.

## isocarboxazid (Marplan)
**CLASS** MAOI
**PREG/CONT** C/NA

**BBW** Increased risk of suicidality in children, adolescents, young adults; monitor accordingly.
**IND & DOSE** **Tx of depression (not a first choice).** *Adult:* Up to 40 mg/d PO.
**ADJUST DOSE** Hepatic, severe renal impairment
**ADV EFF** Constipation, **CV events,** drowsiness, dry mouth
**INTERACTIONS** Anesthetics, antihypertensives, buspirone, caffeine, CNS depressants, dextromethorphan, meperidine, SSRIs, sympathomimetics, TCAs, tyramine-containing foods
**NC/PT** Do not use w/known cerebrovascular disorders, pheochromocytoma. Check complete drug list before giving; many interactions. Pt should avoid foods high in tyramine, use sugarless lozenges for dry mouth, report thoughts of suicide, chest pain.

## isoniazid (generic)
**CLASS** Antituberculotic
**PREG/CONT** C/NA

**BBW** Risk of serious to fatal hepatitis; monitor liver enzymes monthly.
**IND & DOSE** **Tx of active TB.** *Adult:* 5 mg/kg/d (max, 300 mg) PO or IM in single dose w/other effective drugs. Or, 15 mg/kg (max, 900 mg) PO two or three ×/wk. *Child:* 10–15 mg/kg/d (max, 300 mg) PO or IM in single dose w/other effective drugs. Or, 20–40 mg/kg (max, 900 mg/d) two or three ×/wk. **Px for TB.** *Adult:* 300 mg/d PO in single dose. *Child:* 10 mg/kg/d (max, 300 mg) PO in single dose.
**ADV EFF** Epigastric distress, fever, gynecomastia, **hepatitis,** injection-site reactions, peripheral neuropathy, **thrombocytopenia**
**INTERACTIONS** Acetaminophen, alcohol, carbamazepine, enflurane, phenytoin, rifampin, tyramine-containing foods
**NC/PT** Concomitant administration of 10–50 mg/d pyridoxine recommended for pts who are malnourished or predisposed to neuropathy (alcoholics, diabetics). Pt should take on empty stomach; avoid alcohol, foods high in tyramine; get

regular medical checkups; take safety precautions to avoid injury (loss of sensation possible).

**DANGEROUS DRUG**

## isoproterenol hydrochloride (Isuprel)

**CLASS** Antiasthmatic, beta agonist, bronchodilator, vasopressor
**PREG/CONT** C/NA

**IND & DOSE** **Mgt of bronchospasm during anesthesia.** *Adult:* 0.01–0.02 mg (0.5–1 mL diluted sol) by IV bolus; repeat when needed. *Child 7–19 yr:* 0.05–0.17 mcg/kg/min by IV bolus. Max, 1.3–2.7 mcg/kg/min. **Vasopressor as adjunct tx of shock.** *Adult:* 0.5–5 mcg/min; infuse IV at adjusted rate based on hr, CVP, systemic BP, urine flow. **Tx of cardiac standstill, arrhythmias.** *Adult:* 0.02–0.06 mg IV injection using diluted sol. Or, 5 mcg/min IV infusion using diluted sol.
**ADJUST DOSE** Elderly pts
**ADV EFF** Anxiety, apprehension, bronchospasm, cardiac arrhythmias, cough, dyspnea, fear, pallor, palpitations, **pulmonary edema,** respiratory difficulties, sweating
**INTERACTIONS** Antiarrhythmics, ergots, halogenated hydrocarbon anesthetics, oxytocics, TCAs
**NC/PT** Protect from light. Give smallest dose for minimum period. Have beta blocker on hand to reverse effects. Pt should report chest pain, tremor.

## isosorbide dinitrate (Dilatrate SR, Isordil), isosorbide mononitrate (Monoket)

**CLASS** Antianginal, nitrate
**PREG/CONT** C; B (Monoket)/NA

**IND & DOSE** **Tx of angina** (dinitrate). *Adult:* 2.5–5 mg SL or 5- to 20-mg oral tablets; maint, 10–40 mg PO q 6 hr or tid (oral tablets/capsules). SR or ER: Initially, 40 mg, then 40–80 mg PO q 8–12 hr. **Px of angina** (mononitrate). *Adult:* 20 mg PO bid 7 hr apart. ER tablets: 30–60 mg/d PO; may increase to 120 mg/d. **Acute px of angina** (dinitrate). *Adult:* 2.5–5 mg SL q 2–3 hr. Give 15 min before activity that may cause angina.
**ADV EFF** Apprehension, collapse, dizziness, headache, hypotension, orthostatic hypotension, rebound HTN, restlessness, tachycardia, weakness
**INTERACTIONS** Ergots
**NC/PT** Reduce dose gradually when stopping. Headache possible. Pt should place SL form under tongue or in buccal pouch, try not to swallow; take orally on empty stomach; take safety precautions for CNS effects, orthostatic hypotension; report blurred vision, severe headache, more frequent anginal attacks. Name confusion Isordil (isosorbide) and Plendil (felodipine).

## ISOtretinoin (Absorica, Amnesteem, Claravis, Myorisan, Zenatane)

**CLASS** Acne product, retinoid
**PREG/CONT** X/NA

**BBW** Ensure pt reads, signs consent form; place form in pt's permanent record. Rule out preg before tx; test for preg within 2 wk of starting tx. Advise use of two forms of contraception starting 1 mo before tx until 1 mo after tx ends. Pharmacists must register pts in iPLEDGE program before dispensing drug. Pt may obtain no more than 30-day supply.
**IND & DOSE** **Tx of severe recalcitrant nodular acne unresponsive to conventional tx.** *Adult, child ≥12 yr:* 0.5–1 mg/kg/d PO; range, 0.5–2 mg/kg/d divided into two doses for 15–20 wk. Max daily dose, 2 mg/kg. If second course needed, allow rest period of at least 8 wk between courses.

**ADV EFF** Abd pain, bronchospasm, cheilitis, conjunctivitis, dizziness, dry nose/skin, epistaxis, eye irritation, fatigue, headache, hematuria, insomnia, lethargy, lipid changes, n/v, papilledema, skin irritation, **suicidality,** visual changes
**INTERACTIONS** Corticosteroids, phenytoin, tetracycline, vitamin A
**NC/PT** Ensure pt has read, signed consent form. Rule out preg; ensure pt using contraception. Not for use in breastfeeding. Allow 8 wk between tx cycles. Only 1 mo prescription can be given. Pt may be unable to wear contact lenses. Give w/food to improve absorption. Pt should swallow capsule whole and not cut/crush/chew it; avoid donating blood; avoid vitamin supplements; take safety precautions for CNS effects; report visual changes, thoughts of suicide.

## isradipine (generic)
**CLASS** Antihypertensive, calcium channel blocker
**PREG/CONT** C/NA

**IND & DOSE Mgt of HTN.** *Adult:* 2.5 mg PO bid; max, 20 mg/d. CR, 5–10 mg/d PO.
**ADJUST DOSE** Elderly pts; hepatic/renal impairment
**ADV EFF** Dizziness, edema, headache, hypotension, nausea
**INTERACTIONS** Antifungals, atracurium, beta blockers, calcium, carbamazepine, digoxin, fentanyl, $H_2$ antagonists, pancuronium, prazosin, quinidine, rifampin, tubocurarine, vecuronium
**NC/PT** Monitor BP; other antihypertensives may be added as needed. Monitor BP, cardiac rhythm closely when determining dose. Pt should swallow CR tablet whole and not cut/crush/chew it; take safety precautions for CNS effects; treat for headache; report swelling, palpitations.

▶NEW DRUG

## istradefylline (Nourianz)
**CLASS** Adenosine receptor antagonist, antiparkinsonian
**PREG/CONT** High risk/NA

**IND & DOSE Tx of pts w/Parkinson disease experiencing "off" episodes, w/levodopa/carbidopa.** *Adult:* 20 mg PO daily w/ or w/o food; max, 40 mg daily.
**ADV EFF** Compulsive behavior, constipation, dizziness, dyskinesia, hallucinations, insomnia, nausea, psychosis
**INTERACTIONS** Strong CYP3A inducers/inhibitors
**NC/PT** Reduce dose w/hepatic impairment. For smokers (≥20 cigarettes/d, or equivalent of other tobacco product), give 40 mg/d.

## itraconazole (Onmel, Sporanox, Tolsura)
**CLASS** Antifungal
**PREG/CONT** Moderate risk/NA

**BBW** Risk of severe HF; do not give if evidence of cardiac dysfx, HF. Potential for serious CV events (including ventricular tachycardia, QT prolongation, death) w/lovastatin, simvastatin, triazolam, midazolam, pimozide, dofetilide, quinidine due to significant CYP450 inhibition; avoid these combos. Administration w/colchicine/fesoterodine/solifenacin contraindicated in pts w/varying degrees of renal/hepatic impairment (*Tolsura*).
**IND & DOSE Tx of empiric febrile neutropenia.** *Adult:* 200 mg PO bid until clinically significant neutropenia resolves. **Tx of candidiasis.** *Adult:* 200 mg/d PO (oral sol only) for 1–2 wk (oropharyngeal); 100 mg/d PO for at least 3 wk (esophageal); 200 mg/d PO in AIDS/neutropenic pts. **Tx of blastomycosis/chronic histoplasmosis.** *Adult:* 200 mg/d PO for at least 3 mo; max, 400 mg/d; *or* 130–260 mg/d PO

w/ or w/o food (*Tolsura*). **Tx of systemic mycoses.** *Adult:* 100–200 mg/d PO for 3–6 mo. **Tx of dermatophytoses.** *Adult:* 100–200 mg/d PO–bid for 7–28 d. **Tx of fingernail onychomycosis** (not *Tolsura*). *Adult:* 200 mg bid PO for 1 wk, then 3-wk rest period; repeat. **Tx of toenail onychomycosis** (not *Tolsura*). *Adult:* 200 mg/d PO for 12 wk. **Tx of aspergillosis.** *Adult:* 200–400 mg/d PO; *or* 130–260 mg/d PO w/ or w/o food (*Tolsura*).
**ADJUST DOSE** Renal impairment
**ADV EFF** Abd pain, edema, headache, **HF, hepatotoxicity,** n/v/d, rash
**INTERACTIONS** Antacids, benzodiazepines, buspirone, carbamazepine, colas, cyclosporine, digoxin, grapefruit juice, histamine$_2$ antagonists, isoniazid, lovastatin, macrolide antibiotics, nevirapine, oral hypoglycemics, phenobarbital, phenytoin, protease inhibitors, proton pump inhibitors, rifampin, warfarin anticoagulants
**NC/PT** Culture before tx. Monitor LFTs; stop if s&sx of active liver disease. Check all drugs being used; many interactions possible. Not for use in preg (contraceptives advised)/breastfeeding. Give capsules w/food. For oral sol, give 100–200 mg (10–20 mL), have pt rinse and hold, then swallow sol daily for 1–3 wk. Pt should avoid grapefruit juice, colas; report difficulty breathing, urine/stool color changes.

## ivabradine (Corlanor)
**CLASS** Cyclic nucleotide-gated channel blocker, HF drug
**PREG/CONT** High risk/NA

**IND & DOSE** **To reduce hospitalization for worsening HF; tx of stable symptomatic HF due to dilated cardiomyopathy.** *Adult, child >40 kg:* 2.5 or 5 mg PO bid w/food. Adjust based on HR; max, 7.5 mg PO bid. *Child <40 kg:* 0.05 mg/kg PO bid w/ food. Adjust based on HR; max, 0.2 mg/kg (child 6 mo to <1 yr) or 0.3 mg/kg (child ≥1 yr), up to 7.5 mg bid.
**ADJUST DOSE** Conduction defects
**ADV EFF** Atrial fibrillation, **bradycardia,** dizziness, HTN, luminous phenomena, syncope
**INTERACTIONS** CYP3A4 inducers/inhibitors, grapefruit juice, negative chronotropes, St. John's wort
**NC/PT** Do not use w/pacemaker set at 60 or higher, second-degree AV block, hypotension, severe hepatic impairment. Monitor HR, BP regularly. Not for use in preg (contraceptives advised)/breastfeeding. Pt should take bid w/meals; learn to take P; use caution in situations where light-intensity changes may occur; avoid grapefruit juice, St. John's wort; report rapid P, chest pain, difficulty breathing, dizziness.

## ivacaftor (Kalydeco)
**CLASS** Cystic fibrosis transmembrane conductance regulator potentiator
**PREG/CONT** B/NA

**IND & DOSE** **Tx of cystic fibrosis in pts ≥6 mo w/mutation in *CFTR* gene responsive to ivacaftor.** *Adult, child ≥6 yr:* 150 mg PO q 12 hr w/fat-containing food. *Child 6 mo to <6 yr and ≥14 kg:* 1 75-mg packet mixed w/1 tsp (5 mL) soft food or liquid PO q 12 hr w/fat-containing food. *Child 6 mo to <6 yr and <14 kg:* 50-mg packet mixed w/1 tsp (5 mL) soft food or liquid PO q 12 hr w/fat-containing food.
**ADJUST DOSE** Moderate to severe hepatic impairment
**ADV EFF** Abd pain, congestion, dizziness, headache, **hepatic impairment,** nasopharyngitis, n/v, rash, URI
**INTERACTIONS** Grapefruit juice, moderate to strong CYP3A inhibitors, St. John's wort
**NC/PT** Obtain FDA-cleared CF mutation test to detect *CFTR* mutation if genotype unkn. Monitor LFTs before and q 3 mo during first yr, then yearly. Give w/fat-containing food; use safety precautions if dizziness occurs. Pt

should take q 12 hr w/fat-containing food; use caution w/dizziness; avoid grapefruit juice, St. John's wort; report yellowing of eyes or skin, urine/stool color changes.

## **ivermectin** (Soolantra, Stromectol)

**CLASS** Anthelmintic, anti-inflammatory
**PREG/CONT** C/NA

**IND & DOSE Tx of intestinal strongyloidiasis** (*Stromectol*). *Adult:* 200 mcg/kg PO as single dose. **Tx of onchocerciasis** (*Stromectol*). *Adult:* 150 mcg/kg PO as single dose; may repeat in 3–12 mo. **Tx of inflammatory lesions of rosacea** (*Soolantra*). *Adult:* Apply pea-size amount to affected areas of face once daily.
**ADV EFF** Abd pain, dizziness, nausea, rash
**NC/PT** Culture before tx. Not for use in breastfeeding. Pt should take *Stromectol* on empty stomach w/water; will need repeat stool cultures; may need repeat tx.

## **ixabepilone** (Ixempra)

**CLASS** Antineoplastic, microtubular inhibitor
**PREG/CONT** D/NA

**BBW** Risk of severe liver failure, severe bone marrow suppression, neurotoxicities, cardiotoxicities; select pt carefully, monitor closely.
**IND & DOSE Tx of metastatic or locally advanced breast cancer in pts who have failed on anthracycline, taxane.** *Adult:* 40 mg/m$^2$ IV over 3 hr q 3 wk; may combine w/capecitabine.
**ADV EFF** Alopecia, anorexia, asthenia, **bone marrow suppression,** fatigue, n/v/d, **peripheral neuropathy, severe hypersensitivity reactions,** stomatitis
**INTERACTIONS** CYP3A4 inducers/inhibitors
**NC/PT** Follow CBC, LFTs closely. Premedicate w/corticosteroids. Not for use in preg (barrier contraceptives advised)/breastfeeding. Pt should mark calendar for tx days; cover head at temp extremes (hair loss possible); avoid exposure to infections; perform mouth care (for stomatitis); take safety precautions (for neuropathies); report chest pain, palpitations, difficulty breathing, numbness/tingling.

## **ixazomib** (Ninlaro)

**CLASS** Antineoplastic, proteasome inhibitor
**PREG/CONT** High risk/NA

**IND & DOSE Tx of multiple myeloma in pts who have received at least one prior therapy.** *Adult:* 4 mg/d PO on days 1, 8, 15 of a 28-day cycle given w/lenalidomide, dexamethasone.
**ADJUST DOSE** Hepatic/renal impairment
**ADV EFF** Back pain, constipation, diarrhea, edema, **hepatotoxicity,** n/v/d, peripheral neuropathy, rash, **thrombocytopenia**
**INTERACTIONS** Strong CYP3A inducers; do not combine.
**NC/PT** Ensure dx. Give w/lenalidomide, dexamethasone. Monitor liver function, platelets at least monthly. Assess for severe GI effects, peripheral neuropathy, dose adjustment may be needed. Pt should avoid preg (contraceptives advised)/breastfeeding; report easy bruising, numbness/tingling/burning, severe GI effects, urine/stool color changes.

## **ixekizumab** (Taltz)

**CLASS** Interleukin antagonist, monoclonal antibody
**PREG/CONT** Low risk/NA

**IND & DOSE Tx of moderate to severe plaque psoriasis.** *Adult:* 160 mg subcut (as two 80-mg injections) at wk 0; then 80 mg subcut wk 2, 4, 6, 8,

10, 12; then 80 mg subcut q 4 wk. **Tx of active psoriatic arthritis/ankylosing spondylitis.** *Adult:* 160 mg subcut (as two 80-mg injections) at wk 0; then 80 mg subcut q 4 wk.
**ADV EFF** **Allergic reactions,** infections, inflammatory bowel disease, injection-site reactions, tinea infections, URI
**INTERACTIONS** Live vaccines
**NC/PT** Monitor for TB before use. Exacerbation risk in pts w/Crohn disease, inflammatory bowel disease. Monitor for hypersensitivity (stop drug) and s&sx of infection (could be severe). Teach pt/caregiver proper use of auto injector; proper technique for subcut injection; rotation of injection sites; proper disposal of injector. Pt should report difficulty breathing, unusual swelling, rash, fever, s&sx of infection, difficulty giving injection.

**DANGEROUS DRUG**

## ketamine (Ketalar)
**CLASS** Nonbarbiturate anesthetic
**PREG/CONT** B/C-III

**BBW** Emergence reaction (confusion, hallucinations, delirium) possible; lessened w/smallest effective dose and use of tactile, verbal, or visual stimuli. Severe cases require small dose of short-acting barbiturate.
**IND & DOSE** **Induction of anesthesia.** *Adult:* 1–4.5 mg/kg IV slowly or 1–2 mg/kg IV at 0.5 mg/kg/min, or 6.5–13 mg/kg IM (10 mg/kg IM produces 12–25 min anesthesia). **Induction of anesthesia in cardiac surgery.** *Adult:* 0.5–1.5 mg/kg IV at 20 mg q 10 sec. **Maint of general anesthesia.** *Adult:* Repeat dose in increments of ½ to full induction dose.
**ADV EFF** Anorexia, confusion, diplopia, dreamlike state, emergence reaction, hallucinations, hypertension, nausea, pain at injection site, vomiting
**INTERACTIONS** Halothane, NMJ blockers, other sedative/hypnotics, thyroid hormones
**NC/PT** Administered by anesthesia specialist. Ensure oxygen, oximetry, cardiac monitoring; have emergency equipment nearby. Warn pt about sedative effect: Pt should avoid driving after receiving drug, tasks requiring mental alertness/coordination, making important decisions. Pt should report difficulty breathing, pain at injection site, changes in thinking.

## ketoconazole (Extina, Nizoral A-D, Xolegel)
**CLASS** Antifungal
**PREG/CONT** C/NA

**BBW** Risk of serious to fatal hepatotoxicity; monitor closely.
**IND & DOSE** **Tx of susceptible, systemic fungal infections; recalcitrant dermatophytosis.** *Adult:* 200 mg PO daily; for severe infections, 400 mg/d PO for 1 wk–6 mo. *Child >2 yr:* 3.3–6.6 mg/kg/d PO as single dose. **To reduce scaling due to dandruff.** *Adult, child:* Moisten hair, scalp thoroughly w/water; apply sufficient shampoo to produce lather; leave on for 5 min. Shampoo twice/wk for 4 wk w/at least 3 d between shampooing. **Topical tx of tinea pedis/corporis/cruris; cutaneous candidiasis.** *Adult, child >12 yr:* Apply thin film of gel, foam, cream once daily to affected area for 2 wk; do not wash area for 3 hr after applying. Wait 20 min before applying makeup, sunscreen. May need 6 wk of tx. **Tx of seborrheic dermatitis.** *Adult, child >12 yr:* Apply foam bid for 4 wk.
**ADV EFF** **Anaphylaxis,** dizziness, **hepatotoxicity,** local stinging on application, n/v, pruritus
**INTERACTIONS** Antacids, corticosteroids, cyclosporine, histamine$_2$ blockers, proton pump inhibitors, rifampin, tacrolimus, warfarin
**NC/PT** Culture before tx. Have epinephrine on hand for anaphylaxis. Monitor LFTs closely. Review proper administration. Pt may need long-term tx. Pt should use proper hygiene

to prevent infection spread; avoid drugs that alter stomach acid level (if needed, pt should take ketoconazole at least 2 hr after these drugs); take safety precautions for CNS effects; report urine/stool changes, unusual bleeding, difficulty breathing.

## ketoprofen (generic)

**CLASS** NSAID

**PREG/CONT** High risk/NA

**BBW** Increased risk of CV events, GI bleeding; monitor accordingly. Contraindicated for tx of periop pain after CABG surgery; serious adverse effects have occurred.

**IND & DOSE Relief of pain from RA, osteoarthritis.** *Adult:* 75 mg PO tid or 50 mg PO qid. Maint, 150–300 mg PO in three or four divided doses; max, 300 mg/d. ER form, 200 mg/d PO; or max, 200 mg/d ER. **Tx of mild to moderate pain, primary dysmenorrhea:** *Adult:* 25–50 mg PO q 6–8 hr as needed.

**ADJUST DOSE** Elderly pts; hepatic, renal impairment

**ADV EFF Anaphylaxis,** dizziness, dyspepsia, edema, **gastric/duodenal ulcer,** GI pain, headache, insomnia, nausea, **renal impairment**

**INTERACTIONS** Aminoglycosides, aspirin, cyclosporine, diuretics, warfarin

**NC/PT** Monitor renal function. Give w/food. Not for use in preg/breastfeeding. Pt should avoid OTC products that might contain NSAIDs; report swelling, difficulty breathing, black tarry stools.

## ketorolac tromethamine

(Acular LS, Acuvail, Sprix)

**CLASS** Antipyretic, NSAID

**PREG/CONT** Moderate risk (1st, 2nd trimesters); high risk (3rd trimester)/NA

**BBW** Increased risk of CV events, GI bleeding, renal failure; monitor accordingly. Do not use during labor/delivery or in breastfeeding; serious adverse effects in fetus/baby possible. May increase risk of bleeding; do not use w/high risk of bleeding or as px before surgery. Increased risk of severe hypersensitivity w/known hypersensitivity to aspirin, NSAIDs. Increased risk of GI bleeding; not for use in setting of CABG surgery.

**IND & DOSE Short-term pain mgt (up to 5 d).** *Adult:* 60 mg IM or 30 mg IV as single dose, or 30 mg IM or IV q 6 hr to max 120 mg/d. Or, 1 spray in one nostril q 6–8 hr; max, 63 mg/d (>65 yr); 1 spray (15.75 mg) in each nostril q 6–8 hr; max, 126 mg/d (<65 yr). *Transfer to oral:* 20 mg PO as first dose for pts who received 60 mg IM or 30 mg IV as single dose or 30-mg multiple dose, then 10 mg PO q 4–6 hr; max, 40 mg/24 hr. *Child 2–16 yr:* 1 mg/kg IM to max 30 mg, or 0.5 mg/kg IV to max 15 mg as single dose. **Relief of itching of allergic conjunctivitis.** *Adult:* 1 drop in affected eye(s) qid. **Relief of cataract postop pain, inflammation.** *Adult:* Dose varies by product; check manufacturer info.

**ADJUST DOSE** Elderly pts, renal impairment, weight <50 kg

**ADV EFF Anaphylaxis,** dizziness, dyspepsia, edema, fluid retention, **gastric/duodenal ulcer,** GI pain, headache, HF, insomnia, nausea, **renal impairment, SJS, thrombotic events**

**INTERACTIONS** Aminoglycosides, aspirin, cyclosporine, diuretics, NSAIDs, warfarin

**NC/PT** Protect vials from light. Monitor renal function. Give to maintain serum levels, control pain. Not for use in preg/breastfeeding. Do not use ophthal drops w/contact lenses. Pt should take w/food; use safety precautions for CNS effects; avoid OTC products that might contain NSAIDs; report swelling, difficulty breathing, black tarry stools, chest pain.

**DANGEROUS DRUG**

## labetalol hydrochloride
(Trandate)
**CLASS** Antihypertensive, sympathetic blocker
**PREG/CONT** C/NA

**IND & DOSE** **Tx of HTN.** *Adult:* 100 mg PO bid; maint, 200–400 mg bid PO; up to 2,400 mg/d has been used. **Tx of severe HTN.** *Adult:* 20 mg (0.25 mg/kg) IV injection slowly over 2 min; can give additional doses of 40 or 80 mg at 10-min intervals until desired BP achieved or 300-mg dose has been injected. Transfer to oral therapy as soon as possible.
**ADJUST DOSE** Elderly pts
**ADV EFF** **Bronchospasm,** constipation, cough, dizziness, dyspnea, ED, flatulence, gastric pain, **HF,** n/v/d, **stroke,** vertigo
**INTERACTIONS** Calcium channel blockers, isoflurane, nitroglycerin
**NC/PT** Taper after long-term tx. Keep pt supine during infusion. Pt should not stop taking suddenly (needs to be tapered); take w/meals; use safety precautions for CNS effects; report difficulty breathing, swelling, chest pain.

## lacosamide (Vimpat)
**CLASS** Antiepileptic
**PREG/CONT** C/NA

**IND & DOSE** **Monotherapy or adjunct tx for partial-onset seizures.** *Adult, child ≥17 yr:* 50 mg PO bid (initial for adjunct therapy), 100 mg PO bid (initial for monotherapy); 200 mg/d recommended dose for both. IV dosing is same as oral, injected over 15–60 min; for short-term use if oral not possible. *Child 4–<17 yr:* PO dose based on body weight and given bid; IV dosing contraindicated.
**ADJUST DOSE** Hepatic/renal impairment
**ADV EFF** Ataxia, prolonged PR interval, diplopia, dizziness, headache, hypersensitivity, n/v, seizure, syncope
**INTERACTIONS** Other PR-prolonging drugs
**NC/PT** Monitor for suicidal behavior/ideation. Obtain ECG before tx, after titration in pts w/underlying proarrhythmic conditions or who are on concomitant drugs affecting cardiac conduction. Taper after long-term tx. Not for use in preg (barrier contraceptives advised)/breastfeeding. Pt should not stop taking suddenly, taper to minimize seizures, take safety precautions for CNS effects, report thoughts of suicide, personality changes.

## lactulose (Cholac, Constilac, Enulose, Generlac)
**CLASS** Ammonia-reducing drug, laxative
**PREG/CONT** B/NA

**IND & DOSE** **Tx of portal-systemic encephalopathy.** 30–45 mL (20–30 g) PO tid or qid. Adjust q 1–2 d to produce two or three soft stools/d. May use 30–45 mL/hr PO if needed. Or, 300 mL (20 g) lactulose mixed w/700 mL water or physiologic saline as retention enema retained for 30–60 min; may repeat q 4–6 hr. *Child:* 2.5–10 mL/d PO in divided dose for small child or 40–90 mL/d for older child suggested. Goal: Two or three soft stools daily. **Laxative.** *Adult:* 15–30 mL/d (10–20 g) PO; up to 60 mL/d has been used.
**ADV EFF** Belching, distention, intestinal cramping, transient flatulence
**NC/PT** Give laxative syrup orally w/fruit juice, water, milk to increase palatability. Monitor serum ammonia levels. Monitor for electrolyte imbalance w/long-term tx. Pt should not use other laxatives, not use as laxative for longer than 1 wk unless prescribed, have ready access to bathroom facilities, report diarrhea.

## lamiVUDine (Epivir, Epivir-HBV)

**CLASS** Antiviral, reverse transcriptase inhibitor
**PREG/CONT** Low risk/NA

**BBW** Monitor hematologic indices, LFTs q 2 wk during tx; severe hepatomegaly w/steatosis, lactic acidosis possible. Counsel, periodically test pts receiving *Epivir-HBV;* severe, acute HBV exacerbations have occurred in pts w/both HIV and HBV infection who stop taking lamivudine.
**IND & DOSE** **Tx of chronic HBV.** *Adult:* 100 mg PO daily. *Child 2–17 yr:* 3 mg/kg PO daily; max, 100 mg daily. **Tx of HIV, w/other drugs.** *Adult, child ≥16 yr:* 150 mg PO bid or 300 mg/d PO as single dose, or 150 mg PO bid. *Child 3 mo–16 yr:* 4 mg/kg PO bid; max, 300 mg/d. *>30 kg:* 150 mg PO bid. *>21 kg–<30 kg:* 75 mg PO in a.m. and 150 mg PO in p.m. *14–21 kg:* 75 mg PO bid.
**ADJUST DOSE** Renal impairment
**ADV EFF** Agranulocytosis, asthenia, diarrhea, GI pain, headache, **hepatomegaly w/lactic acidosis,** nasal s&sx, nausea, **pancreatitis, steatosis**
**INTERACTIONS** Trimethoprim-sulfamethoxazole, zalcitabine
**NC/PT** Give w/other antiretrovirals for HIV. Risk of emergence of lamivudine-resistant HBV; monitor. Monitor for s&sx of pancreatitis; stop immediately if evident. Monitor for opportunistic infections. Not for use in preg/breastfeeding. Pt should use protection to prevent transmission (drug not a cure); get frequent blood tests; report severe headache, severe n/v, urine/stool color changes.

## lamoTRIgine (Lamictal)

**CLASS** Antiepileptic
**PREG/CONT** C/NA

**BBW** Risk of serious, life-threatening rash, including SJS; monitor accordingly. Stop immediately if rash appears; have appropriate life support on hand.
**IND & DOSE** **Tx of partial-onset seizures, primary generalized tonic-clonic seizures, Lennox-Gastaut syndrome.** *Adult taking enzyme-inducing antiepileptics (ie, carbamazepine, phenobarbital, phenytoin) but not valproic acid:* 50 mg PO daily for 2 wk, then 100 mg PO daily in two divided doses for 2 wk. Then may increase by 100 mg/d q wk to maint of 300–500 mg/d PO in two divided doses. ER form: wk 1–2, 50 mg/d PO; wk 3–4, 100 mg/d PO; wk 5, 200 mg/d PO; wk 6, 300 mg/d PO; wk 7, 400 mg/d PO. Range, 400–600 mg/d. *Adult, child >12 yr taking enzyme-inducing antiepileptics and valproic acid:* 25 mg PO q other day for 2 wk, then 25 mg PO daily for 2 wk. Then may increase by 25–50 mg q 1–2 wk to maint 100–400 mg/d PO in two divided doses. *Child 2–12 yr taking non-enzyme-inducing antiepileptics and valproic acid:* 0.15 mg/kg/d PO in one–two divided doses for 2 wk. Then 0.3 mg/kg/d PO in one–two divided doses, rounded down to nearest 5 mg for 2 wk. Maint, 1–5 mg/kg/d in one–two divided doses to max of 200 mg/d. *Child 2–12 yr taking single enzyme-inducing antiepileptic w/o valproic acid:* 0.6 mg/kg/d PO in two divided doses for 2 wk, then 1.2 mg/kg/d PO in two divided doses for 2 wk. Maint, 5–15 mg/kg/d in two divided doses to max 400 mg/d. **Tx of bipolar I disorder.** *Adult taking valproic acid:* 25 mg PO q other day for 2 wk, then 25 mg PO once daily for 2 wk. After 4 wk, may double dose at wkly intervals to target 100 mg/d. *Adult taking enzyme-inducing antiepileptics but not valproic acid:* 50 mg/d PO for 2 wk; then 100 mg PO daily in two divided doses for 2 wk. After 4 wk, may increase dose in 100-mg increments at wkly intervals to target maint of 400 mg/d PO in two divided doses. *Adult taking neither enzyme-inducing antiepileptics nor valproic acid:* 25 mg/d PO for

2 wk, then 50 mg PO daily for 2 wk. After 4 wk, may double dose at wkly intervals to maint of 200 mg/d.
**ADV EFF** Aseptic meningitis, ataxia, **blood dyscrasias,** dizziness, hemophagocytic lymphohistiocytosis, **hepatotoxicity, multiorgan hypersensitivity reactions,** nausea, **rash, SJS, toxic epidermal necrosis w/multiorgan failure, suicidality**
**INTERACTIONS** Carbamazepine, phenobarbital, phenytoin, primidone, valproic acid
**NC/PT** Monitor LFTs, renal function closely. Monitor for aseptic meningitis. Monitor for rash; stop if rash evident. Taper slowly over 2 wk when stopping. Ensure pt. Not for use in preg. Pt should swallow ER tablet whole and not cut/crush/chew it; wear medical ID; take safety precautions for CNS effects; report rash, urine/stool color changes. Name confusion between Lamictal (lamotrigine) and Lamisil (terbinafine).

**▶NEW DRUG**

## lanadelumab-flyo
(Takhzyro)
**CLASS** Monoclonal antibody, prophylaxis
**PREG/CONT** Unkn/NA

**IND & DOSE Px of hereditary angioedema attacks.** *Adult, child ≥12 yr:* 300 mg subcut q 2 or 4 wk.
**ADV EFF** Diarrhea, dizziness, headache, **hypersensitivity,** injection-site reactions, myalgia, respiratory infections
**NC/PT** Store in refrigerator; remove 15 min before injection. Pt/caregiver may give injection after learning proper technique.

## lanreotide acetate
(Somatuline Depot)
**CLASS** Growth hormone (GH) inhibitor
**PREG/CONT** C/NA

**IND & DOSE Long-term tx of acromegaly in pts unresponsive to other tx.** *Adult:* 90 mg deep subcut q 4 wk for 3 mo; then adjust based on growth hormone (GH) and/or insulin-like growth factor (IGF)-1 levels. **Tx of unresectable, differentiated, advanced gastroenteropancreatic neuroendocrine tumors.** *Adult:* 120 mg deep subcut q 4 wk. **Tx of pts w/carcinoid syndrome to reduce frequency of short-acting somatostatin analog rescue therapy.** *Adult:* 120 mg deep subcut q 4 wk.
**ADJUST DOSE** Hepatic/renal impairment
**ADV EFF** Abd pain, cholelithiasis, diarrhea, flatulence, hyperglycemia, hypoglycemia, injection-site reactions, sinus bradycardia, thyroid dysfx
**INTERACTIONS** Antidiabetics, beta blockers, cyclosporine, insulin
**NC/PT** Drug injected into buttocks by provider, alternating left and right; monitor for injection-site reactions. Monitor GH, IGF-1. Monitor serum glucose, thyroid function; intervene as indicated. Monitor for bradycardia. Not for use in preg/breastfeeding. Pt should mark calendar of tx days; keep frequent follow-up appointments; report upper gastric pain, injection-site reactions.

## lansoprazole (Prevacid, Prevacid 24 hr)
**CLASS** Proton pump inhibitor
**PREG/CONT** Low risk/NA

**IND & DOSE Tx of active duodenal ulcer.** *Adult:* 15 mg PO daily for 4 wk; maint, 15 mg/d PO. **Tx of gastric ulcer.** *Adult:* 30 mg/d PO for up to 8 wk. **To reduce risk of gastric ulcer w/NSAIDs.** *Adult:* 15 mg/d PO for up to 12 wk. **Tx of duodenal ulcers associated w/*Helicobacter pylori*.** *Adult:* 30 mg lansoprazole, 500 mg clarithromycin, 1 g amoxicillin, all PO bid for 10–14 d; or 30 mg lansoprazole, 1 g amoxicillin PO tid for 14 d. **GERD.** *Adult, child 12–17 yr:* 15 mg/d PO for up to 8 wk. *Child 1–11 yr:* >30 kg,

30 mg/d PO for up to 12 wk. 30 kg or less, 15 mg/d PO for up to 12 wk. **Tx of erosive esophagitis, poorly responsive GERD.** *Adult, child 12–17 yr:* 30 mg/d PO daily for up to 8 wk. Additional 8-wk course may be helpful for pts not healed after 8-wk tx. Maint, 15 mg/d PO. **Tx of pathological hypersecretory conditions.** *Adult:* 60 mg/d PO; up to 90 mg bid have been used. **Short-term tx of erosive esophagitis (all grades).** *Adult:* 30 mg/d IV over 30 min for up to 7 d; switch to oral form as soon as possible for total of 8 wk. **Tx of heartburn.** *Adult:* 1 capsule *Prevacid 24 hr* PO w/ full glass of water in a.m. before eating for 14 d; may repeat 14-day course q 4 mo.
**ADJUST DOSE** Hepatic impairment
**ADV EFF** Abd pain, bone loss, CDAD, dizziness, headache, hypocalcemia, hypomagnesemia, n/v/d, pneumonia, rash, URI
**INTERACTIONS** Ketoconazole, sucralfate, theophylline
**NC/PT** Give w/meals. May open capsule, sprinkle on applesauce, *Ensure,* yogurt, cottage cheese, strained pears. For NG tube, place 15- or 30-mg tablet in syringe, draw up 4 or 10 mL water; shake gently for quick dispersal. After dispersal, inject through NG tube into stomach within 15 min. If using capsules w/NG tube, mix granules from capsule w/40 mL apple juice, inject through tube, then flush tube w/more apple juice. For orally disintegrating tablet, place on tongue, follow w/water after it dissolves. For IV, switch to oral form as soon as feasible. Arrange for further evaluation if no symptom improvement. Not for use in breastfeeding. Pt should swallow capsule whole and not cut/crush/chew it; take safety precautions for CNS effects; report severe diarrhea.

## lanthanum carbonate
(Fosrenol)
**CLASS** Phosphate binder
**PREG/CONT** C/NA

**IND & DOSE To reduce serum phosphate level in pts w/ESRD.** *Adult:* 1,500–3,000 mg/d PO in divided doses w/meals; base dose on serum phosphate level.
**ADJUST DOSE** Hepatic impairment
**ADV EFF** Abd pain, allergic skin reactions, dyspepsia, **GI obstruction,** n/v/d, tooth injury
**INTERACTIONS** Antacids, levothyroxine, quinolone antibiotics
**NC/PT** Monitor serum phosphate (target, 6 mg/dL or lower). Pt should chew/crush tablets, not swallow whole. Consider powder form if pt cannot chew tablets (sprinkle powder over applesauce and have pt consume immediately). Give w/meals; separate from other oral drugs by 2 hr. Not for use in preg/breastfeeding. Pt should report severe abd pain, constipation.

**DANGEROUS DRUG**

## lapatinib (Tykerb)
**CLASS** Antineoplastic, kinase inhibitor
**PREG/CONT** D/NA

**BBW** Severe to fatal hepatotoxicity has occurred; monitor LFTs closely.
**IND & DOSE Tx of advanced/metastatic breast cancer w/tumors that overexpress HER2 in women who have received other tx.** *Adult:* 1,250 mg/d PO on days 1–21 w/ capecitabine 2,000 mg/m$^2$/d PO on days 1–14, given 12 hr apart. Repeat 21-day cycle. **Tx of HER2-positive metastatic breast cancer.** *Adult:* 1,500 mg/d PO w/letrozole 2.5 mg/d PO.
**ADJUST DOSE** Cardiotoxicities, concomitant CYP3A4 inducers/inhibitors, hepatic impairment

**ADV EFF Anaphylaxis, decreased left ventricular function,** diarrhea, fatigue, **hepatotoxicity, interstitial pneumonitis,** n/v, **prolonged QT, serious to fatal cutaneous reactions**
**INTERACTIONS** Antacids, carbamazepine, digoxin, grapefruit juice, ketoconazole, midazolam, paclitaxel, QT-prolonging drugs, St. John's wort
**NC/PT** Monitor LFTs before and regularly during tx. Monitor cardiac/respiratory function; evaluate lungs for pneumonitis. Not for use in preg (contraceptives advised)/breastfeeding. Pt should take 1 hr before or after meals; avoid grapefruit juice, St. John's wort, antacids; report difficulty breathing, swelling, dizziness, rash, urine/stool color changes.

## laronidase (Aldurazyme)

**CLASS** Enzyme
**PREG/CONT** Unkn/NA

**BBW** Life-threatening anaphylaxis has occurred; have medical support on hand.
**IND & DOSE Tx of pts w/Hurler, Hurler-Scheie forms of mucopolysaccharidosis 1; Scheie forms w/ moderate to severe sx.** *Adult, child ≥6 yr:* 0.58 mg/kg IV infused over 3–4 hr once/wk.
**ADV EFF Anaphylaxis,** fever, HTN, hyperreflexia, injection-site reactions, paresthesia, tachycardia, UTI
**NC/PT** Pretreat w/antipyretics, antihistamines; monitor continually during infusion. Have emergency equipment on hand. Pt should mark calendar of tx days; report injection-site pain/swelling, difficulty breathing.

## larotrectinib (Vitrakvi)

**CLASS** Antineoplastic, tropomyosin receptor kinase inhibitor
**PREG/CONT** High risk/NA

**IND & DOSE Tx of pts w/solid tumors that have a neurotrophic receptor tyrosine kinase gene fusion w/o a known acquired resistance mutation or are metastatic; when surgical resection is likely to result in severe morbidity; that have no satisfactory alternative tx or have progressed after tx.** *Adult, child w/ BSA of at least 1.0 m²:* 100 mg PO bid. *Child w/BSA <1.0 m²:* 100 mg/m² PO bid.
**ADV EFF** Constipation, diarrhea, dizziness, fatigue
**INTERACTIONS** CYP3A inducers/inhibitors/substrates
**NC/PT** Monitor LFTs; reduce dose for moderate to severe hepatic impairment. Risk of hepatotoxicity, especially if combined w/certain drugs. Drug may impair fertility. Women should use nonhormonal contraceptives/avoid breastfeeding and men should use contraceptives during and for at least 1 wk after tx. Pt should report all concomitant drugs, new/worsening neurotoxicity s&sx; avoid driving/operating hazardous machinery.

**▶NEW DRUG**

## lefamulin acetate (Xenleta)

**CLASS** Antibacterial, pleuromutilin anti-infective
**PREG/CONT** High risk/NA

**IND & DOSE Tx of community-acquired bacterial pneumonia.** *Adult:* 120 mg IV q 12 hr over 60 min for 5–7 d or 600 mg PO q 12 hr for 5 d.
**ADV EFF** *Clostridium difficile* diarrhea, headache, hepatic enzyme elevation, hypokalemia, insomnia, nausea, **prolonged QT,** vomiting
**INTERACTIONS** Strong CYP3A/P-gp inducers (reduce efficacy); strong CYP3A/P-gp inhibitors, drugs that prolong QT
**NC/PT** Reduce dose w/hepatic impairment. Pt should take tablets at least 1 hr before or 2 hr after meal; swallow whole w/6–8 oz water. Breastfeeding pt should pump and

discard milk during tx and for 2 d after final dose.

## leflunomide (Arava)

**CLASS** Antiarthritic, pyrimidine synthesis inhibitor
**PREG/CONT** High risk/NA

**BBW** Advise women of childbearing age of risks of preg; provide counseling for appropriate contraceptive use during tx. If pt decides to become preg, withdrawal program to rid body of leflunomide recommended. May use cholestyramine to rapidly decrease serum level if unplanned preg occurs. Risk of severe liver injury; monitor LFTs before, periodically during tx. Not recommended w/preexisting liver disease or liver enzymes >2 × ULN. Use caution w/other drugs that cause liver injury; start cholestyramine washout if ALT increases to 3 × ULN.
**IND & DOSE** **Tx of active RA; to relieve s&sx, improve functioning.** *Adult:* Loading dose, 100 mg/d PO for 3 d; maint, 20 mg/d PO. May reduce to 10 mg/d PO.
**ADJUST DOSE** Hepatic impairment
**ADV EFF** Alopecia, drowsiness, diarrhea, erythematous rashes, headache, **hepatotoxicity**
**INTERACTIONS** Charcoal, cholestyramine, hepatotoxic drugs, rifampin
**NC/PT** Monitor LFTs. If ALT rise between 2 and 3 × ULN, monitor closely if continued tx desired. If ALT ≥3 × ULN, cholestyramine may decrease absorption; consider stopping. Not for use in preg (barrier contraceptives advised)/breastfeeding. Pt should continue other RA tx; get regular medical follow-up; cover head at temp extremes (hair loss possible); take safety precautions for CNS effects; report urine/stool color changes.

## lenalidomide (Revlimid)

**CLASS** Antianemic, immunomodulator
**PREG/CONT** High risk/NA

**BBW** Thalidomide derivative associated w/birth defects; rule out preg before tx. Available under limited access program. Can cause significant bone marrow suppression. Increased risk of DVT, PE.
**IND & DOSE** **Tx of multiple myeloma (MM), w/dexamethasone.** *Adult:* 25 mg/d PO days 1–21 of repeated 28-day cycle. **Tx of transfusion-dependent anemia due to low- or intermediate-risk myelodysplastic syndromes.** *Adult:* 10 mg/d PO. **Tx of mantle cell lymphoma in pts who progress after two prior therapies.** *Adult:* 25 mg/d PO on days 1–21 of repeated 28-day cycle. **Tx of previously treated follicular lymphoma/ marginal zone lymphoma, w/rituximab.** *Adult:* 20 mg/d PO on d 1–21 of 28-d cycle for up to 12 cycles.
**ADJUST DOSE** Renal impairment
**ADV EFF** Anemia, back pain, **bone marrow suppression, cancer,** constipation, diarrhea, dizziness, dyspnea, edema, fatigue, fever, **hepatotoxicity, hypersensitivity,** nausea, rash, **serious to fatal cardiac events, serious to fatal skin reactions,** thrombocytopenia, TLS, URI
**INTERACTIONS** Digoxin, erythropoietin-stimulating tx, estrogens; increased mortality in pts w/MM when pembrolizumab was added to dexamethasone and thalidomide analog
**NC/PT** Monitor CBC; adjust dose as needed. Rule out preg; ensure contraceptive use. Not for use in breastfeeding. Pt should take safety precautions for CNS effects; avoid exposure to infection; get cancer screening; report s&sx of infection, unusual bleeding, muscle pain, difficulty breathing, chest pain, rash.

**lenvatinib** (Lenvima)
**CLASS** Antineoplastic, kinase inhibitor
**PREG/CONT** High risk/NA

**IND & DOSE** **Tx of locally recurrent or metastatic, progressive, radioactive iodine-refractory differentiated thyroid cancer.** *Adult:* 24 mg/d PO. **Tx of renal cell cancer w/everolimus after prior antiangiogenic therapy.** *Adult:* 18 mg/d PO w/5 mg everolimus. **Tx of unresectable hepatocellular carcinoma.** *Pts ≥60 kg:* 12 mg/d PO. *Pts <60 kg:* 8 mg/d PO. **Tx of advanced endometrial carcinoma w/ disease progression despite tx in pts who are not candidates for curative surgery or radiation, w/pembrolizumab.** *Adult:* 20 mg/d PO.
**ADJUST DOSE** Hepatic/renal impairment
**ADV EFF** Cholecystitis, **GI perforation, HF,** hemorrhage, **hepatotoxicity,** HTN, hypocalcemia, **n/v/d,** pancreatitis, proteinuria, prolonged QT, **renal impairment, RPLS,** stomatitis, thrombotic events
**NC/PT** Control BP before start of tx or withhold if HTN cannot be treated. Monitor hepatic/renal function. Watch for s&sx of intestinal perforation. Not for use in preg (contraceptives advised)/breastfeeding. Pt should take once a day; report severe abd pain, unusual bleeding, chest pain, calf pain, urine/stool color changes.

**letermovir** (Prevymis)
**CLASS** Antiviral
**PREG/CONT** Moderate risk/NA

**IND & DOSE** **Px of cytomegalovirus (CMV) infection/disease in adult CMV-seropositive recipients [R+] of an allogeneic hematopoietic stem cell transplant.** *Adult:* 480 mg PO or IV q d through 100 d post transplant. If administered w/cyclosporine, decrease to 240 mg q d.
**ADV EFF** Abd pain, cough, diarrhea, fatigue, headache, n/v, peripheral edema
**INTERACTIONS** Cyclosporine, ergot alkaloids, pimozide, pitavastatin/simvastatin if w/cyclosporine; risk of adverse reactions/reduced effectiveness
**NC/PT** Monitor serum creatinine in pt w/CrCl <50 mL/min. Not recommended for pt w/severe hepatic impairment. Pt should report all concomitant drugs; significant interactions common.

**letrozole** (Femara)
**CLASS** Antiestrogen, antineoplastic, aromatase inhibitor
**PREG/CONT** X/NA

**IND & DOSE** **Tx of advanced breast cancer in postmenopausal women progressing after antiestrogen tx; adjuvant tx of early receptor-positive breast cancer; extended adjuvant tx of breast cancer in postmenopausal women who have had 5 yr of tamoxifen; tx of postmenopausal women w/hormone receptor–positive or unkn advanced breast cancer.** *Adult:* 2.5 mg/d PO; continue until tumor progression evident.
**ADJUST DOSE** Hepatic impairment
**ADV EFF** Decreased bone density, dizziness, fatigue, GI upset, headache, hot flashes, nausea, somnolence, **thromboembolic events**
**NC/PT** Not for use in preg (contraceptives advised)/breastfeeding. Give comfort measures for adverse effects. Pt should take safety precautions for CNS effects; report, chest pain, leg pain, urine/stool color changes.

**leucovorin calcium** (generic)
**CLASS** Folic acid derivative
**PREG/CONT** C/NA

**IND & DOSE** **Leucovorin rescue, after high-dose methotrexate.** *Adult:*

Start within 24 hr of methotrexate dose; 10 mg/m² PO q 6 hr for 10 doses or until methotrexate <0.05 micromolar. If serum creatinine is 100% greater than pretreatment level 24 hr after methotrexate dose, or based on methotrexate level, increase leucovorin to 150 mg IV q 3 hr until serum methotrexate <1.0 micromolar; then 15 mg IV q 3 hr until methotrexate is <0.05 micromolar. **Tx of megaloblastic anemia NOT due to lack of vitamin $B_{12}$.** *Adult:* 1 mg/d IM; max, 1 mg/d. **Palliative tx of metastatic colon cancer.** *Adult:* 100 mg/m² by slow IV injection over 3 min, then 5-FU 370 mg/m² IV. Or, 10 mg/m² IV, then 5-FU 425 mg/m² IV. Repeat daily for 5 d; may repeat at 4-wk intervals.
**ADV EFF** Hypersensitivity reactions, pain/discomfort at injection site
**INTERACTIONS** 5-FU
**NC/PT** Give orally if possible. Monitor for hypersensitivity reactions; have emergency support on hand. Do not use intrathecally. Pt should report rash, difficulty breathing. Name confusion between *Leukeran* (chlorambucil) and leucovorin; use care.

## leuprolide acetate

(Eligard, Lupron Depot)
**CLASS** GnRH analog
**PREG/CONT** High risk/NA

**IND & DOSE** **Palliative tx of advanced prostate cancer.** *Adult:* 1 mg/d subcut, or depot 7.5 mg IM monthly (q 28–33 d), or 22.5 mg depot IM or subcut q 3 mo (84 d), or 30 mg depot IM or subcut q 4 mo, or 45 mg depot subcut q 6 mo (*Eligard*). **Tx of endometriosis.** *Adult:* 3.75 mg as single monthly IM injection, or 11.25 mg IM q 3 mo. Continue for 6 mo (*Lupron*). **Tx of uterine leiomyomata.** *Adult:* 3.75 mg as single monthly injection for 3 mo, or 11.25 mg IM once; give w/concomitant iron tx (*Lupron*). **Tx of central precocious puberty.** *Child:* 50 mcg/kg/d subcut; may increase by 10-mcg/kg/d increments. Or, 0.3 mg/kg IM depot q 4 wk. Round to nearest depot size; minimum, 7.5 mg (*Lupron*).
**ADV EFF** Anorexia, constipation, dizziness, headache, hematuria, hot flashes, hyperglycemia, injection-site reactions, **MI**, n/v, peripheral edema, **prolonged QT**, sweating, tumor flare
**NC/PT** Give only w/syringe provided. Give depot injections deep into muscle. Obtain periodic tests of testosterone, PSA. Not for use in preg (contraceptives advised)/breastfeeding. Stop if precocious puberty before 11 yr (girls), 12 yr (boys). Teach proper administration/disposal of needles/syringes. Pt should take safety precautions for CNS effects, report injection-site reaction, chest pain, hyperglycemia.

## levalbuterol hydrochloride (Xopenex), levalbuterol tartrate

(Xopenex HFA)
**CLASS** Antiasthmatic, beta agonist, bronchodilator
**PREG/CONT** Unkn/NA

**IND & DOSE** **Tx/px of bronchospasm.** *Adult, child ≥12 yr (Xopenex):* 0.63 mg tid, q 6–8 hr by nebulization; may increase up to 1.25 mg tid by nebulization. *Child 6–11 yr (Xopenex):* 0.31 mg tid by nebulization; max, 0.63 mg tid. *Adult, child ≥4 yr (Xopenex HFA):* 2 inhalations (90 mcg) repeated q 4–6 hr; some pts may respond to 1 inhalation (45 mcg) q 4 hr.
**ADV EFF** Anxiety, apprehension, BP changes, **bronchospasm**, CNS stimulation, CV events, fear, headache, hypokalemia, nausea
**INTERACTIONS** Aminophylline, beta blockers, MAOIs, sympathomimetics, theophylline
**NC/PT** Keep unopened drug in foil pouch until ready to use; protect from heat, light. Once foil pouch open, use vial within 2 wk, protected from heat, light. Once vial is removed from pouch, use immediately. If not used, protect

from light, use within 1 wk. Discard vial if sol not colorless. Teach proper use of inhaler/nebulizer. Overuse may be fatal; explain dosing regimen. Pt should take safety precautions for CNS effects; not exceed recommended dose; report chest pain, difficulty breathing, worsening of condition, more frequent need for drug.

## levETIRAcetam (Elepsia XR, Keppra, Spritam)

**CLASS** Antiepileptic
**PREG/CONT** C/NA

**IND & DOSE** **Tx of partial-onset seizures.** *Adult, child >16 yr:* 500 mg PO or IV bid; max, 3,000 mg/d. ER tablets: 1,000 mg/d PO; max, 3,000 mg/d. *Child 4–16 yr:* 10 mg/kg PO bid; may increase q 2 wk in 20-mg/kg increments to 30 mg/kg bid. Daily dose of oral sol: total dose (mL/d) = daily dose (mg/kg/d) × pt weight (kg) ÷ 100 mg/mL PO. *Child 6 mo–<4 yr:* 10 mg/kg PO bid; may increase q 2 wk in 10-mg/kg increments to 25 mg/kg PO bid. *Child 1 mo–<6 mo:* 7 mg/kg PO bid; may increase q 2 wk in 7-mg/kg increments to 21 mg/kg PO bid. **Tx of generalized tonic-clonic seizures.** *Adult, child >16 yr:* 500 mg PO bid; increase by 1,000 mg/d q 2 wk to recommended 3,000 mg/d. *Child 6–15 yr:* 10 mg/kg PO bid; increase q 2 wk by 20-mg/kg increments to recommended 60 mg/kg/d given as 30 mg/kg bid. **Tx of myoclonic seizures.** *Adult, child ≥12 yr:* 500 mg PO bid; slowly increase to recommended max, 3,000 mg/d.
**ADJUST DOSE** Renal impairment
**ADV EFF** Behavioral abnormalities, dizziness, dyspepsia, fatigue, headache, psychiatric reactions, **seizures w/withdrawal,** somnolence, **suicidality,** vertigo, vision changes
**NC/PT** Taper when stopping to minimize withdrawal seizures. Give w/food. Not for use in preg (barrier contraceptives advised)/breastfeeding. Pt should swallow ER tablet whole and not cut/crush/chew it; take safety precautions for CNS effects; wear medical ID; report severe headache, thoughts of suicide. Name confusion between *Keppra* (levetiracetam) and *Kaletra* (lopinavir/ritonavir).

## levocetirizine dihydrochloride (Xyzal)

**CLASS** Antihistamine
**PREG/CONT** Low risk/NA

**IND & DOSE** **Sx relief of seasonal, perennial allergic rhinitis in pts ≥6 mo; tx of uncomplicated skin effects in chronic idiopathic urticaria in pts ≥2 yr.** *Adult, child ≥12 yr:* 5 mg/d PO in evening. *Child 6–11 yr:* 2.5 mg/d PO in evening. *Child 6 mo–5 yr:* 1.25 mg (½ tsp oral sol) PO once daily in evening.
**ADJUST DOSE** Renal impairment
**ADV EFF** Dry mouth, fatigue, mental alertness changes, nasopharyngitis, somnolence
**INTERACTIONS** Alcohol, CNS depressants
**NC/PT** Encourage humidifiers, adequate fluid intake to help prevent severe dryness of mucous membranes; skin care for urticaria. Not for use in preg/breastfeeding. Pt should take in evening, use safety precautions for CNS effects, avoid alcohol.

## levodopa (generic); levodopa inhalation (Inbrija)

**CLASS** Antiparkinsonian
**PREG/CONT** C/NA

**IND & DOSE** **Tx of parkinsonism.** *Adult:* 1 g/d PO in two or more doses w/food; increase gradually in increments not exceeding 0.75 g/d q 3–7 d as tolerated. Max, 8 g/d. Only available in combo products. **Tx of "off" episodes in pts w/Parkinson disease treated w/carbidopa/levodopa** (*Inbrija*). *Adult:* 2 capsules as needed for "off" sx up to 5 ×/d.

**ADV EFF** Abd pain, adventitious movements, anorexia, ataxia, dizziness, drowsiness, dry mouth, n/v, numbness, **suicidality,** weakness
**INTERACTIONS** Benzodiazepines, MAOIs, phenytoin, pyridoxine, TCAs
**NC/PT** Ensure 14 d free of MAOIs before use. Give w/meals. Decreased dose needed if tx interrupted. Observe for suicidal tendencies. Limit vitamin $B_6$ intake; check multivitamin use. Pt should take safety precautions for CNS effects, use sugarless lozenges for dry mouth, report uncontrollable movements, difficulty urinating. Only available in combo products.

## levoFLOXacin (generic)
**CLASS** Fluoroquinolone antibiotic
**PREG/CONT** C/NA

**BBW** Risk of tendinitis, tendon rupture. Risk increased in pts >60 yr, w/concurrent corticosteroids use, and w/kidney, heart, lung transplant. Risk of exacerbation of myasthenia gravis w/serious muscle weakness; do not use w/hx of myasthenia gravis. Reserve use for pts w/no other tx option for uncomplicated UTI, acute bacterial sinusitis, acute bacterial bronchitis.
**IND & DOSE** **Tx of community-acquired pneumonia.** *Adults:* 500 mg/d PO or IV for 7–14 d. **Tx of sinusitis.** *Adult:* 500 mg/d PO or IV for 10–14 d, or 750 mg/d PO or IV for 5 d. **Tx of chronic bronchitis.** *Adult:* 500 mg/d PO or IV for 7 d. **Tx of skin infection.** *Adult:* 500–750 mg/d PO or IV for 7–14 d. **Tx of UTIs, pyelonephritis.** *Adults:* 250 mg daily PO or IV for 3–10 d; complicated, 750 mg/d PO or IV for 5 d. **Tx of nosocomial pneumonia.** *Adult:* 750 mg/d PO or IV for 7–14 d. **Tx of chronic prostatitis.** *Adults:* 500 mg/d PO for 28 d, or 500 mg/d by slow IV infusion over 60 min for 28 d. **Postexposure anthrax.** *Adult:* 500 mg/d PO or IV for 60 d. *Child ≥6 mo >50 kg:* 500 mg/d PO for 60 d. *Child ≥6 mo <50 kg:* 8 mg/kg q 12 hr PO for 60 d. Max, 250 mg/dose. **Tx/px of plague due to *Yersinia pestis.*** *Adult, child >50 kg:* 500 mg/d PO for 10–14 d. *Child ≥6 mo <50 kg:* 8 mg/kg PO q 12 hr for 10–14 d; max, 250 mg/dose.
**ADJUST DOSE** Renal impairment
**ADV EFF** Diarrhea, dizziness, headache, **hepatic impairment,** insomnia, muscle/joint tenderness, neuropathy, photosensitivity, **prolonged QT,** rash, renal impairment, **tendon rupture**
**INTERACTIONS** Antacids, iron salts, magnesium, NSAIDs, QT-prolonging drugs, St. John's wort, sucralfate, zinc
**NC/PT** Culture before starting tx. Ensure proper use. Ensure hydration. Stop if hypersensitivity reaction. Separate from antacids by at least 2 hr. Not for use in breastfeeding. Pt should avoid sun exposure/St. John's wort; take safety precautions for CNS effects; report muscle/tendon pain, weakness, numbness/tingling, urine/stool color changes.

## levoleucovorin (Fusilev, Khapzory)
**CLASS** Folate analog
**PREG/CONT** C/NA

**IND & DOSE** **Rescue after high-dose methotrexate; to diminish toxicity from impaired methotrexate elimination.** *Adult:* 7.5 mg IV q 6 hr for 10 doses, starting 24 hr after start of methotrexate infusion. **Palliative tx of advanced metastatic colorectal cancer, w/5-FU.** *Adult:* 100 mg/m² by IV injection over at least 3 min, then 5-FU 370 mg/m² by IV injection. Or, or 10 mg/m² by IV injection, then 5-FU 425 mg/m² by IV injection.
**ADV EFF** Hypersensitivity, n/v/d, stomatitis
**INTERACTIONS** 5-FU, phenobarbital, phenytoin, primidone, trimethoprim-sulfamethoxazole
**NC/PT** Not indicated for tx of anemia due to vitamin $B_{12}$ deficiency. Inject slowly IV, no faster than 160 mg/min because of high calcium content. Give antiemetics if needed, mouth care for

stomatitis. Pt should report pain at injection site, severe n/v/d.

## levomilnacipran (Fetzima)

**CLASS** Antidepressant, serotonin/norepinephrine reuptake inhibitor

**PREG/CONT** High risk/NA

**BBW** Increased risk of suicidality in child, adolescent, young adult; monitor closely.

**IND & DOSE Tx of major depressive disorder.** *Adult:* 20 mg/d PO for 2 d; then 40 mg/d PO. May increase in increments of 40 mg/d q 2 d as needed. Max, 120 mg/d.

**ADJUST DOSE** Severe renal impairment

**ADV EFF** Activation of mania, angle-closure glaucoma, bradycardia, constipation, discontinuation syndrome, ED, HTN, hyponatremia, n/v, palpitations, serotonin syndrome, sweating, urine retention, Takotsubo cardiomyopathy

**INTERACTIONS** Azole antifungals, buspirone, clarithromycin, diuretics, fentanyl, linezolid, lithium, methylene blue (IV), NSAIDs, St. John's wort, tramadol, tryptophan

**NC/PT** Monitor for hypomania, BP periodically, IOP in pts w/glaucoma, serotonin syndrome, discontinuation syndrome. Not for use in preg/breastfeeding. Pt should swallow capsule whole and not cut/crush/chew it. Pt should avoid St. John's wort; empty bladder before taking drug; take safety precautions for CNS effects; report thoughts of suicide, hallucinations, continued rapid HR.

DANGEROUS DRUG

## levorphanol tartrate (generic)

**CLASS** Opioid agonist analgesic

**PREG/CONT** C/C-II

**IND & DOSE Relief of moderate to severe pain.** *Adult:* 2 mg PO q 3–6 hr; range, 8–16 mg/d.

**ADJUST DOSE** Elderly pts, impaired adults

**ADV EFF Bronchospasm, cardiac arrest,** constipation, dizziness, drowsiness, **laryngospasm,** lightheadedness, n/v, **respiratory arrest, shock,** sweating

**INTERACTIONS** Alcohol, antihistamines, barbiturate anesthetics, CNS depressants

**NC/PT** Monitor closely w/first dose. Pt should take safety precautions for CNS effects, use laxative for constipation, take 4–6 hr before next feeding if breastfeeding, report difficulty breathing.

## levothyroxine sodium (Euthyrox, Levo-T, Levoxyl, Synthroid, Tirosint, Unithroid)

**CLASS** Thyroid hormone

**PREG/CONT** A/NA

**BBW** Do not use for weight loss; possible serious adverse effects w/ large doses.

**IND & DOSE Replacement tx in hypothyroidism.** *Adult:* 12.5–25 mcg PO, w/increasing increments of 25 mcg PO q 2–4 wk; maint, up to 200 mcg/d. Can substitute IV or IM injection for oral form when oral route not possible. Usual IV dose is 50% of oral dose. Start at 25 mcg/d or less in pts w/long-standing hypothyroidism, known cardiac disease. Usual replacement, 1.7 mcg/kg/d. **Tx of myxedema coma w/o severe heart disease.** *Adult:* Initially, 200–500 mcg IV. May give additional 100–300 mcg or more second day if needed. **Thyroid suppression tx.** *Adult:* 2.6 mcg/kg/d PO for 7–10 d. **TSH suppression in thyroid cancer, nodules, euthyroid goiters.** Individualize dose based on specific disease and pt; larger amounts than used for normal suppression. **Tx of congenital hypothyroidism.** *Child:* >12 yr, 2–3 mcg/kg/d PO; 6–12 yr, 4–5 mcg/kg/d PO; 1–5 yr, 5–6 mcg/kg/d PO; 6–12 mo, 6–8 mcg/kg/d PO; 3–6 mo, 8–10 mcg/kg/d PO; 0–3 mo, 10–15 mcg/kg/d PO.

**ADJUST DOSE** Elderly pts
**ADV EFF** **Cardiac arrest,** esophageal atresia, n/v/d, tremors
**INTERACTIONS** Aluminum- and magnesium-containing antacids, cholestyramine, colestipol, digoxin, iron, sucralfate, theophylline, warfarin
**NC/PT** Monitor thyroid function. Do not add IV form to other IV fluids. Replaces normal hormone; adverse effects should not occur. Pt should swallow whole w/full glass of water, wear medical ID, report chest pain, unusual sweating.

## L-glutamine (Endari)
**CLASS** Amino acid
**PREG/CONT** Unkn/NA

**IND & DOSE** **To reduce complications of sickle cell disease.** *Adult, child:* 5–15 g PO bid, based on weight.
**ADV EFF** Abd pain, back pain, constipation, cough, headache, nausea
**NC/PT** Monitor severity/frequency of sickle cell episodes. Pt should mix powder in 8 oz of cold or room temperature beverage or 4–8 oz of food (complete dissolving is not necessary; pt should not double doses); report severe constipation, sickle cell episode.

**DANGEROUS DRUG**

## lidocaine hydrochloride (Akten, Glydo, Xylocaine, Zingo)
**CLASS** Antiarrhythmic, local anesthetic
**PREG/CONT** B/NA

**IND & DOSE** **Tx of ventricular arrhythmias.** *Adult:* Use 10% sol for IM injection: 300 mg in deltoid or thigh muscle; may repeat in 60–90 min. Switch to IV or oral form as soon as possible. Or, 1–4 mg/min (20–50 mcg/kg/min) IV; decrease as soon as cardiac rhythm stabilizes. *Child:* Safety/efficacy not established. AHA recommends bolus of 0.5–1 mg/kg IV, then 30 mcg/kg/min w/caution. **Local anesthetic.** *Adult, child:* Conc, diluent should be appropriate to particular local anesthetic use: 5% sol w/glucose for spinal anesthesia, 1.5% sol w/dextrose for low spinal or saddle block anesthesia. Dose varies w/area to be anesthetized and reason for anesthesia; use lowest dose needed to achieve results. **Topical analgesia.** *Adult, child:* Up to 3 transdermal patches to area of pain for up to 12 hr within 24-hr period, or apply cream, ointment, gel, sol, oral patch, spray as directed 1–3 ×/d.
**ADJUST DOSE** Elderly, debilitated pts; HF; hepatic/renal impairment
**ADV EFF** **Anaphylactoid reactions,** back pain, **cardiac arrest,** cardiac arrhythmias, dizziness, drowsiness, fatigue, headache, hypotension, lightheadedness, **respiratory arrest, seizures,** urine retention
**INTERACTIONS** Beta blockers, cimetidine, succinylcholine
**NC/PT** Have life support equipment on hand; continually monitor pt response. Check conc carefully; varies by product. Monitor for safe, effective serum conc (antiarrhythmic: 1–5 mcg/mL); conc of ≥6 mcg/mL usually toxic. Pt should take safety precautions for CNS effects, local anesthesia; report difficulty speaking/breathing, numbness, pain at injection site.

## linaclotide (Linzess)
**CLASS** Guanylate cyclase-C agonist, IBS drug
**PREG/CONT** Unkn/NA

**BBW** Contraindicated in child up to 6 yr; avoid use in child 6–17 yr; caused deaths due to dehydration in juvenile mice.
**IND & DOSE** **Tx of IBS w/constipation.** *Adult:* 290 mcg/d PO. **Tx of chronic idiopathic constipation.** *Adult:* 145 mcg/d PO.

**ADV EFF** Abd pain, diarrhea, distention, flatulence, **severe diarrhea**
**NC/PT** Ensure constipation is main complaint; ensure no GI obstruction. Give on empty stomach at least 30 min before first meal of day. Have pt swallow capsule whole and not cut/crush/chew it. May open capsule and sprinkle contents on 1 tsp applesauce or in 1 oz boiled water in a clean cup; have pt consume immediately; pt should not chew beads. Use caution in preg/breastfeeding. Pt should take on empty stomach; store in original container protected from moisture; report severe diarrhea, severe abd pain, dehydration.

## linagliptin (Tradjenta)
**CLASS** Antidiabetic, DPP-4 inhibitor
**PREG/CONT** Unkn/NA

**IND & DOSE** **Adjunct to diet/exercise to improve glycemic control in pts w/type 2 diabetes; tx of type 2 diabetes in pts w/severe renal impairment w/insulin; add on tx to insulin, diet/exercise to achieve glycemic control in pts w/type 2 diabetes.** *Adult:* 5 mg PO once/d.
**ADV EFF** Hypoglycemia, nasopharyngitis, **pancreatitis, severe debilitating arthralgia**
**INTERACTIONS** Celery, coriander, dandelion root, fenugreek, garlic, ginger, juniper berries, potent CYP3A inhibitors
**NC/PT** Monitor blood glucose, $HbA_{1c}$ before, periodically during tx. Not for use in type 1 diabetes or ketoacidosis. Ensure pt continues diet/exercise, other drugs for diabetes control. Use caution in preg/breastfeeding. Arrange for thorough diabetic teaching program. Consider stopping drug w/ reports of severe joint pain. Monitor for s&sx of HF due to possible risk. Pt should report OTC/herbal use that could alter blood glucose, s&sx of infection, uncontrolled glucose level, joint pain.

## lincomycin hydrochloride (Lincocin)
**CLASS** Lincosamide antibiotic
**PREG/CONT** C/NA

**BBW** Risk of CDAD, pseudomembranous colitis; monitor closely.
**IND & DOSE** **Tx of serious infections caused by susceptible bacteria strains.** *Adult:* 600 mg IM q 12–24 hr, or 600 mg–1 g IV q 8–12 hr. *Child:* 10 mg/kg IM q 12–24 hr, or 10–20 mg/kg/d IV in divided doses.
**ADJUST DOSE** Renal impairment
**ADV EFF** Abd pain, **agranulocytosis, anaphylactic reactions**, anorexia, **cardiac arrest**, CDAD, contact dermatitis, esophagitis, n/v/d, pain after injection, **pseudomembranous colitis**, rash
**INTERACTIONS** Aluminum salts, kaolin, NMJ blockers
**NC/PT** Culture before tx. Do not give IM injection of >600 mg; inject deeply into muscle. Monitor LFTs, renal function. Pt should report severe, watery diarrhea.

## linezolid (Zyvox)
**CLASS** Oxazolidinone antibiotic
**PREG/CONT** C/NA

**IND & DOSE** **Tx of VREF, MRSA, pneumonia, complicated skin/skin-structure infections, including diabetic foot ulcers w/o osteomyelitis.** *Adult, child ≥12 yr:* 600 mg IV or PO q 12 hr for 10–28 d. *Child ≤11 yr:* 10 mg/kg IV or PO q 8 hr for 10–14 d. **Tx of uncomplicated skin/skin-structure infections.** *Adult, child ≥12 yr:* 400 mg PO q 12 hr for 10–14 d. *Child 5–11 yr:* 10 mg/kg PO q 12 hr for 10–14 d.
**ADV EFF** Bone marrow suppression, CDAD, diarrhea, dizziness, hypoglycemia, insomnia, nausea, peripheral/optic neuropathy, **pseudomembranous colitis**, rash, serotonin syndrome

**INTERACTIONS** Aspirin, dipyridamole, MAOIs, NSAIDs, pseudoephedrine, SSRIs, St. John's wort, sympathomimetics, tyramine-containing foods
**NC/PT** Culture before tx. Ensure no MAOIs within 2 wk. Do not mix IV solution w/other solutions. Monitor platelets, CBC wkly; BP w/long-term use. Use caution in preg/breastfeeding. Pt should complete full course; avoid foods high in tyramine; report all OTC and herbal use; report severe GI problems, bloody diarrhea. Name confusion between *Zyvox* (linezolid) and *Zovirax* (acyclovir).

**liothyronine** (Cytomel, Triostat)
**CLASS** Thyroid hormone
**PREG/CONT** A/NA

**BBW** Do not use for weight loss; serious adverse effects w/large doses possible.
**IND & DOSE Replacement tx in hypothyroidism.** *Adult:* 25 mcg PO; maint, 25–75 mcg/d. **Tx of myxedema.** 5 mcg/d PO; maint, 50–100 mcg/d. **Tx of myxedema coma, precoma.** *Adult:* 25–50 mcg IV q 4–12 hr; do not give IM or subcut. Start at 10–20 mcg IV w/heart disease. Max, 100 mcg/24 hr. **Tx of simple goiter.** *Adult:* 5 mcg/d PO; maint, 75 mcg/d. **Thyroid suppression tx.** *Adult:* 75–100 mcg/d PO for 7 d. Repeat $I^{131}$ uptake test; unaffected w/ hyperthyroidism, decreased by 50% w/euthyroidism. **Tx of congenital hypothyroidism.** *Child:* Birth, 5 mcg/d PO. Usual maint, 20 mcg/d up to 1 yr; 50 mcg/d PO for 1–3 yr, adult dose >3 yr.
**ADJUST DOSE** Elderly pts
**ADV EFF** Acute adrenal crisis, **cardiac arrest,** esophageal atresia, hyperthyroidism, n/v/d, tremors
**INTERACTIONS** Antacids containing aluminum or magnesium, cholestyramine, colestipol, digoxin, iron, sucralfate, theophylline, warfarin
**NC/PT** Monitor thyroid function; overreplacement may decrease bone mineral density. May worsen glycemic control. Treat w/glucocorticoids if adrenal insufficiency. Do not add IV form to other IV fluids. Replaces normal hormone; adverse effects should not occur. Pt should swallow whole w/full glass of water, wear medical ID, report chest pain, unusual sweating.

**DANGEROUS DRUG**

**liraglutide** (Saxenda, Victoza)
**CLASS** Antidiabetic, glucagon-like peptide receptor agonist
**PREG/CONT** High risk /NA

**BBW** Causes thyroid medullary cancer in rodents. Not for use w/personal, family hx of thyroid medullary cancer, multiple endocrine neoplasia syndrome type 2; monitor closely.
**IND & DOSE Adjunct to diet/exercise to improve glycemic control in type 2 diabetes; to reduce risk of CV events in pts w/type 2 diabetes and CV disease** (*Victoza*). *Adult, child:* Initially, 0.6 mg/d by subcut injection; may increase to 1.2 mg/d after 1 wk if needed. Max, 1.8 mg/d. **Adjunct to diet/exercise for chronic weight mgt in adults w/BMI of 30 kg/m² or greater (obese) or 27 kg/m² or greater (overweight) w/at least one weight-related comorbidity** (*Saxenda*). *Adult:* Initially, 0.6 mg/wk subcut; increase gradually to 3 mg/wk.
**ADV EFF** Dizziness, gallbladder disease, headache, hypersensitivity reactions, **hypoglycemia,** n/v/d, **pancreatitis, papillary thyroid carcinoma, renal impairment, suicidality**
**INTERACTIONS** Antidiabetic secretagogues, celery, coriander, dandelion root, drugs that would be affected by delayed GI emptying, garlic, ginseng, fenugreek, juniper berries
**NC/PT** Not for tx of type 1 diabetes, ketoacidosis; not for first line tx. Monitor blood glucose, $HbA_{1c}$ before, periodically during tx. Ensure pt

continues diet/exercise, other drugs for diabetes. Provide complete diabetic teaching program. Teach proper administration/disposal of needles/syringes; should inject once/d subcut in abdomen, thigh, or upper arm. Not for use in preg/breastfeeding. Pt should report OTC/herb use; difficulty swallowing; lump in throat; severe abd pain radiating to back; lack of glycemic control; thoughts of suicide.

**lisdexamfetamine dimesylate** (Vyvanse)
**CLASS** Amphetamine, CNS stimulant
**PREG/CONT** High risk/C-II

**BBW** High risk of abuse; could lead to drug dependence. Amphetamine misuse has caused serious CV events, sudden death. Assess risk of abuse before to use; monitor continually.
**IND & DOSE Tx of ADHD as part of integrated tx plan.** *Adult, child ≥6 yr:* 30 mg/d PO in a.m.; may increase at wkly intervals in increments of 10–20 mg/d. Max, 70 mg/d. **Tx of moderate to severe binge eating disorder.** *Adult, child ≥6 yr:* 30 mg PO q a.m.; titrate at rate of 20 mg/wk. Range, 50–70 mg/d; max, 70 mg/d.
**ADJUST DOSE** Renal impairment
**ADV EFF** Abd pain, **cardiac events,** decreased appetite, dizziness, dry mouth, fever, headache, insomnia, irritability, n/v/d, peripheral vascular disease, **psychiatric adverse reactions, sudden death,** tachycardia, weight loss
**INTERACTIONS** Chlorpromazine, haloperidol, MAOIs, meperidine, methenamine, norepinephrine, sympathomimetics, TCAs, urine acidifiers/alkalinizers
**NC/PT** Ensure proper dx. Baseline ECG before tx. Not indicated for weight loss. Part of comprehensive tx plan. Controlled substance; needs to be secured. Monitor growth in child. If pt cannot swallow whole, empty contents into glass of water, have pt drink right away. Stop periodically to validate use. Not for use in preg/breastfeeding. Pt should avoid MAOI use within 14 d; take in a.m. to prevent insomnia; store in dry place; secure drug (controlled substance); report vision changes, manic sx, marked weight loss, chest pain.

**lisinopril** (Prinivil, Qbrelis, Zestril)
**CLASS** ACE inhibitor, antihypertensive
**PREG/CONT** High risk/NA

**BBW** Contraceptives advised. If preg occurs, stop drug as soon as possible; fetal injury/death possible.
**IND & DOSE Tx of HTN.** *Adults:* 10 mg/d PO; range, 20–40 mg/d. If also taking diuretic, start at 5 mg/d; monitor BP. *Child ≥6 yr:* 0.07 mg/kg/d PO; max, 5 mg/d. **Adjunct tx of HF.** *Adults:* 5 mg/d PO w/diuretics, digitalis. Effective range, 5–20 mg/d (*Prinivil*), 5–40 mg/d (*Zestril*). **To improve survival post-MI.** *Adults:* Start within 24 hr of MI; 5 mg PO, then 5 mg PO in 24 hr; 10 mg PO after 48 hr; then 10 mg/d PO for 6 wk.
**ADJUST DOSE** Elderly pts, renal impairment
**ADV EFF Airway obstruction, angioedema, anaphylactoid reactions,** cough, dizziness, fatigue, gastric irritation, headache, **hepatic failure,** HTN, hyperkalemia, insomnia, **MI,** n/v/d, orthostatic hypotension, **pancytopenia, renal impairment**
**INTERACTIONS** ACE inhibitors, ARBs, capsaicin, diuretics, lithium, NSAIDs, renin inhibitors
**NC/PT** Mark chart if surgery scheduled; fluid replacement may be needed postop. Suspension can be made if pt cannot swallow tablets (see manufacturer guide). Monitor BP; use care in situations that may lead to decreased BP. Maintain hydration, potassium. Not for use in preg (contraceptives advised)/breastfeeding. Pt should take safety precautions

for CNS effects; report swelling, difficulty breathing, chest pain. Name confusion between lisinopril and fosinopril.

**lithium carbonate, lithium citrate** (Lithobid)
**CLASS** Antimanic drug
**PREG/CONT** High risk/NA

**BBW** Monitor clinical status closely, especially during initial tx stages. Monitor for therapeutic serum level (0.6–1.2 mEq/L); toxicity closely related to serum level.
**IND & DOSE Tx of manic episodes of bipolar disorder.** *Adult, child 7≥yr >30 kg:* 300 mg PO tid *or* 900 mg SR form PO bid *or* 8 mEq (5 mL) oral sol tid to produce effective serum level between 1 and 1.5 mEq/L. Maint, 300 mg PO tid–qid to produce serum level of 0.6–1.2 mEq/L (acute episodes) or 0.8–1.2 mEq/L (maint). *Child 20–30 kg:* 300 mg PO bid *or* 8 mEq (5 mL) bid. Determine serum level at least q 2 mo in samples drawn immediately before dose (at least 8–12 hr after previous dose).
**ADJUST DOSE** Elderly pts, renal impairment
**ADV EFF** Related to serum levels: **Death,** lethargy, muscle weakness, **pulmonary complications,** slurred speech, tremor progressing to **CV collapse.** Other: Dizziness, drowsiness, GI upset, thirst, tremor
**INTERACTIONS** ACE inhibitors, antacids, ARBs, carbamazepine, dandelion root, diuretics, haloperidol, indomethacin, iodide salts, juniper, NSAIDs, SSRIs, tromethamine, urinary alkalinizers
**NC/PT** Before tx, evaluate renal/thyroid function, vital signs, electrolytes, concurrent drugs, preg status. Monitor serum level regularly; therapeutic range, 0.8–1.2 mEq/L. Avoid use if CrCl <30 mL/min. Maintain salt, fluid intake. Not for use in preg (contraceptives advised)/breastfeeding. Teach toxicity warning s&sx. Pt should take w/food, milk; take safety precautions for CNS effects; report diarrhea, unsteady walking, slurred speech, difficulty breathing.

**lixisenatide** (Adlyxin)
**CLASS** Antidiabetic, glucagon-like peptide-1 receptor agonist
**PREG/CONT** Moderate risk/NA

**IND & DOSE W/diet, exercise to improve glycemic control in type 2 diabetes.** *Adult:* 10 mcg/d subcut for 14 d; then increase to 20 mcg/d subcut.
**ADV EFF** Dizziness, headache, hypoglycemia, n/v/d, renal impairment
**INTERACTIONS** Oral medications, oral contraceptives
**NC/PT** Do not use w/pancreatitis, type 1 diabetes, ketoacidosis. Pt must continue diet/exercise program. Pt should inject into abdomen, thigh, or upper arm; never share pen; take oral drugs 1 hr before injection; take oral contraceptives 1 hr before or 11 hr after this drug; take safety precautions for CNS effects; report difficulty breathing, severe GI effects; worsening of glycemic control.

**lofexidine** (Lucemyra)
**CLASS** Central $alpha_2$ adrenergic agonist
**PREG/CONT** Unkn/NA

**IND & DOSE Tx of opioid withdrawal sx to facilitate abrupt opioid discontinuation.** *Adult:* Three 0.18-mg tablets PO 4 ×/day at 5- to 6-hr intervals up to 14 d w/gradual dose reduction over 2–4 d.
**ADV EFF** Bradycardia, dizziness, dry mouth, hypotension, **prolonged QT, sedation,** somnolence, syncope
**INTERACTIONS** CNS depressants, CYP2D6 inhibitors, methadone, oral naltrexone
**NC/PT** Adjust dose w/moderate or severe hepatic/renal impairment. Opioid withdrawal s&sx may still exist

even w/tx. Taking other CNS depressants may increase adverse effects. After a period of not using opioids, pt may be more sensitive to effects of opioids and at greater risk for overdose. Pt should report s&sx of low BP, avoid driving/operating heavy machinery.

**DANGEROUS DRUG**

**lomitapide** (Juxtapid)
**CLASS** Antitriglyceride
**PREG/CONT** High risk/NA

**BBW** Increased transaminase elevations; monitor LFTs closely. Stop drug at s&sx of hepatotoxicity; risk of hepatic steatosis, cirrhosis. Only available through Juxtapid REMS program.
**IND & DOSE** **Adjunct to low-fat diet, other lipid-lowering tx to reduce LDL, total cholesterol, apolipoprotein B, non-HDL cholesterol in pts w/homozygous familial hypercholesterolemia.** *Adult:* Initially 5 mg/d PO; increase after 2 wk to 10 mg/d PO, then at 4-wk intervals to 20, 40, and 60 mg/d PO.
**ADJUST DOSE** Hepatic/renal impairment
**ADV EFF** Abd pain, dyspepsia, **hepatotoxicity,** myalgia, n/v/d
**INTERACTIONS** Bile acid sequestrants, lovastatin, simvastatin, strong or moderate CYP3A4 inhibitors, warfarin
**NC/PT** Available only through restricted access program. Ensure negative preg test before tx and continued use of low-fat diet other lipid-lowering agents. Ensure appropriate dx. Monitor LFTs regularly. Consider supplemental vitamin E, and fatty acids, tx for severe GI effects. Not for use in preg (barrier contraceptives advised)/breastfeeding. Pt should take as prescribed (dosage will be slowly increased); take w/water (not food) in evening; swallow capsule whole and not cut/crush/chew it; continue low-fat diet, other lipid-lowering drugs; take vitamin E, fatty acids if prescribed; report severe GI complaints, urine/stool color changes, extreme fatigue.

**DANGEROUS DRUG**

**lomustine** (generic)
**CLASS** Alkylating agent, antineoplastic
**PREG/CONT** D/NA

**BBW** Arrange for blood tests to evaluate hematopoietic function before tx, then wkly for at least 6 wk; severe bone marrow suppression possible. Delayed suppression at or beyond 6 wk also possible.
**IND & DOSE** **Tx of primary/metastatic brain tumors, secondary tx of Hodgkin disease in pts who relapse after primary tx w/other drugs.** *Adult, child:* 130 mg/m² PO as single dose q 6 wk. Must make adjustments w/bone marrow suppression: Initially, reduce to 100 mg/m² PO q 6 wk; do not give repeat dose until platelets >100,000/mm² and leukocytes >4,000/mm².
**ADV EFF** Alopecia, ataxia, **bone marrow suppression,** n/v, **pulmonary fibrosis, renal toxicity**
**NC/PT** Monitor CBC, respiratory function. Do not give full dose within 2–3 wk of radiation therapy. Not for use in preg (barrier contraceptives advised)/breastfeeding. Antiemetics may be ordered. Pt should avoid exposure to infection, report unusual bleeding, difficulty breathing, s&sx of infection.

**loperamide hydrochloride** (Imodium A-D)
**CLASS** Antidiarrheal
**PREG/CONT** B/NA

**IND & DOSE** **Tx of acute/chronic diarrhea/traveler's diarrhea.** *Adult:* 4 mg PO, then 2 mg after each unformed stool; max, 16 mg/d. *Child:* 8–12 yr (>30 kg): 2 mg PO tid; 6–8 yr (20–30 kg): 2 mg PO bid; 2–5 yr (13–20 kg): 1 mg PO tid. For traveler's

diarrhea, 6–11 yr (22–43 kg): 2 mg PO after loose stool, then 1 mg w/each subsequent stool; max, 4 mg/d PO (6–8 yr) or 6 mg/d PO (9–11 yr) for 2 d.
**ADV EFF** Abd pain, constipation, distention, dry mouth, nausea, **pulmonary infiltrates, toxic megacolon**
**NC/PT** Stools may be dark. Pt should take drug after each stool; stop if no response in 48 hr; drink clear fluids to prevent dehydration; report fever, continued diarrhea, abd pain/distention, severe constipation.

## loratadine (Alavert, Claritin)

**CLASS** Antihistamine
**PREG/CONT** B/NA

**IND & DOSE Sx relief of allergic rhinitis; tx of rhinitis/urticaria.** *Adult, child ≥6 yr:* 10 mg/d PO. *Child 2–5 yr:* 5 mg PO daily (syrup, chewable tablets).
**ADJUST DOSE** Elderly pts; hepatic/renal impairment
**ADV EFF Bronchospasm,** dizziness, headache, increased appetite, nervousness, thickened bronchial secretions, weight gain
**INTERACTIONS** Alcohol, CNS depressants
**NC/PT** Pt should place orally disintegrating tablet on tongue, swallow after it dissolves; avoid alcohol; use humidifier for dry mucous membranes; take safety precautions for CNS effects; report difficulty breathing.

## LORazepam (Ativan, Lorazepam Intensol)

**CLASS** Anxiolytic, benzodiazepine, sedative-hypnotic
**PREG/CONT** D/C-IV

**IND & DOSE Mgt of anxiety disorders; short-term relief of anxiety sx.** *Adults:* 2–6 mg/d PO; range, 1–10 mg/d in divided doses w/largest dose at bedtime. **Insomnia due to transient stress.** *Adult:* 2–4 mg PO at bedtime. **Preanesthetic sedation, anxiolytic.** *Adult:* 0.05 mg/kg IM; max, 4 mg at least 2 hr before procedure. Or, 2 mg total IV or 0.044 mg/kg, whichever smaller; may give doses as high as 0.05 mg/kg to total of 4 mg 15–20 min before procedure. **Tx of status epilepticus.** *Adult:* 4 mg slowly IV at 2 mg/min. May give another 4 mg IV after 10–15 min if needed.
**ADJUST DOSE** Hepatic/renal impairment
**ADV EFF** Apathy, confusion, depression, disorientation, drowsiness, dry mouth, **CV collapse,** gynecomastia, hostility, light-headedness, nausea, restlessness
**INTERACTIONS** Alcohol, CNS depressants, kava, probenecid, theophyllines
**NC/PT** Do not give intra-arterially. Give IM injection deep into muscle. Protect sol from light. May mix oral sol w/water, juice, soda, applesauce, pudding. Taper gradually after long-term tx. Pt should take safety precautions for CNS effects, report vision changes, chest pain, fainting. Name confusion between lorazepam and alprazolam.

## lorcaserin hydrochloride (Belviq, Belviq XR)

**CLASS** Serotonin receptor agonist, weight-loss drug
**PREG/CONT** High risk/NA

**IND & DOSE Adjunct to diet/exercise for long-term weight management in adults w/initial body mass index of ≥30 kg/m² or ≥27 kg/m² w/at least one weight-related condition.** *Adult:* 10 mg PO bid or 20 mg/d PO ER tablets.
**ADV EFF** Back pain, cognitive changes, constipation, dizziness, dry mouth, fatigue, headache, hypoglycemia, **NMS, priapism, pulmonary HTN, serotonin syndrome, suicidality, valvular heart disease**

**INTERACTIONS** Bupropion, dextromethorphan, linezolid, lithium, MAOIs, selected serotonin norepinephrine reuptake inhibitors, SSRIs, St. John's wort, TCAs, tramadol, tryptophan; avoid these combos
**NC/PT** Ensure appropriate use of drug; if 5% of body weight is not lost within 12 wk, stop drug. Be aware of risk of cognitive changes, suicidality; monitor for s&sx of valvular heart disease, NMS. Not for use in preg/breastfeeding. Pt should take immediate-release form bid, and not change dosage; take ER form once a day; continue diet/exercise program; avoid combining w/other weight-loss drugs; avoid St. John's wort; use safety precautions w/dizziness, sugarless candy for dry mouth; watch for slowed thinking, sleepiness; report thoughts of suicide, changes in HR, mental status.

## lorlatinib (Lorbrena)
**CLASS** Anaplastic lymphoma kinase inhibitor, antineoplastic, tyrosine kinase inhibitor
**PREG/CONT** High risk/NA

**IND & DOSE** **Tx of pts w/anaplastic lymphoma kinase (ALK)-positive metastatic NSCLC whose disease has progressed on crizotinib and at least one other ALK inhibitor for metastatic disease; or on alectinib or ceritinib as first ALK inhibitor therapy for metastatic disease.** *Adult:* 100 mg PO q d.
**ADV EFF** Arthralgia, **AV block,** cognitive effects, diarrhea, dyspnea, edema, fatigue, hallucinations, **hepatotoxicity** (especially if combined w/certain drugs), hyperlipidemia, ILD/pneumonitis, mood effects, peripheral neuropathy, **seizures,** weight gain
**INTERACTIONS** CYP3A inducers/inhibitors/substrates
**NC/PT** Monitor for hyperlipidemia regularly. Risk of hepatotoxicity. Women should use nonhormonal contraceptives during and for at least 6 mo after tx, avoid breastfeeding during and for at least 7 d after tx. Men should use contraceptives during and for at least 3 mo after tx. Tx may transiently impair fertility. Pt should report all concomitant drugs, new/worsening CNS effects, cardiac/respiratory sx.

## losartan potassium
(Cozaar)
**CLASS** Antihypertensive, ARB
**PREG/CONT** D/NA

**BBW** Rule out preg before starting tx. Suggest barrier contraceptives during tx; fetal injury/death have occurred.
**IND & DOSE** **Tx of HTN.** *Adult:* 50 mg/d PO; range, 25–100 mg/d PO once or bid. *Child ≥6 yr:* 0.7 mg/kg/d PO; max, 50 mg/d. **Tx of diabetic nephropathy.** *Adult:* 50 mg/d PO; may increase to 100 mg/d based on BP response. **Tx of HTN w/left ventricular hypertrophy.** *Adult:* 50–100 mg/d PO w/12.5–25 mg/d hydrochlorothiazide.
**ADV EFF** Abd pain, cough, diarrhea, dizziness, drowsiness, hyperkalemia, nausea, URI
**INTERACTIONS** ACE inhibitors, ARBs, fluconazole, indomethacin, ketoconazole, phenobarbital, renin inhibitors, rifamycin
**NC/PT** If surgery needed, alert surgeon to drug use; volume replacement may be needed. Monitor potassium w/long-term use. Not for use in preg (barrier contraceptives advised)/breastfeeding. Pt should use caution in situations that could lead to fluid loss, maintain hydration, take safety precautions for CNS effects.

## lovastatin (Altoprev)
**CLASS** Antihyperlipidemic, statin
**PREG/CONT** X/NA

**IND & DOSE** **Tx of familial hypercholesterolemia, type II hyperlipidemia (ER only); to slow progression**

**of atherosclerosis in pts w/CAD; tx of primary hypercholesterolemia.** *Adult:* 20 mg/d PO in evening w/ meals. Maint, 10–80 mg/d PO; max, 80 mg/d. For ER tablets, 10–60 mg/d PO single dose in evening. **As adjunct to diet to reduce total cholesterol, LDLs, apolipoprotein B in heterozygous familial hypercholesterolemia.** *Adolescent boy, postmenarchal girl, 10–17 yr:* 10–40 mg/d PO; may increase to max 40 mg/d.
**ADJUST DOSE** Renal impairment
**ADV EFF** Abd pain, cataracts, cramps, constipation, flatulence, headache, hepatic impairment, nausea, **rhabdomyolysis**
**INTERACTIONS** Amiodarone, azole antifungals, cyclosporine, erythromycin, gemfibrozil, grapefruit juice, itraconazole, ketoconazole, other statins, verapamil
**NC/PT** Monitor LFTs. Stop drug if myopathy occurs. Not for use in preg (barrier contraceptives advised)/ breastfeeding. Pt should not cut/ crush/chew ER tablets; take in evening for best effects; continue diet/ exercise program; get periodic eye exams; report muscle pain w/fever, unusual bleeding.

## loxapine hydrochloride, loxapine succinate (Adasuve)

**CLASS** Antipsychotic, dopaminergic blocker
**PREG/CONT** High risk/NA

**BBW** Increased risk of mortality when antipsychotics used in elderly pts w/dementia-related psychosis. Avoid this use; not approved for this use. Increased risk of potentially fatal bronchospasm w/inhaled form; available only through limited release program; monitor pt closely.
**IND & DOSE Tx of schizophrenia.** *Adult:* 10 mg PO bid; max, 50 mg/d. Increase fairly rapidly over first 7–10 d until sx controlled; range, 60–100 mg/d PO. Dosage >250 mg/d PO not recommended. For maint: range, 20–60 mg/d PO. **Acute tx of agitation associated w/schizophrenia, bipolar disorder.** *Adult:* 10 mg/ 24 hr by oral inhalation using inhaler.
**ADJUST DOSE** Elderly pts
**ADV EFF Bone marrow suppression, bronchospasm,** drowsiness, dry mouth, extrapyramidal sx, gynecomastia, hypotension, **laryngospasm, NMS,** photosensitivity, rash, **refractory arrhythmias, TIA**
**INTERACTIONS** CNS drugs, drugs that affect airway disease (inhaled form)
**NC/PT** Ensure hydration of elderly pts. Monitor CBC; stop if suppressed. Screen pulmonary hx and examine pt before using inhaled form; inhaled form available only through restricted access program. Not for use in preg/ breastfeeding. Monitor infants born to mothers using drug for extrapyramidal/withdrawal symptoms. Pt should take safety precautions for CNS effects; avoid sun exposure; report unusual bleeding, infections, palpitations. Name confusion w/ *Loxitane* (loxapine), *Lexapro* (escitalopram), *Soriatane* (acitretin).

## lurasidone hydrochloride (Latuda)

**CLASS** Atypical antipsychotic
**PREG/CONT** High risk/NA

**BBW** Increased risk of mortality when antipsychotics used in elderly pts w/dementia-related psychosis. Avoid this use; not approved for this use. Increased risk of suicidality in child, adolescent, young adult; monitor accordingly.
**IND & DOSE Tx of schizophrenia.** *Adult, adolescent 13–17 yr:* 40 mg/d PO w/food; may titrate to max 160 (adult) or 80 (adolescent) mg/d PO. **Tx of bipolar depression.** *Adult:* 20 mg/d PO; may titrate to max 120 mg/d. *Child 10–17 yr:* 20 mg/d PO; may titrate to max 80 mg/d.

**ADJUST DOSE** Hepatic/renal impairment
**ADV EFF** Akathisia, dystonia, hyperglycemia, hyperprolactinemia, **NMS**, n/v/d, parkinsonism, **suicidality**, weight gain
**INTERACTIONS** Alcohol, grapefruit juice, strong CYP3A4 inducers/inhibitors
**NC/PT** Dispense least amount possible to suicidal pt. Obtain CBC in pt w/preexisting low WBC count or history of leukopenia/neutropenia; consider stopping if significant decrease in counts. Monitor HR/BP in pt w/CV disease. Not for use in preg/breastfeeding. Monitor infant born to mother using drug for extrapyramidal/withdrawal symptoms. Pt should take safety measures for CNS effects; monitor serum glucose/weight gain; avoid alcohol; report increased thirst/appetite, thoughts of suicide.

**▶NEW DRUG**

**lusutrombopag** (Mulpleta)
**CLASS** Hematopoietic, thrombopoietin receptor agonist
**PREG/CONT** Unkn/NA

**IND & DOSE** **Preprocedure tx of thrombocytopenia in pts w/chronic liver disease.** *Adult:* 3 mg PO daily w/ or w/o food for 7 d 2–8 d before procedure.
**ADV EFF** Headache, **thrombotic/thromboembolic complications**
**NC/PT** Obtain platelet count before giving; monitor count again ≤2 d before procedure.

**lutetium Lu 177 dotatate** (Lutathera)
**CLASS** Radiolabeled somatostatin analog
**PREG/CONT** High risk/NA

**IND & DOSE** **Tx of somatostatin receptor–positive gastroenteropancreatic neuroendocrine tumors, including foregut, midgut, hindgut tumors.** *Adult:* 7.4 GBq (200 mCi) IV q 8 wk for four doses.
**ADV EFF** **Hepatotoxicity**, hyperglycemia/hypokalemia, increased liver enzymes, **infertility**, lymphopenia, **myelosuppression, neuroendocrine hormonal crisis**, n/v, **renal toxicity**
**INTERACTIONS** Somatostatin analogs; must discontinue before each dose (24 hr before for short-acting, 4 wk before for long-acting)
**NC/PT** High risk of embryo-fetal toxicity and risk of infertility; obtain preg status. Premedicate w/antiemetics 30 min before; octreotide used post administration. Minimize radiation exposure during/after tx. Monitor blood counts; may need to withhold doses if low levels. Monitor for renal/hepatic toxicity. Pt should avoid breastfeeding, report fever, chills, dizziness, shortness of breath, increased bleeding/bruising.

**macimorelin** (Macrilen)
**CLASS** Growth hormone (GH) receptor agonist
**PREG/CONT** Unkn/NA

**IND & DOSE** **Dx of adult GH deficiency.** *Adult:* 0.5 mg/kg once after fasting for at least 8 hr.
**ADV EFF** Bradycardia, diarrhea, dizziness, fatigue, headache, hunger, hyperhidrosis, nasopharyngitis, nausea, **prolonged QT**, respiratory tract infection
**INTERACTIONS** CYP3A4 inducers, GHs
**NC/PT** Discontinue strong CYP3A4 inducers, GH before use. Avoid use w/drugs known to affect pituitary GH secretion. Safety has not been established for pt w/body mass index >40 kg/m$^2$. For pt w/sex hormone, thyroid hormone, and/or glucocorticoid deficiencies, adequately replace each missing hormone before giving Macrilen. Pt must fast at least 8 hr before dose.

## macitentan (Opsumit)

**CLASS** Endothelin receptor blocker, pulmonary HTN drug

**PREG/CONT** High risk/NA

**BBW** Known teratogen; life-threatening birth defects possible. Available by limited access program for women. Monthly preg tests required.

**IND & DOSE Tx of pulmonary artery HTN.** *Adult:* 10 mg/d PO.

**ADV EFF** Anemia, bronchitis, decreased Hgb, fluid retention, headache, **hepatotoxicity,** nasopharyngitis, **pulmonary edema,** reduced sperm count, UTI

**INTERACTIONS** Ketoconazole, rifampin, ritonavir; avoid these combos

**NC/PT** Ensure proper dx, negative monthly preg test. Monitor LFTs, Hgb, respiratory status. Pt should avoid preg (contraceptives required)/breastfeeding; males should be aware of reduced sperm count. Pt should monitor activity tolerance; report difficulty breathing, urine/stool color changes, extreme fatigue.

## magnesium salts, magnesia, magnesium citrate, magnesium hydroxide (Milk of Magnesia), magnesium oxide (Mag-Ox)

**CLASS** Antacid, laxative

**PREG/CONT** C; A (antacids); B (laxative)/NA

**IND & DOSE Laxative.** *Adult:* 300 mL (citrate) PO w/full glass of water, or 15–60 mL (hydroxide) PO w/liquid. *Child ≥12 yr:* 30–60 mL (400 mg/5 mL) (hydroxide) PO w/water or 15–30 mL/d (800 mg/5 mL) PO once daily at bedtime, or eight 311-mg tablets PO once daily at bedtime or in divided doses. *Child 6–11 yr:* 15–30 mL (400 mg/5 mL) (hydroxide) PO once daily at bedtime, or 7.5–15 mL/d (800 mg/5 mL) PO once daily at bedtime, or four 311-mg tablets/d PO at bedtime. *Child 2–5 yr:* 5–15 mL (400 mg/5 mL) (hydroxide) PO once daily at bedtime, or two 311-mg tablets/d PO at bedtime. **Antacid.** *Adult:* 5–15 mL (hydroxide) liquid or 622–1,244-mg tablets PO qid (adult, child >12 yr). **Supplemental magnesium replacement.** *Adult:* Magnesium oxide capsules, 140 mg PO tid–qid. Tablets, 400–800 mg/d PO.

**ADV EFF** Dizziness, hypermagnesemia, n/v/d, perianal irritation

**INTERACTIONS** Fluoroquinolones, ketoconazole, nitrofurantoin, penicillamine, tetracyclines

**NC/PT** Pt should avoid other oral drugs within 1–2 hr of antacids, take between meals and at bedtime, chew antacid tablet thoroughly, avoid long-term laxative use, avoid laxatives if abd pain, n/v occur, maintain hydration, report rectal bleeding, weakness.

**DANGEROUS DRUG**

## magnesium sulfate (generic)

**CLASS** Antiepileptic, electrolyte, laxative

**PREG/CONT** D; B (laxative)/NA

**IND & DOSE Control of HTN w/ acute nephritis.** *Child:* 100 mg/kg (0.8 mEq/kg or 0.2 mL/kg of 50% sol) IM q 4–6 hr as needed. Or, 20–40 mg/kg (0.16–0.32 mEq/kg or 0.1–0.2 mL/kg of 20% sol) IM. Or, for severe sx, 100–200 mg/kg of 1%–3% sol IV over 1 hr w/half of dose given in first 15–20 min (seizure control). **Laxative.** *Adult:* 10–30 g/d PO. *Child 6–11 yr:* 5–10 g/d PO; 15–30 mL/d PO. *Child 2–5 yr:* 2.5–5 g/d PO; 5–15 mL/d PO. **Tx of arrhythmias.** *Adult:* 3–4 g IV over several min; then 3–20 mg/min continuous infusion for 5–48 hr. **Tx of eclampsia, severe preeclampsia.** *Adult:* 10–14 g IV. May infuse 4–5 g in 250 mL 5% dextrose injection or normal saline while giving IM doses up to 10 g (5 g or 10 mL of undiluted 50% sol in each buttock). Or, may give initial 4 g IV by diluting 50% sol to 10%

or 20%; may inject diluted fluid (40 mL of 10% or 20 mL of 20% sol) IV over 3–4 min. Then inject 4–5 g (8–10 mL of 50% sol) IM into alternate buttocks q 4 hr as needed depending on patellar reflex, respiratory function. Or, after initial IV dose, may give 1–2 g/hr by constant IV infusion. Continue until paroxysms stop. To control seizures, optimal serum magnesium is 6 mg/100 mL; max, 30–40 g/24 hr. **Correction of hypomagnesemia.** *Adult:* 1 g IM or IV q 6 hr for four doses (32.5 mEq/24 hr); up to 246 mg/kg IM within 4 hr or 5 g (40 mEq)/1,000 mL $D_5W$ or normal saline IV infused over 3 hr for severe cases. **Parenteral nutrition.** *Adult:* 8–24 mEq/d IV.
**ADJUST DOSE** Renal impairment
**ADV EFF** Dizziness, excessive bowel activity, fainting, magnesium intoxication, perianal irritation, weakness
**INTERACTIONS** Alcohol, aminoglycosides, amphotericin B, cisplatin, cyclosporine, digoxin, diuretics, NMJ blockers
**NC/PT** Monitor serum magnesium during parenteral tx; normal limits, 1.5–3 mEq/L. Fetal harm can occur if used beyond 5 d; use shortest time possible for preterm tx. Save IV use in eclampsia for life-threatening situations. Monitor knee-jerk reflex before repeated parenteral administration. If knee-jerk reflex suppressed, do not give. Use as temporary relief of constipation; stop if diarrhea occurs.

## mannitol (Osmitrol)
**CLASS** Diagnostic agent, osmotic diuretic, urinary irrigant
**PREG/CONT** Unkn/NA

**IND & DOSE** **Px of oliguria in renal failure.** *Adult:* 50–100 g IV as 5%–25% sol. **Tx of oliguria in renal failure.** *Adult:* 50–100 g IV as 15%–25% sol. **To reduce intracranial pressure, cerebral edema.** *Adult:* 1.5–2 g/kg IV as 15%–25% sol over 30–60 min. Reduced pressure should be evident in 15 min. **Reduction of IOP.** *Adult:* 1.5–2 g/kg IV infusion as 25%, 20%, or 15% sol over 30 min. If used preop, give 60–90 min before surgery for max effect. **Adjunct tx to promote diuresis in intoxication.** *Adult:* Max 200 g IV mannitol w/other fluids, electrolytes. **To measure GFR.** *Adult:* Dilute 100 mL of 20% sol w/180 mL sodium chloride injection. Infuse this 280 mL of 7.2% sol IV at 20 mL/min. Collect urine w/catheter for specified time to measure mannitol excreted in mg/min. Draw blood at start and end of time for mannitol measurement in mg/mL plasma. **Test dose of mannitol in pts w/inadequate renal function.** *Adult:* 0.2 g/kg IV (about 50 mL of 25% sol, 75 mL of 20% sol) in 3–5 min to produce urine flow of 30–50 mL/hr. If urine flow not increased, repeat dose. If no response to second dose, reevaluate situation.
**ADV EFF** Anorexia, CNS toxicity, diuresis, dizziness, dry mouth, hyperosmolarity, infusion reactions, n/v, **seizures,** thirst
**INTERACTIONS** Nephrotoxic/neurotoxic drugs, renally eliminated drugs
**NC/PT** Do not give electrolyte-free mannitol w/blood. If blood must be given, add at least 20 mEq sodium chloride to each liter mannitol sol; use filter. Monitor serum electrolytes periodically. Pt should use sugarless lozenges for dry mouth, take safety precautions for CNS effects.

## maprotiline hydrochloride (generic)
**CLASS** TCA
**PREG/CONT** B/NA

**BBW** Increased risk of suicidal thinking, behavior in child, adolescent, young adult; monitor accordingly.
**IND & DOSE** **Tx of mild to moderate depression.** *Adult:* 75 mg/d PO in outpts; after 2 wk may increase gradually in 25-mg increments. Usual dose, 150 mg/d. **Tx of severe depression.** *Adult:* 100–150 mg/d PO in

inpts; may gradually increase to 225 mg/d. **Maint tx of depression.** *Adult:* Use lowest effective dose, usually 75–150 mg/d PO.
**ADJUST DOSE** Elderly pts
**ADV EFF** Confusion, constipation, disturbed conc, dry mouth, gynecomastia, **MI,** orthostatic hypotension, peripheral neuropathy, photosensitivity, rash, restlessness, sedation, **stroke,** urine retention
**INTERACTIONS** Alcohol, anticholinergics, phenothiazines, sympathomimetics, thyroid medication
**NC/PT** Limit access to depressed/potentially suicidal pts. Expect clinical response in 3 wk. Give at bedtime if orthostatic hypotension occurs. Not for use in preg (barrier contraceptives advised). Pt should avoid alcohol, sun exposure; report numbness/tingling, chest pain, thoughts of suicide.

## maraviroc (Selzentry)

**CLASS** Antiviral, CCR5 coreceptor antagonist
**PREG/CONT** B/NA

**BBW** Risk of severe hepatotoxicity, possibly preceded by systemic allergic reaction (rash, eosinophilia, elevated IgE). Immediately evaluate, support pt w/s&sx of hepatitis, allergic reaction.
**IND & DOSE Combo antiretroviral tx of pts infected only w/detectable CCR5-tropic HIV-1.** *Adult, child>16 yr:* W/strong CYP3A inhibitors, protease inhibitors (except tipranavir/ritonavir), delavirdine, 150 mg PO bid. W/tipranavir/ritonavir, nevirapine, enfuvirtide, nucleoside reverse transcriptase inhibitors, other drugs that are not strong CYP3A inhibitors, 300 mg PO bid. W/potent CYP3A inducers including efavirenz, 600 mg PO bid. *Child≥2 yr ≥10 kg:* Base dose on body weight bid; do not exceed recommended adult dose.
**ADJUST DOSE** Renal impairment
**ADV EFF** Abd pain, cough, CV events, dizziness, fever, headache, **hepatotoxicity,** musculoskeletal sx, rash to **potentially fatal SJS**
**INTERACTIONS** CYP3A inducers/inhibitors, St. John's wort
**NC/PT** Give w/other antiretrovirals. Monitor LFTs, CD4. Use caution in preg; not for use in breastfeeding. Pt should swallow tablet whole and not cut/crush/chew it; take precautions to prevent spread (drug not a cure); avoid St. John's wort; take safety precautions for CNS effects; report chest pain, rash, urine/stool color changes.

## mecasermin (Increlex)

**CLASS** Insulin-like growth factor-1
**PREG/CONT** Unkn/NA

**IND & DOSE Long-term tx of growth failure in child w/severe primary insulin growth factor-1 deficiency or w/growth hormone gene deletion who has developed neutralizing antibodies to growth hormone.** *Child≥2 yr:* Initially, 0.04–0.08 mg/kg (40–80 mcg/kg) bid by subcut injection shortly before meal or snack; may be increased by 0.04 mg/kg/dose to max of 0.12 mg/kg bid.
**ADV EFF** Hypersensitivity reactions, hypoglycemia, **intracranial HTN, malignant neoplasm,** progression of scoliosis, slipped capital femoral epiphysis, tonsillar hypertrophy
**NC/PT** Not a substitute for growth hormone. Monitor blood glucose, tonsils. Ensure given just before meal or snack. Pt should avoid preg/breastfeeding; learn proper administration/disposal of needles/syringes; report difficulty breathing/swallowing, sudden limb or hip/knee pain, injection-site pain, rash.

DANGEROUS DRUG

**mechlorethamine hydrochloride** (Valchlor)
**CLASS** Alkylating agent, antineoplastic, nitrogen mustard
**PREG/CONT** D/NA

**BBW** Handle drug w/caution; use chemo-safe nonpermeable gloves. Drug highly toxic and a vesicant. Avoid inhaling dust, vapors; avoid contact w/skin, mucous membranes (especially eyes). If eye contact, immediately irrigate w/copious amount of ophthal irrigating sol, get ophthalmologic consultation. If skin contact, irrigate w/copious amount of water for 15 min, then apply 2% sodium thiosulfate. Monitor injection site for extravasation. Painful inflammation/induration, skin sloughing possible. If leakage, promptly infiltrate w/ sterile isotonic sodium thiosulfate (1/6M), apply ice compress for 6–12 hr. Notify physician.
**IND & DOSE** **Palliative tx of bronchogenic carcinoma, Hodgkin disease, lymphosarcoma, CML, chronic lymphocytic leukemia, mycosis fungoides, polycythemia vera.** *Adult:* Total 0.4 mg/kg IV for each course as single dose or in two–four divided doses of 0.1–0.2 mg/kg/d. Give at night if sedation needed for side effects. Interval between courses usually 3–6 wk. **Palliative tx of effusion secondary to metastatic carcinoma.** *Adult:* Dose, preparation for intracavity use vary greatly; usual dose, 0.2–0.4 mg/kg. **Tx of stage 1A, 1B mycosis fungoides–type T-cell lymphoma after direct skin tx.** *Adult:* Apply thin film to affected areas of skin; avoid eyes and mucous membranes.
**ADV EFF** Anorexia, **bone marrow suppression**, dizziness, drowsiness, impaired fertility, n/v/d, thrombophlebitis, weakness
**INTERACTIONS** Adalimumab, denosumab, infliximab, leflunomide, natalizumab, pimecrolimus, roflumilast
**NC/PT** Avoid skin contact w/powder for injection. Premedicate w/ antiemetics, sedatives. Monitor CBC closely, injection site for extravasation. Maintain hydration. Not for use in preg (contraceptives advised)/ breastfeeding. Pt should take safety precautions for CNS changes; avoid smoking, open flames when using topical gel until gel dries (very flammable); dispose of tube appropriately; report burning at IV site, fever.

**meclizine hydrochloride** (Antivert, Bonine, Dramamine)
**CLASS** Anticholinergic, antiemetic, antihistamine, anti–motion sickness
**PREG/CONT** Low risk/NA

**IND & DOSE** **Px, tx of motion sickness.** *Adult, child >12 yr:* 25–50 mg/d PO 1 hr before travel. **Tx of vertigo.** *Adult, child >12 yr:* 25–100 mg/d PO.
**ADJUST DOSE** Elderly pts
**ADV EFF** Anorexia, confusion, drowsiness, dry mouth, nausea, **respiratory depression to death**, urinary difficulty/frequency
**INTERACTIONS** Alcohol, CNS depressants
**NC/PT** For anti–motion sickness, works best if used before motion. Pt should avoid alcohol, take safety precautions for CNS depression, use sugarless lozenges for dry mouth, report difficulty breathing.

DANGEROUS DRUG

**medroxyPROGESTERone acetate** (Depo-Provera, depo-subQ provera 104, Provera)
**CLASS** Antineoplastic, contraceptive, hormone, progestin
**PREG/CONT** X/NA

**BBW** Before tx, rule out preg; caution pt to avoid preg and have frequent medical follow-up. Alert pt using

contraceptive injections that drug does not protect from HIV, other STDs, and to take precautions. *Depo-Provera* use may result in significant bone density loss; drug should not be used for longer than 2 yr unless no other contraception form is adequate.
**IND & DOSE** **Contraception.** *Adult:* 150 mg IM q 3 mo. For *depo-subQ provera:* 104 mg subcut into thigh or abdomen q 12–14 wk. **Tx of secondary amenorrhea.** *Adult:* 5–10 mg/d PO for 5–10 d. **Tx of abnormal uterine bleeding.** *Adult:* 5–10 mg/d PO for 5–10 d, starting on 16th or 21st day of menstrual cycle. **Tx of endometrial, renal carcinoma.** *Adult:* 400–1,000 mg/wk IM. **To reduce endometrial hyperplasia.** *Adult:* 5–10 mg/d PO for 12–14 consecutive days/mo. Start on 1st or 16th day of cycle. **Mgt of endometriosis-associated pain.** *Adult:* 104 mg subcut *(depo-subQ Provera)* into anterior thigh or abdomen q 12–14 wk for no longer than 2 yr.
**ADV EFF** Amenorrhea, anaphylaxis, bone loss, breakthrough bleeding, **breast cancer, ectopic preg,** edema, fluid retention, hepatic impairment, menstrual flow changes, rash, **thromboembolic events,** vision changes, weight changes
**INTERACTIONS** CYP3A4 inducers, HIV protease and nonnucleoside reverse transcriptase inhibitors, St. John's wort
**NC/PT** Arrange for pretreatment, periodic (at least annual) complete hx, physical. Monitor bone density. Do not use w/active thrombophlebitis. Not for use in preg. Pt should know drug does not protect against STDs, HIV; protection is still required. Use second form of contraception w/antibiotics, CYP3A4 inducers. Limit use to 2 yr as contraceptive. Pt should mark calendar for tx days; report sudden vision loss, swelling, severe headache, chest pain, urine/stool color changes, severe abd pain.

## mefenamic acid (Ponstel)

**CLASS** NSAID
**PREG/CONT** Moderate risk (1st, 2nd trimesters); high risk (3rd trimester)/NA

**BBW** Increased risk of CV events, GI bleeding; monitor accordingly. Do not use for periop pain in CABG surgery.
**IND & DOSE** **Tx of acute pain.** *Adult, child >14 yr:* 500 mg PO, then 250 mg q hr as needed for up to 1 wk. **Tx of primary dysmenorrhea.** *Adult, child >14 yr:* 500 mg PO, then 250 mg q 6 hr starting w/bleeding onset. Can initiate at start of menses, then for 2–3 d.
**ADJUST DOSE** Elderly pts, renal impairment (not recommended)
**ADV EFF** **Anaphylactoid reactions to anaphylactic shock, bone marrow suppression,** constipation, diarrhea, dizziness, dyspepsia, edema, GI pain, headache, HTN, nausea, rash, **renal impairment**
**INTERACTIONS** ASA, anticoagulants, methotrexate, NSAIDs
**NC/PT** Not for use in preg/breastfeeding. Pt should take w/food; use safety precautions for CNS effects; stop drug and report rash, diarrhea, black tarry stools, difficulty breathing, edema.

**DANGEROUS DRUG**
**(AS ANTINEOPLASTIC)**

## megestrol acetate
(Megace ES)

**CLASS** Antineoplastic, hormone, progestin
**PREG/CONT** High risk/NA

**BBW** Caution pt not to use if preg; fetal risks. Advise barrier contraceptives. Risk of thromboembolic events, stop drug at sx of thrombosis.
**IND & DOSE** **Palliative tx of breast cancer.** *Adult:* 160 mg/d PO (40 mg qid). **Palliative tx of endometrial cancer.** *Adult:* 40–320 mg/d PO. **Tx of cachexia w/HIV.** *Adult:* 800 mg/d PO;

range, 400–800 mg/d (suspension only) or 625 mg/d PO (ES suspension).
**ADV EFF** Amenorrhea, breakthrough bleeding, dizziness, edema, fluid retention, menstrual flow changes, photosensitivity, rash, somnolence, **thromboembolic events,** vision changes, weight changes
**NC/PT** Obtain negative preg test before tx. Stop if thromboembolic events. Store suspension in cool place; shake well before use. Not for use in preg (barrier contraceptives advised)/breastfeeding. Pt should avoid sun exposure; take safety precautions for CNS effects; report chest/leg pain, swelling, numbness/tingling, severe headache.

**meloxicam** (Mobic, Qmiiz ODT, Vivlodex)
**CLASS** NSAID
**PREG/CONT** Moderate risk (1st, 2nd trimesters); high risk (3rd trimester)/NA

**BBW** Increased risk of CV events, GI bleeding; monitor accordingly. Do not use for periop pain in CABG surgery.
**IND & DOSE** **Relief of s&sx of osteoarthritis, RA.** *Adult:* 7.5 mg/d PO. Max, 15 mg/d. **Management of osteoarthritis pain.** *Adult:* 5 mg/d PO; max, 10 mg/d (*Vivlodex*). **Relief of s&sx of pauciarticular/polyarticular course juvenile RA.** *Child ≥2 yr:* 0.125 mg/kg/d PO; max, 7.5 mg (oral suspension).
**ADV EFF** **Anaphylactic shock, bone marrow suppression,** diarrhea, dizziness, dyspepsia, edema, GI pain, headache, hepatic impairment, HTN, insomnia, nausea, rash, renal injury, serious skin events including **SJS**
**INTERACTIONS** ACE inhibitors, aspirin, anticoagulants, diuretics, lithium, methotrexate, oral corticosteroids, other NSAIDs, warfarin
**NC/PT** *Vivlodex* and *Mobic* not interchangeable w/other formulations. Pt should take w/food, use safety precautions for CNS effects, report difficulty breathing, swelling, black tarry stools, rash.

**DANGEROUS DRUG**

**melphalan** (Alkeran, Evomela)
**CLASS** Alkylating agent, antineoplastic, nitrogen mustard
**PREG/CONT** High risk/NA

**BBW** Arrange for blood tests to evaluate hematopoietic function before and wkly during tx; severe bone marrow suppression possible. Caution pt to avoid preg during tx; drug considered mutagenic.
**IND & DOSE** **Tx of multiple myeloma.** *Adult:* 6 mg/d PO. After 2–3 wk, stop for up to 4 wk, monitor blood counts. When counts rising, start maint of 2 mg/d PO. Or, 16 mg/$m^2$ as single IV infusion over 15–20 min at 2-wk intervals for four doses, then at 4-wk intervals. **Palliative tx of multiple myeloma (*Evomela*).** 16 mg/$m^2$ IV over 15–20 min at 2- to 4-wk intervals. **Conditioning tx before autologous stem cell transplant (*Evomela*).** 100 mg/$m^2$/d IV over 30 min for 2 consecutive d before transplant. **Tx of epithelial ovarian carcinoma.** *Adult:* 0.2 mg/kg/d PO for 5 d as single course. Repeat courses q 4–5 wk.
**ADJUST DOSE** Renal impairment
**ADV EFF** Alopecia, amenorrhea, **anaphylaxis, bone marrow suppression, cancer,** n/v, **pulmonary fibrosis,** rash
**NC/PT** Refrigerate tablets in glass bottle. Monitor CBC regularly; dose adjustment may be needed. Monitor respiratory function. Maintain hydration. Give antiemetics for severe nausea. Not for use in preg (barrier contraceptives advised)/breastfeeding. Pt should cover head at temp extremes (hair loss possible); avoid exposure to infection; report bleeding, s&sx of infection, difficulty breathing.

**memantine hydrochloride** (Namenda, Namenda XR)
**CLASS** Alzheimer drug; *N*-methyl-*D*-aspartate receptor antagonist
**PREG/CONT** Unkn/NA

**IND & DOSE** **Tx of moderate to severe Alzheimer-type dementia.** *Adult:* 5 mg/d PO. Increase at wkly intervals to 5 mg PO bid (10 mg/d), 15 mg/d PO (5-mg and 10-mg doses) w/at least 1 wk between increases. Target, 20 mg/d (10 mg bid). ER form: 7 mg/d PO; may increase by 7 mg/d after at least 1 wk. Maint, 28 mg/d.
**ADJUST DOSE** Renal impairment
**ADV EFF** Confusion, constipation, cough, dizziness, fatigue, headache
**INTERACTIONS** Amantadine, carbonic anhydrase inhibitors, dextromethorphan, ketamine, sodium bicarbonate, urine alkalinizers
**NC/PT** Obtain baseline functional profile. Not a cure; medical follow-up needed. Pt should swallow ER tablet whole and not cut/crush/chew it; take safety precaution for CNS effects; report lack of improvement, swelling, respiratory problems.

**menotropins** (Menopur)
**CLASS** Fertility drug, hormone
**PREG/CONT** X/NA

**IND & DOSE** **To induce ovulation in anovulatory women, w/HCG.** *Adult:* 225 units/d subcut; **ADJUST DOSE** after 5 d by no more than 150 units each time; max, 450 units/d for no longer than 20 d.
**ADV EFF** Congenital malformations, dizziness, ectopic preg, febrile reactions, multiple births, ovarian enlargement, ovarian neoplasms, **ovarian overstimulation, ovarian torsion, thromboembolic events**
**NC/PT** Must follow w/HCG when clinical evidence shows sufficient follicular maturation based on urine excretion of estrogens. Give subcut into abdomen. Not for use in preg/breastfeeding. Monitor for ovarian overstimulation; admit pt to hospital for tx. Risk of multiple births. Teach proper administration/disposal of needles/syringes. Pt should mark calendar of tx days; report severe abd pain, fever, chest pain.

DANGEROUS DRUG

**meperidine hydrochloride** (Demerol)
**CLASS** Opioid agonist analgesic
**PREG/CONT** Low risk (short-term use; high risk (long-term use)/C-II

**BBW** Medication errors/accidental ingestion can be fatal. Risk of addiction, abuse, misuse. Life-threatening respiratory depression and death can occur, especially if used w/drugs utilizing CYP450 3A4 system, benzodiazepines, other CNS depressants/MAOIs. Risk of neonatal opioid withdrawal syndrome if used in preg. The FDA has required a REMS to ensure benefits outweigh risks.
**IND & DOSE** **Relief of moderate to severe acute pain.** *Adult:* 50–150 mg IM, subcut, or PO q 3–4 hr as needed. May give diluted sol by slow IV injection. IM route preferred for repeated injections. *Child:* 1.1–1.75 mg/kg IM, subcut, or PO up to adult dose q 3–4 hr as needed. **Preop medication.** *Adult:* 50–100 mg IM or subcut 30–90 min before anesthesia. *Child:* 1.1–2.2 mg/kg IM or subcut, up to adult dose, 30–90 min before anesthesia. **Anesthesia support.** *Adult:* Dilute to 10 mg/mL; give repeated doses by slow IV injection. Or, dilute to 1 mg/mL; infuse continuously. **Obstetric analgesia.** *Adult:* When contractions regular, 50–100 mg IM or subcut; repeat q 1–3 hr.
**ADJUST DOSE** Elderly, debilitated pts; hepatic, renal impairment
**ADV EFF** **Apnea, cardiac arrest, circulatory depression,** constipation,

dizziness, light-headedness, n/v, **respiratory arrest/depression, shock,** sweating
**INTERACTIONS** Alcohol, barbiturate anesthetics, CNS depressants, MAOIs, phenothiazines. Incompatible w/sols of barbiturates, aminophylline, heparin, iodide, morphine sulfate, methicillin, phenytoin, sodium bicarbonate, sulfadiazine, sulfisoxazole
**NC/PT** Contraindicated in preterm infants and in pts w/GI obstruction. May give diluted sol by slow IV injection. IM route preferred for repeated injections. Oral tablet/sol only indicated for severe pain; use lowest effective dose. Have opioid antagonist, facilities for assisted or controlled respiration on hand during parenteral administration. Pt should take safety precautions for CNS effects; use laxative if constipated; take drug 4–6 hr before next feeding if breastfeeding; report difficulty breathing, chest pain.

## mepolizumab (Nucala)
**CLASS** Antiasthmatic, interleukin antagonist monoclonal antibody
**PREG/CONT** Unkn/NA

**IND & DOSE** **Adjunct maint tx of pts ≥6 yr w/severe asthma w/eosinophilic phenotype.** *Adult, child ≥12 yr:* 100 mg subcut once q 4 wk. *Child 6–11 yr:* 40 mg subcut once q 4 wk. **Tx of eosinophilic granulomatosis w/polyangiitis.** *Adult:* 300 mg subcut as three separate 100-mg injections q 4 wk.
**ADV EFF** Back pain, fatigue, headache, **hypersensitivity reaction,** injection-site reaction, opportunistic infections
**NC/PT** Not for use in acute bronchospasm, status asthmaticus. Discontinue systemic/inhaled corticosteroids gradually w/initiation of therapy. Monitor for opportunistic infections, herpes zoster, helminth infections. Pt should learn proper administration of subcut injections, proper disposal of needles/syringes; rotate injection sites. Pt should enroll in preg registry (risks unkn); continue other therapies for asthma as indicated; report difficulty breathing, swelling, rash, s&sx of infection.

## meprobamate (generic)
**CLASS** Anxiolytic
**PREG/CONT** High risk/C-IV

**IND & DOSE** **Mgt of anxiety disorders.** *Adult:* 1,200–1,600 mg/d PO in three or four divided doses. Max, 2,400 mg/d. *Child 6–12 yr:* 100–200 mg PO bid–tid.
**ADJUST DOSE** Elderly pts
**ADV EFF** Ataxia, **bone marrow suppression,** dependence w/withdrawal reactions, dizziness, drowsiness, headache, impaired vision, **hypotensive crisis,** n/v/d, rash, **suicidality,** vertigo
**INTERACTIONS** Alcohol, CNS depressants, barbiturates, opioids
**NC/PT** Dispense least amount possible to depressed/addiction-prone pts. Withdraw gradually over 2 wk after long-term use. Not for use in preg (barrier contraceptives advised)/breastfeeding. Pt should avoid alcohol, take safety precautions for CNS effects, report thoughts of suicide.

**DANGEROUS DRUG**

## mercaptopurine (Purinethol, Purixan)
**CLASS** Antimetabolite, antineoplastic
**PREG/CONT** High risk/NA

**BBW** Reserve for pts w/established dx of acute lymphatic leukemia; serious adverse effects possible.
**IND & DOSE** **Tx of acute leukemia (lymphocytic, lymphoblastic) as part of combo therapy.** *Adult, child:* Induction, 1.5–2.5 mg/kg/d PO (50–75 mg/m$^2$).
**ADJUST DOSE** Renal impairment

**ADV EFF Bone marrow depression, hepatosplenic T-cell lymphoma, hepatotoxicity,** hyperuricemia, immunosuppression, n/v, stomatitis
**INTERACTIONS** Allopurinol, TNF blockers, warfarin
**NC/PT** Monitor CBC, LFTs regularly; dose adjustment may be needed. Oral suspension available. Not for use in preg (barrier contraceptives advised)/ breastfeeding. Maintain hydration. Pt should get regular checkups, report night sweats, fever, abd pain, weight loss.

## meropenem (Merrem IV)

**CLASS** Carbapenem antibiotic
**PREG/CONT** Unkn/NA

**IND & DOSE Tx of meningitis, intra-abd infections caused by susceptible strains.** *Adult:* 1 g IV q 8 hr. *Child ≥3 mo:* For meningitis: >50 kg, 2 g IV q 8 hr; <50 kg, 40 mg/kg IV q 8 hr. For intra-abd infections: >50 kg, 1 g IV q 8 hr; <50 kg, 20 mg/kg IV q 8 hr. *Child >32 wk:* 20 mg/kg IV q 8 hr if gestational age (GA) and postnatal age (PNA) <2 wk; 30 mg/kg IV q 8 hr if GA and PNA >2 wk. *Child <33 wk:* 20 mg/kg IV q 12 hr if GA and PNA <2 wk; q 8 hr if GA and PNA ≥2 wk. **Tx of skin/skin-structure infections caused by susceptible strains.** *Adult:* 500 mg IV q 8 hr. *Child ≥3 mo:* >50 kg, 500 mg IV q 8 hr; <50 kg, 10 mg/kg IV q 8 hr.
**ADJUST DOSE** Renal impairment
**ADV EFF** Abd pain, anorexia, CDAD, **cutaneous reactions,** flatulence, headache, **hypersensitivity reactions,** n/v/d, phlebitis, **pseudomembranous colitis,** rash, superinfections
**INTERACTIONS** Probenecid, valproic acid
**NC/PT** Culture before tx. Do not mix in sol w/other drugs. Stop if s&sx of colitis. Pt should report severe or bloody diarrhea, pain at injection site, difficulty breathing.

## mesalamine (Apriso, Asacol HD, Canasa, Delzicol, Lialda, Pentasa, Rowasa, Sfrowasa)

**CLASS** Anti-inflammatory
**PREG/CONT** Low risk/NA

**IND & DOSE Tx of active mild to moderate ulcerative colitis.** *Adult:* 2–4 1.2-g tablets PO once daily w/ food for total 2.4–4.8 g (*Lialda*). Or, 1.5 g/d PO (4 capsules) in a.m. for up to 6 mo (*Apriso*). Or, 1 g PO qid for total daily dose of 4 g for up to 8 wk (*Pentasa*). Or, 800 mg PO tid for 6 wk (*Asacol HD, Delzicol*). *Child ≥5 yr:* Base dose on weight bid for 6 wk (*Delzicol*). **Maint of remission of mild to moderate ulcerative colitis.** *Adult:* 1.6 g/d PO in two to four divided doses. **Tx of active, distal, mild to moderate ulcerative colitis/proctitis, proctosigmoiditis.** *Adult:* 60-mL units in 1 rectal instillation (4 g) once/d, preferably at bedtime, retained for approx 8 hr for 3–6 wk. Effects may occur within 3–21 d. Usual course, 3–6 wk. Or, 1,000 mg rectal instillation/d at bedtime for 3–6 wk (*Canasa*).
**ADJUST DOSE** Renal impairment
**ADV EFF** Abd pain, cramps, fatigue, fever, flatulence, flulike sx, gas, headache, hypersensitivity reactions, **liver failure,** malaise, renal impairment
**INTERACTIONS** Azathioprine, 6-mercaptopurine, nephrotoxic drugs, NSAIDs
**NC/PT** Products vary; use caution to differentiate doses. Monitor CBC, renal/hepatic function. Teach proper retention enema administration. Pt should swallow tablet whole and not cut/crush/chew it; report severe abd pain, difficulty breathing. Name confusion w/mesalamine, methenamine, memantine.

## mesna (Mesnex)

**CLASS** Cytoprotective
**PREG/CONT** Unkn/NA

**IND & DOSE Px to reduce incidence of ifosfamide-induced hemorrhagic cystitis.** *Adult:* 20% ifosfamide dose IV at time of ifosfamide infusion and at 4 and 8 hr after; timing must be exact.
**ADV EFF** Abd pain, alopecia, **anaphylaxis,** anemia, anorexia, constipation, fatigue, fever, n/v, **rash to SJS,** thrombocytopenia
**NC/PT** Not indicated to reduce risk of hematuria due to pathologic conditions. Contains benzyl alcohol; contraindicated in neonates, premature and low-birth-weight infants. Not for use in breastfeeding. Helps prevent chemo complications; timing critical to balance chemo effects. May give antiemetics. Monitor skin; stop if rash occurs. Pt should report severe abd pain, difficulty breathing, rash.

## metaproterenol sulfate (generic)

**CLASS** Antiasthmatic, $beta_2$-selective agonist, bronchodilator
**PREG/CONT** C/NA

**IND & DOSE Px, tx of bronchial asthma, reversible bronchospasm.** *Adult, child ≥12 yr:* 20 mg PO tid–qid. *Child >9–<12 yr, >27 kg:* 20 mg PO tid–qid. *Child 6–9 yr, <27 kg:* 10 mg PO tid–qid.
**ADJUST DOSE** Elderly pts
**ADV EFF** Anxiety, apprehension, CNS stimulation, fear, flushing, heartburn, n/v, pallor, sweating, tachycardia
**NC/PT** Switch to syrup if swallowing difficult. Protect tablets from moisture. Do not exceed recommended dose. Pt should take safety precautions for CNS effects; report chest pain, difficulty breathing.

## metaxalone (Skelaxin)

**CLASS** Skeletal muscle relaxant (centrally acting)
**PREG/CONT** C/NA

**IND & DOSE Adjunct for relief of discomfort associated w/acute, painful musculoskeletal disorders.** *Adult, child ≥12 yr:* 800 mg PO tid–qid.
**ADV EFF** Dizziness, drowsiness, **hemolytic anemia, leukopenia,** light-headedness, nausea
**INTERACTIONS** Alcohol, CNS depressants
**NC/PT** Arrange for other tx for muscle spasm relief. Pt should take safety precautions for CNS effects, avoid alcohol, report rash, yellowing of skin/eyes.

**DANGEROUS DRUG**

## metFORMIN hydrochloride (Glumetza, Riomet)

**CLASS** Antidiabetic
**PREG/CONT** Low risk/NA

**BBW** Risk of severe lactic acidosis. Monitor pt; treat if suspicion of lactic acidosis. Risk factors include renal/hepatic impairment, concomitant use of certain drugs, >65 yr, radiologic studies w/contrast, surgery/other procedures, hypoxic states, excessive alcohol intake.
**IND & DOSE Adjunct to diet to lower blood glucose in type 2 diabetes, alone or w/sulfonylurea.** *Adult:* 500 mg PO bid or 850 mg PO once daily; max, 2,550 mg/d in divided doses. ER tablet: 1,000 mg/d PO w/evening meal; max, 2,000 mg/d. *Child 10–16 yr:* 500 mg bid w/meals. Max, 2,000 mg/d in divided doses. ER form not recommended for child.
**ADJUST DOSE** Elderly pts, renal impairment
**ADV EFF** Allergic skin reactions, anorexia, gastric discomfort, heartburn, hypoglycemia, **lactic acidosis,** n/v/d, vitamin $B_{12}$ deficiency

**INTERACTIONS** Alcohol, amiloride, celery, cimetidine, coriander, dandelion root, digoxin, fenugreek, furosemide, garlic, ginseng, iodinated contrast media, juniper berries, nifedipine, sulfonylureas, vancomycin **NC/PT** Monitor serum glucose frequently to determine drug effectiveness, dose. Arrange for transfer to insulin during high-stress periods. Not for use in preg/breastfeeding. Pt should swallow ER tablet whole and not cut/crush/chew it; take at night if GI problems; avoid alcohol; continue diet/exercise program; report all herbs used (so dose adjustment can be made), hypoglycemic episodes, urine/stool color changes, difficulty breathing.

**DANGEROUS DRUG**

## methadone hydrochloride (Dolophine, Methadose)

**CLASS** Opioid agonist analgesic
**PREG/CONT** High risk/C-II

**BBW** Use for opioid addiction should be part of approved program; deaths have occurred during start of tx for opioid dependence. Carefully determine all drugs pt taking; respiratory depression and death have occurred. Have emergency services on standby. Monitor for prolonged QT, especially at higher doses. Neonatal withdrawal syndrome if used in preg.

Accidental ingestion, especially by child, can cause fatal overdose. Many drug interactions w/methadone can result in death (especially other CNS depressants; CYP3A4, 2B6, 2C9, 2C19, 2D6 inhibitors; discontinuation of concomitantly used CYP3A4 2B6, 2C9, 2C19 inducers).

**IND & DOSE** **Relief of severe pain, requiring around-the-clock tx, unresponsive to nonopioid analgesics.** *Adult:* 2.5–10 mg IM, subcut, or PO q 8–12 hr as needed. **Detoxification, temporary maint tx of opioid addiction.** *Adult:* 20–30 mg PO or parenteral; PO preferred. Increase to suppress withdrawal s&sx; 40 mg/d in single or divided doses is usual stabilizing dose. Continue stabilizing doses for 2–3 d, then gradually decrease q 1 or 2 d. Provide sufficient amount to keep withdrawal sx tolerable. Max, 21 days' tx; do not repeat earlier than 4 wk after completion of previous course. For maint tx: For heavy heroin users up until hospital admission, initially 20 mg PO 4–8 hr after heroin stopped or 40 mg PO in single dose; may give additional 10-mg doses if needed to suppress withdrawal syndrome. Adjust dose to max 120 mg/d PO.
**ADJUST DOSE** Elderly pts, impaired adults
**ADV EFF** **Apnea, cardiac arrest, circulatory depression,** constipation, dizziness, light-headedness, hypotension, n/v, **prolonged QT, respiratory arrest, respiratory depression, shock,** sweating
**INTERACTIONS** Barbiturate anesthetics, CNS depressants, CYP3A4 inducers/inhibitors, HIV antiretrovirals, hydantoins, protease inhibitors, QT-prolonging drugs, rifampin, urine acidifiers
**NC/PT** Have opioid antagonist, equipment for assisted or controlled respiration on hand during parenteral administration. Do not stop suddenly in physically dependent pt. Not for use in preg (barrier contraceptives advised); neonatal opioid withdrawal syndrome expected outcome of prolonged opioid use during preg. Not for use w/impaired consciousness or coma w/head injury. Pt should take drug 4–6 hr before next feeding if breastfeeding, avoid alcohol, take safety precautions for CNS effects, report difficulty breathing, severe n/v.

## methazolamide (generic)

**CLASS** Carbonic anhydrase inhibitor, glaucoma drug
**PREG/CONT** C/NA

**IND & DOSE** **Tx of ocular conditions where lowering IOP is beneficial.** *Adult:* 50–100 mg PO bid–tid.

**ADJUST DOSE** Hepatic, renal impairment
**ADV EFF** Anorexia, **bone marrow suppression,** dizziness, drowsiness, fatigue, GI disturbances, kidney stones, photosensitivity, **SJS,** taste alteration, tingling, tinnitus
**INTERACTIONS** Aspirin, corticosteroids
**NC/PT** Monitor IOP regularly. Pt should take safety precautions for CNS effects; avoid exposure sun, infection; report fever, rash.

**methenamine** (generic), **methenamine hippurate** (Hiprex, Urex)
**CLASS** Antibacterial, urinary tract anti-infective
**PREG/CONT** C/NA

**IND & DOSE To suppress, eliminate bacteriuria associated w/UTIs.** *Adult:* 1 g methenamine PO qid after meals and at bedtime, or 1 g hippurate PO bid. *Child 6–12 yr:* 500 mg methenamine PO qid, or 0.5–1 g hippurate PO bid. *Child <6 yr:* 50 mg/kg/d PO methenamine divided into three doses.
**ADV EFF** Bladder irritation, dysuria, **hepatotoxicity** (hippurate), nausea, rash
**NC/PT** Culture before tx. Maintain hydration. Monitor LFTs w/hippurate form. Use additional measures for UTIs. Pt should take w/food, report rash, urine/stool color changes. Name confusion between methimazole and mesalamine.

**methIMAzole** (Tapazole)
**CLASS** Antithyroid drug
**PREG/CONT** D/NA

**IND & DOSE Tx of hyperthyroidism; palliation in certain thyroid cancers.** *Adult:* 15–60 mg/d PO in three equal doses q 8 hr. Maint, 5–15 mg/d PO. *Child:* 0.4 mg/kg/d PO, then maint of approx ½ initial dose. Or, initially, 0.5–0.7 mg/kg/d or 15–20 mg/m²/d PO in three divided doses, then maint of ⅓–⅔ initial dose, starting when pt becomes euthyroid. Max, 30 mg/24 hr.
**ADV EFF Bone marrow suppression,** dizziness, neuritis, paresthesia, rash, vertigo, weakness
**INTERACTIONS** Cardiac glycosides, metoprolol, oral anticoagulants, propranolol, theophylline
**NC/PT** Monitor CBC, thyroid function. Tx will be long-term. Not for use in preg (barrier contraceptives advised)/breastfeeding. Pt should take safety precautions for CNS effects, report unusual bleeding/bruising, s&sx of infection.

**methocarbamol** (Robaxin)
**CLASS** Skeletal muscle relaxant
**PREG/CONT** C/NA

**IND & DOSE Relief of discomfort associated w/acute, painful musculoskeletal conditions.** *Adult:* 1.5 g PO qid. For first 48–72 hr, 6 g/d or up to 8 g/d recommended. Maint, 1 g PO qid, or 750 mg q 4 hr, or 1.5 g tid for total 4–4.5 g/d. Or, 1 g IM or IV; may need 2–3 g in severe cases. Do not use 3 g/d for >3 d. **Control of neuromuscular manifestations of tetanus.** *Adult:* Up to 24 g/d PO or 1 g IM or IV; may need 2–3 g for no longer than 3 d. *Child:* 15 mg/kg IV repeated q 6 hr as needed.
**ADV EFF** Bradycardia, discolored urine, dizziness, drowsiness, headache, nausea, urticaria
**NC/PT** Have pt remain recumbent during and for at least 15 min after IV injection. For IM, do not inject >5 mL into each gluteal region; repeat at 8-hr intervals. Switch from parenteral to oral route as soon as possible. Not for use in preg/breastfeeding. Urine may darken to green, brown, black on standing. Pt should take safety precautions for CNS effects; avoid alcohol.

DANGEROUS DRUG

**methotrexate** (Otrexup, Rasuvo, Reditrex, Trexall, Xatmep)
**CLASS** Antimetabolite, antineoplastic, antipsoriatic, antirheumatic
**PREG/CONT** High risk/NA

**BBW** Arrange for CBC, urinalysis, LFTs/renal function tests, chest X-ray before, during, and for several wk after tx; severe toxicity possible. Rule out preg before tx; counsel pt on severe risks of fetal abnormalities. Reserve use for life-threatening neoplastic diseases, severe psoriasis/RA unresponsive to other tx. Monitor LFTs carefully w/long-term use; serious hepatotoxicity possible. High risk of serious opportunistic infections, interstitial pneumonitis, serious to fatal skin reactions, intestinal perforation; monitor closely during tx. Use cautiously w/malignant lymphomas, rapidly growing tumors; worsening of malignancy possible.
**IND & DOSE Tx of choriocarcinoma, other trophoblastic diseases.** *Adult:* 15–30 mg PO or IM daily for 5-day course. Repeat course three–five times w/rest periods of 1 wk or longer between courses until toxic sx subside. **Tx of leukemia.** *Adult:* Induction: 3.3 mg/m$^2$ methotrexate PO or IM w/60 mg/m$^2$ prednisone daily for 4–6 wk. Maint, 30 mg/m$^2$ methotrexate PO or IM twice wkly or 2.5 mg/kg IV q 14 d. *Child:* 20 mg/m$^2$ PO as component of combo chemo (*Xatmep*). **Tx of meningeal leukemia.** *Adult:* Give methotrexate intrathecally as px in lymphocytic leukemia. 12 mg/m$^2$ (max, 15 mg) intrathecally at intervals of 2–5 d; repeat until CSF cell count normal, then give one additional dose. *Child:* ≥3 yr, 12 mg intrathecally q 2–5 d. 2–3 yr, 10 mg intrathecally q 2–5 d. 1–2 yr, 8 mg intrathecally q 2–5 d. <1 yr, 6 mg intrathecally q 2–5 d. **Tx of lymphomas.** *Adult:* Burkitt tumor (stages I, II), 10–25 mg/d PO for 4–8 d. Stage III, use w/other neoplastic drugs. All usually require several courses of tx w/7- to 10-day rest periods between doses. **Tx of mycosis fungoides.** *Adult:* 2.5–10 mg/d PO for wks or mos, or 50 mg IM once wkly, or 25 mg IM twice wkly. Can also give IV w/combo chemo regimens in advanced disease. **Tx of osteosarcoma.** *Adult:* 12 g/m$^2$ or up to 15 g/m$^2$ IV to give peak serum conc of 1,000 micromol. Must use as part of cytotoxic regimen w/leucovorin rescue. **Tx of severe psoriasis.** *Adult:* 10–25 mg/wk PO, IM, subcut, or IV as single wkly dose; max, 30 mg/wk. Or, 2.5 mg PO at 12-hr intervals for three doses each wk. **Tx of severe RA.** *Adult:* Single doses of 7.5 mg/wk PO or subcut (*Otrexup, Rasuvo, Reditrex*) or divided dose of 2.5 mg PO at 12-hr intervals for three doses as a course once wkly. Max, 20 mg/wk. **Tx of polyarticular course juvenile RA.** *Child 2–16 yr:* 10 mg/m$^2$ PO wkly; max, 20 mg/m$^2$/wk. Or 10 mg/m$^2$/wk subcut (*Otrexup, Reditrex, Xatmep*).
**ADV EFF** Alopecia, **anaphylaxis,** blurred vision, chills, dizziness, fatigue, fertility alterations, fever, **interstitial pneumonitis,** n/v/d, rash, **renal failure, serious to fatal skin reactions, severe bone marrow depression, sudden death,** ulcerative stomatitis
**INTERACTIONS** Alcohol, digoxin, NSAIDs (serious to fatal reactions), phenytoin, probenecid, salicylates, sulfonamides, theophylline
**NC/PT** Monitor CBC, LFTs, renal/pulmonary function regularly. Have leucovorin or levoleucovorin on hand as antidote for methotrexate overdose or when large doses used. Not for use in preg (men, women should use contraceptives during, for 3 mo after tx)/breastfeeding. Give antiemetic for n/v. Autoinjector for adults/juveniles using home injections. Pt should avoid alcohol, NSAIDs; cover head at temp extremes (hair loss possible); perform frequent mouth care; take safety precautions for CNS effects; report

urine changes, abd pain, black tarry stools, unusual bleeding, difficulty breathing, rash, s&sx of infection.

**methoxsalen** (Oxsoralen-Ultra, Uvadex)
**CLASS** Psoralen
**PREG/CONT** C/NA

**BBW** Reserve use for severe/disabling disorders unresponsive to traditional tx; risk of eye/skin damage, melanoma. Brand names not interchangeable; use extreme caution.
**IND & DOSE** **Tx of disabling psoriasis; repigmentation of vitiliginous skin; cutaneous T-cell lymphoma.** *Adult:* Dose varies by weight. Must time tx w/UV exposure; see manufacturer's details.
**ADV EFF** Depression, dizziness, headache, itching, leg cramps, **melanoma, ocular/skin damage,** swelling
**INTERACTIONS** Anthralin, coal tar/coal tar derivatives, fluoroquinolones, griseofulvin, methylene blue, nalidixic acid, phenothiazines, sulfonamides, tetracyclines, thiazides/certain organic staining dyes
**NC/PT** Do not use w/actinic degeneration; basal cell carcinomas; radiation, arsenic tx; hepatic, cardiac disease. Alert pt to adverse effects, including ocular damage, melanoma. Must time tx w/UV light exposure. Pt should mark calendar for tx days, take safety precautions if dizzy, report vision changes.

**methscopolamine bromide** (generic)
**CLASS** Anticholinergic, antispasmodic
**PREG/CONT** C/NA

**IND & DOSE** **Adjunct tx of peptic ulcer.** *Adult:* 2.5 mg PO 30 min before meals, 2.5–5 mg PO at bedtime.
**ADV EFF** Altered taste perception, blurred vision, decreased sweating, dry mouth, dysphagia, n/v, urinary hesitancy, urine retention
**INTERACTIONS** Anticholinergics, antipsychotics, haloperidol, TCAs
**NC/PT** Pt should maintain adequate hydration, empty bladder before each dose, avoid hot environments, use sugarless lozenges for dry mouth, take safety precautions w/vision changes, report difficulty swallowing, palpitations.

**methsuximide** (Celontin)
**CLASS** Antiepileptic, succinimide
**PREG/CONT** C/NA

**IND & DOSE** **Control of absence seizures.** *Adult:* 300 mg/d PO for first wk; titrate to max 1.2 g/d.
**ADV EFF** Aggression, ataxia, **blood dyscrasias,** blurred vision, dizziness, drowsiness, headache, nervousness **hepatotoxicity,** n/v/d, **SJS, SLE, suicidality**
**INTERACTIONS** Other antiepileptics
**NC/PT** Monitor CBC, LFTs w/long-term tx. Not for use in preg (barrier contraceptives advised)/breastfeeding. Pt should take safety precaution for CNS effects; report rash, urine/stool color changes, thoughts of suicide.

**methyldopa, methyldopate hydrochloride** (generic)
**CLASS** Antihypertensive, sympatholytic
**PREG/CONT** B (oral); C (IV)/NA

**IND & DOSE** **Tx of HTN.** *Adult:* 250 mg PO bid–tid in first 48 hr; maint, 500 mg–2 g/d PO in two–four doses. If given w/other antihypertensives, limit initial dose to 500 mg/d in divided doses. *Child:* 10 mg/kg/d PO in two–four doses. Max, 65 mg/kg/d PO or 3 g/d PO, whichever less. **Tx of hypertensive crisis.** *Adult:* 250–500 mg IV q 6 hr as needed; max, 1 g q 6 hr. Switch to oral tx as soon as

control attained. *Child:* 20–40 mg/kg/d IV in divided doses q 6 hr. Max, 65 mg/kg or 3 g/d, whichever less.
**ADJUST DOSE** Elderly pts, renal impairment
**ADV EFF** Asthenia, bradycardia, constipation, decreased mental acuity, distention, headache, **hemolytic anemia, hepatotoxicity, HF, myocarditis,** n/v, rash, sedation, weakness
**INTERACTIONS** General anesthetics, levodopa, lithium, sympathomimetics
**NC/PT** Give IV slowly over 30–60 min; monitor injection site. Monitor CBC, LFTs periodically. Monitor BP carefully when stopping; HTN usually returns within 48 hr. Pt should take safety precautions for CNS effects; report urine/stool color changes, rash, unusual tiredness.

## methylene blue (generic)

**CLASS** Antidote, diagnostic agent, urinary tract anti-infective
**PREG/CONT** C/NA

**BBW** Avoid use w/serotonergic drugs due to possible serious or fatal serotonin syndrome.
**IND & DOSE Tx of cyanide poisoning, drug-induced methemoglobinemia; GU antiseptic for cystitis, urethritis.** *Adult, child:* 65–130 mg PO tid w/full glass of water. Or, 1–2 mg/kg IV or 25–50 mg/m$^2$ IV injected over several min. May repeat after 1 hr.
**ADV EFF** Blue-green stool, confusion, discolored urine, dizziness, n/v
**INTERACTIONS** SSRIs
**NC/PT** Give IV slowly over several min; do not give subcut or intrathecally. Contact w/skin will dye skin blue; may remove stain w/hypochlorite sol. Use other measures to decrease UTI incidence. Urine/stool may turn blue-green. Pt should take safety measures for CNS effects, report severe n/v.

## methylergonovine maleate (Methergine)

**CLASS** Ergot derivative, oxytocic
**PREG/CONT** C/NA

**IND & DOSE Routine mgt after delivery of placenta; tx of postpartum atony, hemorrhage; subinvolution of uterus; uterine stimulation during second stage of labor after delivery of anterior shoulder.** *Adult:* 0.2 mg IM or IV slowly over at least 60 sec, after delivery of placenta/anterior shoulder, or during puerperium. May repeat q 2–4 hr, then 0.2 mg PO three or four ×/d in puerperium for up to 1 wk.
**ADV EFF** Dizziness, headache, HTN, nausea
**INTERACTIONS** CYP3A4 inhibitors, ergot alkaloids, vasoconstrictors
**NC/PT** Reserve IV use for emergency; monitor BP/bleeding postpartum; use for no longer than 1 wk. Pt should report increased vaginal bleeding, numb/cold extremities.

## methylnaltrexone bromide (Relistor)

**CLASS** Opioid receptor antagonist, laxative
**PREG/CONT** High risk/NA

**IND & DOSE Tx of opioid-induced constipation (OIC) in adults w/chronic noncancer pain, including pts w/chronic pain related to prior cancer or its treatment who do not need frequent (eg, wkly) opioid dosage escalation.** *Adult:* 12 mg subcut daily; 450 mg PO once daily in a.m. **Tx of OIC in adults w/advanced illness or pain caused by active cancer who need opioid dosage escalation for palliative care.** *Adult:* 62–114 kg, 12 mg subcut q other day; 38–<62 kg, 8 mg subcut q other day. If weight not in above range, 0.15 mg/kg subcut q other day.
**ADJUST DOSE** Renal impairment

**ADV EFF** Abd pain, diarrhea, dizziness, flatulence, **GI perforation,** hyperhidrosis, nausea
**INTERACTIONS** Opioid antagonists
**NC/PT** Avoid use in preg/breastfeeding. Teach proper administration/disposal of needles/syringes. Discontinue laxatives before start of therapy; may resume after 3 d if needed. Pt should inject in upper arm, abdomen, or thigh; take tablets w/water on empty stomach at least 30 min before first meal of day; take safety precautions w/dizziness; report acute abd pain, severe diarrhea.

**methylphenidate hydrochloride** (Adhansia XR, Aptensio XR, Concerta, Daytrana, Metadate, Methylin, Quillichew ER, Quillivant XR, Ritalin)
**CLASS** CNS stimulant
**PREG/CONT** Moderate risk/C-II

**BBW** Potential for abuse; use caution w/emotionally unstable pts, pts w/hx of drug dependence or alcoholism.
**IND & DOSE** **Tx of narcolepsy (*Ritalin, Ritalin SR, Metadate ER, Methylin*); tx of attention-deficit disorders, hyperkinetic syndrome, minimal brain dysfx in child, adult w/behavioral syndrome.** *Adult:* Range, 10–60 mg/d PO. ER: 18 mg/d PO in a.m. May increase by 18 mg/d at 1-wk intervals; max, 54 mg/d (*Concerta*). *Adhansia XR: Adult, child ≥6 yr:* Initially, 25 mg PO (in a.m.)/d; may increase in 10- to 15-mg increments. *Aptensio XR:* 10 mg/d PO; titrate to max 60 mg/d. Or, 10- to 20-mg/d increments to max 60 mg/d (*Metadate CD, Ritalin LA*). *Child 13–17 yr:* 18 mg/d PO in a.m. Titrate to max 72 mg/d PO; do not exceed 2 mg/kg/d. Or, 10–30 mg/d transdermal patch; apply 2 hr before effect needed, remove after 9 hr. *Child 6–12 yr:* 5 mg PO before breakfast, lunch w/gradual increments of 5–10 mg wkly; max, 60 mg/d. ER: Use adult dose up to max 54 mg/d or 60 mg/d (*Aptensio XR, Quillichew ER, Quillivant XR*) PO. Or, 10–30 mg/d transdermal patch; apply 2 hr before effect needed, remove after 9 hr.
**ADV EFF** Abd pain, angina, anorexia, cardiac arrhythmias, changes in P/BP, chemical leukoderma, contact sensitization w/transdermal patch, growth changes, insomnia, nausea, nervousness, rash, visual disturbances
**INTERACTIONS** Alcohol, MAOIs, oral anticoagulants, phenytoin, SSRIs, TCAs
**NC/PT** Ensure proper dx; rule out underlying cardiac problems. Baseline ECG recommended. Stop tx periodically to evaluate sx. Used as part of overall tx program. Monitor growth in child. Not for use in breastfeeding. Alert pts that *Quillichew ER* contains phenylalanine; risk in phenylketonurics. Monitor BP frequently when starting tx. Pt should swallow ER tablet whole and not cut/crush/chew it; take before 6 p.m. to avoid sleep disturbances; apply patch to clean, dry area of hip (remove old patch before applying new one); avoid heating pads on patch; shake bottle vigorously before each use (suspension); keep in secure place; report chest pain, nervousness, insomnia. Controlled substance; secure drug.

**methyLPREDNISolone** (Medrol), **methyLPREDNISolone acetate** (Depo-Medrol), **methyLPREDNISolone sodium succinate** (Solu-Medrol)
**CLASS** Corticosteroid, hormone
**PREG/CONT** High risk/NA

**IND & DOSE** **Short-term mgt of inflammatory/allergic disorders, thrombocytopenic purpura, erythroblastopenia, ulcerative colitis, acute exacerbations of MS, trichinosis w/neuro/cardiac involvement; px of n/v w/chemo.** *Adult:* 4–48 mg/d PO. Alternate-day tx: twice usual dose

q other a.m. Or, 10–40 mg IV over several min. Or, high-dose tx: 30 mg/kg IV infused over 10–30 min; repeat q 4–6 hr but not longer than 72 hr. *Child:* Minimum dose, 0.5 mg/kg/d PO; base dose on actual response. **Maint tx of RA.** *Adult:* 40–120 mg/wk IM. **Adrenogenital syndrome.** *Adult:* 40 mg IM q 2 wk. **Dermatologic lesions.** *Adult:* 40–120 mg/wk IM for 1–4 wk. **Asthma, allergic rhinitis.** *Adult:* 80–120 mg IM. **Intralesional.** *Adult:* 20–60 mg. **Intra-articular.** *Adult:* Dose depends on site of injection: 4–10 mg (small joints); 10–40 mg (medium); 20–80 mg (large).
**ADV EFF** Aggravation of infections, amenorrhea, **anaphylactic reactions,** edema, fluid retention, headache, hyperglycemia, hypotension, immunosuppression, impaired healing, increased appetite, **shock,** vertigo
**INTERACTIONS** Azole antifungals, edrophonium, erythromycin, live vaccines, neostigmine, phenytoin, potassium-depleting drugs, pyridostigmine, rifampin, salicylates, troleandomycin
**NC/PT** Individualize dose based on severity, response. Give daily dose before 9 a.m. to minimize adrenal suppression. For maint, reduce initial dose in small increments at intervals until lowest satisfactory clinical dose reached. If long-term tx needed, consider alternate-day therapy w/short-acting corticosteroid. After long-term tx, withdraw slowly to prevent adrenal insufficiency. Use caution in preg (monitor newborn carefully for hypoadrenalism). Not for use in breastfeeding. Monitor serum glucose. Pt should avoid exposure to infections; report difficulty breathing, s&sx of infection, black tarry stools.

## metoclopramide (Reglan)
**CLASS** Antiemetic, dopaminergic, GI stimulant
**PREG/CONT** Low risk/NA

**BBW** Long-term tx associated w/ permanent tardive dyskinesia; risk increases w/pts >60 yr, especially women. Use smallest dose possible. Max, 3 mo of tx.
**IND & DOSE** **Relief of gastroparesis sx.** *Adult:* 10 mg PO 30 min before each meal and at bedtime for 2–8 wk; severe, 10 mg IM or IV for up to 10 d until sx subside. **Tx of symptomatic gastroesophageal reflux.** *Adult:* 10–15 mg PO up to four ×/d 30 min before meals and at bedtime for max 12 wk. **Px of postop n/v.** *Adult:* 10–20 mg IM at end of surgery. **Px of chemo-induced vomiting.** *Adult:* IV infusion over at least 15 min. First dose 30 min before chemo; repeat q 2 hr for two doses, then q 3 hr for three doses. For highly emetogenic drugs (cisplatin, dacarbazine), initial two doses, 1–2 mg/kg. If extrapyramidal sx, give 50 mg diphenhydramine IM. **Facilitation of small-bowel intubation, gastric emptying.** *Adult:* 10 mg (2 mL) by direct IV injection over 1–2 min. *Child 6–14 yr:* 2.5–5 mg by direct IV injection over 1–2 min. *Child <6 yr:* 0.1 mg/kg by direct IV injection over 1–2 min.
**ADV EFF** Diarrhea, drowsiness, extrapyramidal reactions, fatigue, lassitude, nausea, restlessness
**INTERACTIONS** Alcohol, CNS depressants, cyclosporine, digoxin, succinylcholine
**NC/PT** Monitor BP w/IV use. Give diphenhydramine for extrapyramidal reactions. Pt should take safety precautions for CNS effects, avoid alcohol, report involuntary movements, severe diarrhea.

## metOLazone (Zaroxolyn)
**CLASS** Thiazide diuretic
**PREG/CONT** B/NA

**BBW** Do not interchange *Zaroxolyn* w/other formulations; not therapeutically equivalent.
**IND & DOSE** **Tx of HTN.** *Adult:* 2.5–5 mg/d PO. **Tx of edema from systemic disease.** *Adult:* 5–20 mg/d PO.
**ADV EFF** Anorexia, **bone marrow depression,** dizziness, dry mouth,

nocturia, n/v/d, orthostatic hypotension, photophobia, polyuria, vertigo
**INTERACTIONS** Antidiabetics, cholestyramine, colestipol, diazoxide, dofetilide, lithium
**NC/PT** Withdraw drug 2–3 d before elective surgery; for emergency surgery, reduce preanesthetic/anesthetic dose. Pt should take early in day to avoid sleep interruption; avoid sun exposure; weigh self daily, report changes of ≥3 lb/d; report unusual bleeding.

**DANGEROUS DRUG**

## metoprolol, metoprolol succinate, metoprolol tartrate (Lopressor)

**CLASS** Antihypertensive, selective beta blocker
**PREG/CONT** Low risk/NA

**BBW** Do not stop abruptly after long-term tx (hypersensitivity to catecholamines possible, causing angina exacerbation, MI, ventricular arrhythmias). Taper gradually over 2 wk w/ monitoring. Pts w/bronchospastic diseases should not, in general, receive beta blockers. Use w/caution only in pts unresponsive to or intolerant of other antihypertensives.
**IND & DOSE** **Tx of HTN.** *Adult:* 100 mg/d PO; maint, 100–450 mg/d. Or, 25–100 mg/d ER tablet PO; max, 400 mg/d. **Tx of angina pectoris.** *Adult:* 100 mg/d PO in two divided doses; range, 100–400 mg/d. Or, 100 mg/d ER tablet PO. **Early tx of MI.** *Adult:* 3 IV boluses of 5 mg each at 2-min intervals, then 50 mg PO 15 min after last IV dose and q 6 hr for 48 hr. Then maint of 100 mg PO bid. **Late tx of MI.** *Adult:* 100 mg PO bid as soon as possible after infarct, continuing for at least 3 mo–3 yr. **Tx of HF.** *Adult:* 12.5–25 mg/d ER tablet PO for 2 wk; max, 200 mg/d.
**ADV EFF** ANA development, **bronchospasm,** cardiac arrhythmias, constipation, decreased exercise tolerance/libido, dizziness, ED, flatulence, gastric pain, HF, **laryngospasm,** n/v/d, paresthesia
**INTERACTIONS** Barbiturates, cimetidine, clonidine, epinephrine, hydralazine, lidocaine, methimazole, NSAIDs, prazosin, propylthiouracil, rifampin, verapamil
**NC/PT** Monitor cardiac function w/ IV use. Pt should swallow ER tablet whole and not cut/crush/chew it; take safety precautions for CNS effects; report difficulty breathing, swelling.

## metreleptin (Myalept)

**CLASS** Leptin analog
**PREG/CONT** Unkn/NA

**BBW** Risk of development of antimetreleptin antibodies, w/loss of drug efficacy and worsening metabolic issues, severe infections; test for antibodies in pts w/severe infection or loss of efficacy. Risk of T-cell lymphoma; assess risk in pts w/hematologic abnormalities and/or acquired generalized lipodystrophy. Available only through restricted access program.
**IND & DOSE** **Adjunct to diet as replacement tx in leptin deficiency in pts w/congenital or acquired lipodystrophy.** *Adult, child ≤40 kg:* 0.06 mg/kg/d subcut; max, 0.13 mg/kg. *Males >40 kg:* 2.5 mg/d subcut; max 10 mg/d. *Females >40 kg:* 5 mg/d subcut; max 10 mg/d.
**ADV EFF** Abd pain, autoimmune disorder progression, **benzyl alcohol toxicity,** headache, hypersensitivity reactions, hypoglycemia, **T-cell lymphoma,** weight loss
**NC/PT** Ensure proper use of drug; only use for approved indication. Monitor for infections; test for antibody development. Dilute w/Bacteriostatic Water for Injection or Sterile Water for Injection; avoid benzyl alcohol when using drug in neonates, infants. Pt should learn proper reconstitution, subcut administration, proper disposal of syringes; avoid preg/breastfeeding; report difficulty

breathing, dizziness, fever, sx of infection.

**metroNIDAZOLE** (Flagyl, MetroCream, MetroGel, Nuvessa)
**CLASS** Amebicide, antibiotic, antiprotozoal
**PREG/CONT** Unkn/NA

**BBW** Avoid use unless needed; possibly carcinogenic.
**IND & DOSE** **Tx of amebiasis.** *Adult:* 750 mg PO tid for 5–10 d. *Child:* 35–50 mg/kg/d PO in three divided doses for 10 d. **Tx of antibiotic-associated pseudomembranous colitis.** *Adult:* 1–2 g/d PO in three–four divided doses for 7–10 d. **Tx of *Gardnerella vaginalis* infection.** *Adult:* 500 mg PO bid for 7 d. **Tx of giardiasis.** *Adult:* 250 mg PO tid for 7 d. **Tx of trichomoniasis.** *Adult:* 2 g PO in 1 d (1-d tx) or 250 mg PO tid for 7 d. **Tx of bacterial vaginosis.** Nonpreg women, 750 mg PO daily for 7 d, or 1 applicator intravaginally one–two ×/d for 5 d. Preg women, 750 mg/d PO for 7 d; avoid in first trimester. **Tx of anaerobic bacterial infection.** *Adult:* 15 mg/kg IV infused over 1 hr, then 7.5 mg/kg infused over 1 hr q 6 hr for 7–10 d; max, 4 g/d. **Preop, intraop, postop px for pts undergoing colorectal surgery.** *Adult:* 15 mg/kg infused IV over 30–60 min, completed about 1 hr before surgery; then 7.5 mg/kg infused over 30–60 min at 6- to 12-hr intervals after initial dose during day of surgery only. **Tx of inflammatory papules, pustules, erythema of rosacea.** Apply, rub in thin film bid (a.m. and p.m.) to entire affected areas after washing; for 9 wk.
**ADV EFF** Anorexia, ataxia, darkened urine, dizziness, dry mouth, headache, injection-site reactions, n/v/d, superinfections, unpleasant metallic taste
**INTERACTIONS** Alcohol, barbiturates, disulfiram, oral anticoagulants
**NC/PT** Not for use in breastfeeding. Urine may darken. Pt should take full course; take orally w/food; avoid alcohol or alcohol-containing preparations during and for 24–72 after tx (severe reactions possible); use sugarless lozenges for dry mouth/metallic taste; report severe GI problems, fever.

**metyrosine** (Demser)
**CLASS** Enzyme inhibitor
**PREG/CONT** C/NA

**IND & DOSE** **Mgt of pheochromocytoma.** *Adult, child >12 yr:* 250–500 mg PO qid. **Preop preparation for pheochromocytoma surgery.** *Adult, child >12 yr:* 2–3 g/d PO for 5–7 d; max, 4 g/d.
**ADV EFF** Anxiety, diarrhea, dysuria, extrapyramidal effects, gynecomastia, hypotension, insomnia, sedation
**INTERACTIONS** Alcohol, CNS depressants, haloperidol, phenothiazines
**NC/PT** Maintain hydration. Antidiarrheals may be needed. Give supportive care throughout surgery. Monitor for hypotension. Pt should avoid alcohol.

**DANGEROUS DRUG**

**mexiletine hydrochloride** (generic)
**CLASS** Antiarrhythmic
**PREG/CONT** C/NA

**BBW** Reserve for life-threatening arrhythmias; possible serious proarrhythmic effects.
**IND & DOSE** **Tx of documented life-threatening ventricular arrhythmias.** *Adult:* 200 mg PO q 8 hr. Increase in 50- to 100-mg increments q 2–3 d until desired antiarrhythmic effect. Max, 1,200 mg/d PO. Rapid control, 400 mg loading dose, then 200 mg PO q 8 hr. Transferring from other antiarrhythmics: Lidocaine, stop lidocaine w/first mexiletine dose; leave IV line open until adequate arrhythmia suppression ensured. Quinidine sulfate, initially 200 mg PO 6–12 hr after last

quinidine dose. Disopyramide, 200 mg PO 6–12 hr after last disopyramide dose.
**ADV EFF** **Cardiac arrhythmias,** chest pain, coordination difficulties, dizziness, dyspnea, headache, heartburn, light-headedness, n/v, rash, tremors, visual disturbances
**INTERACTIONS** Hydantoins, propafenone, rifampin, theophylline
**NC/PT** Monitor for safe, effective serum level (0.5–2 mcg/mL); monitor cardiac rhythm frequently. Pt should not stop w/o consulting prescriber, take safety precautions for CNS effects, report chest pain, excessive tremors, lack of coordination.

**DANGEROUS DRUG**

## micafungin sodium
(Mycamine)
**CLASS** Antifungal, echinocandin
**PREG/CONT** Moderate risk/NA

**IND & DOSE** **Tx of esophageal candidiasis.** *Adult:* 150 mg/d by IV infusion over 1 hr for 10–30 d. *Child >30 kg and ≥4 mo:* 2.5 mg/kg/d IV; max, 150 mg/d. *Child ≤30 kg and ≥4 mo:* 3 mg/kg/d IV. **Px of candidal infections in pts undergoing hematopoietic stem-cell transplantation.** *Adult:* 50 mg/d by IV infusion over 1 hr for about 19 d. *Child ≥4 mo:* 1 mg/kg/d IV; max, 50 mg/d. **Tx of systemic candidal infections, *Candida* peritonitis, abscesses.** *Adult:* 100 mg/d by IV infusion over 1 hr for 10–47 d based on infection. *Child ≥4 mo:* 2 mg/kg/d IV.
**ADV EFF** Headache, **hemolytic anemia, hepatotoxicity,** nausea, phlebitis, **renal toxicity, serious hypersensitivity reaction**
**INTERACTIONS** Itraconazole, nifedipine, sirolimus
**NC/PT** Obtain baseline, periodic CBC, LFTs, renal function tests. Monitor injection site for phlebitis. Not for use in preg (contraceptives advised)/breastfeeding. Pt should get periodic blood tests, report difficulty breathing, urine/stool color changes, pain at IV site.

**DANGEROUS DRUG**

## miconazole nitrate
(Fungoid Tincture, Lotrimin AF, Monistat)
**CLASS** Antifungal
**PREG/CONT** B/NA

**IND & DOSE** **Local tx of vulvovaginal candidiasis (moniliasis).** *Adult:* 1 suppository intravaginally once daily at bedtime for 3 d (*Monistat*). Or, 1 applicator cream or 1 suppository intravaginally daily at bedtime for 7 d (*Monistat 7*). Repeat course if needed. Alternatively, one 1,200-mg vaginal suppository at bedtime for 1 dose. **Topical tx of susceptible fungal infections.** *Adult, child >2 yr:* Cream/lotion, cover affected areas a.m. and p.m. Powder, spray or sprinkle powder liberally over affected area a.m. and p.m.
**ADV EFF** Local irritation/burning, nausea, rash
**NC/PT** Culture before tx. Monitor response. Pt should take full tx course; insert vaginal suppositories high into vagina; practice good hygiene to prevent spread, reinfection; report rash, pelvic pain.

**DANGEROUS DRUG**

## midazolam hydrochloride (Seizalam)
**CLASS** Benzodiazepine, CNS depressant
**PREG/CONT** Unkn/C-IV

**BBW** Only personnel trained in general anesthesia should give. Have equipment for maintaining airway, resuscitation on hand; respiratory depression/arrest possible. Give IV w/ continuous monitoring of respiratory, CV function. Individualize dose; use lower dose in elderly/debilitated pts. Adjust according to other premedication use.
**IND & DOSE** **Preop sedation, anxiety, amnesia.** *Adult:* >60 yr or debilitated, 20–50 mcg/kg IM 1 hr

before surgery; usual dose, 1–3 mg. < 60 yr, 70–80 mcg/kg IM 1 hr before surgery; usual dose, 5 mg. *Child 6 mo–16 yr:* 0.1–0.15 mg/kg IM; max, 10 mg/dose. **Conscious sedation for short procedures.** *Adult:* >60 yr, 1–1.5 mg IV initially. Maint, 25% initial dose; total dose, 3.5 mg. <60 yr, 1–2.5 mg IV initially. Maint, 25% of initial dose; total dose, 5 mg. *Child >12 yr:* 1–2.5 mg IV; maint, 25% of initial dose. **Conscious sedation for short procedures before anesthesia.** *Child 6–12 yr:* Initially, 25–50 mcg/kg IV. May give up to 400 mcg/kg; max, 10 mg/dose. *6 mo–5 yr:* 50–100 mcg/kg IV; max, 6 mg total dose. **Induction of anesthesia.** *Adult:* >55 yr, 150–300 mcg/kg IV as initial dose. <55 yr, 300–350 mcg/kg IV (to total 600 mcg/kg). Debilitated adult, 200–250 mcg/kg IV as initial dose. **Sedation in critical care areas.** *Adult:* 10–50 mcg/kg (0.5–4 mg usual dose) as loading dose. May repeat q 10–15 min; continuous infusion of 20–100 mcg/kg/hr to sustain effect. **Sedation in critical care areas for intubated child.** *Neonates >32 wks' gestation:* 60 mcg/kg/hr IV. *Neonates <32 wks' gestation:* 30 mcg/kg/hr IV. **Tx of status epilepticus (*Seizalam*).** *Adult:* 10 mg IM in mid outer thigh.
**ADV EFF** Amnesia, bradycardia, confusion, disorientation, drowsiness, sedation, incontinence, injection-site reactions, n/v/d, rash, **respiratory depression,** slurred speech
**INTERACTIONS** Alcohol, antihistamines, carbamazepine, CNS depressants, grapefruit juice, opioids, phenobarbital, phenytoin, protease inhibitors, rifabutin, rifampin
**NC/PT** Do not give intra-arterially; may cause arteriospasm, gangrene. Keep resuscitative facilities on hand; have flumazenil available as antidote if overdose. Monitor P, BP, R during administration. Monitor level of consciousness for 2–6 hr after use. Do not let pt drive after use. Provide written information (amnesia likely). Pt should take safety precautions for CNS effects; avoid alcohol, grapefruit juice before receiving drug; report visual/hearing disturbances, persistent drowsiness, difficulty breathing.

## midodrine (Orvaten)
**CLASS** Antihypotensive, alpha agonist
**PREG/CONT** C/NA

**BBW** Use only w/firm dx of orthostatic hypotension that interferes w/daily activities; systolic pressure increase can cause serious problems.
**IND & DOSE** **Tx of severe orthostatic hypotension.** *Adult:* 10 mg PO tid while upright.
**ADJUST DOSE** Renal impairment
**ADV EFF** Bradycardia, dizziness, increased IOP, paresthesia, pruritus, supine HTN, syncope, urine retention
**INTERACTIONS** Corticosteroids, digoxin, sympathomimetics, vasoconstrictors
**NC/PT** Monitor BP, orthostatic BP carefully. Monitor IOP w/long term use. Pt should take safety precautions for CNS effects, empty bladder before taking, avoid OTC cold/allergy remedies, report headache, fainting, numbness/tingling.

## midostaurin (Rydapt)
**CLASS** Antineoplastic, kinase inhibitor
**PREG/CONT** High risk/NA

**IND & DOSE** **Tx of newly diagnosed AML that is FLT3 mutation-positive.** *Adult:* 50 mg PO bid w/food, given w/other drugs. **Tx of aggressive systemic mastocytosis, systemic mastocytosis w/hematologic neoplasm, mast cell leukemia.** *Adult:* 100 mg PO bid w/food.
**ADV EFF** Abd pain, constipation, dyspnea, fever, hyperglycemia, infection, n/v/d, **pulmonary toxicity,** URI
**INTERACTIONS** Strong CYP3A4 inhibitors/inducers; avoid use

**NC/PT** Ensure proper dx. Monitor lung function. Stop drug for s&sx of pneumonitis; fatalities have occurred. Pt should avoid preg (contraceptives advised)/breastfeeding; report difficulty breathing, chest pain, fever, s&sx of infection.

**mifepristone** (Korlym, Mifeprex)
**CLASS** Abortifacient
**PREG/CONT** High risk/NA

**BBW** Serious, fatal infection possible after abortion; monitor for sustained fever, prolonged heavy bleeding, severe abd pain. Urge pt to seek emergency medical help if these occur. Rule out preg before tx and if tx stopped for 14 d or longer (w/*Korlym*).
**IND & DOSE** **Preg termination through 70 d gestational age.** *Adult:* Day 1, 200 mg (*Mifeprex*) followed in 24–48 hr by 800 mcg buccal misoprostol (*Cytotec*). **To control hyperglycemia secondary to hypercortisolism in adults w/Cushing syndrome and type 2 diabetes or glucose intolerance who have failed other tx and are not candidates for surgery.** *Adult:* 300 mg/d PO w/meal; max, 1,200 mg/d (*Korlym*).
**ADV EFF** Abd pain, dizziness, headache, n/v/d, **potentially serious to fatal infection,** heavy uterine bleeding
**INTERACTIONS** Anticoagulants, CYP3A4 inducers/inhibitors (limit to 600 mg daily w/inhibitors)
**NC/PT** Exclude ectopic preg before use. Alert pt that menses usually begins within 5 d of tx and lasts for 1–2 wk; arrange to follow drug within 48 hr w/ prostaglandin (*Cytotec*) as appropriate. Ensure abortion complete or that other measures are used to complete abortion if drug effects insufficient. Give analgesic, antiemetic as needed for comfort. Ensure pt follow-up; serious to fatal infections possible. Pt treated for hyperglycemia should take w/meals; continue other tx for Cushing syndrome. Not for use in preg w/ this indication (contraceptives advised). Pt should swallow tablet whole and not cut/crush/chew it; immediately report sustained fever, severe abd pain, prolonged heavy bleeding, dizziness on arising, persistent malaise. Name confusion between mifepristone and misoprostol, *Mifeprex* and *Mirapex* (pramipexole).

▶NEW DRUG

**migalastat hydrochloride** (Galafold)
**CLASS** Alpha-galactosidase A chaperone, metabolic agent
**PREG/CONT** Unkn/NA

**IND & DOSE** **Tx of pts w/Fabry disease and an amenable galactosidase alpha gene (GLA) variant.** *Adult:* 123 mg PO daily q other d at same time of d on empty stomach.
**ADV EFF** Headache, nasopharyngitis, nausea, pyrexia, UTI
**NC/PT** Consult clinical genetics professional before dosing. Pt should fast for at least 2 hr before to 2 hr after taking (4 hr total); swallow capsules whole; not take 2 d in a row.

DANGEROUS DRUG

**miglitol** (Glyset)
**CLASS** Alpha-glucosidase inhibitor, antidiabetic
**PREG/CONT** B/NA

**IND & DOSE** **Adjunct to diet/exercise to lower blood glucose in type 2 diabetes as monotherapy or w/sulfonylurea.** *Adult:* 25 mg PO tid at first bite of each meal. After 4–8 wk, start maint: 50 mg PO tid at first bite of each meal. Max, 100 mg PO tid. If combined w/sulfonylurea, monitor blood glucose; adjust doses accordingly.
**ADV EFF** Abd pain, anorexia, flatulence, hypoglycemia, n/v/d
**INTERACTIONS** Celery, charcoal, coriander, dandelion root, digestive enzymes, fenugreek, garlic, ginseng, juniper berries, propranolol, ranitidine

**NC/PT** Ensure thorough diabetic teaching, diet/exercise program. Pt should take w/first bite of each meal, monitor blood glucose, report severe abd pain.

**miglustat** (Zavesca)
**CLASS** Enzyme inhibitor
**PREG/CONT** High risk/NA

**IND & DOSE** **Tx of mild to moderate type 1 Gaucher disease.** *Adult:* 100 mg PO tid.
**ADJUST DOSE** Elderly pts, renal impairment
**ADV EFF** Diarrhea, GI complaints, male infertility, peripheral neuropathy, reduced platelet count, tremor, weight loss
**NC/PT** Not for use in preg/breastfeeding; men should use barrier contraceptives during tx. Pt should use antidiarrheals for severe diarrhea, report unusual bleeding, increasing tremors.

**milnacipran** (Savella)
**CLASS** Selective serotonin and norepinephrine reuptake inhibitor
**PREG/CONT** Moderate risk/NA

**BBW** Increased risk of suicidality; monitor accordingly. Not approved for use in child.
**IND & DOSE** **Mgt of fibromyalgia.** *Adult:* 12.5 mg/d PO; increase over 1 wk to target 50 mg PO bid.
**ADJUST DOSE** Elderly pts, renal impairment
**ADV EFF** Angle-closure glaucoma, bleeding, constipation, dizziness, dry mouth, headache, HTN, insomnia, nausea, **NMS**, palpitations, **seizures, serotonin syndrome, suicidality,** Takotsubo cardiomyopathy
**INTERACTIONS** Alcohol, clonidine, digoxin, epinephrine, MAOIs, norepinephrine, tramadol, triptans
**NC/PT** Not for use in breastfeeding. Monitor newborns for respiratory complications. Taper when stopping to avoid withdrawal reactions. Pt should avoid alcohol; take safety precautions for CNS effects; report bleeding, rapid HR, thoughts of suicide.

DANGEROUS DRUG

**milrinone lactate** (generic)
**CLASS** Inotropic
**PREG/CONT** C/NA

**IND & DOSE** **Short-term mgt of pts w/acute decompensated HF.** *Adult:* 50 mcg/kg IV bolus over 10 min. Maint infusion, 0.375–0.75 mcg/kg/min IV. Max, 1.13 mg/kg/d.
**ADJUST DOSE** Renal impairment
**ADV EFF** Headache, hypotension, **death,** ventricular arrhythmias
**INTERACTIONS** Furosemide in sol
**NC/PT** Do not mix in sol w/other drugs. Monitor rhythm, BP, P, I & O, electrolytes carefully. Pt should report pain at injection site, chest pain.

**miltefosine** (Impavido)
**CLASS** Antileishmanial drug
**PREG/CONT** High risk/NA

**BBW** May cause fetal harm; not for use in preg. Negative preg test required before use; contraceptives advised. Pt should not become preg during and for 5 mo after tx.
**IND & DOSE** **Tx of visceral, cutaneous, mucosal leishmaniasis caused by susceptible strains.** *Adult, child ≥12 yr:* ≥45 kg: 50 mg PO tid for 28 d; 30–44 kg: 50 mg PO bid for 28 d.
**ADV EFF** Abd pain, dizziness, hepatotoxicity, n/v/d, rash, renal toxicity, somnolence, **SJS**
**NC/PT** Culture to ensure proper use. Not for use in preg (negative preg test required, barrier contraceptives advised)/breastfeeding. Monitor for dehydration, fluid loss w/GI effects. Pt should avoid preg during and for 5 mo after tx; use safety precautions for

CNS effects; report severe diarrhea, dehydration, rash.

**minocycline hydrochloride** (Amzeeq, Arestin, Dynacin, Minocin, Minolira, Solodyn, Ximino)
**CLASS** Tetracycline
**PREG/CONT** High risk/NA

**IND & DOSE Infections caused by susceptible bacteria.** *Adult:* Initially, 200 mg PO or IV, then 100 mg q 12 hr PO or IV. Or, 100–200 mg PO initially, then 50 mg PO qid. *Adult (ER):* 91–136 kg, 135 mg/d PO; 60–90 kg, 90 mg/d PO; 45–59 kg, 45 mg/d PO. *Child >8 yr:* 4 mg/kg PO, then 2 mg/kg PO q 12 hr. **Tx of syphilis.** *Adult:* 100 mg PO q 12 hr for 10–15 d. **Tx of urethral, endocervical, rectal infections.** *Adult:* 100 mg PO q 12 hr for 7 d. **Tx of gonococcal urethritis in men.** *Adult:* 100 mg PO bid for 5 d. **Tx of gonorrhea.** *Adult:* 200 mg PO, then 100 mg q 12 hr for 4 d. Obtain post-tx cultures within 2–3 d. **Tx of meningococcal carrier state.** *Adult:* 100 mg PO q 12 hr for 5 d. **Tx of periodontitis.** *Adult:* Unit dose cartridge discharged in subgingival area. **Tx of moderate to severe acne vulgaris.** *Adult, child ≥12 yr:* 1 mg/kg/ day PO for up to 12 wk (ER form). *Adult, child ≥9 yr (Amzeeq):* Apply to affected areas once daily by rubbing into skin.
**ADJUST DOSE** Elderly pts, renal impairment
**ADV EFF** Anorexia; **bone marrow depression;** discoloring/inadequate calcification of primary teeth of fetus if used by preg women, of permanent teeth if used during dental development; glossitis; **liver failure;** n/v/d; phototoxic reactions; rash; superinfections
**INTERACTIONS** Alkali, antacids, dairy products, food, digoxin, hormonal contraceptives, iron, penicillin
**NC/PT** Culture before tx; ensure proper use. Give w/food for GI upset (avoid dairy products). Use IV only if oral not possible; switch to oral as soon as feasible. Not for use in preg/breastfeeding. Additional form of contraception advised; hormonal contraceptives may be ineffective. Pt should avoid sun exposure; report rash, urine/stool color changes, watery diarrhea.

**minoxidil** (Rogaine)
**CLASS** Antihypertensive, vasodilator
**PREG/CONT** C/NA

**BBW** Arrange for echocardiographic evaluation of possible pericardial effusion if using oral drug; more vigorous diuretic therapy, dialysis, other tx (including minoxidil withdrawal) may be needed. Increased risk of exacerbation of angina, malignant HTN. When first administering, hospitalize pt, monitor closely; use w/beta blocker and/or diuretic to decrease risk.
**IND & DOSE Tx of severe HTN.** *Adult, child ≥12 yr:* 5 mg/d PO as single dose. Range, usually 10–40 mg/d PO; max, 100 mg/d. Concomitant therapy w/diuretics: Add hydrochlorothiazide 50 mg PO bid, or chlorthalidone 50–100 mg/d PO, or furosemide 40 mg PO bid. Concomitant therapy w/beta-adrenergic blockers, other sympatholytics: Add propranolol 80–160 mg/d PO; other beta blockers (dose equivalent to above); methyldopa 250–750 mg PO bid (start methyldopa at least 24 hr before minoxidil); clonidine 0.1–0.2 mg PO bid. *Child <12 yr:* General guidelines: 0.2 mg/kg/d PO as single dose. Range, 0.25–1 mg/kg/d; max, 50 mg/d. **Topical tx of alopecia areata, male-pattern alopecia.** *Adult:* 1 mL to total affected scalp areas bid. Total daily max, 2 mL. May need 4 mo of tx to see results; balding returns if untreated 3–4 mo.
**ADJUST DOSE** Elderly pts, renal impairment
**ADV EFF** Bronchitis, dry scalp, eczema, edema, fatigue, headache, hypertrichosis, local irritation, pruritus, **SJS,** tachycardia, URI

**NC/PT** Monitor pt closely. Withdraw slowly w/systemic use. Do not apply other topical drugs to topically treated area. Enhanced/darkening of body, facial hair possible w/topical use. Twice-daily use will be needed to maintain hair growth; baldness will return if drug stopped. Pt should take P, report increase >20 beats above normal; report weight gain of >3 lb in 1 d; wash hands thoroughly after applying topical form; avoid applying more than prescribed; not apply to inflamed or broken skin; report rash, difficulty breathing (w/oral drug).

## mipomersen sodium (Kynamro)

**CLASS** Lipid-lowering drug, oligonucleotide inhibitor
**PREG/CONT** Unkn/NA

**BBW** May cause transaminase increases, hepatotoxicity, hepatic steatosis; available only through restricted access program.
**IND & DOSE** **Adjunct to other lipid-lowering drugs, diet to reduce LDL, total cholesterol, non-HDL cholesterol in pts w/familial hypercholesterolemia.** *Adult:* 200 mg/wk subcut.
**ADJUST DOSE** Hepatic impairment
**ADV EFF** Arthralgia, chills, fatigue, flulike sx, injection-site reactions, **hepatotoxicity**, malaise, myalgia
**NC/PT** Available only through limited access program. Ensure dx before use; not for tx of other hypercholesterolemias. Monitor LFTs before and frequently during therapy. Rotate injection sites; ensure continued diet/exercise, other drugs to lower lipids. Not for use in preg (contraceptives advised)/breastfeeding. Pt should learn proper injection technique, disposal of syringes; rotate injection sites; refrigerate drug, protect from light; report urine/stool color changes, extreme fatigue.

## mirabegron (Myrbetriq)

**CLASS** Beta-adrenergic agonist
**PREG/CONT** High risk/NA

**IND & DOSE** **Tx of overactive bladder.** *Adult:* 25 mg/d PO; max, 50 mg/d.
**ADJUST DOSE** Hepatic, renal impairment
**ADV EFF** Angioedema, dizziness, headache, HTN, nasopharyngitis, UTI, urine retention
**INTERACTIONS** Anticholinergics, desipramine, digoxin, drugs metabolized by CYP2D6, flecainide, metoprolol, propafenone
**NC/PT** Ensure dx; rule out obstruction, infection. Monitor BP; check for urine retention. Not for use in preg/breastfeeding. Pt should swallow tablet whole and not cut/crush/chew it; take w/full glass of water; use safety precautions w/dizziness; report swelling of face, urinary tract sx, fever, persistent headache.

## mirtazapine (Remeron)

**CLASS** Antidepressant
**PREG/CONT** Unkn/NA

**BBW** Ensure depressed/potentially suicidal pts have access only to limited quantities. Increased risk of suicidality in child, adolescent, young adult. Observe for clinical worsening of depressive disorders, suicidality, unusual changes in behavior, especially when starting tx or changing dose.
**IND & DOSE** **Tx of major depressive disorder.** *Adult:* 15 mg/d PO as single dose in evening. May increase up to 45 mg/d as needed. Change dose only at intervals of >1–2 wk. Continue tx for up to 6 mo for acute episodes.
**ADJUST DOSE** Elderly pts; hepatic, renal impairment
**ADV EFF** **Agranulocytosis,** confusion, constipation, dry mouth, disturbed concentration, dizziness, dysphagia, gynecomastia, **heart block,** increased appetite, **MI,** neutropenia,

photosensitivity, prolonged QT, **stroke,** urine retention, weight gain
**INTERACTIONS** Alcohol, CNS depressants, MAOIs, QT-prolonging drugs
**NC/PT** Do not give within 14 d of MAOIs; serious reactions possible. CBC needed if fever, s&sx of infection. Pt should take safety precautions for CNS effects; avoid alcohol, sun exposure; use sugarless lozenges for dry mouth; report s&sx of infection, chest pain, thoughts of suicide.

## misoprostol (Cytotec)

**CLASS** Prostaglandin
**PREG/CONT** X/NA

**BBW** Arrange for serum preg test for women of childbearing age. Women must have negative test within 2 wk of starting tx; drug possible abortifacient.
**IND & DOSE Px of NSAID (including aspirin)-induced gastric ulcers in pts at high risk for gastric ulcer complications.** *Adult:* 100–200 mcg PO four ×/d w/food.
**ADJUST DOSE** Elderly pts, renal impairment
**ADV EFF** Abd pain, dysmenorrhea, flatulence, miscarriage, n/v/d
**NC/PT** Explain high risk of miscarriage if used in preg (contraceptives advised). Pt should take drug w/ NSAID, not share drug w/others, report severe diarrhea, preg. Name confusion between misoprostol and mifepristone.

**DANGEROUS DRUG**

## mitoMYcin (Mitosol)

**CLASS** Antineoplastic antibiotic
**PREG/CONT** High risk/NA

**BBW** Monitor CBC, renal/pulmonary function tests frequently at start of tx; risk of bone marrow suppression, hemolytic uremic syndrome w/renal failure. Adverse effects may require decreased dose or drug stoppage; consult physician.
**IND & DOSE Palliative tx of disseminated adenocarcinoma of stomach, pancreas, w/other drugs.** *Adult:* 20 mg/m$^2$ IV as single dose q 6–8 wk; adjust according to hematologic profile.
**ADV EFF Acute respiratory distress syndrome,** alopecia, anorexia, **bone marrow toxicity,** confusion, drowsiness, fatigue, **hemolytic uremic syndrome,** injection-site reactions, n/v/d, **pulmonary toxicity**
**NC/PT** Do not give IM, subcut. Monitor CBC regularly, injection site for extravasation. Not for use in preg (barrier contraceptives advised)/ breastfeeding. Pt should mark calendar for tx days; cover head at temp extremes (hair loss possible); take safety precautions for CNS effects; report difficulty breathing, unusual bleeding.

## mitotane (Lysodren)

**CLASS** Antineoplastic
**PREG/CONT** High risk/NA

**BBW** Stop temporarily during stress (adrenal crisis possible); adrenal hormone replacement may be needed.
**IND & DOSE Tx of inoperable adrenocortical carcinoma.** *Adult:* 2–6 g/d PO in divided doses; gradually increase to target blood conc of 14–20 mg/L.
**ADV EFF** Anorexia, dizziness, lethargy, n/v, orthostatic hypotension, rash, somnolence, visual disturbances
**INTERACTIONS** Warfarin
**NC/PT** Give antiemetics if needed. Not for use in preg/breastfeeding. Stop drug in stress, surgery, etc. Premenopausal women should seek medical advice for vaginal bleeding/ pelvic pain due to ovarian macrocysts. Pt should take safety precautions for CNS effects, hypotension.

DANGEROUS DRUG

**mitoXANTRONE hydrochloride** (generic)
**CLASS** Antineoplastic, MS drug
**PREG/CONT** High risk/NA

**BBW** Monitor CBC and LFTs carefully before and frequently during tx; dose adjustment possible if myelosuppression severe. Monitor IV site for extravasation; if extravasation occurs, stop and immediately restart at another site. Evaluate left ventricular ejection fraction (LVEF) before each dose when treating MS. Evaluate yearly after tx ends to detect late cardiac toxic effects; decreased LVEF, frank HF possible. Monitor BP, P, cardiac output regularly during tx; start supportive care for HF at first sign of failure.
**IND & DOSE** **Tx of acute nonlymphocytic leukemia as part of comb tx.** *Adult:* 12 mg/m²/d IV on days 1–3, w/100 mg/m² cytarabine for 7 d as continuous infusion on days 1–7. Consolidation tx: Mitoxantrone 12 mg/m² IV on days 1, 2, w/cytarabine 100 mg/m² as continuous 24-hr infusion on days 1–5. First course given 6 wk after induction tx if needed. Second course generally given 4 wk after first course. **Tx of pain in advanced prostate cancer.** *Adult:* 12–14 mg/m² as short IV infusion q 21 d. **Tx of MS.** *Adult:* 12 mg/m² IV over 5–15 min q 3 mo; max cumulative lifetime dose, 140 mg/m².
**ADV EFF** Alopecia, **bone marrow depression,** cough, fever, headache, **HF,** hyperuricemia, n/v/d
**NC/PT** Handle drug w/great care; gloves, gowns, goggles recommended. If drug contacts skin, wash immediately w/warm water. Clean spills w/ calcium hypochlorite sol. Monitor CBC, uric acid level, LFTs. Not for use in preg (barrier contraceptives advised)/breastfeeding. Urine, whites of eyes may appear blue; should pass w/time. Pt should avoid exposure to infection; mark calendar for tx days; cover head at temp extremes (hair loss possible); report swelling, s&sx of infection, unusual bleeding.

**modafinil** (Provigil)
**CLASS** CNS stimulant, narcolepsy drug
**PREG/CONT** High risk/C-IV

**IND & DOSE** **Tx of narcolepsy; improvement in wakefulness in pts w/obstructive sleep apnea/ hypopnea syndrome.** *Adult:* 200 mg/d PO. Max, 400 mg/d. **Tx of shift-work sleep disorder.** *Adult:* 200 mg/d PO 1 hr before start of shift.
**ADJUST DOSE** Elderly pts, hepatic impairment
**ADV EFF** **Anaphylaxis,** angioedema, anorexia, anxiety, dry mouth, headache, insomnia, nervousness, persistent sleepiness, psychiatric sx, **SJS**
**INTERACTIONS** Cyclosporine, diazepam, hormonal contraceptives, omeprazole, phenytoin, TCAs, triazolam, warfarin
**NC/PT** Ensure accurate dx. Distribute least feasible amount of drug at any time to decrease risk of overdose. Monitor LFTs. Monitor pt w/CV disease closely. Consider stopping drug if psychiatric sx occur. Not for use in preg (barrier contraceptives advised)/ breastfeeding; pt using hormonal contraceptives should use second method (drug affects hormonal contraceptives). Pt should take safety precautions for CNS effects; report rash, difficulty breathing, persistent sleeping.

**moexipril** (generic)
**CLASS** ACE inhibitor, antihypertensive
**PREG/CONT** High risk/NA

**BBW** Do not give during preg; serious fetal injury or death possible.
**IND & DOSE** **Tx of HTN.** *Adult:* 7.5 mg/d PO 1 hr before meal; maint, 7.5–30 mg/d PO 1 hr before meals. If

pt receiving diuretic, stop diuretic for 2 or 3 d before starting moexipril. If diuretic cannot be stopped, start w/3.75 mg; monitor for symptomatic hypotension.
**ADJUST DOSE** Elderly pts, renal impairment
**ADV EFF** Aphthous ulcers, cough, diarrhea, dizziness, dysgeusia, flulike sx, flushing, gastric irritation, hyperkalemia, **MI, pancytopenia,** peptic ulcers, proteinuria, pruritus, rash
**INTERACTIONS** ACE inhibitors, ARBs, diuretics, lithium, potassium supplements, renin inhibitors
**NC/PT** Alert surgeon if surgery required; volume support may be needed. Monitor for BP fall w/drop in fluid volume; potassium w/long-term use. Not for use in preg (barrier contraceptives advised)/breastfeeding. Pt should perform mouth care for mouth ulcers; take safety precautions for CNS effects; report chest pain, s&sx of infection.

## mogamulizumab-kpkc
(Poteligeo)
**CLASS** Anti-CC chemokine receptor 4 antibody, antineoplastic, monoclonal antibody
**PREG/CONT** Moderate risk/NA

**IND & DOSE** **Tx of relapsed or refractory mycosis fungoides or Sézary syndrome after at least one prior systemic therapy.** *Adult:* 1 mg/kg IV over 60 min on days 1, 8, 15, and 22 of first 28-d cycle and on days 1 and 15 of subsequent cycles.
**ADV EFF** Acute GVHD, diarrhea, fatigue, infection, infusion reactions, musculoskeletal pain, **severe rashes,** URI
**NC/PT** Risk of posttransplant complications. Contraceptives advised during and for 3 mo after tx. Pt should report history of autoimmune disease, new/worsening rash, infusion reactions.

## montelukast sodium
(Singulair)
**CLASS** Antiasthmatic, leukotriene receptor antagonist
**PREG/CONT** B/NA

**IND & DOSE** **Px, long-term tx of asthma in pts ≥12 mo; relief of seasonal allergic rhinitis sx in pts ≥2 yr; relief of perennial allergic rhinitis sx in pts ≥6 mo; px of exercise-induced bronchoconstriction in pts ≥6 yr.** *Adult, child ≥15 yr:* 10 mg/d PO in p.m. For exercise-induced bronchoconstriction, dose taken 2 hr before exercise, not repeated for at least 24 hr. *Child 6–14 yr:* 5 mg/d chewable tablet PO in p.m. *Child 2–5 yr:* 4 mg/d chewable tablet PO in p.m. *Child 6–23 mo:* 1 packet (4 mg)/d PO. For asthma only, 4 mg granules/d PO in p.m.
**ADV EFF** Abd pain, behavior/mood changes, dizziness, fatigue, headache, nausea, systemic eosinophilia, URI
**INTERACTIONS** Phenobarbital
**NC/PT** Chewable tablets contain phenylalanine; alert pt w/phenylketonuria. Give in p.m. continually for best results. Not for acute asthma attacks. Pt should have rescue medication for acute asthma; take safety precautions for CNS effects; report increased incidence of acute attacks, changes in behavior/mood.

**DANGEROUS DRUG**

## morphine sulfate
(Duramorph PF, Infumorph, Kadian, Mitigo, Morphabond ER, MS Contin, Roxanol)
**CLASS** Opioid agonist analgesic
**PREG/CONT** High risk/C-II

**BBW** Caution pt not to chew/crush CR, ER, SR forms; ensure appropriate use of forms. Do not substitute *Infumorph for Duramorph;* conc differs significantly, serious overdose possible. Ensure pt observed for at least 24 hr in fully equipped, staffed

environment if given by epidural, intrathecal route; risk of serious adverse effects. Liposome preparation for lumbar epidural injection only; do not give liposome intrathecally, IV, IM. **IND & DOSE Relief of moderate to severe pain; analgesic adjunct during anesthesia; preop medication.** *Adult:* 5–30 mg PO q 4 hr. CR, ER, SR: 30 mg q 8–12 hr PO or as directed by physician. *Kadian,* 20–100 mg/d PO. *MS Contin,* 200 mg PO q 12 hr. **Relief of intractable pain.** *Adult:* 5 mg injected in lumbar region provides relief for up to 24 hr; max, 10 mg/24 hr. For continuous infusion, initial dose of 2–4 mg/24 hr recommended. Or, intrathecally, w/dosage 1/10 epidural dosage; single injection of 0.2–1 mg may provide satisfactory relief for up to 24 hr. Do not inject >2 mL of 5 mg/10-mL ampule or >1 mL of 10 mg/10-mL ampule. Use only in lumbar area. Repeated intrathecal injections not recommended. **Tx of pain after major surgery.** *Adult:* 10–15 mg liposome injection by lumbar epidural injection using catheter or needle before major surgery or after clamping umbilical cord during cesarean birth.
**ADJUST DOSE** Elderly pts, impaired adults
**ADV EFF Apnea, bronchospasm, cardiac arrest, circulatory depression,** dizziness, drowsiness, hypotension, impaired mental capacity, injection-site irritation, **laryngospasm,** light-headedness, n/v, **respiratory arrest/depression,** sedation, **shock,** sweating
**INTERACTIONS** Alcohol, barbiturate anesthetics, CNS depressants, MAOIs
**NC/PT** Have opioid antagonist, facilities for assisted or controlled respiration on hand during IV administration. Pt should lie down during IV use. Use caution when injecting IM, subcut into chilled areas and in pts w/hypotension, shock; impaired perfusion may delay absorption. Excessive amount may be absorbed w/repeated doses when circulation restored. Use caution in preg; not for use in breastfeeding. Pt should swallow CR, ER, SR forms whole and not cut/crush/chew them; store in secure place; take safety precautions for CNS effects; report difficulty breathing.

**DANGEROUS DRUG**

## moxetumomab pasudotox-tdfk (Lumoxiti)
**CLASS** Anti-CD22 recombinant immunotoxin, antineoplastic
**PREG/CONT** High risk/NA

**BBW** Risk of capillary leak syndrome and hemolytic uremic syndrome, including life-threatening cases. May need to delay or discontinue drug.
**IND & DOSE Tx of pts w/relapsed or refractory hairy cell leukemia who received at least two prior systemic therapies, including tx w/a purine nucleoside analog.** *Adult:* 0.04 mg/kg as IV infusion over 30 min on days 1, 3, and 5 of each 28-day cycle.
**ADV EFF** Anemia, constipation, diarrhea, edema, electrolyte disturbance, fatigue, fever, headache, infusion reactions, nausea, **renal toxicity**
**NC/PT** Monitor weight/BP before each infusion; serum electrolytes before each dose and day 8 of tx cycle; renal function. Maintain adequate hydration. Consider low-dose aspirin on days 1 through 8 of 28-d cycle. May need to premedicate w/acetaminophen, antipyretic, antihistamine, and $H_2$-receptor antagonist to decrease discomfort. Contraceptives advised during tx and for at least 30 d after tx.

## moxifloxacin hydrochloride (Avelox, Moxeza, Vigamox)
**CLASS** Fluoroquinolone
**PREG/CONT** High risk/NA

**BBW** Increased risk of tendonitis, tendon rupture, especially in pts >60 yr,

pts taking corticosteroids, pts w/kidney, heart, lung transplant. Risk of peripheral neuropathy and CNS effects. Risk of exacerbated weakness in pts w/myasthenia gravis; avoid use w/hx of myasthenia gravis. Reserve use for pts w/no other tx option for bacterial sinusitis, chronic bronchitis.
**IND & DOSE Tx of bacterial infections in adults caused by susceptible strains.** *Pneumonia:* 400 mg/d PO, IV for 7–14 d. *Sinusitis:* 400 mg/d PO, IV for 10 d. *Acute exacerbation of chronic bronchitis:* 400 mg/d PO, IV for 5 d. *Uncomplicated skin/skin-structure infections:* 400 mg/d PO for 7 d. *Complicated skin/skin-structure infections:* 400 mg/d PO, IV for 7–21 d. *Complicated intra-abd infections:* 400 mg PO, IV for 5–14 d. *Plaque:* 400 mg IV or PO for 10–14 d.
**ADV EFF Aortic aneurysm/dissection,** blood glucose disturbance, **bone marrow suppression,** cough, dizziness, drowsiness, headache, insomnia, n/v/d, photosensitivity, **prolonged QT,** psychiatric adverse reactions, rash, seizures, vision changes
**INTERACTIONS** Risk of prolonged QT w/amiodarone other QT-prolonging drugs, phenothiazines, procainamide, quinidine, sotalol; do not combine. Antacids, didanosine, NSAIDs, sucralfate
**NC/PT** Culture before tx. Reserve use for situations in which no other tx possible. Pt should take oral drug 4 hr before or 8 hr after antacids; stop if severe diarrhea, rash; take safety precautions for CNS effects; avoid sun exposure; report rash, unusual bleeding, severe GI problems.

## mycophenolate mofetil (CellCept), mycophenolate sodium (Myfortic)

**CLASS** Immunosuppressant
**PREG/CONT** High risk/NA

**BBW** Risk of serious to life-threatening infection. Protect from exposure to infections; maintain sterile technique for invasive procedures. Monitor for possible lymphoma development related to drug action. Risk of preg loss/congenital abnormalities; contraceptives strongly advised.
**IND & DOSE Px of organ rejection in allogeneic transplants. Renal.** *Adult:* 1 g bid PO, IV (over at least 2 hr) as soon as possible after transplant. Or, 720 mg PO bid on empty stomach (*Myfortic*). *Child:* 600 mg/m$^2$ oral suspension PO bid; max daily dose, 2 g/10 mL. Or, 400 mg/m$^2$ PO bid; max, 720 mg bid (*Myfortic*). **Cardiac.** *Adult:* 1.5 g PO bid, or IV (over at least 2 hr). **Hepatic.** *Adult:* 1 g IV bid over at least 2 hr, or 1.5 g PO bid.
**ADJUST DOSE** Elderly pts; hepatic, renal impairment; cardiac dysfx
**ADV EFF** Anorexia, **bone marrow suppression,** constipation, headache, **hepatotoxicity,** HTN, infection, insomnia, n/v/d, photosensitivity, **renal impairment**
**INTERACTIONS** Antacids, cholestyramine, cyclosporine, hormonal contraceptives, phenytoin, sevelamer, theophylline; avoid live vaccines
**NC/PT** Intended for use w/corticosteroids, cyclosporine. Do not mix w/ other drugs in infusion. Monitor LFTs, renal function regularly. Do not confuse two brand names; not interchangeable. Not for use in preg (barrier contraceptives advised)/ breastfeeding. Pt should swallow DR form whole and not cut/crush/chew it; avoid exposure to sun, infection; get cancer screening; avoid donating blood/semen during and for 6 wk (blood) or 90 d (semen) after tx; report s&sx of infection, unusual bleeding, urine/stool color changes.

## nabilone (Cesamet)

**CLASS** Antiemetic, cannabinoid
**PREG/CONT** C/C-II

**IND & DOSE** **Tx of n/v associated w/chemo in pts unresponsive to conventional antiemetics.** *Adult:* 1–2 mg PO bid. Give initial dose 1–3 hr before chemo. Max, 6 mg/d PO divided tid. May give daily during each chemo cycle and for 48 hr after last dose in cycle, if needed. Risk of altered mental state; supervise pt closely.
**ADV EFF** Ataxia, concentration difficulties, drowsiness, dry mouth, euphoria, orthostatic hypotension, vertigo
**INTERACTIONS** Alcohol, amitriptyline, amoxapine, amphetamines, anticholinergics, antihistamines, atropine, barbiturates, benzodiazepines, buspirone, CNS depressants, cocaine, desipramine, lithium, muscle relaxants, opioids, scopolamine, sympathomimetics, TCAs
**NC/PT** Risk of altered mental state; supervise pt closely; stop w/sx of psychotic reaction. Use caution in preg/breastfeeding. Warn pt possible altered mental state may persist for 2–3 d after use. Pt should take safety measures for CNS effects, avoid alcohol, report all drugs used (interactions possible), chest pain, psychotic episodes.

## nabumetone (generic)

**CLASS** NSAID
**PREG/CONT** C (1st, 2nd trimesters); D (3rd trimester)/NA

**BBW** Increased risk of CV events, GI bleeding; monitor accordingly. Not for use for periop pain after CABG surgery.
**IND & DOSE** **Tx of s&sx of RA, osteoarthritis.** *Adult:* 1,000 mg PO as single dose w/ or w/o food; 1,500–2,000 mg/d has been used.
**ADJUST DOSE** Renal impairment
**ADV EFF** **Anaphylactic shock, bone marrow suppression, bronchospasm,** dizziness, dyspepsia, GI pain, headache, insomnia, n/v/d, rash, **renal impairment**
**INTERACTIONS** Aspirin, warfarin
**NC/PT** Not for use in preg/breastfeeding. Pt should take w/food; take safety precautions for CNS effects; report swelling, s&sx of infection, difficulty breathing.

## nadolol (Corgard)

**CLASS** Antianginal, antihypertensive, beta blocker
**PREG/CONT** High risk/NA

**IND & DOSE** **Tx of HTN; mgt of angina.** *Adult:* 40 mg/d PO; gradually increase in 40- to 80-mg increments. Maint, 40–80 mg/d.
**ADJUST DOSE** Elderly pts, renal failure
**ADV EFF** Cardiac arrhythmias, constipation, decreased exercise tolerance/libido, diarrhea, dizziness, ED, flatulence, gastric pain, HF, **laryngospasm,** n/v/d, **pulmonary edema, stroke**
**INTERACTIONS** Alpha-adrenergic blockers, clonidine, dihydroergotamine, epinephrine, ergotamine, lidocaine, NSAIDs, theophylline, verapamil
**NC/PT** To discontinue, reduce gradually over 1–2 wk, risk of exacerbation of CAD. Alert surgeon if surgery required; volume replacement may be needed. Pt should take safety precautions for CNS effects; report difficulty breathing, numbness, confusion.

## nafarelin acetate (Synarel)

**CLASS** GnRH
**PREG/CONT** High risk/NA

**IND & DOSE** **Tx of endometriosis.** *Adult:* 400 mcg/d: One spray (200 mcg) into one nostril in a.m., 1 spray into other nostril in p.m. Start tx between d 2, 4 of menstrual cycle.

May give 800-mcg dose as 1 spray into each nostril in a.m. (total of 2 sprays) and again in p.m. for pts w/persistent regular menstruation after 2 mo of tx. Tx for 6 mo recommended. Retreatment not recommended. **Tx of central precocious puberty.** *Child:* 1,600 mcg/d: Two sprays (400 mcg) in each nostril in a.m., 2 sprays in each nostril in p.m.; may increase to 1,800 mcg/d. If 1,800 mcg needed, give 3 sprays into alternating nostrils three ×/d. Continue until resumption of puberty desired.
**ADV EFF** Acne, androgenic effects, dizziness, headache, hot flashes, hypoestrogenic effects, nasal irritation, rash, vaginal bleeding
**NC/PT** Not for use in preg (rule out before tx/advise barrier contraceptives)/breastfeeding. Risk of seizures/serious psychiatric adverse events in pts being treated for central precocious puberty. Store upright, protected from light. Begin endometriosis tx during menstrual period, between d 2, 4. Low estrogen effects, masculinizing effects possible (some may not be reversible). If nasal decongestant used, use at least 2 hr before dose. Pt should not interrupt tx; report nasal irritation, unusual bleeding.

DANGEROUS DRUG

## nalbuphine hydrochloride (generic)

**CLASS** Opioid agonist-antagonist analgesic
**PREG/CONT** High risk/NA

**BBW** Risk of addiction/abuse. Assess pt for addiction risk; monitor accordingly. Risk of life-threatening respiratory depression; monitor respiratory status. Risk of neonatal opioid withdrawal syndrome; ensure support available at delivery if long-term use during preg.
**IND & DOSE Relief of moderate to severe pain.** *Adult, 70 kg:* 10 mg IM, IV, subcut q 3–6 hr as needed. **Supplement to anesthesia.** *Adult:* Induction, 0.3–3 mg/kg IV over 10–15 min; maint, 0.25–0.5 mg/kg IV.
**ADJUST DOSE** Hepatic/renal impairment
**ADV EFF** Bradycardia, dizziness, drowsiness, dry mouth, headache, hypotension, n/v, **respiratory depression,** sweating, vertigo
**INTERACTIONS** Barbiturate anesthetics
**NC/PT** Taper when stopping after prolonged use to avoid withdrawal sx. Have opioid antagonist, facilities for assisted or controlled respiration on hand for respiratory depression. Not for use in preg (prepare for neonate support if used). Use caution in breastfeeding. Pt should take safety precautions for CNS effects, report difficulty breathing.

## naldemedine (Symproic)

**CLASS** Antidiarrheal, opioid antagonist
**PREG/CONT** High risk/C-II

**IND & DOSE Tx of opioid-induced constipation in adults w/chronic noncancer pain.** *Adult:* 0.2 mg/d PO.
**ADJUST DOSE** Hepatic impairment
**ADV EFF** Abd pain, diarrhea, **GI perforation,** nausea, opioid withdrawal
**INTERACTIONS** Strong CYP3A inducers (avoid use); opioid antagonists, moderate CYP3A4 inhibitors, P-gp inhibitors
**NC/PT** Monitor for possible opioid withdrawal; discontinue drug if opioid is stopped. Monitor pt w/hx of GI obstruction for possible perforation. Pt should take once daily; take only if still using opioid for pain; avoid preg (contraceptives advised)/breastfeeding; report severe abd pain, flushing, fever, sweating, diarrhea.

## naloxegol (Movantik)

**CLASS** Laxative, opioid antagonist
**PREG/CONT** Unkn/NA

**IND & DOSE Tx of opioid-induced constipation in adults w/chronic noncancer pain, including pts w/**

**chronic pain due to prior cancer or its tx.** *Adult:* 25 mg/d PO 1 hr before or 2 hr after first meal of day. If not tolerated, decrease to 12.5 mg/d PO.
**ADJUST DOSE** CYP3A4 inhibitor/inducer use, hepatic/renal impairment
**ADV EFF** Abd pain, diarrhea, flatulence, **GI perforation,** n/v/d, opioid withdrawal
**INTERACTIONS** CYP3A4 inducers/inhibitors
**NC/PT** Effective in pts using opioids for at least 4 wk. Stop drug if opioid for pain is stopped. Stop other laxative tx before naloxegol; may restart if constipation remains after 3 d. Monitor for possible opioid withdrawal; stop if opioids are withdrawn. Monitor for possible GI obstruction. Not for use in preg/breastfeeding. Pt should swallow tablet whole; not cut/crush/chew it. If pt cannot swallow, crush tablet, mix w/120 mL water, have pt drink immediately, refill glass, and have pt drink again; or crush to a powder and mix w/60 mL water, inject into NG tube, add 60 mL to container, and inject that fluid. Pt should take on empty stomach; avoid grapefruit/grapefruit juice; report worsening or severe abd pain, severe diarrhea, difficulty breathing.

## naloxone hydrochloride
(Evzio, Narcan Nasal Spray)
**CLASS** Opioid antagonist
**PREG/CONT** High risk/NA

**IND & DOSE** **Emergency tx of known or suspected opioid overdose.** *Adult, child:* 0.4 mg IM or subcut, or 4 mg intranasally sprayed into one nostril. May repeat q 2–3 min until emergency care available.
**ADV EFF** HTN, hypotension, n/v, **pulmonary edema,** sweating, tachycardia, tremors, **ventricular fibrillation**
**NC/PT** Monitor continually after use. Maintain open airway; provide life support as needed. Not a substitute for emergency care. Monitor fetus for distress if used during preg. Teach household members of pts w/potential opioid addiction and first responders stocked w/autoinjector how to identify overdose s&sx, proper use of autoinjector (may be used through clothes, etc)/disposal of autoinjector, proper use of nasal spray, need for immediate emergency medical care. Report difficulty breathing.

## naltrexone hydrochloride (generic)
**CLASS** Opioid antagonist
**PREG/CONT** High risk/NA

**IND & DOSE** **Naloxone challenge.** *Adult:* Draw 2 mL (0.8 mg) into syringe; inject 0.5 mL (0.2 mg) IV. Leave needle in vein; observe for 30 sec. If no withdrawal s&sx, inject remaining 1.5 mL (0.6 mg); observe for 20 min for withdrawal s&sx. Or, 2 mL (0.8 mg) naloxone subcut; observe for withdrawal s&sx for 20 min. If withdrawal s&sx occur or if any doubt pt opioid free, do not administer naltrexone. **Adjunct to tx of alcohol/opioid dependence.** *Adult:* 50 mg/d PO. Or, 380 mg IM q 4 wk into upper outer quadrant of gluteal muscle (*Vivitrol*); alternate buttock w/each dose. **Px of relapse to opioid dependence after opioid detoxification.** *Adult:* 25 mg PO. Observe for 1 hr. If no s&sx, complete dose w/25 mg; maint, 50 mg/24 hr PO. Can use flexible dosing schedule w/100 mg q other day or 150 mg q third day.
**ADV EFF** Abd pain, anxiety, chills, delayed ejaculation, joint/muscle pain, headache, **hepatocellular injury,** increased thirst, insomnia, n/v, nervousness
**INTERACTIONS** Opioid-containing products
**NC/PT** Do not use until pt opioid free for 7–10 d; check urine opioid levels. Do not give until pt has passed naloxone challenge. Keep *Vivitrol* at room temp, not frozen or exposed to heat. Ensure active participation in comprehensive tx program. Large opioid

doses may overcome blocking effect but could cause serious injury/death. Not for use in breastfeeding. Pt should wear medical alert tag; take safety precautions for CNS effects; report unusual bleeding, urine/stool color changes.

**naproxen** (EC-Naprosyn, Naprelan, Naprosyn), **naproxen sodium** (Aleve, Anaprox DS)
**CLASS** Analgesic, NSAID
**PREG/CONT** High risk/NA

**BBW** Increased risk of CV events, GI bleeding; monitor accordingly. Contraindicated for periop pain after CABG surgery; serious complications possible.
**IND & DOSE** **Tx of RA, osteoarthritis, ankylosing spondylitis.** *Adult:* 375–500 mg DR tablet PO bid; or 750–1,000 mg/d CR tablet PO; or 275–550 mg naproxen sodium PO bid (may increase to 1.65 g/d for limited time); or 250–500 mg naproxen PO bid; or 250 mg (10 mL), 375 mg (15 mL), 500 mg (20 mL) naproxen suspension PO bid. **Tx of acute gout.** *Adult:* 1,000–1,500 mg/d CR tablet PO; or 825 mg naproxen sodium PO then 275 mg q 8 hr until attack subsides; or 750 mg naproxen PO then 250 mg q 8 hr until attack subsides. **Tx of mild to moderate pain.** *Adult:* 1,000 mg/d CR tablet PO; or 550 mg naproxen sodium PO then 275 mg q 6–8 hr; or 500 mg naproxen PO then 500 mg q 12 hr; or 250 mg naproxen PO q 6–8 hr; or OTC products 200 mg PO q 8–12 hr w/full glass of liquid while sx persist (max, 600 mg/24 hr). **Tx of juvenile arthritis.** *Child:* 10 mg/kg/d naproxen PO in two divided doses.
**ADJUST DOSE** Elderly pts
**ADV EFF** **Anaphylactoid reactions to anaphylactic shock, bone marrow suppression, bronchospasm,** dizziness, dyspepsia, edema, GI pain, headache, HF, insomnia, nausea, somnolence, **thrombotic events**
**INTERACTIONS** Antihypertensives, lithium
**NC/PT** Pt should not cut/crush/chew DR, CR forms; take w/food for GI upset; take safety precautions for CNS effects; report difficulty breathing, swelling, chest pain, black tarry stools.

**naratriptan** (Amerge)
**CLASS** Antimigraine, triptan
**PREG/CONT** C/NA

**IND & DOSE** **Tx of acute migraine attacks.** *Adult:* 1 or 2.5 mg PO; may repeat in 4 hr if needed. Max, 5 mg/24 hr.
**ADJUST DOSE** Hepatic/renal impairment
**ADV EFF** Chest pain, **CV events,** dizziness, drowsiness, headache, neck/throat/jaw discomfort
**INTERACTIONS** Ergots, hormonal contraceptives, SSRIs
**NC/PT** For acute attack only; not for px. Monitor BP w/known CAD. Not for use in preg (barrier contraceptives advised)/breastfeeding. Pt should take safety measures for CNS effects; continue usual migraine measures; report chest pain, visual changes, severe pain.

**natalizumab** (Tysabri)
**CLASS** Monoclonal antibody, MS drug
**PREG/CONT** Unkn/NA

**BBW** Increased risk of possibly fatal PML. Monitor closely for PML; stop drug immediately if s&sx occur. Drug available only to prescribers and pts in TOUCH prescribing program; pts must understand risks, need for close monitoring. Risk increases w/duration of therapy, prior immunosuppressant use, presence of anti-JCV antibodies. Risk of immune reconstitution inflammatory syndrome in pts who developed PML and stopped drug.

**IND & DOSE Tx of relapsing MS; tx of Crohn disease in pts unresponsive to other tx.** *Adult:* 300 mg by IV infusion over 1 hr q 4 wk.
**ADV EFF** Abd pain, **anaphylactic reactions,** arthralgia, depression, diarrhea, dizziness, **encephalitis,** fatigue, gastroenteritis, **hepatotoxicity,** hypersensitivity reactions, infections, increased WBCs, lower respiratory tract infections, **meningitis, PML**
**INTERACTIONS** Corticosteroids, TNF blockers
**NC/PT** Withhold drug at s&sx of PML. Ensure pt not immune-suppressed or taking immunosuppressants. Refrigerate vials, protect from light; give within 8 hr of preparation. Monitor continually during and for 1 hr after infusion. Not for use in preg (barrier contraceptives advised)/breastfeeding. Pt should mark calendar of tx days; avoid exposure to infection; report difficulty breathing, s&sx of infection, changes in vision/thinking, severe headache, urine/stool color changes.

DANGEROUS DRUG

## nateglinide (generic)

**CLASS** Antidiabetic, meglitinide
**PREG/CONT** C/NA

**IND & DOSE Adjunct to diet/exercise to lower blood glucose in type 2 diabetes, alone or w/metformin, a thiazolidinedione.** *Adult:* 120 mg PO tid 1–30 min before meals; may try 60 mg PO tid if pt near $HbA_{1c}$ goal.
**ADV EFF** Dizziness, headache, hypoglycemia, nausea, URI
**INTERACTIONS** Beta blockers, MAOIs, NSAIDs, salicylates
**NC/PT** Monitor serum glucose, $HbA_{1c}$ frequently to determine effectiveness of drug, dose being used. Arrange for thorough diabetic teaching program; ensure diet/exercise protocols. Pt should take safety precaution for dizziness, report unusual bleeding, severe abd pain.

## nebivolol (Bystolic)

**CLASS** Antihypertensive, beta blocker
**PREG/CONT** Unkn/NA

**IND & DOSE Tx of HTN.** *Adult:* 5 mg/d PO; may increase at 2-wk intervals to max 40 mg/d PO
**ADJUST DOSE** Hepatic/renal impairment
**ADV EFF** Bradycardia, chest pain, dizziness, dyspnea, headache, hypotension
**INTERACTIONS** Antiarrhythmics, beta blockers, catecholamine-depleting drugs, clonidine, CYP2D6 inducers/inhibitors, digoxin, diltiazem, verapamil
**NC/PT** Do not stop abruptly after long-term tx; taper gradually over 2 wk while monitoring pt. Use caution in preg, especially 3rd trimester; not recommended w/breastfeeding. Pt should take safety precautions for CNS effects; report difficulty breathing, fainting.

## necitumumab (Portrazza)

**CLASS** Antineoplastic, epidermal growth factor antagonist
**PREG/CONT** High risk/NA

**BBW** Increased risk of cardiopulmonary arrest, sudden death; closely monitor magnesium, potassium, calcium, w/aggressive replacement if needed. Risk of hypomagnesemia; monitor electrolytes before each dose and at least 8 wk after tx ends.
**IND & DOSE First-line tx of metastatic squamous NSCLC, w/gemcitabine and cisplatin.** *Adult:* 800 mg IV over 60 min on days 1, 8 of each 3-wk cycle.
**ADV EFF Cardiopulmonary arrest, dermatologic reactions, hypomagnesemia, infusion reactions, thromboembolic events**
**NC/PT** Not for use in nonsquamous NSCLC; ensure dx. Monitor electrolytes

before, closely during, and for 8 wk after tx ends; aggressive replacement may be needed. Not for use in preg (contraceptives advised)/breastfeeding. Pt should mark calendar for tx days, avoid sunlight, wear protective clothing, report difficulty breathing, fever, chills, chest pain, muscle pain.

## nefazodone (generic)

**CLASS** Antidepressant
**PREG/CONT** C/NA

**BBW** Increased risk of suicidality in child, adolescent, young adult; monitor accordingly. Risk of severe to fatal liver failure; do not use if s&sx of hepatic impairment. Monitor closely; stop at first sign of liver failure.
**IND & DOSE Tx of depression.** *Adult:* 200 mg/d PO in divided doses; range, 300–600 mg/d.
**ADJUST DOSE** Elderly pts, hepatic impairment
**ADV EFF** Abnormal vision, agitation, asthenia, confusion, constipation, dizziness, dry mouth, **hepatic failure,** insomnia, light-headedness, mania, nausea, orthostatic hypotension, priapism, **seizures, suicidality**
**INTERACTIONS** MAOIs, triazolam. Contraindicated w/astemizole, carbamazepine, cisapride, pimozide, terfenadine
**NC/PT** Monitor LFTs before, regularly during tx. Ensure no MAOI use within 14 d. Use caution in preg/breastfeeding. Pt should avoid antihistamines, take safety precautions for CNS effects, report all drugs being used, urine/stool color changes, thoughts of suicide.

**DANGEROUS DRUG**

## nelarabine (Arranon)

**CLASS** Antimitotic, antineoplastic
**PREG/CONT** High risk/NA

**BBW** Monitor for neurotoxicity, including neuropathies, demyelinating disorders. Stop if neurotoxicity; effects may not be reversible.
**IND & DOSE Tx of T-cell acute lymphoblastic anemia, T-cell lymphoblastic lymphoma.** *Adult:* 1,500 mg/m² IV over 2 hr on days 1, 3, 5; repeat q 21 d. *Child:* 650 mg/m²/d IV over 1 hr for 5 consecutive d; repeat q 21 d.
**ADJUST DOSE** Hepatic/renal impairment
**ADV EFF Bone marrow suppression,** constipation, cough, dizziness, fatigue, fever, **neurotoxicity,** n/v/d, somnolence
**INTERACTIONS** Live vaccines, pentostatin
**NC/PT** Monitor neuro function before, regularly during tx; stop if sign of neurotoxicity. Not for use in preg (barrier contraceptives advised)/breastfeeding. Somnolence may decrease ability to drive, use machinery. Pt should avoid exposure to infection; take safety precautions for CNS effects; report numbness/tingling, unusual bleeding, s&sx of infection.

## nelfinavir mesylate (Viracept)

**CLASS** Antiviral, protease inhibitor
**PREG/CONT** B/NA

**IND & DOSE Tx of HIV infection w/ other drugs.** *Adult, child>13 yr:* 750 mg PO tid, or 1,250 mg PO bid. Max, 2,500 mg/d. *Child 2–13 yr:* 45–55 mg/kg PO bid, or 25–35 mg/kg PO tid.
**ADV EFF** Anorexia, anxiety, bleeding, diarrhea, dizziness, fat redistribution, GI pain, hyperglycemia, immune reconstitution syndrome, nausea, rash, **seizures,** sexual dysfx
**INTERACTIONS** Carbamazepine, dexamethasone, grapefruit juice, hormonal contraceptives, phenobarbital, phenytoin, rifabutin, St. John's wort. Avoid use w/CYP3A-dependent drugs: amiodarone, ergot derivatives, lovastatin, midazolam, pimozide, rifampin, quinidine, simvastatin, triazolam; serious reactions can occur

**NC/PT** Given w/other antivirals. Monitor drug list to avoid serious interactions. Interferes w/hormonal contraceptives (barrier contraceptives advised). Not for use in breastfeeding. Pt should take w/light meal, snack; avoid grapefruit juice, St. John's wort; take safety precautions for CNS effects; use precautions to avoid infections, prevent transmission (drug not a cure). Name confusion between *Viracept* (nelfinavir) and *Viramune* (nevirapine).

## neomycin sulfate
(generic)
**CLASS** Aminoglycoside
**PREG/CONT** D/NA

**IND & DOSE Preop suppression of GI bacteria for colorectal surgery.** *Adult:* See manufacturer's recommendations for complex 3-day regimen that includes oral erythromycin, bisacodyl, magnesium sulfate, enemas, dietary restrictions. **Adjunct tx in hepatic coma to reduce ammonia-forming bacteria in GI tract.** *Adult:* 12 g/d PO in divided doses for 5–6 d as adjunct to protein-free diet, supportive tx. *Child:* 50–100 mg/kg/d PO in divided doses for 5–6 d as adjunct to protein-free diet, supportive tx.
**ADJUST DOSE** Elderly pts, renal failure
**ADV EFF** Anorexia, leukemoid reaction, n/v, ototoxicity, pain, rash, superinfection
**INTERACTIONS** Beta-lactam antibiotics, citrate-anticoagulated blood, carbenicillin, cephalosporins, digoxin, diuretics, NMJ blockers, other aminoglycosides, penicillins, succinylcholine, ticarcillin
**NC/PT** Ensure hydration. Pt should report hearing changes, dizziness, s&sx of infection.

## neostigmine methylsulfate (Bloxiverz)
**CLASS** Antidote, parasympathomimetic, urinary tract drug
**PREG/CONT** High risk/NA

**IND & DOSE Control of myasthenia gravis sx.** *Adult:* 1 mL 1:2,000 sol (0.5 mg) subcut, IM. Use w/atropine to counteract adverse muscarinic effects. *Child:* 0.01–0.04 mg/kg per dose IM, IV, subcut q 2–3 hr as needed. **Antidote for NMJ blockers.** *Adult, child:* 0.6–1.2 mg atropine IV several min before slow neostigmine bromide IV injection of 0.03–0.07 mg/kg. Repeat as needed. Max, 0.07 mg/kg or total of 5 mg.
**ADV EFF** Abd cramps, bradycardia, **bronchospasm, cardiac arrest,** cardiac arrhythmias, dizziness, drowsiness, dysphagia, increased peristalsis, increased pharyngeal/tracheobronchial secretions, increased salivation/lacrimation, **laryngospasm,** miosis, nausea, urinary frequency/incontinence, vomiting
**INTERACTIONS** Aminoglycosides, corticosteroids, succinylcholine
**NC/PT** Have atropine sulfate on hand as antidote and antagonist in case of cholinergic crisis, hypersensitivity reaction. Stop drug, consult physician for excessive salivation, emesis, frequent urination, diarrhea. Give IV slowly. Pt should take safety precautions for CNS effects; report excessive sweating/salivation, difficulty breathing, muscle weakness.

## neratinib (Nerlynx)
**CLASS** Antineoplastic, kinase inhibitor
**PREG/CONT** High risk/NA

**IND & DOSE Extended adjunct tx of early-stage HER2-overexpressed breast cancer after trastuzumab tx.** *Adult:* 240 mg/d PO w/food for 1 year.

May reduce/interrupt due to pt safety and tolerability.
**ADJUST DOSE** Hepatic impairment
**ADV EFF** Abd pain, decreased appetite, **hepatotoxicity,** muscle spasms, n/v/d, rash, UTI, weight loss
**INTERACTIONS** Strong or moderate CYP3A inducers/inducers (avoid use); gastric acid–reducing drugs, P-gp inhibitors
**NC/PT** Monitor LFTs regularly. Start loperamide to ensure 1–2 bowel movements/d. Teach pt antidiarrheal regimen. Pt should take once daily w/ food for 1 year; avoid preg (contraceptives advised) breastfeeding; monitor diarrhea and adhere to antidiarrheal regimen; report >2 bowel movements/d, urine/stool color changes, rash, consistent weight loss.

## nesiritide (Natrecor)

**CLASS** Human B-type natriuretic peptide, vasodilator
**PREG/CONT** Unkn/NA

**IND & DOSE** **Tx of acutely decompensated HF.** *Adult:* 2 mcg/kg IV bolus, then 0.01 mcg/kg/min IV infusion for no longer than 48 hr.
**ADV EFF** Azotemia, headache, hypotension, tachycardia
**INTERACTIONS** ACE inhibitors
**NC/PT** Not for use w/persistent hypotension, shock. Replace reconstituted drug q 24 hr. Monitor continuously during administration. Monitor renal function regularly. Maintain hydration.

## nevirapine (Viramune, Viramune XR)

**CLASS** Antiviral, nonnucleoside reverse transcriptase inhibitor
**PREG/CONT** B/NA

**BBW** Monitor LFTs, renal function before, during tx. Stop if s&sx of hepatic impairment; severe to life-threatening hepatotoxicity possible (greatest risk at 6–18 wk of tx). Monitor closely. Do not give if severe rash occurs, especially w/fever, blisters, lesions, swelling, general malaise; stop if rash recurs on rechallenge. Severe to life-threatening reactions possible; risk greatest at 6–18 wk of tx. Monitoring during first 18 wk essential.
**IND & DOSE** **Tx of HIV-1 infection, w/other drugs.** *Adult:* 200 mg/d PO for 14 d; if no rash, then 200 mg PO bid. Or, 400 mg/d PO ER tablet. Max, 400 mg/d. *Child ≥15 d:* 150 mg/m² PO once daily for 14 d, then 150 mg/m² PO bid.
**ADV EFF** Fat redistribution, headache, **hepatic impairment including hepatitis, hepatic necrosis,** n/v/d, rash, **SJS, toxic epidermal necrolysis**
**INTERACTIONS** Clarithromycin, hormonal contraceptives, itraconazole, ketoconazole, protease inhibitors, rifampin, St. John's wort
**NC/PT** Give w/nucleoside analogs. Do not switch to ER form until pt stabilized on immediate-release form (14 d). Shake suspension gently before use; rinse oral dosing cup and have pt drink rinse. Not for use in preg (barrier contraceptives advised)/ breastfeeding. Pt should swallow ER tablet whole and not cut/crush/chew it; be aware drug not a cure, continue preventive measures, other drugs for HIV; report rash, urine/stool color changes. Name confusion between *Viramune* (nevirapine) and *Viracept* (nelfinavir).

## niacin (Niacor, Niaspan)

**CLASS** Antihyperlipidemic, vitamin
**PREG/CONT** C/NA

**IND & DOSE** **Tx of dyslipidemias.** *Adult, child >16 yr:* 100 mg PO tid, increased to 1,000 mg PO tid (immediate-release form); 500 mg/d PO at bedtime for 4 wk, then 1,000 mg/d PO at bedtime for another 4 wk (ER form); titrate to pt response, tolerance. Max,

2,000 mg/d; 1,000–2,000 mg/d PO (SR form). *Child<16 yr:* 100–250 mg/d PO in three divided doses w/meals; may increase at 2- to 3-wk intervals to max 10 mg/kg/d (immediate-release form). **Tx of CAD, post-MI.** *Adult:* 500 mg/d PO at bedtime, titrated at 4-wk intervals to max 1,000–2,000 mg/d. **Tx of pellagra.** *Adult, child:* 50–100 mg PO tid to max 500 mg/d.
**ADV EFF** Flushing, GI upset, glucose intolerance, hyperuricemia, n/v/d, rash
**INTERACTIONS** Anticoagulants, antihypertensives, bile acid sequestrants, statins, vasoactive drugs
**NC/PT** Do not substitute ER form for immediate-release form at equivalent doses; severe hepatotoxicity possible. ASA 325 mg 30 min before dose may help flushing. Do not combine w/a statin. Pt should take at bedtime; avoid hot foods/beverages, alcohol around dose time to decrease flushing; maintain diet/exercise program; report rash, unusual bleeding/bruising.

## niCARdipine hydrochloride (generic)

**CLASS** Antianginal, antihypertensive, calcium channel blocker
**PREG/CONT** High risk/NA

**IND & DOSE Tx of chronic, stable angina.** *Adult:* Immediate-release only, 20 mg PO tid; range, 20–40 mg PO tid. **Tx of HTN.** *Adult:* Immediate-release, 20 mg PO tid; range, 20–40 mg tid. SR, 30 mg PO bid; range, 30–60 mg bid. Or, 5 mg/hr IV. Increase by 2.5 mg/hr IV q 15 min to max 15 mg/hr. For rapid reduction, begin infusion at 5 mg/hr; switch to oral form as soon as possible.
**ADJUST DOSE** Hepatic/renal impairment
**ADV EFF** Asthenia, bradycardia, dizziness, flushing, headache, heart block, light-headedness, nausea
**INTERACTIONS** Cimetidine, cyclosporine, nicardipine, nitrates
**NC/PT** Monitor closely when titrating to therapeutic dose. Not for use in preg/breastfeeding. Pt should have small, frequent meals for GI complaints; take safety precautions for CNS effects; report irregular heartbeat, shortness of breath.

## nicotine (Habitrol, Nicoderm CQ, Nicotrol)

**CLASS** Smoking deterrent
**PREG/CONT** High risk/NA

**IND & DOSE Temporary aid to give up cigarette smoking.** *Adult:* Apply transdermal system, 5–21 mg, q 24 hr. *Nicoderm CQ:* 21 mg/d for first 6 wk; 14 mg/d for next 2 wk; 7 mg/d for next 2 wk. *Nicotrol:* 15 mg/d for first 6 wk; 10 mg/d for next 2 wk; 5 mg/d for last 2 wk. Or nasal spray, 1 spray in each nostril as needed, one–two doses/hr; max, five doses/hr, 40 doses/d. Or nasal inhaler, 1 spray in each nostril, one–two doses/hr. Max, five doses/hr, 40 doses/d; use for no longer than 6 mo. Treat for 12 wk, then wean over next 6–12 wk.
**ADV EFF** Cough, dizziness, GI upset, headache, insomnia, light-headedness, local reaction to patch
**INTERACTIONS** Adrenergic agonists, adrenergic blockers, caffeine, furosemide, imipramine, pentazocine, theophylline
**NC/PT** Ensure pt has stopped smoking, is using behavioral modification program. Not for use in preg/breastfeeding. Protect dermal system from heat. Apply to nonhairy, clean, dry skin. Remove old system before applying new one; rotate sites. Wrap old system in foil pouch, fold over, dispose of immediately. If nasal spray contacts skin, flush immediately. Dispose of bottle w/cap on. Pt should take safety precautions for CNS effects, report burning/swelling at dermal system site, chest pain.

## nicotine polacrilex
(Nicorette, Nicotine Gum)
**CLASS** Smoking deterrent
**PREG/CONT** High risk/NA

**IND & DOSE Temporary aid to give up cigarette smoking.** *Adult:* Chewing gum—<25 cigarettes/d, 2 mg; >25 cigarettes/d, 4 mg. Have pt chew one piece when urge to smoke occurs; 10 pieces daily often needed for first month. Max, 24 pieces/d no longer than 4 mo. Lozenge—2 mg if first cigarette over 30 min after waking; 4 mg if first cigarette within 30 min of waking. Wk 1–6, 1 lozenge q 1–2 hr; wk 7–9, 1 lozenge q 2–4 hr; wk 10–12, 1 lozenge q 4–8 hr. Max, 5 lozenges in 6 hr or 20/d.
**ADV EFF** Dizziness, GI upset, headache, hiccups, light-headedness, mouth/throat soreness, n/v
**INTERACTIONS** Adrenergic agonists, adrenergic blockers, caffeine, furosemide, imipramine, pentazocine, theophylline
**NC/PT** For gum, have pt chew each piece slowly until it tingles, then place between cheek and gum. When tingle gone, have pt chew again, repeat process. Gum usually lasts for about 30 min to promote even, slow, buccal absorption of nicotine. For lozenge, have pt place in mouth, let dissolve over 20–30 min. Pt should avoid eating, drinking anything but water for 15 min before use. Taper use at 3 mo. Not for use in preg/breastfeeding. Pt should not smoke (behavioral tx program advised), take safety precautions for CNS effects, report hearing/vision changes, chest pain.

## NIFEdipine (Adalat CC, Procardia, Procardia XL)
**CLASS** Antianginal, antihypertensive, calcium channel blocker
**PREG/CONT** C/NA

**IND & DOSE Tx of angina.** *Adult:* 10 mg PO tid; range, 10–20 mg tid. Max, 180 mg/d. **Tx of HTN.** *Adult:* 30–60 mg/d ER tablet PO; max, 90–120 mg/d.
**ADV EFF** Angina, asthenia, AV block, constipation, cough, dizziness, fatigue, flushing, headache, hypotension, light-headedness, mood changes, nasal congestion, nervousness, n/v, peripheral edema, tremor, weakness
**INTERACTIONS** Beta blockers, cimetidine, CYP3A inhibitors/inducers, digoxin, grapefruit juice
**NC/PT** Monitor closely while adjusting dose. Pt should swallow ER tablet whole and not cut/crush/chew it; avoid grapefruit juice; take safety precautions for CNS effects; report irregular heartbeat, swelling of hands/feet.

## nilotinib (Tasigna)
**CLASS** Antineoplastic, kinase inhibitor
**PREG/CONT** High risk/NA

**BBW** Risk of prolonged QT, sudden death. Increased risk w/hypokalemia, hypomagnesemia, known prolonged QT, use of strong CYP3A4 inhibitors; avoid these combos.
**IND & DOSE Tx of Philadelphia chromosome–positive CML.** *Adult:* 300–400 mg PO bid 12 hr apart on empty stomach. *Child ≥1 yr:* 230 mg/$m^2$ PO bid, rounded to nearest 50-mg dose (max single dose, 400 mg).
**ADJUST DOSE** Hepatic impairment
**ADV EFF** Abd pain, anorexia, bleeding, **bone marrow suppression,** constipation, electrolyte abnormalities, fatigue, fluid retention, growth retardation in child, headache, **hepatic dysfx,** nasopharyngitis, n/v/d, pain, pancreatitis, **prolonged QT,** rash, **sudden death, TLS**
**INTERACTIONS** Proton pump inhibitors, QT-prolonging drugs, strong CYP3A4 inducers/inhibitors, St. John's wort
**NC/PT** Obtain baseline, periodic ECG, QT measurement, LFTs, lipase level. Not for use in preg (barrier

contraceptives advised)/breastfeeding, long-term tx. Consider discontinuing after 3 yr if sustained molecular response; monitor BCR-ABL transcript level to determine eligibility for discontinuation. Monitor growth/development in child. Pt should avoid exposure to infection; report all concomitant drugs/herbs, urine/stool color changes, s&sx of infection, unusual bleeding.

## nimodipine (Nymalize)

**CLASS** Calcium channel blocker
**PREG/CONT** Moderate risk/NA

**BBW** Do not give parenterally; serious to fatal reactions have occurred.
**IND & DOSE To improve neuro outcomes after subarachnoid hemorrhage from ruptured aneurysm.** *Adult:* 60 mg PO q 4 hr for 21 d.
**ADJUST DOSE** Hepatic impairment
**ADV EFF** Bradycardia, hypotension, diarrhea
**INTERACTIONS** Antihypertensives, CYP3A4 inducers/inhibitors
**NC/PT** If pt unable to swallow capsule, may extract drug from capsule using syringe, give through NG or PEG tube, then flush w/normal saline. Do not give parenterally. Monitor carefully; provide life support as needed.

## nintedanib (Ofev)

**CLASS** Kinase inhibitor
**PREG/CONT** High risk/NA

**IND & DOSE Tx of idiopathic pulmonary fibrosis; to slow rate of decline in pulmonary function in pts w/systemic sclerosis-associated ILD.** *Adult:* 150 mg PO bid 12 hr apart w/food.
**ADJUST DOSE** Hepatic/renal impairment, mgt of adverse reactions
**ADV EFF** Bleeding, GI perforation, hepatotoxicity, n/v/d, renal toxicity, **thrombotic events**
**INTERACTIONS** CYP3A4 inhibitors, P-gp inhibitors, smoking
**NC/PT** Assess lung function, LFTs before, regularly during tx. Not for use in preg/breastfeeding. Monitor hydration; consider antiemetics, antidiarrheals if needed. Pt should report severe dehydration, vomiting, bleeding, chest pain.

## niraparib (Zejula)

**CLASS** Antineoplastic, poly (ADP-ribose) polymerase inhibitor
**PREG/CONT** High risk/NA

**IND & DOSE Maint tx of recurrent epithelial ovarian, fallopian tube, or primary peritoneal cancer responding to platinum-based therapy or if at ≥3 prior chemo regimens and if cancer is associated w/homologous recombo deficiency positive status.** *Adult:* 300 mg/d until progression or unacceptable adverse effects.
**ADV EFF** Abd pain, **bone marrow suppression, CV stimulation,** headache, hepatic impairment, insomnia, **myelodysplastic syndrome/AML**, n/v/d
**NC/PT** Regularly monitor blood counts. Monitor P, BP; manage w/antihypertensives if needed. Pt should avoid preg (contraceptives advised)/breastfeeding; report palpitations, chest pain, unusual bleeding, extreme fatigue, urine/stool color changes.

## nisoldipine (Sular)

**CLASS** Antihypertensive, calcium channel blocker
**PREG/CONT** C/NA

**IND & DOSE Tx of HTN.** *Adult:* 17 mg/d PO; increase in wkly increments of 8.5 mg/wk until BP controlled; range, 17–34 mg/d PO. Max, 34 mg/d.
**ADJUST DOSE** Elderly pts, hepatic impairment

**ADV EFF** **Angina,** asthenia, dizziness, edema, fatigue, headache, high-fat meals, light-headedness, **MI,** nausea
**INTERACTIONS** Cimetidine, cyclosporine, grapefruit juice, quinidine
**NC/PT** Monitor closely when titrating to therapeutic dose. Not for use in breastfeeding. Pt should swallow tablet whole and not cut/crush/chew it; take w/meals; avoid grapefruit juice, high-fat meals; report chest pain, shortness of breath.

## nitazoxanide (Alinia)

**CLASS** Antiprotozoal
**PREG/CONT** Unkn/NA

**IND & DOSE** **Tx of diarrhea caused by *Giardia lamblia*.** *Adult, child ≥12 yr:* 500 mg PO q 12 hr w/food, or 25 mL (500 mg) suspension PO q 12 hr w/food. *Child 4–11 yr:* 10 mL (200 mg) suspension PO q 12 hr w/food. *Child 1–3 yr:* 5 mL (100 mg) suspension PO q 12 hr w/food. **Tx of diarrhea caused by *Cryptosporidium parvum*.** *Child 4–11 yr:* 10 mL (200 mg) PO q 12 hr w/food. *Child 1–3 yr:* 5 mL (100 mg) suspension PO q 12 hr w/food.
**ADV EFF** Abd pain, diarrhea, headache, vomiting
**NC/PT** Culture before tx. Ensure hydration. Use caution w/breastfeeding. Pt should take w/food; report continued diarrhea, vomiting.

## nitisinone (Nityr, Orfadin)

**CLASS** Hydroxyphenyl-pyruvate dioxygenase inhibitor
**PREG/CONT** Moderate risk/C-II

**IND & DOSE** **Tx of hereditary tyrosinemia type 1 w/dietary restriction of tyrosine and phenylalanine.** *Adult, child:* 0.5 mg/kg/d PO or bid; titrate based on response. Max dose, 2 mg/kg PO.
**ADV EFF** Alopecia; blepharitis; cataracts; conjunctivitis; dry skin; **elevated tyrosine w/ocular problems, developmental delays, hyperkeratotic plaques; leukopenia; severe thrombocytopenia;** rash
**INTERACTIONS** CYP2C9 substrates
**NC/PT** Monitor tyrosine, blood counts. Obtain slit-lamp exam as baseline; reexamine if s&sx occur. For pt w/swallowing difficulties, may disintegrate tablet in water and give w/syringe or crush and mix w/applesauce. Ensure dietary restriction of tyrosine/phenylalanine. Pt should take bid; have periodic blood tests to monitor tyrosine; report vision changes, eye pain or discharge, rash or skin lesions, unusual bleeding, developmental delays in child.

## nitrofurantoin (Furadantin, Macrobid, Macrodantin)

**CLASS** Antibacterial, urinary tract anti-infective
**PREG/CONT** B/NA

**IND & DOSE** **Tx of UTIs.** *Adult:* 50–100 mg PO qid for 10–14 d, or 100 mg PO bid for 7 d (*Macrobid*). Max, 400 mg/d. *Child >1 mo:* 5–7 mg/kg/d in four divided doses PO. **Long-term suppression of UTIs.** *Adult:* 50–100 mg PO at bedtime. *Child:* 1 mg/kg/d PO in one or two doses.
**ADV EFF** Abd pain, **bone marrow suppression,** dizziness, drowsiness, **hepatotoxicity,** n/v/d, **pulmonary hypersensitivity,** rash, **SJS,** superinfections
**NC/PT** Culture before tx. Monitor CBC, LFTs regularly. Monitor pulmonary function. Urine may be brown or yellow-green. Pt should take w/food or milk, complete full course, take safety precautions for CNS effects, report difficulty breathing.

**nitroglycerin** (Gonitro, Minitran, Nitro-Dur, Nitrolingual Pumpspray, Nitromist, Nitrostat, Rectiv)
**CLASS** Antianginal, nitrate
**PREG/CONT** Low risk/NA

**IND & DOSE Tx of acute anginal attack.** *Adult:* 1 SL tablet under tongue or in buccal pouch at first sign of anginal attack, let dissolve; repeat q 5 min until relief obtained. No more than 3 tablets/15 min. Or, for translingual spray: Spray preparation delivers 0.4 mg/metered dose. At onset of attack, one–two metered doses sprayed into oral mucosa; no more than three doses/15 min. **Px of angina attacks.** *Adult:* SL, 1 tablet or 1 packet (*Gonitro*) 5–10 min before activities that might precipitate attack. Buccal, 1 tablet between lip, gum; allow to dissolve over 3–5 min. Tablet should not be chewed/swallowed. Initial dose, 1 mg q 5 hr while awake; maint, 2 mg tid. SR tablet, 2.5–9 mg q 12 hr; max, 26 mg qid. Topical, ½ inch q 8 hr. Increase by ½ inch to achieve desired results. Usual dose, 1–2 inches q 8 hr; max 4–5 inches q 4 hr has been used. 1 inch ½ 15 mg nitroglycerin. Transdermal, one patch applied each day. Translingual spray, one–two metered doses sprayed into oral mucosa 5–10 min before activity that might precipitate attack. **Tx of moderate to severe pain associated w/anal fissure.** *Adult:* 1 inch ointment intra-anally q 12 hr for 3 wk (*Rectiv*). **Tx of periop HTN, HF associated w/MI, angina unresponsive to nitrates, beta blockers.** *Adult:* 5 mcg/min IV through infusion pump. Increase by 5-mcg/min increments q 3–5 min as needed. If no response at 20 mcg/min, increase increments to 10–20 mcg/min.
**ADV EFF** Abd pain, angina, apprehension, faintness, headache, **hypotension,** local reaction to topical use, n/v, rash
**INTERACTIONS** Ergots, heparin, sildenafil, tadalafil, vardenafil
**NC/PT** Review proper administration of each form; pt should sprinkle powder form under tongue. If chest pain persists after three doses, pt should seek medical attention. SL should "fizzle" under tongue; replace q 6 mo. Withdraw gradually after long-term use. Pt may relieve headache by lying down. Pt should not cut/crush/chew SR tablet; apply topical to clean, dry, hair-free area (remove old patch before applying new one); take safety precautions for CNS effects; report unrelieved chest pain, severe headache.

**nitroprusside sodium** (Nitropress)
**CLASS** Antihypertensive, vasodilator
**PREG/CONT** C/NA

**BBW** Monitor BP closely. Do not let BP drop too rapidly; do not lower systolic BP below 60 mm Hg. Monitor blood acid-base balance (metabolic acidosis early sign of cyanide toxicity), serum thiocyanate daily during prolonged tx, especially w/renal impairment.
**IND & DOSE Tx of hypertensive crises; controlled hypotension during anesthesia; tx of acute HF.** *Adult, child:* Not on antihypertensive: Average dose, 3 mcg/kg/min IV; range, 0.3–10 mcg/kg/min. At this rate, diastolic BP usually lowered by 30%–40% below pretreatment diastolic level. Use smaller doses in pts on antihypertensive. Max infusion rate, 10 mcg/kg/min. If this rate does not reduce BP within 10 min, stop drug.
**ADJUST DOSE** Elderly pts, renal impairment
**ADV EFF** Abd pain, apprehension, **cyanide toxicity,** diaphoresis, faintness, headache, **hypotension,** muscle twitching, n/v, restlessness
**NC/PT** Do not mix in sol w/other drugs. Monitor BP, IV frequently. Have amyl nitrate inhalation, materials to make 3% sodium nitrite sol, sodium

thiosulfate on hand for nitroprusside overdose and depletion of body stores of sulfur, leading to cyanide toxicity. Pt should report chest pain, pain at injection site.

## nivolumab (Opdivo)

**CLASS** Antineoplastic, human programmed death receptor-1 blocking antibody
**PREG/CONT** High risk/NA

**IND & DOSE Tx of unresectable or metastatic melanoma w/progression after ipilimumab and BRAF inhibitor if BRAF V600 mutation–positive; advanced, metastatic NSCLC w/ progression after platinum-based chemo; tx of metastatic or recurrent squamous cell carcinoma of head/neck after platinum-based tx; advanced renal cell carcinoma after antiangiogenic therapy; classic Hodgkin lymphoma w/relapse after stem cell transplant and brentuximab tx.** *Adult:* 3 mg/kg IV over 60 min q 2 wk.
**ADV EFF** Immune-mediated reactions (pneumonitis, colitis, hepatitis, thyroiditis), rash
**NC/PT** Give corticosteroids based on immune reaction severity; withhold drug if reaction is severe. Not for use in preg (contraceptives advised)/ breastfeeding. Pt should mark calendar w/return dates for infusion; report difficulty breathing, severe diarrhea, urine/stool color changes.

## nizatidine (Axid AR)

**CLASS** Histamine-2 antagonist
**PREG/CONT** B/NA

**IND & DOSE Short-term tx of active duodenal ulcer, benign gastric ulcer.** *Adult:* 300 mg PO daily at bedtime. **Maint tx of healed duodenal ulcer; tx of GERD.** *Adult:* 150 mg PO daily at bedtime. **Px of heartburn/acid indigestion.** *Adult:* 75 mg PO w/water 30–60 min before problematic food, beverages.
**ADJUST DOSE** Elderly pts; hepatic/ renal impairment
**ADV EFF Bone marrow suppression, cardiac arrest,** cardiac arrhythmias, confusion, diarrhea, dizziness, ED, gynecomastia, hallucinations, headache, **hepatic dysfx,** somnolence
**INTERACTIONS** Aspirin
**NC/PT** Monitor LFTs, renal function, CBC w/long-term use. Switch to oral sol if swallowing difficult. Pt should take drug at bedtime; avoid OTC drugs that may contain same ingredients; have regular medical follow-up; report unusual bleeding, dark tarry stools.

**DANGEROUS DRUG**

## norepinephrine bitartrate (Levophed)

**CLASS** Cardiac stimulant, sympathomimetic, vasopressor
**PREG/CONT** C/NA

**BBW** Have phentolamine on standby for extravasation (5–10 mg phentolamine in 10–15 mL saline to infiltrate affected area).
**IND & DOSE To restore BP in controlling certain acute hypotensive states; adjunct in cardiac arrest.** *Adult:* Add 4 mL sol (1 mg/mL) to 1,000 mL 5% dextrose sol for conc of 4 mcg base/mL. Give 8–12 mcg base/ min IV. Adjust gradually to maintain desired BP (usually 80–100 mm Hg systolic). Average maint, 2–4 mcg base/min.
**ADV EFF** Bradycardia, headache, HTN
**INTERACTIONS** Methyldopa, phenothiazines, reserpine, TCAs
**NC/PT** Give whole blood, plasma separately, if indicated. Give IV infusions into large vein, preferably antecubital fossa, to prevent extravasation. Monitor BP q 2 min from start of infusion until desired BP achieved, then monitor q 5 min if infusion continued. Do not give pink, brown sols. Monitor for extravasation.

## norethindrone acetate
(generic)
**CLASS** Progestin
**PREG/CONT** High risk/NA

**IND & DOSE** **Tx of amenorrhea; abnormal uterine bleeding.** *Adult:* 2.5–10 mg PO for 5–10 d during second half of theoretical menstrual cycle. **Tx of endometriosis.** *Adult:* 5 mg/d PO for 2 wk; increase in increments of 2.5 mg/d q 2 wk to max 15 mg/d.
**ADV EFF** Acne, amenorrhea, breakthrough bleeding/spotting, dizziness, edema, insomnia, menstrual changes, **PE,** photosensitivity, rash, **thromboembolic disorders,** vision changes/blindness, weight increase
**NC/PT** Not for use in preg/breastfeeding. Stop if sudden vision loss, s&sx of thromboembolic event. Pt should mark calendar of tx days; avoid sun exposure; take safety precautions for CNS effects; report calf swelling/pain, chest pain, vision changes, difficulty breathing.

## nortriptyline hydrochloride (Pamelor)
**CLASS** TCA
**PREG/CONT** High risk/NA

**BBW** Limit access in depressed, potentially suicidal pts. Risk of suicidality in child, adolescent, young adult; monitor accordingly.
**IND & DOSE** **Tx of depression.** *Adult:* 25 PO mg tid–qid. Max, 150 mg/d. *Child ≥12 yr:* 30–50 mg/d PO in divided doses.
**ADJUST DOSE** Elderly pts
**ADV EFF** Atropine-like effects, **bone marrow depression,** constipation, disturbed concentration, dry mouth, glossitis, gynecomastia, hyperglycemia, orthostatic hypotension, photosensitivity, **seizures, stroke,** urine retention
**INTERACTIONS** Alcohol, cimetidine, clonidine, fluoxetine, MAOIs, sympathomimetics
**NC/PT** Monitor CBC. Alert pt to risks if used in preg/breastfeeding. Pt should take at bedtime if drowsiness an issue; avoid sun exposure, alcohol; take safety precautions for CNS effects; use sugarless lozenges for dry mouth; report thoughts of suicide, unusual bleeding, numbness/tingling

## nusinersen (Spinraza)
**CLASS** Survival motor neuron-2–directed antisense oligonucleotide
**PREG/CONT** Low risk/NA

**IND & DOSE** **Tx of spinal muscle atrophy.** *Adult, child:* 12 mg intrathecally. Four loading doses: first three at 14-day intervals, fourth loading dose given 40 d after third dose, then given q 4 mo.
**ADV EFF** Bleeding, constipation, **renal toxicity,** respiratory infections, **thrombocytopenia**
**NC/PT** Allow to warm to room temperature; use within 4 hr of removal from vial. Remove 5 mL cerebrospinal fluid before dosing. Inject over 1–3 min. Monitor platelets, coagulation. Spot urine testing. Pt should mark calendar for tx days; report s&sx of bleeding; supply regular spot urine tests.

## nystatin (Nystop)
**CLASS** Antifungal
**PREG/CONT** C/NA

**IND & DOSE** **Local tx of vaginal candidiasis (moniliasis).** *Adult:* 1 tablet (100,000 units) or 1 applicator cream (100,000 units) vaginally daily–bid for 2 wk. **Tx of cutaneous/mucocutaneous mycotic infections caused by *Candida albicans,* other *Candida* sp.** *Adult:* Apply to affected area two–three ×/d until healing complete. For fungal foot infection, dust powder on feet, in shoes/socks. **Tx of oropharyngeal candidiasis.** *Adult, child >1 yr:* 500,000–1,000,000 units PO tid for at

least 48 hr after clinical cure, or 400,000–600,000 units suspension four ×/d for 14 d and for at least 48 hr after sx subside.
**ADV EFF** GI distress, local reactions at application site, n/v/d
**NC/PT** Culture before tx. Pt should complete full course of tx; hold suspension in mouth as long as possible (can be made into popsicle for longer retention); clean affected area before topical application; use appropriate hygiene to prevent reinfection; report worsening of condition.

## obeticholic acid (Ocaliva)

**CLASS** Farnesoid X receptor agonist
**PREG/CONT** Low risk/NA

**BBW** Risk of hepatic decompensation/failure, possibly fatal, in pts w/ Child-Pugh class B or C or decompensated cirrhosis. Starting dose 5 mg once/wk in these pts.
**IND & DOSE Tx of primary biliary cholangitis, w/ursodeoxycholic acid, or as monotherapy if ursodeoxycholic acid not tolerated.** *Adult:* 5 mg/d PO for 3 mo; may titrate up to 10 mg/d.
**ADJUST DOSE** Hepatic impairment
**ADV EFF** Abd pain, arthralgia, constipation, dizziness, eczema, **hepatic injury,** reduced HDL, **severe pruritus,** throat pain, thyroid dysfx
**INTERACTIONS** CYP1A2 substrates, warfarin
**NC/PT** Monitor LFTs; adjust/stop drug accordingly. Consider antihistamines, bile acid–binding resins for severe pruritus. Regularly monitor alkaline phosphatase/total bilirubin; consider increase to max dose if goal not reached in first 3 mo. Pt should take drug at least 4 hr before or 4 hr after any bile acid–binding resin; return for frequent blood tests. Report urine/stool color changes, rash.

**DANGEROUS DRUG**

## obiltoxaximab (Anthim)

**CLASS** Antibacterial, monoclonal antibody
**PREG/CONT** Low risk/NA

**BBW** Risk of anaphylaxis; premedicate w/diphenhydramine. Administer only in monitored setting. Stop drug and immediately treat s&sx of hypersensitivity/anaphylaxis.
**IND & DOSE Tx of inhalational anthrax, w/appropriate antibiotics; px of inhalational anthrax when other tx not appropriate.** *Adult:* 16 mg/kg IV over 90 min. *Child >40 kg:* 16 mg/kg IV over 90 min; *15–40 kg:* 24 mg/kg IV over 90 min; *≤15 kg:* 32 mg/kg IV over 90 min.
**ADV EFF Anaphylaxis,** cough, headache, infusion-site pain/swelling, pain in extremities, urticaria
**NC/PT** Administer only in monitored setting w/trained personnel. Premedicate w/diphenhydramine; monitor for hypersensitivity/anaphylactic reaction. Do not use for px unless benefit outweighs risk. Pt should report difficulty breathing, swelling of face, pain/swelling at injection site, rash.

## obinutuzumab (Gazyva)

**CLASS** Antineoplastic, monoclonal antibody
**PREG/CONT** High risk/NA

**BBW** Risk of reactivation of HBV, fulminant hepatitis, PML, death. Monitor closely.
**IND & DOSE Tx of previously untreated chronic lymphocytic leukemia, w/chlorambucil.** *Adult:* 6-day cycle: 100 mg IV on day 1, cycle 1; 900 mg IV on day 2, cycle 1; 1,000 mg IV on day 8 and 15, cycle 1; 1,000 mg IV on day 1 of cycles 2–6. **Tx of follicular lymphoma in pts w/relapse after or who are refractory to rituximab regimen, w/bendamustine.** *Adult:* 1,000 mg IV on days 1, 8, 15 of cycle 1; 1,000 mg IV on day 1 of cycles 2–6, then once q 2 mo for 2 yr.

**ADV EFF** Cough, bone marrow suppression, fever, **hepatotoxicity,** hypersensitivity including serum sickness, infusion reactions, n/v/d, PML, thrombocytopenia, TLS
**INTERACTIONS** Live vaccines
**NC/PT** Premedicate w/glucocorticoids, acetaminophen, antihistamine. For pt w/large tumor load, premedicate w/antihyperuricemics, ensure adequate hydration. Dilute and administer as IV infusion, not IV push or bolus. Do not give live vaccines before or during tx. Monitor LFTs; stop drug w/sx of hepatotoxicity. Monitor CBC; watch for PML, infection, bleeding; hemorrhage may require blood products. Pt should avoid preg during and for 12 mo after tx; avoid breastfeeding; take safety measures for drug reaction; report urine/stool color changes, severe n/v/d, fever, dizziness, CNS changes, unusual bleeding.

## ocrelizumab (Ocrevus)

**CLASS** CD20-directed cytolytic antibody, MS drug
**PREG/CONT** High risk/NA

**IND & DOSE Tx of relapsing or primary progressive MS.** *Adult:* 300 mg IV followed in 2 wk by 300 mg IV, then 600 mg IV q 6 mo.
**ADV EFF** Infusion reaction, **infections, malignancies,** skin infections, URI
**INTERACTIONS** Live or live-attenuated vaccines
**NC/PT** Screen for HBV before use; contraindicated w/active HBV. Premedicate w/methylprednisolone and antihistamine before each infusion; monitor pt closely during and for at least 1 hr postinfusion for possible infusion reactions. Monitor for infections/malignancies during tx. Pt should avoid preg (contraceptive use for men and women advised during and for 6 mo after tx)/breastfeeding; maintain routine cancer screening procedures; mark calendar for infusion days; report difficulty breathing, fever, s&sx of infection, rash.

## octreotide acetate
(Sandostatin, Sandostatin LAR)

**CLASS** Antidiarrheal, hormone
**PREG/CONT** Low risk/NA

**IND & DOSE Symptomatic tx of carcinoid tumors.** *Adult:* First 2 wk: 100–600 mcg/d subcut in two to four divided doses; mean daily dose, 300 mcg. **Tx of watery diarrhea of VIPomas.** *Adult:* 200–300 mcg subcut in two to four divided doses during first 2 wk to control sx. Depot injection, 20 mg IM q 4 wk. *Child:* 1–10 mcg/kg/d subcut. Range, 150–750 mcg subcut. **Tx of acromegaly.** *Adult:* 50 mcg tid subcut, adjusted up to 100–500 mcg tid. Withdraw for 4 wk once yrly. Depot injection: 20 mg IM intragluteally q 4 wk.
**ADV EFF** Abd pain, asthenia, anxiety, bradycardia, cholelithiasis, dizziness, fatigue, flushing, injection-site pain, hyperglycemia, hypoglycemia, light-headedness, n/v/d
**NC/PT** Give subcut; rotate sites. Give depot injections deep IM; avoid deltoid region. Arrange to withdraw for 4 wk (8 wk for depot injection) once yrly for acromegaly. Monitor blood glucose, gallbladder ultrasound. Teach pt proper injection technique/disposal of needles/syringes. Pt should take safety precautions for CNS effects, report severe abd pain, severe pain at injection site. Name confusion between *Sandostatin* (octreotide) and *Sandimmune* (cyclosporine).

## ofatumumab (Arzerra)

**CLASS** Antineoplastic, cytotoxic
**PREG/CONT** High risk/NA

**BBW** Risk of HBV reactivation, fulminant hepatitis, PML, death. Monitor closely.
**IND & DOSE Tx of chronic lymphocytic leukemia (CLL) refractory to standard tx, w/chlorambucil; tx of**

**relapsed CLL, w/cyclophosphamide, fludarabine.** *Adult:* 300 mg IV, then 1,000 mg/wk IV on day 8, followed by 1,000 mg IV on day 1 of subsequent 28-day cycles. Minimum of 3 cycles, max of 12 cycles. **Tx of CLL refractory to fludarabine, alemtuzumab.** *Adult:* 300 mg IV, followed in 1 wk by 2,000 mg/wk IV in seven doses, followed in 4 wk by 2,000 mg IV q 4 wk for four doses.
**ADV EFF** Anemia, ataxia, **bone marrow suppression,** bronchitis, cough, diarrhea, dizziness, dyspnea, fatigue, fever, **HBV reactivation,** infusion reactions, intestinal obstruction, nausea, **PML,** TLS, URI, vision problems
**INTERACTIONS** Live vaccines
**NC/PT** Premedicate w/acetaminophen, IV antihistamine, IV corticosteroids. Monitor CBC regularly. Not for use in preg (contraceptives advised)/breastfeeding. Pt should avoid exposure to infection, take safety precautions for CNS effects, report difficulty breathing, unusual bleeding, s&sx of infection, difficulty breathing.

## ofloxacin (Ocuflox)
**CLASS** Fluoroquinolone
**PREG/CONT** C/NA

**BBW** Increased risk of tendinitis, tendon rupture. Risk higher in pts >60 yr, women, pts w/kidney/heart/lung transplant. Risk of exacerbated muscle weakness, sometimes severe, w/myasthenia gravis; do not give w/hx of myasthenia gravis. Reserve use in bronchitis, sinusitis, UTIs for severe cases not responsive to other tx.
**IND & DOSE Tx of infections caused by susceptible bacteria strains.** Uncomplicated UTIs: *Adult:* 200 mg q 12 hr PO for 3–7 d. Complicated UTIs: *Adult:* 200 mg PO bid for 10 d. **Bacterial exacerbations of COPD, community-acquired pneumonia, mild to moderate skin infections.** *Adult:* 400 mg PO q 12 hr for 10 d. **Prostatitis.** *Adult:* 300 mg PO q 12 hr for 6 wk. **Acute, uncomplicated gonorrhea.** *Adult:* 400 mg PO as single dose. **Cervicitis, urethritis.** *Adult:* 300 mg PO q 12 hr for 7 d. **Ocular infections.** *Adult:* 1–2 drops/eye as indicated. **Otic infections.** *Adult, child >13 yr:* 10 drops/d in affected ear for 7 d. *Child 6 mo–13 yr:* 5 drops/d in affected ear for 7 d. *Child 1–12 yr w/tympanostomy tubes:* 5 drops in affected ear bid for 10 d. **Swimmer's ear.** *Adult:* 10 drops/d (1.5 mg) in affected ear for 7 d. *Child ≥12 yr:* 10 drops in affected ear bid for 10 d. *Child 6 mo–<12 yr:* 5 drops in affected ear bid for 10 d. **Chronic suppurative otitis media.** *Adult, child:* 10 drops in affected ear bid for 14 d.
**ADJUST DOSE** Elderly pts, renal impairment
**ADV EFF Bone marrow suppression,** dizziness, drowsiness, headache, **hepatic impairment,** insomnia, n/v/d, photosensitivity, **prolonged QT,** tendinitis, **tendon rupture**
**INTERACTIONS** Antacids, iron salts, QT-prolonging drugs, St. John's wort, sucralfate, zinc
**NC/PT** Culture before tx. Reserve use of systemic drug for severe infections. Teach proper administration of eye/eardrops. Pt should take oral drug 1 hr before or 2 hr after meals on empty stomach; avoid antacids within 2 hr of ofloxacin; drink plenty of fluids; avoid sun exposure; take safety precautions for CNS effects; report tendon pain, severe GI upset, unusual bleeding.

## OLANZapine (Zyprexa)
**CLASS** Antipsychotic, dopaminergic blocker
**PREG/CONT** Unkn/NA

**BBW** Increased risk of death when used in elderly pts w/dementia-related psychosis; drug not approved for this use. Risk of severe sedation, including coma/delirium, after each injection of *Zyprexa Relprevv.* Monitor pt for at least 3 hr after each injection, w/ready access to emergency services.

Because of risk, drug available only through *Zyprexa Relprevv* Patient Care Program.
**IND & DOSE** **Tx of schizophrenia.** *Adult:* 5–10 mg/d PO. Increase to 10 mg/d PO within several d; max, 20 mg/d. Or long-acting injection (*Zyprexa Relprevv*): 150, 210, or 300 mg IM q 2 wk, or 300 or 405 mg IM q 4 wk. *Child 13–17 yr:* 2.5–5 mg/d PO; target, 10 mg/d. **Tx of bipolar mania.** *Adult:* 10–15 mg/d PO. Max, 20 mg/d; maint, 5–20 mg/d PO. *Child 13–17 yr:* 2.5–5 mg/d PO; target, 10 mg/d. **Tx of agitation associated w/schizophrenia, mania.** *Adult:* 10 mg IM; range, 5–10 mg. May repeat in 2 hr if needed; max, 30 mg/24 hr. **Tx-resistant depression.** *Adult:* 5 mg/d PO w/fluoxetine 20 mg/d PO; range, 5–12.5 mg/d olanzapine w/20–50 mg/d PO fluoxetine.
**ADJUST DOSE** Elderly/debilitated pts
**ADV EFF** Constipation, diabetes mellitus, dizziness, **DRESS,** dyslipidemia, fever, gynecomastia, headache, hyperglycemia, hyperprolactinemia, **NMS,** orthostatic hypotension, somnolence, weight gain
**INTERACTIONS** Alcohol, anticholinergics, antihypertensives, benzodiazepines, carbamazepine, CNS drugs, dopamine agonists, fluoxetine, fluvoxamine, levodopa, omeprazole, rifampin, smoking
**NC/PT** Dispense 1 wk at a time. Use care to distinguish short-term from long-term IM form. Monitor serum glucose, lipids; watch for metabolic changes, weight gain, hyperglycemia. Not for use in preg/breastfeeding. Discontinue for s&sx of DRESS. Alert pt of risk of gynecomastia. Pt should peel back (not push through) foil on blister pack of disintegrating tablet, remove w/dry hands; avoid alcohol; report all drugs being used (many interactions possible); take safety precautions for CNS effects, orthostatic hypotension; report fever, flulike sx. Name confusion between *Zyprexa* (olanzapine) and *Zyrtec* (cetirizine).

## olaratumab (Lartruvo)

**CLASS** Antineoplastic, platelet-derived growth factor receptor alpha blocker
**PREG/CONT** High risk/NA

**IND & DOSE** **W/doxorubicin for tx of soft tissue sarcoma for which an anthracycline regimen is appropriate, not curable by surgery or radiation.** *Adult:* 15 mg/kg IV over 60 min days 1, 8 of each 21-day cycle; give w/doxorubicin for first eight cycles
**ADV EFF** Abd pain, alopecia, bone marrow suppression, fatigue, headache, **infusion reaction,** mucositis, muscle pain, n/v/d
**NC/PT** Premedicate w/diphenhydramine, dexamethasone IV. Give by IV infusion only; not for push or bolus. Monitor for infusion reaction. Not for use in preg (contraceptives advised)/breastfeeding. Pt should mark calendar for tx days; report difficulty breathing, fever, chills.

## olmesartan medoxomil (Benicar)

**CLASS** Antihypertensive, ARB
**PREG/CONT** High risk/NA

**BBW** Rule out preg before tx; suggest barrier contraceptives. Fetal injury, death has occurred.
**IND & DOSE** **Tx of HTN.** *Adult, child 6–16 yr, ≥35 kg:* 20 mg/d PO; may titrate to 40 mg/d after 2 wk. *Child 6–16 yr, 20–<35 kg:* 10 mg/d PO; max, 20 mg/d PO.
**ADV EFF** Abd/back pain, **angioedema,** bronchitis, cough, dizziness, drowsiness, flulike sx, headache, hyperkalemia, n/v/d, URI
**INTERACTIONS** ACE inhibitors, ARBs, colesevelam, lithium, NSAIDs, renin inhibitors
**NC/PT** Alert surgeon if surgery scheduled; fluid volume expansion may be needed. Not for use in preg (barrier contraceptives advised)/breastfeeding. Pt should use caution

in situations that may lead to BP drop (excessive hypotension possible); take safety precautions for CNS effects; report swelling.

**olodaterol** (Striverdi Respimat)
**CLASS** Long-acting beta-2 adrenergic agonist
**PREG/CONT** C/NA

**IND & DOSE** **Long-term maint bronchodilator for COPD.** *Adult:* 2 inhalations once daily at same time each day.
**ADV EFF** Abd pain, arrhythmias, arthralgia, bronchitis, **bronchospasm**, cough, diarrhea, dizziness, HTN, hypokalemia, tachycardia, URI, UTI
**INTERACTIONS** Adrenergics, beta blockers, MAOIs, steroids, xanthines
**NC/PT** Not for use in asthma; risk of serious asthma-related events w/o tx w/inhaled corticosteroid. Not for acute attacks. Teach proper use/care of inhaler. Should be used w/inhaled corticosteroid. Pt should report difficulty breathing, worsening of sx, palpitations, chest pain.

**olsalazine sodium** (Dipentum)
**CLASS** Anti-inflammatory
**PREG/CONT** C/NA

**IND & DOSE** **Maint of remission of ulcerative colitis in pts resistant to sulfasalazine.** *Adult:* 1 g/d PO in divided doses w/meals.
**ADJUST DOSE** Renal impairment
**ADV EFF** Abd pain, diarrhea, headache, itching, rash
**INTERACTIONS** Heparin, 6-mercaptopurine, thioguanine, varicella vaccine, warfarin
**NC/PT** Use caution in preg; not for use in breastfeeding. Pt should always take w/food, report severe diarrhea.

**omacetaxine mepesuccinate** (Synribo)
**CLASS** Antineoplastic, protein synthesis inhibitor
**PREG/CONT** High risk/NA

**IND & DOSE** **Tx of adult w/accelerated CML w/resistance or intolerance to two or more kinase inhibitors.** *Adult:* 1.25 mg/m$^2$ subcut bid for 14 consecutive d of 28-d cycle, then 1.25 mg/m$^2$ subcut bid for 7 consecutive d of 28-d cycle.
**ADV EFF** **Bleeding**, fatigue, fever, hair loss, hyperglycemia, injection-site reactions, n/v/d, **severe myelosuppression**
**NC/PT** Monitor bone marrow function frequently; dosage adjustment may be needed. Monitor blood glucose. Not for use in preg/breastfeeding. Pt should avoid exposure to infections; be aware fatigue, bleeding, hair loss possible; report unusual bleeding, fever, s&sx of infection, rash.

**omadacycline** (Nuzyra)
**CLASS** Antibiotic, tetracycline
**PREG/CONT** High risk/NA

**IND & DOSE** **Tx of community-acquired bacterial pneumonia (CABP), acute bacterial skin/skin-structure infections (ABSSSI) caused by susceptible microorganisms.** *Adult:* CABP or ABSSSI: Load, 200 mg IV over 60 min *or* 100 mg IV over 30 min twice; maint, 100 mg IV over 30 min daily *or* 300 mg PO daily. ABSSSI only: 450 mg PO daily for 2 d, then 300 mg PO daily.
**ADV EFF** **Bone growth inhibition, CDAD,** constipation, diarrhea, headache, HTN, infusion-site reactions, insomnia, n/v, **teeth discoloration/enamel hypoplasia**
**INTERACTIONS** Anticoagulants; antacids (impair absorption)
**NC/PT** Due to potential for teeth discoloration/growth inhibition, not recommended for child (<8 yr) or

preg pt. Pt should not ingest food 4 hr before and 2 hr after taking drug or consume dairy products, antacids, multivitamins for 4 hr after taking drug.

## omalizumab (Xolair)

**CLASS** Antiasthmatic, monoclonal antibody
**PREG/CONT** Unkn/NA

**BBW** Anaphylaxis w/bronchospasm, hypotension, syncope, urticaria, edema possible. Monitor closely after each dose; have emergency equipment on hand.
**IND & DOSE** **To decrease asthma exacerbation in pts w/moderate to severe asthma, positive skin test to perennial airborne allergens.** *Adult, child>6 yr:* 75–375 mg subcut q 2–4 wk. **Tx of chronic idiopathic urticaria in pts who remain symptomatic w/ antihistamines.** *Adult, child≥12:* 150–300 mg subcut q 4 wk.
**ADV EFF** Acute asthma sx, **anaphylaxis, cancer,** eosinophilic conditions, fever, injection-site reactions, pain, rash
**NC/PT** Base dose on weight, pretreatment IgE level for asthma. Only 150 mg per site. Monitor after each injection for anaphylaxis. Not for use in breastfeeding. Pt should have appropriate cancer screening, report difficulty breathing, tongue swelling, rash, chest tightness, fever.

## omega-3-acid ethyl esters (Lovaza)

**CLASS** Lipid-lowering drug, omega-3 fatty acid
**PREG/CONT** C/NA

**IND & DOSE** **Adjunct to diet to reduce very high (>500 mg/dL) triglycerides.** *Adult:* 4 g/d PO as single dose (4 capsules) or divided into two doses (2 capsules PO bid).
**ADV EFF** Back pain, eructation, dyspepsia, flulike sx, infection, taste changes
**INTERACTIONS** Anticoagulants
**NC/PT** Monitor serum triglycerides. Ensure use of diet/exercise program. Use caution w/hx of fish, shellfish sensitivity. Not for use in preg/breastfeeding. Name confusion between *Omacor* (former brand name of omega-3-acid ethyl esters) and *Amicar* (aminocaproic acid). Although *Omacor* has been changed to *Lovaza,* confusion possible.

## omega-3-carboxylic acids (Epanova)

**CLASS** Lipid-lowering drug, omega-3 fatty acid
**PREG/CONT** Low risk/NA

**IND & DOSE** **Adjunct to diet to reduce very high (>500 mg/dL) triglycerides.** *Adult:* 2–4 g/d PO as single dose.
**ADV EFF** Abd pain, eructation, dyspepsia, n/v/d
**INTERACTIONS** Drugs affecting coagulation
**NC/PT** Ensure proper use of drug. Monitor serum triglycerides. Ensure use of diet/exercise program. Use caution w/hx of fish, shellfish sensitivity. Not for use in preg/breastfeeding.

## omeprazole (Prilosec, Zegerid)

**CLASS** Proton pump inhibitor
**PREG/CONT** Low risk/NA

**IND & DOSE** **Tx of active duodenal ulcer.** *Adult:* 20 mg/d PO for 2–8 wk. **Tx of active gastric ulcer.** *Adult:* 40 mg/d PO for 4–8 wk. **Tx of severe erosive esophagitis, poorly responsive GERD.** *Adult:* 20 mg/d PO for 4–8 wk. *Child 1–16 yr:* 20 kg and above: 20 mg/d PO; 10–<20 kg: 10 mg/d PO; 5–<10 kg: 5 mg/d PO. *Child 1 mo–1 yr:* ≥10 kg: 10 mg/d PO; 5–<10 kg: 5 mg/d PO; 3–<5 kg: 2.5 mg/d PO. **Tx of pathologic hypersecretory conditions.** *Adult:* 60 mg/d PO. Up to 120 mg tid has been used.

**Tx of frequent heartburn.** 20 mg/d (*Prilosec OTC* tablet) PO in a.m. before eating for 14 d. May repeat 14-day course q 4 mo. **Upper GI bleeding in critically ill pts.** *Adult:* 40 mg PO then 40 mg PO in 6–8 hr on day 1, then 40 mg/d for up to 14 d (*Zegerid*). **GERD, other acid-related disorders.** *Adult, child ≥1 yr:* ≥20 kg, 20 mg daily PO; 10–<20 kg, 10 mg daily PO; 5–10 kg, 5 mg daily PO.
**ADV EFF** Abd pain, **acute interstitial nephritis,** bone fractures, CDAD, dizziness, fundic gland polyps, headache, hypomagnesemia, n/v/d, pneumonia, rash, SLE, URI, vitamin $B_{12}$ deficiency
**INTERACTIONS** Atazanavir, benzodiazepines, cilostazol, clopidogrel, methotrexate, nelfinavir, phenytoin, rifampin, saquinavir, St. John's wort, sucralfate, tacrolimus, warfarin
**NC/PT** If sx persist after 8 wk, reevaluate. Pt should take w/meals; swallow capsule whole and not cut/crush/chew it (if cannot swallow, open capsules, sprinkle contents on applesauce, swallow immediately); avoid St. John's wort; take safety precautions for CNS effects; report severe diarrhea, fever.

## onabotulinumtoxinA

(Botox, Botox Cosmetic)
**CLASS** Neurotoxin
**PREG/CONT** C/NA

**BBW** Drug not for tx of muscle spasticity; toxin may spread from injection area and cause s&sx of botulism (CNS alterations, difficulty speaking and swallowing, loss of bladder control). Use only for approved indications.
**IND & DOSE To improve glabellar/lateral canthal/forehead lines.** *Adult:* 0.1 mL (4 units) injected into multiple sites; total dose, number, location of injections depend on diagnosis; repetition usually needed q 3–4 mo to maintain effect. **Cervical dystonia.** *Adult:* 236 units (range, 198–300 units) divided among affected muscles and injected into each muscle in pts w/known tolerance. In pts w/o prior use, 100 units or less, then adjust dose based on pt response. **Primary axillary hyperhidrosis.** *Adult:* 50 units/axilla injected intradermally 0.1–0.2 mL aliquots at multiple sites (10–15), about 1–2 cm apart. Repeat as needed. **Blepharospasm associated w/dystonia.** *Adult:* 1.25–2.5 units injected into medial and lateral pretarsal orbicularis oculi of lower and upper lids. Repeat about q 3 mo. **Strabismus associated w/dystonia.** *Adult:* 1.25–50 units injected in any one muscle. **Upper/lower limb spasticity.** *Adult, child 2–17 yr:* Base dose on muscles affected and severity of activity; electromyographic guidance recommended. Use no more than 50 units per site. **Px of chronic migraine.** *Adult:* 155 units IM as 0.1 mL (5 units) at each site; divide into seven head/neck muscle areas. **Tx of urinary incontinence in pts w/neuro conditions.** *Adult:* 200 units as 1-mL injection across 30 sites into detrusor muscle. **Tx of overactive bladder.** *Adult:* 100 units as 0.5-mL injections across 20 sites into detrusor muscle.
**ADV EFF Anaphylactic reactions,** dizziness, headache, injection-site infections, local reactions, **MI, spread of toxin that can lead to death,** urine retention (w/detrusor injections)
**INTERACTIONS** Aminoglycosides, anticholinesterases, lincosamides, magnesium sulfate, NMJ blockers, polymyxin, quinidine, succinylcholine
**NC/PT** Not interchangeable w/other botulinum toxins. Store in refrigerator. Have epinephrine available in case of anaphylactic reactions. Effects may not appear for 1–2 d; will persist for 3–4 mo. Not for use in preg; use caution w/breastfeeding. Pt should report difficulty breathing, s&sx of infection.

▶NEW DRUG

## onasemnogene abeparvovec-xioi
(Zolgensma)
**CLASS** CNS agent, gene therapy
**PREG/CONT** Unkn/NA

**BBW** Acute serious liver injury can occur, especially in pts w/preexisting hepatic impairment. Assess liver function before infusion. Give systemic corticosteroid to all pts before and after infusion. Monitor liver function for ≥3 mo after infusion.
**IND & DOSE** **Tx of spinal muscular atrophy w/bi-allelic mutations in survival motor neuron 1 gene.** *Child <2 yr:* 1.1 × $10^{14}$ vector genomes (vg)/kg of body weight IV over 60 min.
**ADV EFF** Elevated troponin I/transferases, **thrombocytopenia,** vomiting
**NC/PT** Do not use until full-term gestational age is reached. Give systemic corticosteroids starting 1 d before infusion and continuing for total of 30 d. Check liver function after 30 d. If liver function abnormalities persist, continue systemic corticosteroids (equivalent to oral prednisolone at 1 mg/kg/d) until findings unremarkable; then taper steroid over 28 d. Consult expert if pt unresponsive to steroid. Monitor platelet count and troponin I.

## ondansetron hydrochloride (Zofran, Zuplenz)
**CLASS** Antiemetic
**PREG/CONT** Low risk/NA

**IND & DOSE** **Px of chemo-induced n/v.** *Adult:* Three 0.15-mg/kg doses IV: First dose over 15 min starting 30 min before chemo; subsequent doses at 4 and 8 hr. Or, single 32-mg dose infused over 15 min starting 30 min before chemo. Or, 8 mg PO 30 min before chemo, then 8 mg PO 8 hr later; give 8 mg PO q 12 hr for 1–2 d after chemo. For highly emetogenic chemo, 24 mg PO 30 min before chemo. *Child 6 mo–18 yr:* Three 0.15-mg/kg doses IV over 15 min starting 30 min before chemo, then 4 and 8 hr later. *Child 4–11 yr:* 4 mg PO 30 min before chemo, 4 mg PO at 4 and 8 hr, then 4 mg PO tid for 1–2 d after chemo. **Px of n/v associated w/radiotherapy.** *Adult:* 8 mg PO tid. For total-body radiotherapy, give 1–2 hr before radiation each day. For single high-dose radiotherapy to abdomen, give 1–2 hr before radiotherapy, then q 8 hr for 1–2 d after therapy. For daily fractionated radiotherapy to abdomen, give 1–2 hr before tx, then q 8 hr for each day tx given. **Px of postop n/v.** *Adult:* 4 mg undiluted IV, preferably over 2–5 min, or as single IM dose immediately before anesthesia induction. Or, 16 mg PO 1 hr before anesthesia. *Child 1 mo–12 yr:* Single dose of 4 mg IV over 2–5 min if >40 kg, 0.1 mg/kg IV over 2–5 min if <40 kg.
**ADJUST DOSE** Hepatic impairment
**ADV EFF** Abd pain, diarrhea, dizziness, drowsiness, headache, myalgia, pain at injection site, **prolong QT,** serotonin syndrome, weakness
**INTERACTIONS** QT-prolonging drugs
**NC/PT** Obtain baseline ECG for QT interval. Ensure timing to correspond w/surgery, chemo. For *Zofran* orally disintegrating tablet, pt should peel foil back over (do not push through) one blister, immediately place on tongue, swallow w/saliva. For *Zuplenz,* pt should use dry hands, fold pouch along dotted line, carefully tear pouch along edge, remove film, place on tongue, swallow after it dissolves, then wash hands. Pt should take safety precautions for CNS effects; report pain at injection site, palpitations.

## oritavancin (Orbactiv)
**CLASS** Lipoglycopeptide antibiotic
**PREG/CONT** Unkn/NA

**IND & DOSE** **Tx of acute bacterial skin/skin-structure infections caused by susceptible strains of**

**gram-positive bacteria.** *Adult:* 1,200 mg IV over 3 hr as single dose.
**ADV EFF** CDAD, **hypersensitivity reactions,** infusion reactions, n/v/d, limb/subcutaneous abscesses, osteomyelitis
**INTERACTIONS** Warfarin
**NC/PT** Culture to ensure proper use. Monitor for infusion reactions; slow infusion. Check for skin abscesses; treat appropriately. Use of IV heparin contraindicated for 5 d (120 hr) after use of drug. Use caution in preg/breastfeeding. Pt should report difficulty breathing, diarrhea w/blood or mucus, skin sores.

## orlistat (Alli, Xenical)

**CLASS** Lipase inhibitor, weight loss drug
**PREG/CONT** High risk/NA

**IND & DOSE Tx of obesity as part of weight loss program; to reduce risk of weight gain after prior weight loss.** *Adult:* 120 mg PO tid w/each fat-containing meal. OTC, 60 mg PO w/each fat-containing meal; max, 3 capsules/d. *Child ≥12 yr:* 120 mg PO tid w/fat-containing meals. OTC not for use in child.
**ADV EFF** Dry mouth, flatulence, incontinence, loose stools, **severe hepatic injury,** vitamin deficiency
**INTERACTIONS** Amiodarone, antiepileptics, cyclosporine, fat-soluble vitamins, levothyroxine, oral anticoagulants
**NC/PT** Increased risk of severe hepatic injury; monitor LFTs before, periodically during tx. Ensure diet, exercise program. Not for use in preg (contraceptives advised); use caution w/breastfeeding. Pt should use sugarless lozenges for dry mouth; use fat-soluble vitamins (take separately from orlistat doses); report right upper quadrant pain, urine/stool color changes.

## orphenadrine citrate (generic)

**CLASS** Skeletal muscle relaxant
**PREG/CONT** C/NA

**IND & DOSE Relief of discomfort associated w/acute, painful musculoskeletal conditions.** *Adult:* 60 mg IV, IM. May repeat q 12 hr. Inject IV over 5 min. Or, 100 mg PO q a.m. and p.m.
**ADJUST DOSE** Elderly pts
**ADV EFF** Confusion, constipation, decreased sweating, dizziness, dry mouth, flushing, gastric irritation, headache, n/v, tachycardia, urinary hesitancy, urine retention
**INTERACTIONS** Alcohol, anticholinergics, haloperidol, phenothiazines
**NC/PT** Ensure pt supine during IV injection and for at least 15 min after; assist from supine position after tx. Pt should swallow SR tablet whole and not cut/crush/chew it; empty bladder before each dose; use caution in hot weather (sweating reduced); avoid alcohol; take safety precautions for CNS effects; use sugarless lozenges for dry mouth; report difficulty swallowing, severe GI upset.

## oseltamivir phosphate (Tamiflu)

**CLASS** Antiviral, neuraminidase inhibitor
**PREG/CONT** Low risk/NA

**IND & DOSE Tx of uncomplicated illness due to influenza virus (A or B).** *Adult, child ≥13 yr:* 75 mg PO bid for 5 d, starting within 2 d of sx onset. *Child 1–12 yr:* 30–75 mg suspension PO bid for 5 d based on weight. *Child 2 wk–<1 yr:* 3 mg/kg PO bid for 5 d. **Px of influenza A and B infection.** *Adult, child ≥13 yr:* 75 mg/d PO for at least 10 d; begin within 2 d of exposure. *Child 1–12 yr:* >40 kg, 75 mg/d PO; 23–40 kg, 60 mg/d PO; 15–23 kg, 45 mg/d PO; ≤15 kg, 30 mg/d PO. Continue for 10 d.

**ADJUST DOSE** Renal impairment
**ADV EFF** Anorexia, confusion, dizziness, headache, n/v, neuropsychiatric events, rhinitis, **SJS**
**NC/PT** Give within 2 d of exposure or sx onset. Do not use intranasal flu vaccine until 48 hr after stopping oseltamivir; do not give oseltamivir until 2 wk after live nasal flu vaccine. Pt should complete full course; refrigerate sol, shake well before each use; take safety precautions w/dizziness, CNS changes; report severe GI problems, rash.

## osimertinib (Tagrisso)

**CLASS** Antineoplastic, kinase inhibitor
**PREG/CONT** High risk/NA

**IND & DOSE** **Tx of metastatic epidermal growth factor receptor (EGFR) T790M mutation–positive NSCLC after tyrosine kinase inhibitor therapy or first-line tx of metastatic NSCLC w/EGFR exon 19 deletions or exon 21 L858R mutations.** *Adult:* 80 mg/d PO.
**ADV EFF** Cardiomyopathy, diarrhea, dry skin, erythema multiforme, **interstitial pneumonitis, prolonged QT, SJS**
**INTERACTIONS** QT-prolonging drugs; strong CYP3A inducers/inhibitors (avoid combo)
**NC/PT** Ensure proper dx. Perform left ventricular function tests before use and then q 3 mo. Monitor lung function. Not for use in preg (contraceptives advised during and for 6 wk after tx)/breastfeeding during and for 2 wk after tx; males should use contraceptives for 4 mo after tx. Pt should place dose in 2 oz water, stir until dissolved, drink right away, then add 4–8 oz water to container and drink (tablet will not completely dissolve); pt should not crush or heat tablet. Pt should report difficulty breathing, swelling, shortness of breath, palpitations, dizziness.

## ospemifene (Osphena)

**CLASS** Estrogen modulator
**PREG/CONT** High risk/NA

**BBW** Increased risk of endometrial cancer in women w/uterus and unopposed estrogens; addition of progestin strongly advised. Increased risk of stroke, DVT; monitor accordingly.
**IND & DOSE** **Tx of moderate to severe dyspareunia/vaginal dryness related to vulvar/vaginal atrophy due to menopause.** *Adult:* 60 mg once/d w/food.
**ADV EFF** **DVT, endometrial cancer**, hot flashes, hyperhidrosis, muscle spasms, **PE**, vaginal discharge
**INTERACTIONS** Estrogen, fluconazole, other estrogen modulators, rifampin
**NC/PT** Rule out preg (contraceptives advised). Not for use in breastfeeding. Combine w/progestin in women w/intact uterus; ensure annual pelvic/breast exam, mammogram. Monitor for DVT, PE, other thrombotic events. Reevaluate need for drug q 3–6 mo. Pt should take once/d, schedule annual complete exam and mammogram, report vision/speech changes, difficulty breathing, vaginal bleeding, chest pain, severe leg pain.

## oxacillin sodium (generic)

**CLASS** Penicillinase-resistant penicillin
**PREG/CONT** B/NA

**BBW** Increased risk of infection by multiple drug-resistant strains; weigh benefit/risk before use.
**IND & DOSE** **Infections due to penicillinase-producing staphylococci; to initiate tx when staphylococcal infection suspected.** *Adult, child ≥40 kg:* 250–500 mg IV q 4–6 hr; up to 1 g q 4–6 hr in severe infections. Max, 6 g/d. *Child <40 kg:* 50–100 mg/kg/d IV in equally divided doses q 4–6 hr. *Neonates ≥2 kg:* 25–50 mg/kg

IV q 8 hr. *Neonates <2 kg:* 25–50 mg/kg IV q 12 hr.
**ADV EFF** **Anaphylaxis, bone marrow suppression,** fever, gastritis, nephritis, n/v/d, pain, phlebitis, rash, **seizures,** sore mouth, superinfections, wheezing
**INTERACTIONS** Aminoglycosides, tetracyclines
**NC/PT** Culture before tx. Do not mix in same IV sol as other antibiotics. Be prepared for serious hypersensitivity reactions. Treat superinfections. Pt should avoid exposure to infection, use mouth care for sore mouth, report rash, difficulty breathing, s&sx of infection.

DANGEROUS DRUG

## oxaliplatin (Eloxatin)

**CLASS** Antineoplastic
**PREG/CONT** High risk/NA

**BBW** Risk of serious to fatal anaphylactic reactions.
**IND & DOSE** **In combo w/5-FU/leucovorin as adjunct tx of stage III colon cancer in pts w/complete resection of primary tumor; tx of advanced colorectal cancer.** *Adult:* 85 mg/m² IV infusion in 250–500 mL $D_5W$ w/leucovorin 200 mg/m² in $D_5W$ both over 2 hr followed by 5-FU 400 mg/m² IV bolus over 2–4 min, followed by 5-FU 600 mg/m² IV infusion in 500 mL $D_5W$ as 22-hr continuous infusion on day 1. Then leucovorin 200 mg/m² IV infusion over 2 hr followed by 5-FU 400 mg/m² bolus over 2–4 min, followed by 5-FU 600 mg/m² IV infusion in 500 mL $D_5W$ as 22-hr continuous infusion on day 2. Repeat cycle q 2 wk.
**ADJUST DOSE** Severe renal impairment
**ADV EFF** Abd pain, **anaphylaxis,** anorexia, constipation, cough, dyspnea, fatigue, hyperglycemia, hypokalemia, injection-site reactions, **neuropathy,** n/v/d, paresthesia, **pulmonary fibrosis,** rhabdomyolysis, **RPLS, severe neutropenia**
**INTERACTIONS** Nephrotoxic drugs
**NC/PT** Premedicate w/antiemetics, dexamethasone. Dose adjustment may be needed based on adverse effects. Monitor for potentially dangerous anaphylactic reactions. Monitor respiratory/neuro function. Not for use in preg/breastfeeding. Pt should take safety precautions for CNS effects, report severe headache, vision changes, difficulty breathing, numbness/tingling.

## oxandrolone (generic)

**CLASS** Anabolic steroid
**PREG/CONT** High risk/C-III

**BBW** Monitor LFTs, serum electrolytes periodically. Consult physician for corrective measures; risk of peliosis hepatitis, liver cell tumors. Measure cholesterol periodically in pts at high risk for CAD; lipids may increase.
**IND & DOSE** **Relief of bone pain w/osteoporosis; adjunct tx to promote weight gain after weight loss due to extensive trauma; to offset protein catabolism associated w/prolonged corticosteroid use; HIV wasting syndrome; HIV-associated muscle weakness.** *Adult:* 2.5 mg PO bid–qid; max, 20 mg. May need 2–4 wk to evaluate response. *Child:* Total daily dose, ≤0.1 mg/kg, or ≤0.045 mg/lb PO; may repeat intermittently.
**ADV EFF** Abd fullness, acne, anorexia, blood lipid changes, burning of tongue, excitation, gynecomastia, **hepatitis,** hirsutism in females, **intra-abd hemorrhage, liver cell tumors, liver failure,** virilization of prepubertal males
**NC/PT** May need 2–4 wk to evaluate response. Monitor effect on child w/long-bone X-rays q 3–6 mo; stop drug well before bone age reaches norm for pt's chronologic age. Monitor LFTs, serum electrolytes, blood lipids. Not for use in preg (barrier contraceptives advised)/breastfeeding. Pt should take w/food, report urine/stool color changes, abd pain, severe n/v.

**oxaprozin** (Daypro)
**CLASS** NSAID
**PREG/CONT** High risk/NA

**BBW** Increased risk of CV events, GI bleeding; monitor accordingly. Contraindicated for periop pain associated w/CABG surgery.
**IND & DOSE Tx of osteoarthritis.** *Adult:* 1,200 mg/d PO. Use initial 600 mg w/low body weight or milder disease. **Tx of RA.** *Adult:* 1,200 mg/d PO. **Tx of juvenile RA.** *Child 6–16 yr:* 600–1,200 mg/d PO based on body weight.
**ADJUST DOSE** Renal impairment
**ADV EFF Anaphylactoid reactions to anaphylactic shock,** constipation, dizziness, dyspepsia, edema, GI bleeding, HF, n/v/d, platelet inhibition, rash, **thrombotic events**
**NC/PT** Avoid use in preg from 30 wk on. Not for use in breastfeeding. Pt should take w/food; take safety precautions w/dizziness; report unusual bleeding, difficulty breathing, black tarry stools, chest pain.

**oxazepam** (generic)
**CLASS** Anxiolytic, benzodiazepine
**PREG/CONT** D/C-IV

**IND & DOSE Mgt of anxiety disorders, alcohol withdrawal.** *Adult, child >12 yr:* 10–15 mg PO or up to 30 mg PO tid–qid, depending on severity of anxiety sx. Higher range recommended in alcoholics.
**ADJUST DOSE** Elderly, debilitated pts
**ADV EFF** Apathy, bradycardia, constipation, **CV collapse,** depression, diarrhea, disorientation, dizziness, drowsiness, dry mouth, fatigue, fever, hiccups, lethargy, light-headedness
**INTERACTIONS** Alcohol, CNS depressants, theophylline
**NC/PT** Taper gradually after long-term tx, especially in pts w/epilepsy. Not for use in preg/breastfeeding. Pt should take safety precautions for CNS effects; report vision changes, fainting, rash.

**OXcarbazepine** (Oxtellar XR, Trileptal)
**CLASS** Antiepileptic
**PREG/CONT** High risk/NA

**BBW** Monitor serum sodium before and periodically during tx; serious hyponatremia can occur. Teach pt to report sx (nausea, headache, malaise, lethargy, confusion).
**IND & DOSE Tx of partial seizures.** *Adult:* 300 mg PO bid; may increase to total 1,200 mg PO bid if clinically needed as adjunct tx. Converting to monotherapy: 300 mg PO bid started while reducing dose of other antiepileptics; reduce other drugs over 3–6 wk while increasing oxcarbazepine over 2–4 wk to max 2,400 mg/d. Starting as monotherapy: 300 mg PO bid; increase by 300 mg/d q third day until desired dose of 1,200 mg/d reached. Or 600 mg/d PO ER form; increase at wkly intervals of 600 mg/d to target 2,400 mg/d. **Adjunct tx of partial seizures.** *Child 4–16 yr:* 8–10 mg/kg/d PO in two equally divided doses; max, 600 mg/d. *Child 2–4 yr >20 kg:* 8–10 mg/kg/d PO; max, 600 mg/d. *Child 2–4 yr <20 kg:* 16–20 mg/kg/d PO; max, 600 mg/d. **Monotherapy for partial seizures in epileptic child.** *Child 4–16 yr:* 8–10 mg/kg/d PO in two divided doses. If pt taking another antiepileptic, slowly withdraw that drug over 3–6 wk. Then, increase oxcarbazepine in 10-mg/kg/d increments at wkly intervals to desired level. If pt not taking another antiepileptic, increase dose by 5 mg/kg/d q third day. Or, *child 6–16 yr (Oxtellar XR):* Initially, 8–10 mg/kg PO once daily, not to exceed 600 mg/d in first wk.
**ADJUST DOSE** Elderly pts, renal impairment
**ADV EFF** Bradycardia, **bronchospasm,** confusion, disturbed coordination,

dizziness, drowsiness, HTN, hypersensitivity, hyponatremia, hypotension, impaired fertility, n/v, **pulmonary edema, skin reactions, suicidality,** unsteadiness
**INTERACTIONS** Alcohol, carbamazepine, felodipine, hormonal contraceptives, phenobarbital, phenytoin, valproic acid, verapamil
**NC/PT** Monitor for hyponatremia. Taper slowly if stopping or switching to other antiepileptic. Not for use in preg (barrier contraceptives advised)/ breastfeeding. Pt should swallow ER tablets whole, not cut/crush/chew them; take safety precautions for CNS effects; avoid alcohol; wear medical alert tag; report unusual bleeding, difficulty breathing, thoughts of suicide, headache, confusion, lethargy.

## oxybutynin chloride
(Ditropan XL, Gelnique, Oxytrol)
**CLASS** Anticholinergic, urinary antispasmodic
**PREG/CONT** Low risk/NA

**IND & DOSE Relief of bladder instability sx; tx of overactive bladder** (ER form). *Adult:* 5 mg PO bid or tid; max, 5 mg qid. ER tablets, 5 mg PO daily; max, 30 mg/d. Transdermal patch, 1 patch applied to dry, intact skin on abdomen, hip, or buttock q 3–4 d (twice wkly). (OTC form available for women ≥18 yr.) Topical gel, 1 mL applied to thigh, abdomen, or upper arm q 24 hr. *Child >6 yr:* 5 mg ER tablets PO daily; max, 20 mg/d. *Child >5 yr:* 5 mg PO bid; max, 5 mg tid.
**ADJUST DOSE** Elderly pts
**ADV EFF** Blurred vision, CNS effects, decreased sweating, dizziness, drowsiness, dry mouth, esophagitis, gastric retention, tachycardia, urinary hesitancy
**INTERACTIONS** Amantadine, haloperidol, nitrofurantoin, phenothiazines
**NC/PT** Arrange for cystometry, other diagnostic tests before, during tx. Monitor vision periodically. Periodic bladder exams needed. Pt should swallow ER tablet whole and not cut/crush/chew it; apply gel to thigh, abdomen, or upper arm (rotate sites); apply patch to dry, intact skin on abdomen, hip, or buttock (remove old patch before applying new one); take safety precautions for CNS effects; use sugarless lozenges for dry mouth; report vision changes, vomiting.

**DANGEROUS DRUG**

## oxyCODONE hydrochloride (OxyContin, Roxicodone)
**CLASS** Opioid agonist analgesic
**PREG/CONT** Low risk (short-term use); moderate/high risk (prolonged use)/C-II

**BBW** Risk of addiction/abuse/misuse that can lead to overdose/death. Concurrent use of CYP3A4 inhibitors, benzodiazepines, other CNS depressants may result in increased drug effects, potentially fatal respiratory depression, coma, death. Accidental ingestion by child can be fatal. Prolonged use in preg can result in neonatal opioid withdrawal. FDA requires REMS to ensure benefits outweigh risks.
**IND & DOSE Relief of moderate to moderately severe pain.** *Adult:* Tablets, 5–15 mg PO q 4–6 hr; opioid-naïve, 10–30 mg PO q 4 hr. Capsules, 5 mg PO q 6 hr. Tablets in aversion technology, 5–15 mg PO q 4 hr as needed. Oral sol, 10–30 mg PO q 4 hr as needed. **Mgt of moderate to severe pain when continuous, around-the-clock analgesic needed for extended period.** *Adult:* CR tablets, 10 mg PO q 12 hr for pts taking nonopioid analgesics and requiring around-the-clock tx for extended period. Adjust q 1–2 d as needed by increasing by 25%–50%. *Child ≥11 yr:* Child must have been receiving opioids for at least 5 d w/ minimum 20 mg/d; dosage based on this previous use and conversion to CR oxycontin.
**ADJUST DOSE** Elderly pts, hepatic impairment, impaired adults

**ADV EFF** **Bronchospasm, cardiac arrest,** constipation, dizziness, drowsiness, flushing, **laryngospasm,** light-headedness, n/v, **respiratory arrest,** sedation, **shock,** sweating, ureteral spasm, vision changes
**INTERACTIONS** Barbiturate general anesthetics, opioids, protease inhibitors; avoid these combos
**NC/PT** CR form not for opioid-naïve child. Use pediatric formulas to determine child dose for immediate-release form. Have opioid antagonist, facilities for assisted, controlled respiration on hand. Risk of withdrawal sx, uncontrolled pain, suicide if abruptly stopped in physically dependent pt. Pt should swallow CR form whole and not cut/crush/chew it; take 4–6 hr before next feeding if breastfeeding; take safety precautions for CNS effects; use laxative for constipation; report difficulty breathing, fainting.

## oxymetazoline (Afrin, Dristan, Neo-Synephrine 12 Hour Extra Moisturizing, Vicks Sinex 12-Hour)

**CLASS** Nasal decongestant
**PREG/CONT** C/NA

**BBW** Monitor BP carefully; pts w/ HTN may experience increased HTN related to vasoconstriction. If nasal decongestant needed, pseudoephedrine is drug of choice.
**IND & DOSE** **Sx relief of nasal, nasopharyngeal mucosal congestion.** *Adult, child>6 yr:* 2–3 sprays of 0.05% sol in each nostril bid a.m. and p.m. or q 10–12 hr for up to 3 d.
**ADV EFF** Anxiety, arrhythmias, **CV collapse,** dizziness, drowsiness, dysuria, fear, headache, HTN, light-headedness, nausea, painful urination, rebound congestion, restlessness, tenseness
**INTERACTIONS** MAOIs, methyldopa, TCAs, urine acidifiers/alkalinizers
**NC/PT** Systemic adverse effects less common because drug not generally absorbed systemically. Review proper administration. Rebound congestion possible. Pt should avoid prolonged use (over 3 d), smoky rooms; drink plenty of fluids; use humidifier; take safety precautions for CNS effects; report excessive nervousness.

## oxymetholone

(Anadrol-50)
**CLASS** Anabolic steroid
**PREG/CONT** High risk/C-III

**BBW** Monitor LFTs, serum electrolytes during tx. Consult physician for corrective measures; risk of peliosis hepatis, liver cell tumors. Measure cholesterol in pts at high risk for CAD; lipids may increase.
**IND & DOSE** **Tx of anemias, including congenital aplastic, hypoplastic.** *Adult, child:* 1–5 mg/kg/d PO. Give for minimum trial of 3–6 mo.
**ADV EFF** Abd fullness, acne, anorexia, blood lipid changes, burning of tongue, confusion, excitation, gynecomastia, **intra-abd hemorrhage, hepatitis,** hirsutism in females, hyperglycemia, insomnia, **liver cell tumors, liver failure,** virilization of prepubertal males
**INTERACTIONS** Oral anticoagulants, oral antidiabetics
**NC/PT** Use w/extreme caution; risk of serious disruption of growth/development; weigh benefits, risks. Monitor LFTs, lipids, bone age in child. Not for use in preg (barrier contraceptives advised)/breastfeeding. Pt should take w/food; monitor glucose closely if diabetic; take safety precautions for CNS effects; report severe nausea, urine/stool color changes.

DANGEROUS DRUG

## oxyMORphone hydrochloride (Opana)

**CLASS** Opioid agonist analgesic
**PREG/CONT** High risk/C-II

**BBW** Risk of addiction/abuse misuse that can lead to overdose/death.

Ensure pt swallows ER form whole; cutting, crushing, chewing could cause rapid release and fatal overdose. ER form has abuse potential; monitor accordingly. ER form indicated only for around-the-clock use over extended period. Do not give PRN. Pt must not consume alcohol in any form while taking oxycodone; risk of serious serum drug level increase, potentially fatal overdose. FDA requires REMS to ensure benefits outweigh risks. Accidental ingestion can result in fatal overdose, especially in child. Prolonged use during preg can result in neonatal opioid withdrawal syndrome. Ingestion w/alcohol can result in fatal levels. Concomitant use w/ CNS depressants can increase risk of sedation/respiratory depression/coma/death.
**IND & DOSE Relief of moderate to moderately severe acute pain.** *Adult:* 10–20 mg PO q 4–6 hr. **Relief of moderate to moderately severe pain in pts needing around-the-clock tx.** *Adult:* 5 mg ER tablet PO q 12 hr; may increase in 5- to 10-mg increments q 3–7 d. **Preop medication; anesthesia support; obstetric analgesia; relief of anxiety in pts w/pulmonary edema associated w/left ventricular dysfx.** *Adult:* 0.5 mg IV or 1–1.5 mg IM, subcut q 4–6 hr as needed. For analgesia during labor, 0.5–1 mg IM.
**ADJUST DOSE** Elderly pts, impaired adults, renal impairment
**ADV EFF Cardiac arrest, bronchospasm,** constipation, dizziness, dry mouth, euphoria, flushing, HTN, hypotension, **laryngospasm,** lightheadedness, n/v, **respiratory arrest,** sedation, **shock,** sweating, urine retention
**INTERACTIONS** Alcohol, barbiturate anesthetics, CNS depressants
**NC/PT** Have opioid antagonist, facilities for assisted, controlled respiration on hand during parenteral administration. Risk of serious withdrawal sx, uncontrolled pain, suicide if abruptly stopped in physically dependent pt. Pt should swallow ER tablet whole and not cut/crush/chew it; take 4–6 hr before next feeding if breastfeeding; monitor infant for sedation/respiratory depression; avoid alcohol; use laxative for constipation; take safety precautions for CNS effects; report difficulty breathing.

**DANGEROUS DRUG**

**oxytocin** (Pitocin)
**CLASS** Hormone, oxytocic
**PREG/CONT** X/NA

**BBW** Reserve for medical use, not elective induction.
**IND & DOSE Induction, stimulation of labor.** *Adult:* 0.5–2 milliunits/min (0.0005–0.002 units/min) by IV infusion through infusion pump. Increase in increments of no more than 1–2 milliunits/min at 30- to 60-min intervals until contraction pattern similar to normal labor established. Rates exceeding 9–10 milliunits/min rarely needed. **Control of postpartum uterine bleeding.** *Adult:* Add 10–40 units to 1,000 mL nonhydrating diluent, infuse IV at rate to control uterine atony. Or, 10 units IM after delivery of placenta. **Tx of incomplete, inevitable abortion.** *Adult:* 10 units oxytocin w/500 mL physiologic saline sol or 5% dextrose in physiologic saline IV infused at 10–20 milliunits (20–40 drops)/min. Max, 30 units in 12 hr.
**ADV EFF Afibrinogenemia, anaphylactic reaction,** cardiac arrhythmias, fetal bradycardia, **maternal death,** neonatal jaundice, n/v, **severe water intoxication**
**NC/PT** Ensure fetal position/size, absence of complications. Continuously observe pt receiving IV oxytocin for induction, stimulation of labor; fetal monitoring preferred. Regulate rate to establish uterine contractions. Stop at first sign of hypersensitivity reactions, fetal distress. Pt should report difficulty breathing.

DANGEROUS DRUG

**PACLitaxel** (Abraxane)
**CLASS** Antimitotic, antineoplastic
**PREG/CONT** High risk/NA

**BBW** Do not give unless blood counts within acceptable range. Premedicate w/one of following to prevent severe hypersensitivity reactions: Oral dexamethasone 20 mg 12 hr and 6 hr before paclitaxel, 10 mg if AIDS-related Kaposi sarcoma; diphenhydramine 50 mg IV 30–60 min before paclitaxel; cimetidine 300 mg IV or ranitidine 50 mg IV 30–60 min before paclitaxel. Do not substitute *Abraxane* for other paclitaxel formulations.
**IND & DOSE Tx of metastatic breast cancer after failure of combo tx.** *Adult:* 260 mg/m$^2$ IV over 3 hr q 3 wk. **Tx of NSCLC.** *Adult:* 100 mg/m$^2$ IV over 30 min on days 1, 8, 15 of 21-day cycle, w/carboplatin on day 1 immediately after infusion. **Tx of metastatic adenocarcinoma of pancreas w/gemcitabine.** *Adult:* 125 mg/m$^2$ IV over 30–40 min on days 1, 8, 15 of each 28-day cycle, w/gemcitabine on days 1, 8, 15.
**ADJUST DOSE** Hepatic impairment
**ADV EFF** Alopecia, arthralgia, **bone marrow depression, hepatic impairment, hypersensitivity reactions, infection,** myalgia, n/v, peripheral neuropathies, **pneumonitis,** sepsis
**INTERACTIONS** Cisplatin, cyclosporine, dexamethasone, diazepam, etoposide, ketoconazole, quinidine, teniposide, testosterone, verapamil, vincristine
**NC/PT** Monitor CBC carefully; dose based on response. Premedicate to decrease risk of hypersensitivity reactions. Not for use in preg (barrier contraceptives advised)/breastfeeding. Pt should avoid exposure to infections; mark calendar of tx days; take safety precautions for CNS effects; cover head at temp extremes (hair loss possible); report s&sx of infection, difficulty breathing.

**palbociclib** (Ibrance)
**CLASS** Antineoplastic, kinase inhibitor
**PREG/CONT** High risk/NA

**IND & DOSE Tx of estrogen receptor–positive, HER2-negative advanced breast cancer as initial endocrine tx, w/aromatase inhibitor (postmenopausal); or in disease progression after endocrine tx, w/fulvestrant (regardless of menopausal status).** *Adult:* 125 mg/d PO w/food for 21 d; then 7 rest ds.
**ADV EFF** Alopecia, anemia, **bone marrow suppression,** infections, **ILD/pneumonitis,** n/v/d, peripheral neuropathy, **PE**
**INTERACTIONS** CYP3A inducers/inhibitors, grapefruit juice
**NC/PT** Ensure dx. Give w/aromatase inhibitor or fulvestrant. Monitor CBC; dosage adjustment or tx interruption may be needed due to safety or lack of tolerance. Not for use in preg (contraceptives advised)/breastfeeding. Pt should take w/food; mark calendar w/tx days; swallow capsule whole and not cut/crush/chew it; avoid grapefruit juice; cover head at temp extremes (hair loss possible); report unusual bleeding, difficulty breathing, numbness/tingling, s&sx of infection.

**palifermin** (Kepivance)
**CLASS** Keratinocyte growth factor
**PREG/CONT** Moderate risk/NA

**IND & DOSE To decrease incidence/duration of severe oral mucositis in pts w/hematologic malignancies receiving myelotoxic chemo requiring hematopoietic stem-cell support.** *Adult:* 60 mcg/kg/d by IV bolus for 3 consecutive d before and 3 consecutive d after chemo regimen.

**ADV EFF** Edema, erythema, pruritus, rash, taste alterations, tongue swelling
**INTERACTIONS** Heparin, myelotoxic chemo
**NC/PT** Not for use w/melphalan as a conditioning tx. Risk of tumor growth stimulation; monitor accordingly. Not for use in breastfeeding. Provide nutrition support w/taste changes, skin care for rash. Pt should report pain at infusion site, severe rash.

## paliperidone (Invega, Invega Trinza), paliperidone palmitate (Invega Trinza)

**CLASS** Atypical antipsychotic, benzisoxazole
**PREG/CONT** High risk/NA

**BBW** Avoid use in elderly pts w/ dementia-related psychosis; increased risk of CV death. Drug not approved for this use.
**IND & DOSE** **Tx of schizophrenia, schizoaffective disorder.** *Adult:* 6 mg/d PO in a.m.; max, 12 mg/d PO. **Tx of schizophrenia.** *Adult:* 234 mg IM, then 156 mg IM in 1 wk, both in deltoid; 117 mg IM 1 wk later in gluteal or deltoid. Maint, 39–234 mg/mo IM. Once regulated on monthly injections, can switch to ER injection of 78–234 mg IM q 3 mo (*Invega Trinza*). *Child 12–17 yr:* ≥51 kg, 3 mg/d PO; range, 3–12 mg/d. <56 kg, 3 mg/d PO; range, 3–6 mg/d.
**ADJUST DOSE** Renal impairment
**ADV EFF** Akathisia, **bone marrow suppression,** cognitive/motor impairment, dizziness, dry mouth, dystonia, extrapyramidal disorders, hyperglycemia, impaired thinking, **increased mortality in geriatric pts w/dementia-related psychosis, NMS,** orthostatic hypotension, **prolonged QT, seizures,** tachycardia, tardive dyskinesia, weight gain
**INTERACTIONS** Alcohol, antihypertensives, CNS depressants, divalproex, dopamine agonist, levodopa, QT-prolonging drugs
**NC/PT** For ER injection, deltoid injection: <90 kg, use 1-inch, 22G needle; >90 kg, use 1½-inch, 22G needle; for gluteal injection, use 1½-inch, 22G needle. Shake syringe vigorously for at least 15 sec; administer within 5 min. Monitor for hyperglycemia, weight gain. Tablet matrix may appear in stool. Not for use in preg/breastfeeding. Pt should swallow tablet whole and not cut/crush/chew it; avoid alcohol; take safety precautions for CNS effects; report fever, thoughts of suicide.

## palivizumab (Synagis)

**CLASS** Antiviral, monoclonal antibody
**PREG/CONT** Not indicated for use in females of reproductive potential/NA

**IND & DOSE** **Px of serious lower respiratory tract disease caused by RSV in child at high risk for RSV disease.** *Child:* 15 mg/kg IM as single injection monthly during RSV season; give first dose before start of RSV season.
**ADV EFF** Chills, fever, malaise, pharyngitis, **severe anaphylactoid reaction**
**INTERACTIONS** Immunosuppressants
**NC/PT** Give preferably in anterolateral aspect of thigh; do not use gluteal muscle. For cardiopulmonary bypass pts, give as soon as possible following procedure, even if <1 mo since previous dose. Monitor for anaphylaxis, infection. Caregivers should protect from infection; report fever, difficulty breathing.

## palonosetron hydrochloride (Aloxi)

**CLASS** Antiemetic, selective serotonin receptor antagonist
**PREG/CONT** B/NA

**IND & DOSE** **Px of acute/delayed n/v associated w/chemo.** *Adult:*

0.25 mg IV as single dose over 30 sec 30 min before start of chemo. *Child 1 mo–<17 yr:* 20 mcg/kg IV as single dose over 18 min 30 min before start of chemo. **Px of postop n/v.** *Adult:* 0.075 mg IV as single dose over 10 sec immediately before anesthesia induction.
**ADV EFF** Arrhythmias, constipation, drowsiness, flulike sx, headache, **hypersensitivity reactions, serotonin syndrome,** somnolence
**NC/PT** Coordinate dose timing. Pt should take safety precautions, analgesic for headache; report severe constipation, fever, difficulty breathing.

## pamidronate disodium (Aredia)

**CLASS** Bisphosphonate, calcium regulator
**PREG/CONT** D/NA

**IND & DOSE** **Tx of hypercalcemia.** *Adult:* 60–90 mg IV over 2–24 hr as single dose; max, 90 mg/dose. **Tx of Paget disease.** *Adult:* 30 mg/d IV as 4-hr infusion on 3 consecutive d for total dose of 90 mg; max, 90 mg/dose. **Tx of osteolytic bone lesions.** *Adult:* 90 mg IV as 2-hr infusion q 3–4 wk. For bone lesions caused by multiple myeloma, monthly 4-hr infusion; max, 90 mg/dose.
**ADJUST DOSE** Renal impairment
**ADV EFF** Bone pain, diarrhea, headache, hypocalcemia, long-bone fractures, nausea, **osteonecrosis of jaw**
**NC/PT** Have calcium on hand for hypocalcemic tetany. Monitor serum calcium regularly. Dental exam needed before tx for cancer pts at risk for osteonecrosis of jaw. Not recommended for use beyond 3–5 yr. Maintain hydration, nutrition. Pt should not take foods high in calcium, calcium supplements within 2 hr of dose; report muscle twitching, severe diarrhea.

## pancrelipase (Creon, Pancreaze, Pertyze, Viokace, Zenpep)

**CLASS** Digestive enzyme
**PREG/CONT** C/NA

**IND & DOSE** **Replacement tx in pts w/deficient exocrine pancreatic secretions.** *Adult:* 4,000–20,000 units (usually 1–3 capsules/tablets) PO w/ each meal, snacks; may increase to 8 capsules/tablets in severe cases. *Viokace:* 500 units/kg/meal PO to max 2,500 units/kg/meal. Pts w/pancreatectomy or obstruction, 72,000 units lipase meal PO while consuming 100 g/d fat (*Creon*). *Child ≥4 yr:* 500 units lipase/kg/meal PO to max 2,500 units/kg/meal. *Child 1–<4 yr:* 1,000 units/kg/meal PO to max 2,500 units/kg/meal or 10,000 units/kg/d. *Child up to 1 yr:* 3,000 units lipase PO/120 mL formula or breastfeeding session.
**ADV EFF** Abd cramps, diarrhea, hyperuricemia, nausea
**NC/PT** Do not mix capsules directly into infant formula, human milk; follow dose w/formula, human milk. *Creon* and *Viokace* are not interchangeable. Pt should not crush/chew enteric-coated capsules. Pt should report difficulty breathing, joint pain.

**DANGEROUS DRUG**

## panitumumab (Vectibix)

**CLASS** Antineoplastic, monoclonal antibody
**PREG/CONT** High risk/NA

**BBW** Monitor for possibly severe to life-threatening dermatologic toxicity.
**IND & DOSE** **Tx of wild-type KRAS and NRAS metastatic colorectal carcinoma as first line w/FOLFOX, or as monotherapy post fluoropyrimidine, oxaliplatin, and irinotecan-containing chemo; NOT for tx of RAS-mutant mCRC or unkn RAS mutation status.** *Adult:* 6 mg/kg IV over 60 min q 14 d;

give doses larger than 1,000 mg over 90 min.
**ADV EFF** Abd pain, constipation, **dermatologic toxicity,** diarrhea, **electrolyte depletion,** fatigue, hypomagnesemia, **infusion reactions,** ocular toxicity, **pulmonary fibrosis, tumor progression**
**NC/PT** Ensure appropriate use. Withdraw from vial w/21G or larger needle. Monitor electrolytes, respiratory function; watch for ocular keratitis. Monitor constantly during infusion; stop if infusion reaction. Men, women should use barrier contraceptives during and for 6 mo after tx; not for use in breastfeeding. Pt should report difficulty breathing, pain at injection site, fever, rash, vision changes.

## panobinostat (Farydak)

**CLASS** Antineoplastic, histone deacetylase inhibitor
**PREG/CONT** High risk/NA

**BBW** Risk of severe diarrhea. Ensure antidiarrheal tx; interrupt/stop drug if not controlled. Serious to fatal cardiac events, arrhythmias possible; monitor ECG, electrolytes before and periodically during tx.
**IND & DOSE Tx of melanoma after at least 2 prior tx, w/bortezomib and dexamethasone.** *Adult:* 20 mg PO q other day for three doses/wk on days 1, 3, 5, 8, 10, 12 of wk 1 and 2 of each 21-day cycle for eight cycles.
**ADJUST DOSE** Hepatic impairment
**ADV EFF Bleeding events,** fatigue, fever, **diarrhea, hepatotoxicity,** n/v/d, peripheral edema
**INTERACTIONS** QT-prolonging drugs, strong CYP3A4 inhibitors. Strong CYP3A4 inducers, CYP2D6 substrates, antiarrhythmics; avoid these combos
**NC/PT** Ensure proper dx; use w/ bortezomib, dexamethasone. Baseline ECG, electrolytes; monitor periodically. Monitor LFTs. Monitor for diarrhea. May use antidiarrheals; stop if severe. Ensure nutrition, hydration; small meals for GI problems. Not for use in preg (contraceptives advised)/breastfeeding. Pt should report diarrhea, bleeding, urine/stool color changes, swelling.

## pantoprazole (Protonix)

**CLASS** Proton pump inhibitor
**PREG/CONT** Low risk/NA

**IND & DOSE Tx of GERD; maint tx of erosive esophagitis; tx of pathological hypersecretory disorders.** *Adult:* 40 mg/d PO for ≤8 wk for maint healing of erosive esophagitis. May repeat 8-wk course if no healing. Give continually for hypersecretory disorders: 40 mg/d IV bid up to 240 mg/d (2-yr duration) or 40 mg/d IV for 7–10 d. For severe hypersecretory syndromes, 80 mg q 12 hr (up to 240 mg/d) PO, IV (6-day duration). **Tx of GERD.** *Child ≥5 yr:* ≥40 kg: 40 mg/d PO for up to 8 wk. 15–<40 kg: 20 mg/d PO for up to 8 wk.
**ADJUST DOSE** Hepatic impairment
**ADV EFF** Abd pain, bone loss, CDAD, cutaneous/systemic lupus, dizziness, headache, hypocalcemia, hypomagnesemia, insomnia, interstitial nephritis, n/v/d, pneumonia, URI
**NC/PT** Further evaluation needed after 4 wk of tx for GERD. Switch from IV to oral as soon as possible. Consider zinc replacement w/IV use in pts prone to zinc deficiency. Not for use in breastfeeding. Pt should swallow tablet whole and not cut/crush/chew it; take safety measures for dizziness; report severe diarrhea, headache, fever.

## parathyroid hormone (Natpara)

**CLASS** Hormone
**PREG/CONT** High risk/NA

**BBW** Increased risk of osteosarcoma; do not use in pts w/known risk of osteosarcoma. Available only through restricted program.

**IND & DOSE Adjunct to calcium, vitamin D to control hypocalcemia in hypoparathyroidism.** *Adult:* 50 mcg/d subcut into thigh. Monitor calcium level q 3–7 d; adjust dose to maintain serum calcium level above 7.5 mg/dL.
**ADV EFF** Arthralgia, headache, **hypercalcemia,** hypersensitivity, n/v/d, **osteosarcoma,** paresthesia, **severe hypocalcemia**
**INTERACTIONS** Digoxin
**NC/PT** Screen pt for risk of osteosarcoma. Confirm adequate vitamin D level, serum calcium level above 7.5 mg/dL before starting. Monitor serum levels; adjust vitamin D/calcium dosages based on pt response and presentation. Not for use in preg (contraceptives advised)/breastfeeding. Pt should report difficulty breathing, chest pain.

## paricalcitol (Zemplar)

**CLASS** Vitamin
**PREG/CONT** Unkn/NA

**IND & DOSE Px/tx of secondary hyperparathyroidism associated w/ chronic renal failure.** *Adult:* 0.04–0.1 mcg/kg injected during dialysis, no more often than q other day. Pts not on dialysis: 1–2 mcg/d PO, or 2–4 mcg PO 3 ×/wk based on parathyroid level.
**ADV EFF** Arthralgia, chills, dry mouth, fever, flulike sx, **GI hemorrhage,** n/v
**INTERACTIONS** Aluminum-containing antacids, ketoconazole
**NC/PT** Arrange for calcium supplements; restrict phosphorus intake. Not for use in breastfeeding. Pt should avoid vitamin D; report changes in thinking, appetite/weight loss, increased thirst.

## PARoxetine hydrochloride (Paxil), PARoxetine mesylate (Brisdelle, Pexeva)

**CLASS** Antidepressant, SSRI
**PREG/CONT** High risk/NA

**BBW** Risk of increased suicidality in child, adolescent, young adult; monitor accordingly.
**IND & DOSE Tx of depression.** *Adult:* 20 mg/d PO; range, 20–50 mg/d. Or, 25–62.5 mg/d CR form. **Tx of OCD.** *Adult:* 20 mg/d PO. May increase in 10-mg/d increments; max, 60 mg/d. **Tx of panic disorder.** *Adult:* 10 mg/d PO; range, 10–60 mg/d. Or 12.5–75 mg/d CR tablet; max, 75 mg/d. **Tx of social anxiety disorder.** *Adult:* 20 mg/d PO in a.m. Or, 12.5 mg/d PO CR form; max, 60 mg/d or 37.5 mg/d CR form. **Tx of generalized anxiety disorder.** *Adult:* 20 mg/d PO; range, 20–50 mg/d. **Tx of PMDD.** *Adult:* 12.5 mg/d PO in a.m.; range, 12.5–25 mg/d. May give daily or just during luteal phase of cycle. **Tx of PTSD.** *Adult:* 20 mg/d PO as single dose; range, 20–50 mg/d. **Tx of vasomotor sx of menopause (hot flashes).** *Adult:* 7.5 mg/d PO at bedtime (*Brisdelle*).
**ADJUST DOSE** Elderly pts; hepatic/renal impairment
**ADV EFF** Anxiety, asthenia, bone fractures, constipation, diarrhea, dizziness, dry mouth, ejaculatory disorders, glaucoma, headache, hyponatremia, insomnia, nervousness, serotonin syndrome, somnolence, **suicidality**
**INTERACTIONS** Digoxin, fosamprenavir, MAOIs, phenobarbital, phenytoin, pimozide, procyclidine, ritonavir, serotonergics, St. John's wort, tamoxifen, thioridazine, tryptophan, warfarin
**NC/PT** Do not give within 14 d of MAOIs or give w/pimozide, thioridazine. Not for use in preg/breastfeeding. Pt should take in evening; swallow

CR tablet whole and not cut/crush/ chew it; shake suspension before use; take safety precautions for CNS effects; avoid St. John's wort; report blurred vision, thoughts of suicide.

**pasireotide** (Signifor, Signifor LAR)
**CLASS** Somatostatin analog
**PREG/CONT** Unkn/NA

**IND & DOSE Tx of Cushing disease when pituitary surgery is not an option.** *Adult:* 0.6–0.9 mg subcut bid; titrate based on response. Or, 40 mg IM q 28 d (LAR).
**ADJUST DOSE** Hepatic impairment
**ADV EFF** Bradycardia, cholelithiasis, diabetes, headache, hyperglycemia, hypocortisolism, **prolonged QT**
**INTERACTIONS** Bromocriptine, cyclosporine, QT-prolonging drugs
**NC/PT** Baseline and periodic fasting blood glucose, $HbA_{1c}$, LFTs, ECG, gallbladder ultrasound. Diabetic teaching, intervention may be needed. Use w/ caution in preg; not for use in breastfeeding. Teach proper subcut or IM administration/disposal of needles/ syringes. Pt should mark calendar for IM injection dates; report abd pain, excessive thirst, fatigue, urine/stool color changes.

**▶ NEW DRUG**

**patisiran** (Onpattro)
**CLASS** Anti-transthyretin small interfering RNA agent, metabolic agent
**PREG/CONT** Unkn/NA

**IND & DOSE Tx of polyneuropathy of hereditary transthyretin-mediated amyloidosis.** *Adult ≥100 kg:* 30 mg IV q 3 wk. *Adult <100 kg:* 0.3 mg/kg IV once q 3 wk.
**ADV EFF** Infusion-related reactions, low vitamin A, URI
**NC/PT** Premedicate w/corticosteroid, acetaminophen, antihistamines. Infuse over approx 80 min. Pt should take recommended vitamin A to decrease risk of deficiency.

**patiromer** (Veltassa)
**CLASS** Potassium binder
**PREG/CONT** Low risk/NA

**IND & DOSE Tx of hyperkalemia.** *Adult:* 8.4 g/d PO; may increase at 1-wk intervals by 8.4 g/d to reach target potassium level.
**ADV EFF** Abd discomfort, constipation, flatulence, hypomagnesemia, n/d
**NC/PT** Give other oral drugs at least 6 hr before or after patiromer. Mix drug w/full glass of water, stir well; have pt drink immediately. Do not heat drug or add to heated liquids. Check potassium level before and periodically during tx. Pt should report severe constipation, diarrhea.

**pazopanib** (Votrient)
**CLASS** Antineoplastic, kinase inhibitor
**PREG/CONT** High risk/NA

**BBW** Risk of severe to fatal hepatotoxicity. Monitor LFTs regularly; adjust dose accordingly.
**IND & DOSE Tx of advanced renal cell carcinoma; tx of soft-tissue sarcoma progressed after prior tx.** *Adult:* 800 mg/d PO w/o food.
**ADJUST DOSE** Hepatic impairment
**ADV EFF** Anorexia, **arterial thrombotic events, GI perforation,** hair color changes, **hemorrhagic events, hepatotoxicity, HTN,** hypothyroidism, **impaired wound healing, interstitial pneumonitis,** n/v, **prolonged QT, proteinuria, RPLS, serious infections**
**INTERACTIONS** CYP3A4 inducers/ inhibitors, simvastatin
**NC/PT** Not for use in preg/breastfeeding. Hair may lose pigmentation. Provide nutrition support for n/v. Stop drug w/interstitial pneumonitis, RPLS. Pt should take on empty stomach at least 1 hr before, 2 hr after

meal; report all drugs/OTC/herbs used (many drug interactions possible); urine/stool color changes, yellowing of skin/eyes, severe abd pain, difficulty breathing, chest pain, fever.

**pegaptanib** (Macugen)
**CLASS** Monoclonal antibody
**PREG/CONT** B/NA

**IND & DOSE Tx of neovascular (wet) age-related macular degeneration.** *Adult:* 0.3 mg q 6 wk by intravitreous injection into affected eye.
**ADV EFF Anaphylaxis; endophthalmitis;** eye discharge, pain, infection; increased IOP; retinal detachment; traumatic cataract; vision changes; vitreous floaters
**NC/PT** Monitor IOP. Pt should mark calendar of tx days, report eye redness, sensitivity to light, sudden vision change.

**DANGEROUS DRUG**

**pegaspargase** (Oncaspar)
**CLASS** Antineoplastic
**PREG/CONT** Unkn/NA

**IND & DOSE Tx of ALL.** *Adult, child ≤21 yr:* 2,500 international units/$m^2$ IM, IV no more often than q 14 d. *Adult >21 yr:* 2,000 international units/$m^2$ IM, IV no more often than q 14 d.
**ADV EFF Anaphylaxis, bleeding, bone marrow depression, coagulopathy,** glucose intolerance, **hepatotoxicity**, hypoalbuminemia, hypersensitivity, hypertriglyceridemia, **pancreatitis, renal toxicity**
**NC/PT** Do not use if hx of thrombosis, pancreatitis, severe hepatic impairment, bleeding w/prior L-asparaginase. Limit IM injection volume to 2 mL; if >2 mL, use multiple injection sites. For IV, give over 1–2 hr in 100 mL NSS or 5% dextrose. Monitor LFTs/renal function/amylase. Not for use in preg/breastfeeding. Pt should report excessive thirst, severe headache, acute shortness of breath, difficulty breathing.

**pegfilgrastim** (Fulphila, Neulasta, Udenyca, Ziextenzo)
**CLASS** Colony stimulating factor
**PREG/CONT** Unkn/NA

**IND & DOSE To decrease incidence of infection in pts w/nonmyeloid malignancies receiving myelosuppressive anticancer drugs.** *Adult, child >45 kg:* 6 mg subcut as single dose once per chemo cycle. Do not give within 14 d before and 24 hr after cytotoxic chemo. *Child <45 kg:* Base dosage on wt. **To increase survival in pts exposed to myelosuppressive doses of radiation.** *Adult, child >45 kg:* Two doses of 6 mg each subcut 1 wk apart; give first dose as soon after exposure as possible. *Child <45 kg:* Base dosage on wt.
**ADV EFF Acute respiratory distress syndrome,** alopecia, anorexia, arthralgia, **bone marrow suppression,** bone pain, dizziness, dyspepsia, edema, **fatal sickle cell crisis,** fatigue, fever, generalized weakness, glomerulonephritis, mucositis, n/v/d, **splenic rupture,** stomatitis
**INTERACTIONS** Lithium
**NC/PT** Monitor CBC. Protect from light. Do not shake syringe. Sol should be free of particulate matter, not discolored. Pt should cover head at temp extremes (hair loss possible); avoid exposure to infection; report s&sx of infection, difficulty breathing, pain at injection site. Name confusion between *Neulasta* (pegfilgrastim) and *Neumega* (oprelvekin).

**peginterferon alfa-2a** (Pegasys)
**CLASS** Interferon
**PREG/CONT** C/NA

**BBW** May cause, aggravate life-threatening to fatal neuropsychiatric,

autoimmune, ischemic, infectious disorders. Monitor closely; stop w/ persistent s&sx. Risk of serious fetal defects when used w/ribavirin; men, women should avoid preg.
**IND & DOSE Tx of HCV in pts w/ compensated liver disease as part of combo regimen.** *Adult:* 180 mcg subcut wkly for 48 wk w/other antivirals. *Child ≥5 yr:* 180 mcg/1.73 $m^2$ × BSA subcut per wk w/ribavirin. **Tx of adult, child ≥3 yr w/chronic HBV w/compensated liver disease, evidence of viral replication/liver inflammation.** *Adult:* 180 mcg subcut wkly for 48 wk w/other antivirals. *Child:* 180 mcg/1.73 $m^2$ × BSA/wk w/ribavirin; duration varies.
**ADJUST DOSE** Hepatic/renal impairment
**ADV EFF** Asthenia, **bone marrow suppression, colitis,** fatigue, fever, growth impairment, headache, **hemolytic anemia, hepatic impairment, infections,** myalgia, **neuropsychiatric events, pancreatitis, peripheral neuropathy, pulmonary events, SJS, suicidality**
**INTERACTIONS** Azathioprine, didanosine, methadone, nucleoside analogs, theophylline, zidovudine
**NC/PT** Monitor closely; adverse effects may require stopping. Evaluate use in preg based on other antivirals used. Store in refrigerator. Teach proper administration/disposal of needles/syringes. Pt should avoid exposure to infection; report severe abd pain, bloody diarrhea, s&sx of infection, thoughts of suicide, difficulty breathing, rash.

## peginterferon alfa-2b
(Pegintron, Sylatron)
**CLASS** Antineoplastic, interferon
**PREG/CONT** High risk/NA

**BBW** May cause, aggravate life-threatening to fatal neuropsychiatric, autoimmune, ischemic, infectious disorders. Monitor closely; stop w/ persistent s&sx. Risk of serious fetal defects when used w/ribavirin; men, women should avoid preg.
**IND & DOSE Tx of chronic HCV in pts w/compensated liver disease.** *Adult:* 1.5 mcg/kg/wk subcut w/800–1,400 mg/d PO ribavirin. *Child:* 60 mcg/$m^2$/wk subcut w/15 mg/kg/d PO ribavirin in two divided doses.
**ADJUST DOSE** Hepatic/renal impairment
**ADV EFF** Asthenia, **bone marrow suppression, colitis,** fatigue, fever, headache, **hemolytic anemia, hepatic impairment, infections,** injection-site reactions, **ischemic cerebral events,** myalgia, **neuropsychiatric events, pancreatitis, pericarditis, pulmonary events, suicidality**
**INTERACTIONS** Azathioprine, didanosine, methadone, nucleoside analogs, theophylline, zidovudine
**NC/PT** Monitor closely; adverse effects may require stopping. Not for use in preg (men, women should use two forms of contraception during, for 6 mo after tx)/breastfeeding. Store in refrigerator. Teach proper administration/disposal of needles/syringes. Pt should mark calendar w/tx days; avoid exposure to infection; report severe abd pain, bloody diarrhea, s&sx of infection, suicidal thoughts, difficulty breathing, chest pain.

## pegloticase (Krystexxa)
**CLASS** PEGylated uric-acid specific enzyme
**PREG/CONT** C/NA

**BBW** Severe anaphylaxis, infusion reactions have occurred; premedicate, closely monitor. Monitor serum uric acid level. Screen pt for G6PD deficiency before medicating.
**IND & DOSE Tx of chronic gout in pts refractory to conventional tx.** *Adult:* 8 mg by IV infusion over no less than 120 min q 2 wk.
**ADJUST DOSE** Renal impairment
**ADV EFF Anaphylaxis,** chest pain, constipation, ecchymosis, gout flares,

**HF,** infusion reactions, nasopharyngitis, vomiting
**NC/PT** Monitor serum uric acid level. Discontinue oral urate-lowering agents. Premedicate w/antihistamines, corticosteroids. Contraindicated w/ G6PD deficiencies. Not for use in breastfeeding. Alert pt gout flares may occur up to 3 mo after starting tx. Pt should mark calendar for infusion d; report difficulty breathing, edema.

DANGEROUS DRUG

## pegvaliase-pqpz (Palynziq)

**CLASS** Phenylalanine ammonia lyase enzyme
**PREG/CONT** High risk/NA

**BBW** Anaphylaxis has been reported; may occur at any time during tx. Give initial dose under supervision of health care provider equipped to manage anaphylaxis; closely observe pt for at least 60 min after injection. Before self-injection, confirm pt competency, pt's ability to recognize anaphylaxis s&sx and to self-administer auto-injectable epinephrine; before first dose, instruct pt on its use and to seek immediate medical care after use. Instruct pt to carry auto-injectable epinephrine at all times during tx. Medication available only through Palynziq REMS.
**IND & DOSE To reduce blood phenylalanine conc in pts w/phenylketonuria who have uncontrolled blood phenylalanine conc >600 micromol/L on existing mgt.** *Adult:* 2.4 mg subcut once a wk for 4 wk. May titrate up in step-wise manner to 20 mg subcut daily, or 40 mg subcut daily in some pts.
**ADV EFF** Abd pain, **anaphylaxis,** arthralgia, cough, fatigue, headache, hypersensitivity reactions, injection-site reactions, n/v/d, oropharyngeal pain, pruritus, skin reactions
**NC/PT** May need to premedicate to decrease adverse reactions. Rotate injection sites at least 2 inches apart. Teach pt anaphylaxis s&sx, how to use epinephrine, and that phenylalanine level will be monitored q 4 wk initially. Pt should seek medical attention after epinephrine use, reduce dietary protein and phenylalanine intake.

## pegvisomant (Somavert)

**CLASS** Human growth hormone analog
**PREG/CONT** Moderate risk/NA

**IND & DOSE Tx of acromegaly in pts w/inadequate response to surgery, radiation.** *Adult:* 40 mg subcut as loading dose, then 10 mg/d subcut.
**ADV EFF** Diarrhea, dizziness, edema, **hepatic impairment,** infection, injection-site reactions, nausea, pain, peripheral edema, sinusitis
**INTERACTIONS** Opioids
**NC/PT** Local reactions to injection common; rotate sites regularly. Monitor for infection. Monitor LFTs. Not for use in breastfeeding. Teach proper administration/disposal of needles/ syringes.

## pembrolizumab (Keytruda)

**CLASS** Antineoplastic, human programmed death receptor-1 blocking antibody
**PREG/CONT** High risk/NA

**IND & DOSE Tx of unresectable or metastatic melanoma; adjuvant tx if melanoma w/lymph node involvement.** *Adult:* 200 mg IV over 30 min q 3 wk. **Tx of NSCLC w/PD-L1 expression as first-line therapy or w/progression after platinum therapy; tx of NSCLC as first-line tx w/pemetrexed and carboplatin; tx of head/ neck cancer w/progression during or after platinum-based therapy.** *Adult:* 200 mg IV over 30 min q 3 wk. **Tx of pts w/refractory or relapsed classical Hodgkin lymphoma after three other lines of therapy**. *Adult:* 200 mg IV q 3 wk. *Child:* 2 mg/kg (up to 200 mg) IV q 3 wk. **Tx of pts w/locally**

**advanced or metastatic urothelial carcinoma not eligible for cisplatin therapy, or w/progression during or after platinum-containing therapy.** 200 mg IV q 3 wk. **Tx of pts w/unresectable or metastatic microsatellite instability-high or mismatch repair deficient solid tumors w/other tx choices or colorectal cancer after tx w/a fluoropyrimidine, oxaliplatin, and irinotecan.** *Adult:* 200 mg IV q 3 wk. *Child:* 2 mg/kg (up to 200 mg) q 3 wk. **Tx of recurrent locally advanced or metastatic gastric or gastroesophageal junction adenocarcinoma that expresses PD-L1 and w/progression during or after ≥two lines of tx, including fluoropyrimidine- and platinum-containing therapy.** *Adults:* 200 mg IV q 3 wk.
**ADV EFF** Cough, fatigue, **infusion reactions**, n/v/d, **potentially serious immune-mediated reactions (colitis, endocrinopathies, hepatitis, nephritis, pneumonitis)**, rash
**NC/PT** Ensure dx. Monitor immune-mediated reactions (LFTs, renal/thyroid function); give corticosteroids based on severity; stop if severe. Not for use in preg/breastfeeding. Frequent follow-up needed. Pt should mark calendar w/tx days; report s&sx of infection, difficulty breathing.

**DANGEROUS DRUG**

## PEMEtrexed (Alimta)
**CLASS** Antifolate antineoplastic
**PREG/CONT** High risk/NA

**IND & DOSE Tx of unresectable malignant mesothelioma; tx of locally advanced, metastatic NSCLC.** *Adult:* 500 mg/m² IV infused over 10 min on day 1, then 75 mg/m² cisplatin (tx of mesothelioma only) IV over 2 hr; repeat cycle q 21 d.
**ADJUST DOSE** Renal/hepatic impairment
**ADV EFF** Anorexia, **bone marrow suppression,** constipation, fatigue, interstitial pneumonitis, n/v/d, **renal impairment,** stomatitis, toxicity
**INTERACTIONS** Nephrotoxic drugs, NSAIDs
**NC/PT** Pretreat w/corticosteroids, oral folic acid, IM vitamin $B_{12}$. Monitor CBC; dosage adjustment based on response. Not for use in preg (barrier contraceptives advised)/breastfeeding. Pt should avoid NSAIDs, exposure to infection; report unusual bleeding, severe GI sx.

## penicillamine (Cuprimine, Depen)
**CLASS** Antirheumatic, chelate
**PREG/CONT** D/NA

**BBW** Because of severe toxicity, including bone marrow suppression, renal damage, reserve use for serious cases; monitor closely.
**IND & DOSE Tx of severe, active RA, Wilson disease, cystinuria when other measures fail.** *Adult:* 125–250 mg/d PO; max, 1 g/d.
**ADV EFF** Agitation, anxiety, **bone marrow suppression,** fever, **myasthenia gravis,** paresthesia, rash, **renal toxicity,** tinnitus
**INTERACTIONS** Gold salts, nephrotoxic drugs
**NC/PT** Monitor CBC, renal function twice/wk. Assess neuro functioning; stop if increasing weakness. Not for use in preg (barrier contraceptives advised)/breastfeeding. Pt should avoid exposure to infection; report s&sx of infection, muscle weakness, edema.

## penicillin G benzathine (Bicillin L-A)
**CLASS** Penicillin antibiotic
**PREG/CONT** B/NA

**BBW** Not for IV use. Do not inject or mix w/other IV sols. Inadvertent IV administration has caused cardiorespiratory arrest, death.
**IND & DOSE Tx of streptococcal infections.** *Adult:* 1.2 million units IM. *Older child:* 900,000 units IM. *Child <27 kg:* 300,000–600,000 units IM.

**Tx of early syphilis.** *Adult:* 2.4 million units IM. **Tx of syphilis lasting longer than 1 yr.** *Adult:* 7.2 million units as 2.4 million units IM wkly for 3 wk. **Tx of yaws, bejel, pinta, erysipeloid.** *Adult:* 1.2 million units IM single dose. **Tx of congenital syphilis.** *Child 2–12 yr:* Adjust dose based on adult schedule. *Child <2 yr:* 50,000 units/kg body weight IM. **Px of rheumatic fever, chorea.** *Adult:* 1.2 million units IM q mo; or 600,000 units q 2 wk.
**ADV EFF** **Anaphylaxis, bone marrow suppression,** gastritis, glossitis, n/v/d, pain, phlebitis, rash, superinfections
**INTERACTIONS** Amikacin, gentamicin, neomycin, tetracyclines, tobramycin
**NC/PT** Culture before tx. Use IM only: upper outer quadrant of buttock (adults), midlateral aspect of thigh (infants, small child). Pt should report difficulty breathing, rash, pain at injection site.

## penicillin G potassium, penicillin G sodium

(Pfizerpen)
**CLASS** Penicillin antibiotic
**PREG/CONT** B/NA

**IND & DOSE** **Tx of meningococcal meningitis.** *Adult:* 1–2 million units q 2 hr IM, or 20–30 million units/d by continuous IV infusion. *Child:* 200,000–300,000 units/kg/d IV q 6 hr. Infants <7 d: 50,000 units/kg/d IV in divided doses q 12 hr. **Tx of actinomycosis.** *Adult:* 1–6 million units/d IM in divided doses q 4–6 hr for 6 wk, or IV for cervicofacial cases. Or, 10–20 million units/d IV for thoracic, abd diseases. **Tx of clostridial infections.** *Adult:* 20 million units/d in divided doses q 4–6 hr IM or IV w/ antitoxin. **Tx of fusospirochetal infections (Vincent disease).** *Adult:* 5–10 million units/d IM or IV in divided doses q 4–6 hr. **Tx of rat-bite fever.** *Adult:* 12–20 million units/d IM or IV in divided doses q 4–6 hr for 3–4 wk. **Tx of Listeria infections.** *Adult:* 15–20 million units/d IM or IV in divided doses q 4–6 hr for 2 or 4 wk (meningitis, endocarditis, respectively). **Tx of Pasteurella infections.** *Adult:* 4–6 million units/d IM or IV in divided doses q 4–6 hr for 2 wk. **Tx of erysipeloid endocarditis.** *Adult:* 12–20 million units/d IM or IV in divided doses q 4–6 hr for 4–6 wk. **Tx of diphtheria (adjunct tx w/antitoxin to prevent carrier state).** *Adult:* 2–3 million units/d IM or IV in divided doses q 4–6 hr for 10–12 d. **Tx of anthrax.** *Adult:* Minimum 5 million units/d IM or IV in divided doses. **Tx of streptococcal infections.** *Adult:* 5–24 million units/d IM or IV in divided doses q 4–6 hr. *Child:* 150,000 units/kg/d IM or IV q 4–6 hr. *Child <7 d:* 75,000 units/kg/d IV in divided doses q 8 hr. **Tx of syphilis.** *Adult:* 18–24 million units/d IV q 4–6 hr for 10–14 d, then benzathine penicillin G 2.4 million units IM wkly for 3 wk. **Tx of gonorrhea.** 10 million units/d IV q 4–6 hr until improvement. **Tx of group B streptococci.** *Child:* 100,000 units/kg/d IV.
**ADV EFF** **Anaphylaxis, bone marrow suppression,** gastritis, glossitis, n/v/d, pain, phlebitis, rash, superinfections
**INTERACTIONS** Amikacin, gentamicin, neomycin, tetracyclines, tobramycin
**NC/PT** Culture before tx. Smallest volume possible for IM use. Have emergency equipment on hand w/IV infusion. Monitor serum electrolytes w/penicillin potassium. Pt should report difficulty breathing, rash, unusual bleeding, s&sx of infection.

## penicillin G procaine

(generic)
**CLASS** Penicillin antibiotic
**PREG/CONT** Low risk/NA

**IND & DOSE** **Tx of moderately severe infections caused by sensitive strains of streptococci, pneumococci, staphylococci.** *Adult:* 600,000–1 million units/d IM for

minimum 10 d. **Tx of bacterial endocarditis (group A streptococci).** *Adult:* 600,000–1 million units/d IM. **Tx of fusospirochetal infections, rat-bite fever, erysipeloid, anthrax.** *Adult:* 600,000–1 million units/d IM. **Tx of diphtheria.** *Adult:* 300,000–600,000 units/d IM w/antitoxin. **Tx of diphtheria carrier state.** *Adult:* 300,000 units/d IM for 10 d. **Tx of syphilis.** *Adult, child >12 yr:* 600,000 units/d IM for 8 d, 10–15 d for late-stage syphilis. **Tx of neurosyphilis.** *Adult:* 2.4 million units/d IM w/500 mg probenecid PO qid for 10–14 d, then 2.4 million units benzathine penicillin G IM after completion of tx regimen. **Tx of congenital syphilis.** *Child <32 kg:* 50,000 units/kg/d IM for 10 d. **Tx of group A streptococcal, staphylococcal pneumonia.** *Child <27 kg:* 300,000 units/d IM.
**ADV EFF** **Anaphylaxis, bone marrow suppression,** gastritis, glossitis, n/v/d, pain, phlebitis, rash, superinfections
**INTERACTIONS** Amikacin, gentamicin, neomycin, tetracyclines, tobramycin
**NC/PT** Culture before tx. IM route only in upper outer quadrant of buttock; midlateral aspect of thigh may be preferred for infants, small child. Pt should report difficulty breathing, rash, unusual bleeding, s&sx of infection.

## penicillin V (Penicillin-VK)

**CLASS** Penicillin antibiotic
**PREG/CONT** B/NA

**IND & DOSE** **Tx of fusospirochetal infections, staphylococcal infections of skin, soft tissues.** *Adult, child >12 yr:* 250–500 mg PO q 6–8 hr. **Tx of streptococcal infections.** *Adult, child >12 yr:* 125–250 mg PO q 6–8 hr for 10 d. **Tx of pneumococcal infections.** *Adult, child >12 yr:* 250–500 mg PO q 6 hr until afebrile for 48 hr. **Px of rheumatic fever/chorea recurrence.** *Adult, child >12 yr:* 25–250 mg PO bid. **Tx of Lyme disease.** *Adult, child >12 yr:* 500 mg PO qid for 10–20 d. **Tx of mild, uncomplicated cutaneous anthrax.** *Adult, child >12 yr:* 200–500 mg PO qid. *Child 2–12 yr:* 25–50 mg/kg/d PO in two or four divided doses. **Px of anthrax px.** *Adult, child >9 yr:* 7.5 mg/kg PO qid. *Child <9 yr:* 50 mg/kg/d PO in four divided doses. **Px of Streptococcus pneumoniae septicemia in sickle cell anemia.** *Child 6–9 yr:* 250 mg PO bid. *Child 3 mo–5 yr:* 125 mg PO bid.
**ADV EFF** **Anaphylaxis, bone marrow suppression,** gastritis, glossitis, n/v/d, pain, phlebitis, rash, superinfections
**INTERACTIONS** Tetracyclines
**NC/PT** Culture before tx. Stable for max 14 d. Pt should take w/water, not w/milk, fruit juices, soft drinks; refrigerate suspension; report difficulty breathing, rash, unusual bleeding, s&sx of infection.

## pentamidine isethionate (NebuPent, Pentam)

**CLASS** Antiprotozoal
**PREG/CONT** C/NA

**IND & DOSE** **Tx of *Pneumocystis jiroveci* pneumonia.** *Adult, child:* 4 mg/kg/d for 14–21 d by deep IM injection or IV infusion over 60–120 min. **Px of *P. jiroveci* pneumonia.** *Adult, child:* 300 mg once q 4 wk through *Respirgard II* nebulizer.
**ADV EFF** **Acute renal failure,** anorexia, cough, dizziness, fatigue, fever, hypotension, **laryngospasm,** metallic taste (inhalation), prolonged QT, **severe hypotension,** pain at injection site, rash, **SJS**
**INTERACTIONS** NSAIDs, QT-prolonging drugs
**NC/PT** Culture before tx. Drug a biohazard; use safe handling procedures. Monitor CBC, LFTs, renal function. Have pt in supine position for parenteral administration. Not for use in preg/breastfeeding. Pt should take safety

precautions w/hypotension, CNS effects; learn proper use, care of *Respirgard II*; report difficulty breathing, dizziness, rash.

**DANGEROUS DRUG**

**pentobarbital** (Nembutal Sodium)
**CLASS** Antiepileptic, barbiturate, sedative-hypnotic
**PREG/CONT** D/C-II

**BBW** Do not administer intra-arterially; may produce arteriospasm, thrombosis, gangrene.
**IND & DOSE Sedative-hypnotic, preanesthetic, emergency antiseizure.** *Adult:* Give by slow IV injection (max, 50 mg/min); 100 mg in 70-kg adult. Wait at least 1 min for full effect. Base dose on response. May give additional small increments to max 200–500 mg. Minimize dose in seizure states to avoid compounding possible depression after seizures. Or, 150–200 mg IM. *Child:* Reduce initial adult dose based on age, weight, condition. Or, 25–80 mg or 2–6 mg/kg IM; max, 100 mg.
**ADJUST DOSE** Elderly pts, debilitated adults
**ADV EFF** Agitation, apnea, ataxia, bradycardia, **bronchospasm,** CNS depression, **circulatory collapse,** confusion, dizziness, hallucinations, hyperkinesia, hypotension, hypoventilation, insomnia, **laryngospasm,** pain/necrosis at injection site, **SJS,** somnolence, syncope, **withdrawal syndrome**
**INTERACTIONS** Alcohol, beta-adrenergic blockers, CNS depressants, corticosteroids, doxycycline, estrogens, hormonal contraceptives, metronidazole, oral anticoagulants, phenylbutazones, quinidine, theophylline
**NC/PT** Use caution in child; may produce irritability, aggression, inappropriate tearfulness. Give slowly IV or by deep IM injection. Monitor continuously during IV use; monitor injection site for irritation. Taper gradually w/long-term use. Not for use in preg; use caution w/breastfeeding. Pt should take safety precautions for CNS effects; report difficulty breathing, rash.

**pentosan polysulfate sodium** (Elmiron)
**CLASS** Bladder protectant
**PREG/CONT** B/NA

**IND & DOSE Relief of bladder pain associated w/interstitial cystitis.** *Adult:* 100 mg PO tid on empty stomach.
**ADV EFF** Abd pain, alopecia, bleeding, diarrhea, dizziness, dyspepsia, liver function changes, nausea
**INTERACTIONS** Anticoagulants, aspirin, NSAIDs
**NC/PT** Use caution w/hepatic insufficiency. Drug a heparin; use caution if surgery needed. Pt should cover head at temp extremes (hair loss possible); report unusual bleeding, urine/stool color changes.

**DANGEROUS DRUG**

**pentostatin** (Nipent)
**CLASS** Antineoplastic antibiotic
**PREG/CONT** High risk/NA

**BBW** Associated w/fatal pulmonary toxicity, bone marrow depression.
**IND & DOSE Tx of alpha interferon–refractory hairy cell leukemia, chronic lymphocytic leukemia, cutaneous/peripheral T-cell lymphoma.** *Adult:* 4 mg/m$^2$ IV q other wk.
**ADJUST DOSE** Renal impairment
**ADV EFF** Abd pain, anorexia, **bone marrow suppression,** chills, cough, dizziness, dyspepsia, n/v, **pulmonary toxicity,** rash
**INTERACTIONS** Allopurinol, cyclophosphamide, fludarabine, vidarabine
**NC/PT** Toxic drug; use special precautions in handling. Monitor CBC regularly; monitor pulmonary function. Not for use in preg (contraceptives advised)/breastfeeding. Pt should

mark calendar of tx days; avoid exposure to infection; report difficulty breathing, s&sx of infection.

## pentoxifylline (Pentoxil)

**CLASS** Hemorrheologic, xanthine

**PREG/CONT** C/NA

**IND & DOSE** **Tx of intermittent claudication.** *Adult:* 400 mg PO tid w/ meals for at least 8 wk.

**ADJUST DOSE** Renal impairment

**ADV EFF** Angina, anxiety, dizziness, dyspepsia, headache, nausea, rash

**INTERACTIONS** Anticoagulants, theophylline

**NC/PT** Not for use in breastfeeding. Pt should take w/meals; swallow tablet whole and not cut/crush/chew it; take safety precautions for CNS effects; report chest pain.

## peramivir (Rapivab)

**CLASS** Antiviral, neuraminidase inhibitor

**PREG/CONT** Limited data/NA

**IND & DOSE** **Tx of acute uncomplicated influenza in pts ≥2 yr w/sx for no more than 2 d.** *Adult, adolescent:* 600 mg IV as single dose over 15 min. *Child 2–12 yr:* 12 mg/kg IV up to 600 mg as single dose over 15 min.

**ADJUST DOSE** Renal impairment

**ADV EFF** **Anaphylaxis,** diarrhea, neuropsychiatric events, **serious skin reactions to SJS**

**INTERACTIONS** Live flu vaccine (avoid use 2 wk before or 48 hr after infusion)

**NC/PT** Confirm dx, timing of sx. Use w/caution in preg/breastfeeding. Pt should take safety precaution for CNS effects; report difficulty breathing, rash, abnormal behavior.

## perampanel (Fycompa)

**CLASS** Antiepileptic, glutamate receptor antagonist

**PREG/CONT** High risk/NA

**BBW** Risk of serious to life-threatening psychiatric, behavioral reactions. Monitor pt closely, especially when starting drug or changing dose; reduce dose or stop drug if these reactions occur.

**IND & DOSE** **Tx of partial-onset seizures (≥4 yr); adjunct tx of primary, generalized tonic-clonic seizures (≥12 yr).** *Adult, child ≥4 yr:* Starting dose, 2 mg/d PO at bedtime; 4 mg/d PO at bedtime if pt also on enzyme-inducing antiepileptics. Maint dose, 8–12 mg PO (partial-onset seizures), 8 mg/d PO (tonic-clonic seizures).

**ADJUST DOSE** Elderly pts; mild to moderate hepatic impairment. Severe hepatic/renal impairment, dialysis (not recommended)

**ADV EFF** Ataxia, balance disorders, **DRESS,** falls, fatigue, gait disturbances, irritability, nausea, **serious psychiatric/behavioral reactions,** somnolence, **suicidality,** weight gain

**INTERACTIONS** Alcohol, carbamazepine, CNS depressants, hormonal contraceptives, oxcarbazepine, phenytoin, rifampin, St. John's wort

**NC/PT** Monitor closely when starting tx or changing dose; taper gradually after long-term use. Not for use in preg/breastfeeding. Protect from falls; advise pt to avoid driving, operating dangerous machinery. Pt should take once a day at bedtime; not stop drug suddenly; measure oral suspension using adapter/dosing syringe provided; avoid alcohol/ St. John's wort; use caution to avoid falls/injury; be aware of behavior changes (suicidal thoughts possible); report severe dizziness, trouble walking, suicidal thoughts, behavior changes.

## perindopril erbumine
(generic)
**CLASS** ACE inhibitor, antihypertensive
**PREG/CONT** High risk/NA

**BBW** Serious fetal injury possible; advise barrier contraceptives.
**IND & DOSE Tx of HTN.** *Adult:* 4 mg/d PO; max, 16 mg/d. **Tx of pts w/ stable CAD to reduce risk of CV mortality, nonfatal MI.** *Adult:* 4 mg/d PO for 2 wk; maint, 8 mg/d PO.
**ADJUST DOSE** Elderly pts, renal impairment
**ADV EFF Airway obstruction, angioedema, bone marrow suppression,** cough, diarrhea, dizziness, fatigue, gastric irritation, headache, hyperkalemia, insomnia, nausea, orthostatic hypotension, somnolence
**INTERACTIONS** ACE inhibitors, ARBs, gold, indomethacin, lithium, NSAIDs, potassium-sparing diuretics, potassium supplements, renin inhibitors
**NC/PT** Have epinephrine on hand for angioedema of face, neck. Alert surgeons; volume replacement may be needed if surgery required. Use caution in conditions w/possible BP drop (diarrhea, sweating, vomiting, dehydration). Not for use in preg (barrier contraceptives advised)/breastfeeding. Pt should avoid potassium supplements, OTC drugs that might increase BP; take safety precautions for CNS effects; report difficulty breathing, s&sx of infection, swelling of face/neck.

## pertuzumab (Perjeta)
**CLASS** Antineoplastic, HER2/NEU receptor antagonist
**PREG/CONT** High risk/NA

**BBW** Risk of embryo-fetal and/or birth defects; not for use in preg. Risk of left ventricular dysfx. Evaluate before/during tx.
**IND & DOSE Adjunct tx of pts w/ HER2-positive metastatic breast cancer who have not received prior HER2 therapy or tx for metastatic disease, w/trastuzumab and docetaxel.** *Adult:* 840 mg IV over 60 min, then 420 mg IV over 30–60 min q 3 wk, w/trastuzumab and docetaxel. **Adjunct tx of pts w/HER2-positive early breast cancer w/high risk of recurrence w/trastuzumab and chemo.** *Adult:* 840 mg IV over 60 min, then 420 mg IV over 30–60 min q 3 wk for 1 year w/trastuzumab and chemo. **Neoadjuvant tx of pts w/HER2-positive, locally advanced, inflammatory or early stage w/ trastuzumab and chemo.** *Adult:* 840 mg IV over 60 min, then 420 mg IV over 30–60 min q 3 wk for three–six cycles.
**ADV EFF** Alopecia, fatigue, hypersensitivity, **infusion reaction, left ventricular (LV) dysfx,** neutropenia, n/v, peripheral neuropathy, rash
**NC/PT** Perform HER2 testing before use; ensure concurrent use of trastuzumab/docetaxel. Do not give as bolus. Not for use in preg (contraceptives advised during and for 7 mo after tx)/breastfeeding (avoid for 7 mo after tx). Monitor for infusion reactions, LV dysfx. Pt should mark calendar for injection days; be aware hair loss possible; report difficulty breathing, numbness/tingling, fever, s&sx of infection.

**▶NEW DRUG**

## pexidartinib (Turalio)
**CLASS** Antineoplastic, kinase inhibitor
**PREG/CONT** High risk/NA

**BBW** Risk of serious/potentially fatal liver injury. Monitor LFTs before start/during tx; stop if hepatotoxicity. Only available via REMS program.
**IND & DOSE Tx of tenosynovial giant cell tumor associated w/severe morbidity or functional limitations and not amenable to improvement**

**w/surgery.** *Adult:* 400 mg PO bid on empty stomach.
**ADV EFF** Eye edema, fatigue, increased liver enzymes, rash
**INTERACTIONS** Acid-reducing agents, hepatotoxic products, strong CYP3A inducers/inhibitors. UGT inhibitors
**NC/PT** Give at least 1 hr before or 2 hr after meal/snack. Reduced dose or drug discontinuation may be required based on adverse effects, including hepatotoxicity.

## phenelzine sulfate
(Nardil)
**CLASS** Antidepressant, MAOI
**PREG/CONT** C/NA

**BBW** Increased risk of suicidality in child, adolescent, young adult; monitor accordingly.
**IND & DOSE Tx of depression in pts unresponsive to other tx.** *Adult:* 15 mg PO tid. Rapidly increase to at least 60 mg/d. After max benefit achieved, reduce dose slowly over several wk. Maint, 15 mg/d or q other day PO.
**ADJUST DOSE** Elderly pts
**ADV EFF** Abd pain, anorexia, blurred vision, confusion, constipation, dizziness, drowsiness, dry mouth, headache, hyperreflexia, **hypertensive crisis,** hypomania, hypotension, insomnia, jitteriness, **liver toxicity,** n/v/d, orthostatic hypotension, serotonin syndrome, suicidal thoughts, twitching, vertigo
**INTERACTIONS** Alcohol, amphetamines, antidiabetics, beta blockers, dextromethorphan, meperidine, SSRIs, sympathomimetics, TCAs, thiazides, tyramine-containing foods
**NC/PT** Have phentolamine/other alpha-adrenergic blocker on hand for hypertensive crisis. Monitor LFTs/BP regularly. Pt should avoid diet high in tyramine-containing foods during, for 2 wk after tx; avoid alcohol, OTC appetite suppressants; take safety precautions for CNS effects; change position slowly if orthostatic hypotension; report rash, urine/stool color changes, thoughts of suicide.

## phentermine hydrochloride
Adipex-P, Lomaira
**CLASS** Sympathomimetic
**PREG/CONT** High risk/C-IV

**IND & DOSE Adjunct to diet/exercise for short-term mgt of exogenous obesity w/body mass of ≥30 mg/m² or ≥27 mg/m² w/other risk factors.** *Adult:* 8 mg PO tid ½ hr before meal.
**ADV EFF** Diarrhea, dizziness, drug dependence, dry mouth, **HTN, pulmonary HTN, valvular heart disease**
**INTERACTIONS** Adrenergic blockers, alcohol, **insulin,** MAOIs, oral antidiabetic agents
**NC/PT** Contraindicated w/known cardiac disease, hyperthyroidism, glaucoma, agitated states, hx of drug abuse. Ensure 14 d MAOI-free before use. Pt must use diet/weight-loss program. Drug only for short-term use. Do not combine w/other weight-loss drugs. Not for use in preg (contraceptives advised)/breastfeeding. Pt should avoid alcohol; report difficulty breathing, swelling.

**DANGEROUS DRUG**

## phentolamine mesylate
(OraVerse)
**CLASS** Alpha blocker, diagnostic agent
**PREG/CONT** C/NA

**IND & DOSE Px/control of hypertensive episodes in pheochromocytoma.** *Adult:* For preop reduction of elevated BP, 5 mg IV or IM 1–2 hr before surgery; repeat if necessary. Give 5 mg IV during surgery as indicated to control paroxysms of HTN, other epinephrine toxicity effects. *Child:* 1 mg IV or IM 1–2 hr before surgery; repeat if necessary. Give 1 mg IV during surgery as indicated for epinephrine toxicity. **Px of tissue necrosis, sloughing after IV dopamine extravasation.** *Adult:* Infiltrate 10–15 mL normal saline injection containing 5–10 mg phentolamine. *Child:* Infiltrate 0.1–0.2 mg/kg to max 10 mg. **Px of tissue necrosis, sloughing after IV norepinephrine extravasation.** *Adult:* 10 mg phentolamine added to each liter IV fluids containing norepinephrine. **Dx of pheochromocytoma.** *Adult:* Use only to confirm evidence after risks carefully considered. Usual dose, 5 mg IM or IV. **Reversal of soft-tissue anesthesia.** *Adult:* 0.2–0.8 mg based on amount of local anesthetic given, injected into anesthetized area. *Child ≥3 yr, >30 kg:* Adult dose w/max 0.4 mg. *Child ≥3 yr, 15–30 kg:* Max, 0.2 mg (*OraVerse*).

**ADV EFF** Acute, prolonged hypotension; arrhythmias; dizziness; **MI;** nausea; weakness

**INTERACTIONS** Ephedrine, epinephrine

**NC/PT** Give *OraVerse* after dental procedure, using same location as local anesthetic. Monitor P/BP closely. Pt should take safety precautions for CNS effects, hypotension; report palpitations, chest pain.

**DANGEROUS DRUG**

## phenylephrine hydrochloride (Neo-Synephrine, PediaCare Children's Decongestant, Sudafed PE, Vazculep, Vicks Sinex Ultra Fine Mist)

**CLASS** Alpha agonist, nasal decongestant, ophthal mydriatic, sympathomimetic

**PREG/CONT** C/NA

**BBW** Protect parenteral sol from light. Do not give unless sol is clear; discard unused sol.

**IND & DOSE Tx of mild to moderate hypotension.** *Adult:* 1–10 mg subcut, IM; max initial dose, 5 mg. Or, 0.1 or 0.5 mg IV, max initial dose, 0.5 mg. Do not repeat more often than q 10–15 min; 0.5 mg IV should raise BP for 15 min. **Tx of severe hypotension, shock.** *Adult:* For continuous infusion, add 10 mg to 500 mL dextrose or normal saline injection. Start at 100–180 mcg/min (based on drop factor of 20 drops/mL [100–180 drops/min]). When BP stabilized, maint, 40–60 mcg/min. **Spinal anesthesia.** *Adult:* 2–3 mg subcut or IM 3–4 min before spinal anesthetic injection. **Hypotensive emergencies during anesthesia.** *Adult:* 0.2 mg IV; max, 0.5 mg/dose. *Child:* 0.5–1 mg/11.3 kg subcut, IM. Prolongation of spinal anesthesia. *Adult:* Adding 2–5 mg to anesthetic sol increases motor block duration by as much as 50%. **Vasoconstrictor for regional anesthesia.** *Adult:* 1:20,000 conc (add 1 mg phenylephrine to q 20 mL local anesthetic sol). **Tx of paroxysmal supraventricular tachycardia.** *Adult:* Rapid IV injection (within 20–30 sec) recommended. Max initial dose, 0.5 mg. Subsequent doses should not exceed preceding dose by >0.1–0.2 mg; should never exceed 1 mg. Use only after other tx failed. **Tx of nasal congestion.** *Adult:* 2–3 sprays, drops of 0.25% or 0.5% sol in each nostril q 3–4 hr. In severe cases, may need 0.5% or 1% sol. Or, 10 mg PO bid–qid. Or, 1–2 tablets PO q 4 hr. Or, 1 strip q 4 hr; max, 6 strips/24 hr. Place 1 strip on tongue; let dissolve. Or, 10 mL liquid q 6 hr. *Child ≥6 yr:* 2–3 sprays 0.25% sol in each nostril no more than q 4 hr. Or, 1 tablet PO q 4 hr. *Child 2–5 yr:* 2–3 drops 0.125% sol in each nostril q 4 hr PRN. Or, 1 dropperful (5 mL [2.5 mg]) 0.25% oral drops q 4 hr; max, 6 mL (15 mg)/d. **Vasoconstriction, pupil dilation.** *Adult:* 1 drop 2.5% or 10% sol on upper limbus. May repeat in 1 hr. **Tx of uveitis to prevent posterior synechiae.** *Adult:* 1 drop 2.5% or 10% sol on surface of cornea w/atropine. Max, three times. **Tx of wide-angle glaucoma.** *Adult:* 1 drop 2.5% or 10% sol on upper surface of cornea

repeated as necessary, w/miotics. **Intraocular surgery.** *Adult:* 2.5% or 10% sol in eye 30–60 min before procedure. **Refraction.** *Adult:* 1 drop of cycloplegic then, in 5 min, 1 drop phenylephrine 2.5% sol and, in 10 min, another drop of cycloplegic. **Ophthalmoscopic exam.** *Adult:* 1 drop 2.5% sol in each eye. Mydriasis produced in 15–30 min, lasting 4–6 hr. **Tx of minor eye irritation.** *Adult:* 1–2 drops 0.12% sol in eye bid–qid as needed.
**ADJUST DOSE** Elderly pts
**ADV EFF** Anorexia, anxiety, blurred vision, **cardiac arrhythmias,** decreased urine output, dizziness, drowsiness, dysuria, fear, headache, light-headedness, local stinging w/ ophthal sol, nausea, pallor, rebound congestion w/nasal sol, urine retention
**INTERACTIONS** Halogenated anesthetics, MAOIs, methyldopa, oxytocics, sympathomimetics, TCAs
**NC/PT** Have alpha-adrenergic blocker on hand. If extravasation, infiltrate area w/phentolamine (5–10 mg in 10–15 mL saline) using fine hypodermic needle; usually effective if area infiltrated within 12 hr of extravasation. Five mg IM should raise BP for 1–2 hr; 0.5 mg IV, for 15 min. Do not give within 14 d of MAOIs. Monitor closely during administration. Teach proper administration of nasal sol, eyedrops. Pt should not use longer than prescribed; take safety precautions for CNS effects; report chest pain, palpitations, vision changes.

## phenytoin (Dilantin, Phenytek)

**CLASS** Antiarrhythmic, antiepileptic, hydantoin
**PREG/CONT** High risk/NA

**BBW** Give IV slowly to prevent severe hypotension, venous irritation; small margin of safety between full therapeutic, toxic doses. Continually monitor cardiac rhythm; check BP frequently, regularly during infusion. Suggest use of fosphenytoin sodium if IV route needed.
**IND & DOSE Tx of status epilepticus.** *Adult:* 10–15 mg/kg by slow IV. Maint, 100 mg PO IV q 6–8 hr; max infusion rate, 50 mg/min. *Child:* Dose based on child's formulas; may also calculate infants', child's doses based on 10–15 mg/kg IV in divided doses of 5–10 mg/kg. For neonates, 15–20 mg/kg IV in divided doses of 5–10 mg/kg recommended. **Px of seizures during neurosurgery.** *Adult:* 100–200 mg IM q 4 hr during surgery, postop; not preferred route. **Tx of tonic-clonic, psychomotor seizures.** *Adult:* Loading dose in hospitalized pts: 1 g phenytoin capsules (phenytoin sodium, prompt) divided into three doses (400 mg, 300 mg, 300 mg) and given PO q 2 hr. When control established, may consider once-a-day dosing w/300 mg PO. W/no previous tx: Initially, 100 mg PO tid; maint, 300–400 mg/d. *Child not previously treated:* 5 mg/kg/d PO in two–three equally divided doses. Max, 300 mg/d; maint, 4–8 mg/kg. Child >6 yr may need minimum adult dose (300 mg/d). **IM tx in pt previously stabilized on oral dose.** *Adult:* Increase dose by 50% over oral dose. When returning to oral dose, decrease dose by 50% of original oral dose for 1 wk to prevent excessive plasma level.
**ADJUST DOSE** Elderly pts, hepatic impairment
**ADV EFF Angioedema, aplastic anemia,** ataxia, dizziness, drowsiness, dysarthria, **frank malignant lymphoma, bullous/exfoliative/ purpuric dermatitis, CV collapse,** gum hyperplasia, **hematopoietic complications,** insomnia, irritation, **liver damage, lupus erythematosus,** mental confusion, nausea, nystagmus, **SJS**
**INTERACTIONS** Acetaminophen, alcohol, allopurinol, amiodarone, antineoplastics, atracurium, benzodiazepines, carbamazepine, cardiac glycosides, chloramphenicol, cimetidine,

corticosteroids, cyclosporine, diazoxide, disopyramide, disulfiram, doxycycline, estrogens, fluconazole, folic acid, furosemide, haloperidol, hormonal contraceptives, isoniazid, levodopa, loxapine, methadone, metronidazole, metyrapone, mexiletine, miconazole, nitrofurantoin, omeprazole, pancuronium, phenacemide, phenothiazine, phenylbutazone, primidone, pyridoxine, quinidine, rifampin, sucralfate, sulfonamides, sulfonylureas, theophylline, trimethoprim, valproic acid, vecuronium
**NC/PT** Monitor for therapeutic serum level (10–20 mcg/mL). Enteral tube feedings may delay absorption. Provide 2-hr window between *Dilantin* doses, tube feedings. Reduce dose, stop phenytoin, or substitute other antiepileptic gradually; stopping abruptly may precipitate status epilepticus. Stop if rash, depressed blood count, enlarged lymph nodes, hypersensitivity reaction, s&sx of liver damage, Peyronie disease (induration of corpora cavernosa of penis); start another antiepileptic promptly. Have lymph node enlargement during tx evaluated carefully. Lymphadenopathy that simulates Hodgkin lymphoma has occurred; lymph node hyperplasia may progress to lymphoma. Not for use in preg (contraceptives advised)/breastfeeding. Pt should have regular dental care; take safety precautions for CNS effects; wear medical ID; report rash, unusual bleeding, urine/stool color changes, thoughts of suicide.

## pilocarpine hydrochloride (Salagen)
**CLASS** Parasympathomimetic
**PREG/CONT** C/NA

**IND & DOSE Tx of sx of xerostomia from salivary gland dysfx caused by radiation for head/neck cancer.** *Adult:* 5–10 mg PO tid. **Tx of dry mouth in Sjögren syndrome.** *Adult:* 5 mg PO qid.
**ADJUST DOSE** Severe hepatic impairment
**ADV EFF Bronchospasm,** headache, HTN, hypotension, n/v/d, renal colic, sweating, tearing, visual changes
**INTERACTIONS** Anticholinergics, beta blockers
**NC/PT** Maintain hydration. Not for use in breastfeeding. Pt should take safety precautions w/vision changes, report dehydration, difficulty breathing.

## pimavanserin (Nuplazid)
**CLASS** Atypical antipsychotic
**PREG/CONT** Low risk/NA

**BBW** Risk of death when used in elderly pts w/dementia-related psychosis.
**IND & DOSE Tx of hallucinations/delusions associated w/Parkinson dx.** *Adult:* 34 mg (two 17-mg tablets) once a day PO w/ or w/o food.
**ADJUST DOSE** Hepatic impairment (not recommended); strong CYP3A4 inhibitors (decrease dose)
**ADV EFF** Confusion, nausea, peripheral edema, **prolonged QT**
**INTERACTIONS** CYP3A4 inducers/inhibitors, QT-prolonging drugs
**NC/PT** Ensure correct dx. Obtain baseline, periodic ECG. Pt should report changes in drug regimen; take safety precautions for CNS effects; report edema.

## pimozide (generic)
**CLASS** Antipsychotic, diphenylbutylpiperidine
**PREG/CONT** C/NA

**IND & DOSE To suppress severely compromising motor, phonic tics in Tourette syndrome.** *Adult:* 1–2 mg/d PO; max, 10 mg/d.
**ADJUST DOSE** Severe hepatic impairment
**ADV EFF** Akathisia, asthenia, dry mouth, extrapyramidal effects, fever, headache, increased salivation, motor restlessness, **NMS, prolonged QT,** sedation, somnolence, tardive dyskinesia, weight gain

**INTERACTIONS** Amphetamines, antifungals, citalopram, escitalopram, grapefruit juice, methylphenidate, nefazodone, pemoline, protease inhibitors, QT-prolonging drugs, sertraline, strong CYP2D6 inhibitors
**NC/PT** Ensure correct dx. Obtain baseline, periodic ECG. Not for use in breastfeeding. Check pt's drugs closely; numerous drug interactions w/contraindications. Pt should take safety precautions for CNS effects; avoid grapefruit juice.

---

## **pindolol** (generic)
**CLASS** Antihypertensive, beta blocker
**PREG/CONT** B/NA

**IND & DOSE Tx of HTN.** *Adult:* 5 mg PO bid; max, 60 mg/d. Usual maint, 5 mg PO tid.
**ADV EFF** Arrhythmias, **bronchospasm,** constipation, decreased exercise tolerance/libido, fatigue, flatulence, gastric pain, serum glucose changes, **HF, laryngospasm,** n/v/d
**INTERACTIONS** Clonidine, epinephrine, ergots, ibuprofen, indomethacin, insulin, lidocaine, naproxen, piroxicam, prazosin, sulindac, theophyllines, thioridazine, verapamil
**NC/PT** When stopping, taper gradually over 2 wk w/monitoring. Pt should take safety precautions for CNS effects; report difficulty breathing, swelling. Name confusion between pindolol and *Plendil* (felodipine).

---

## **pioglitazone** (Actos)
**CLASS** Antidiabetic, thiazolidinedione
**PREG/CONT** C/NA

**BBW** Thiazolidinediones cause or worsen HF in some pts; pioglitazone not recommended for pts w/symptomatic HF (contraindicated in NYHA Class III, IV HF). After starting or increasing, watch carefully for HF s&sx. If they occur, manage HF according to current standards of care. Pioglitazone may be reduced or stopped. Increased risk of bladder cancer when used for longer than 1 yr; monitor accordingly.
**IND & DOSE Adjunct to diet/exercise to improve glucose control in type 2 diabetes as monotherapy or w/insulin, sulfonylurea, metformin.** *Adult:* 15–30 mg/d PO; max, 45 mg daily PO.
**ADJUST DOSE** Hepatic impairment
**ADV EFF** Aggravated diabetes, **bladder cancer,** fatigue, fractures, headache, **hepatic injury, HF, hyperglycemia, hypoglycemia,** infections, macular edema, myalgia, pain
**INTERACTIONS** Celery, coriander, dandelion root, fenugreek, garlic, gemfibrozil, ginseng, hormonal contraceptives, juniper berries, rifampin
**NC/PT** Not for use in pts w/type 1 diabetes/ketoacidosis, NYHA Class III or IV HF. Interferes w/hormonal contraceptives; suggest alternative birth control method or consider higher contraceptive dose. Increased risk of bladder cancer when used for longer than 1 yr; monitor accordingly. Monitor blood glucose regularly; ensure complete diabetic teaching/support. Not for use in breastfeeding. Pt should take w/o regard to meals; report infections, difficulty breathing, uncontrolled glucose level. Name confusion between *Actos* (pioglitazone) and *Actonel* (risedronate).

---

## **pirfenidone** (Esbriet)
**CLASS** Pyridone
**PREG/CONT** Unkn/NA

**IND & DOSE Tx of idiopathic pulmonary fibrosis.** *Adult:* Initially, 267 mg PO tid w/food. Titrate over 2 wk to full dose of 801 mg PO tid w/food.
**ADJUST DOSE** Hepatic/renal impairment
**ADV EFF** Abd pain, **bleeding, GI perforation/toxicity,** GERD,

**hepatotoxicity,** insomnia, n/v/d, photosensitivity, sinusitis, rash, URI, weight loss
**INTERACTIONS** Ciprofloxacin, fluvoxamine, smoking
**NC/PT** Monitor LFTs/renal function. Taper over 2 wk to reach therapeutic dose. Use w/caution in preg; not for use in breastfeeding. Pt should avoid sun exposure; use sunscreen/protective clothing; avoid smoking; report severe n/v/d, urine/stool color changes.

## piroxicam (Feldene)

**CLASS** NSAID
**PREG/CONT** High risk/NA

**BBW** Increased risk of CV events, GI bleeding; monitor accordingly. Contraindicated for periop pain after CABG surgery.
**IND & DOSE** **Relief of s&sx of acute/chronic RA, osteoarthritis.** *Adult:* 20 mg/d PO.
**ADJUST DOSE** Elderly pts
**ADV EFF** **Anaphylactoid reactions to anaphylactic shock, bone marrow suppression, bronchospasm,** constipation, dizziness, dyspepsia, edema, fatigue, **GI bleeding/perforation**, GI pain, headache, HF, HTN, insomnia, nausea, rash, somnolence, **thrombotic events**
**INTERACTIONS** Beta blockers, cholestyramine, lithium, oral anticoagulants
**NC/PT** Not for use in preg/breastfeeding. Pt should take w/food or milk; use safety precautions for CNS effects; report swelling, difficulty breathing, rash, chest pain.

## pitavastatin (Livalo, Zypitamag)

**CLASS** Antihyperlipidemic, statin
**PREG/CONT** X/NA

**IND & DOSE** **Adjunct to diet/exercise to reduce elevated total cholesterol, LDLs, apolipoprotein B, triglycerides, increase HDL in primary hyperlipidemia, mixed dyslipidemia; tx of heterozygous familial hypercholesterolemia.** *Adult, child ≥8 yr:* 2 mg/d PO w/ or w/o food; max, 4 mg/d.
**ADJUST DOSE** Renal impairment (pts on dialysis)
**ADV EFF** Back pain, constipation, diarrhea, flulike sx, headache, **liver toxicity,** myalgias, **rhabdomyolysis**
**INTERACTIONS** Alcohol, cyclosporine, erythromycin, fibrates, lopinavir/ritonavir, niacin, rifampin
**NC/PT** Monitor LFTs regularly. Ensure diet/exercise program. Monitor lipid levels after 4 wk; adjust dose accordingly. Not for use in preg (barrier contraceptives advised)/breastfeeding. Pt should get regular blood tests; avoid alcohol; report severe muscle pain w/fever, weakness, urine/stool color changes.

**▶NEW DRUG**

## pitolisant (Wakix)

**CLASS** Histamine-3 receptor antagonist, stimulant
**PREG/CONT** Unkn/NA

**IND & DOSE** **Tx of excessive daytime sleepiness due to narcolepsy.** *Adult:* Initially, 8.9 mg PO daily in a.m.; may increase wkly to max 35.6 mg PO daily.
**ADJUST DOSE** Hepatic/renal impairment. Not recommended if ESRD
**ADV EFF** Anxiety, insomnia, nausea, **prolonged QT**
**INTERACTIONS** Sensitive CYP3A4 substrates, including hormonal contraceptives; strong CYP2D6 inducers/inhibitors
**NC/PT** May reduce efficacy of hormonal contraceptives; alternative nonhormonal contraceptive method advised during and for ≥21 d after tx. Preg exposure registry available to monitor preg outcomes in women exposed to Wakix during preg.

## plasma protein fraction
(Plasmanate, Plasma-Plex, Protenate)
**CLASS** Blood product, plasma protein
**PREG/CONT** C/NA

**IND & DOSE Tx of hypovolemic shock.** *Adult:* Initially, 250–500 mL IV. Max, 10 mL/min; do not exceed 5–8 mL/min as plasma volume nears normal. **Tx of hypoproteinemia.** *Adult:* 1,000–1,500 mL IV daily; max, 5–8 mL/min. Adjust rate based on pt response.
**ADV EFF** Chills, fever, **HF,** hypotension, n/v, **pulmonary edema after rapid infusion,** rash
**INTERACTIONS** Alcohol, cyclosporine, erythromycin, fibrates, lopinavir/ritonavir, niacin, rifampin
**NC/PT** Infusion only provides symptomatic relief of hypoproteinemia; consider need for whole blood based on pt's clinical condition. Give IV w/o regard to blood type. Monitor closely during infusion. Pt should report headache, difficulty breathing.

## plecanatide (Trulance)
**CLASS** Guanylate cyclase-C agonist
**PREG/CONT** Low risk/NA

**BBW** Risk of serious complications/dehydration when used in pt <18 yr. Contraindicated in pt ≤6 yr; use caution in pt 6–18 yr.
**IND & DOSE Tx of adults w/chronic idiopathic constipation.** *Adult:* 3 mg/d PO.
**ADV EFF** Diarrhea
**NC/PT** Not for use w/GI obstruction. Tablet should be swallowed whole. For difficulty swallowing, may crush tablet, mix w/tsp applesauce, and have pt swallow immediately. Or for difficulty swallowing or w/NG or gastric feeding tube, place in 30 mL room temp water, swirl to dissolve, then instill immediately or have pt swallow; add 30 mL water to cup, swirl again, and reinstill or have pt swallow. Use caution in preg; not for use in breastfeeding. Pt should report severe diarrhea (rehydration may be needed).

## plerixafor (Mozobil)
**CLASS** Hematopoietic stem-cell mobilizer
**PREG/CONT** High risk/NA

**IND & DOSE To mobilize hematopoietic stem cells to peripheral blood for collection, subsequent autologous transplantation in pts w/non-Hodgkin lymphoma/multiple myeloma, w/granulocyte-colony stimulating factor (G-CSF).** *Adult:* 0.24 mg/kg subcut for up to 4 consecutive d; start after pt has received G-CSF once daily for 4 d. Give approx 11 hours before apheresis.
**ADJUST DOSE** Renal impairment
**ADV EFF Anaphylactic shock,** dizziness, headache, injection-site reactions, n/v/d, orthostatic hypotension, rash, **splenic rupture, tumor cell mobilization**
**NC/PT** Do not use in leukemia; may mobilize leukemic cells. Not for use in preg (barrier contraceptives advised)/breastfeeding. Pt should report rash, injection-site reactions, difficulty breathing, edema.

**▶ NEW DRUG**

## polatuzumab vedotin-piiq (Polivy)
**CLASS** Antibody-drug conjugate, antineoplastic
**PREG/CONT** Unkn/NA

**IND & DOSE Tx of relapsed/refractory diffuse large B-cell lymphoma not otherwise specified after at least 2 prior tx.** *Adult:* 1.8 mg/kg IV infusion q 21 d for six cycles w/bendamustine and a rituximab product on d 1 of each cycle.
**ADV EFF** Anemia, diarrhea, fatigue, **hepatotoxicity, infections, infusion**

reactions, myelosuppression, peripheral neuropathy, PML, pyrexia, TLS
**INTERACTIONS** Strong CYP3A inducers/inhibitors
**NC/PT** Premedicate w/antihistamine, antipyretic. Effective contraception advised during tx and for at least 3 mo (women) and 5 mo (men) after final dose. Pt should not breastfeed during tx and for at least 2 mo after final dose.

## polidocanol (Asclera, Varithena)
**CLASS** Sclerosing agent
**PREG/CONT** Low risk/NA

**IND & DOSE Tx of uncomplicated spider, reticular veins in lower extremities.** *Adult:* 0.1–0.3 mL as IV injection at varicose vein site; max volume/session, 10 mL.
**ADV EFF Anaphylaxis,** injection-site reactions
**NC/PT** Do not inject intra-arterially. Have emergency equipment on hand. Advise compression stockings, support hose on treated legs continuously for 2–3 d, then for 2–3 wk during the day; walk for 15–20 min immediately after procedure and daily for next few d.

## poly-l-lactic acid (Sculptra)
**CLASS** Polymer
**PREG/CONT** Unkn/NA

**IND & DOSE To restore, correct sx of lipoatrophy in pts w/HIV syndrome.** *Adult:* 0.1–0.2 mL injected intradermally at each injection site. May need up to 20 injections/cheek; retreat periodically.
**ADV EFF** Injection-site reactions
**NC/PT** Do not use if s&sx of skin infection. Apply ice packs to area immediately after injection and for first 24 hr. Massage injection sites daily. Monitor pt on anticoagulants for increased bleeding.

**DANGEROUS DRUG**

## polymyxin B sulfate (generic)
**CLASS** Antibiotic
**PREG/CONT** C/NA

**BBW** Monitor renal function carefully; nephrotoxicity possible. Avoid concurrent use of other nephrotoxics. Neurotoxicity can cause respiratory paralysis; monitor accordingly. IV, intrathecal administration for hospitalized pts only.
**IND & DOSE Tx of acute infections caused by susceptible bacteria strains when less toxic drugs contraindicated.** *Adult, child >2 yr:* 15,000–25,000 units/kg/d IV q 12 hr; max, 25,000 units/kg/d. *Infants:* 40,000 units/kg/d IV, IM. **Tx of meningeal infections caused by *Pseudomonas aeruginosa*.** *Adult, child >2 yr:* 50,000 units/d intrathecally for 3–4 d; then 50,000 units q other day for at least 2 wk after CSF cultures negative, glucose content normal. *Infants:* 20,000 units/d intrathecally for 3–4 d or 25,000 units q other day. Continue w/25,000 units once q other day for at least 2 wk after CSF cultures negative, glucose content normal.
**ADJUST DOSE** Renal impairment
**ADV EFF Apnea, nephrotoxicity, neurotoxicity,** pain at injection site, rash, superinfections, thrombophlebitis
**INTERACTIONS** Aminoglycosides, nephrotoxic drugs, NMJ blockers
**NC/PT** Culture before tx. Monitor renal function regularly. IM route may cause severe pain. Treat superinfections. Use caution in preg/breastfeeding. Pt should take safety precautions for CNS effects; report swelling, difficulty breathing, vision changes.

## pomalidomide (Pomalyst)
**CLASS** Antineoplastic, thalidomide analog
**PREG/CONT** High risk/NA

**BBW** Known human teratogen. Can cause severe, life-threatening birth

defects; not for use in preg. Risk of DVT/PE in pts treated for multiple myeloma.
**IND & DOSE Tx of multiple myeloma in pts who have had disease progression after at least two other therapies.** *Adult:* 4 mg/d PO on d 1–21 of repeated 28-d cycle until progression occurs.
**ADJUST DOSE** Severe hepatic/ renal impairment
**ADV EFF** Anemia, asthenia, back pain, confusion, constipation, diarrhea, dizziness, **DVT,** dyspnea, fatigue, **hepatotoxicity,** hypersensitivity reactions, nausea, neuropathy, **neutropenia, PE,** TLS, URI
**INTERACTIONS** Increased mortality if used w/dexamethasone and thalidomide analog. CYP1A2 inhibitors; combo is contraindicated
**NC/PT** Available only through REMS program. Rule out preg before starting drug. Ensure monthly negative preg test; recommend highly effective contraceptive measures for men, women. Not for use in breastfeeding. Give w/dexamethasone. Monitor for DVT/PE. Obtain baseline, periodic CBC; dosage may need adjustment. Pt should take drug once/d at about same time each day; mark calendar w/tx days; swallow capsule whole w/ water and not cut/crush/chew it; obtain monthly preg test; avoid donating blood during and for 1 mo after tx; take safety precautions for CNS effects; report extreme fatigue, difficulty breathing, calf pain.

DANGEROUS DRUG

## ponatinib (Iclusig)

**CLASS** Antineoplastic, kinase inhibitor
**PREG/CONT** High risk/NA

**BBW** Risk of vascular occlusion, HF, hepatotoxicity, any of which can lead to death.
**IND & DOSE Tx of T3151-positive CML or T3151-positive ALL.** *Adult:* 45 mg/d w/food; adjust based on toxicity.
**ADJUST DOSE** Severe hepatic impairment
**ADV EFF** Abd pain, arrhythmias, arthralgia, compromised wound healing, constipation, fever, fluid retention, **GI perforation, HF, hepatotoxicity,** HTN, myelosuppression, neuropathies, n/v, pancreatitis, **vascular occlusions,** vision changes
**INTERACTIONS** CYP3A inhibitors, CYP3A inducers, avoid use
**NC/PT** Ensure proper dx. Monitor LFTs, lipase, cardiac function, CBC, BP. Ensure comprehensive eye exam, adequate hydration; correct uric acid level. Pt should avoid preg (serious fetal harm possible)/breastfeeding; report fever, extreme fatigue, urine/ stool color changes, headache, vision changes.

## poractant alfa (Curosurf)

**CLASS** Lung surfactant
**PREG/CONT** Unkn/NA

**IND & DOSE Rescue tx of infants w/RDS.** *Infants:* Entire contents of vial (2.5 mL/kg birth weight) intratracheally, ½ of dose into each bronchus. Give first dose as soon as possible after RDS dx and when pt on ventilator. May need up to two subsequent doses of 1.25 mL/kg birth weight at 12-hr intervals. Max total dose, 5 mL/kg (sum of initial, two repeat doses).
**ADV EFF** Bradycardia, flushing, hyperbilirubinemia, hypotension, infections, **intraventricular hemorrhage, patent ductus arteriosus, pneumothorax,** sepsis
**NC/PT** Ensure ET tube in correct position, w/bilateral chest movement, lung sounds. Store in refrigerator; protect from light. Enter vial only once. Instill slowly; inject ¼ of dose over 2–3 sec. Do not suction infant for 1 hr after completion of full dose; do not flush catheter. Maintain appropriate interventions for critically ill infant.

DANGEROUS DRUG

## porfimer sodium

(Photofrin)
**CLASS** Antineoplastic
**PREG/CONT** High risk/NA

**IND & DOSE Photodynamic tx for palliation of pts w/completely/partially obstructing esophageal/transitional cancer who cannot be treated w/laser alone; transitional cell carcinoma in situ of urinary bladder; endobronchial NSCLC; high-grade dysplasia of Barrett esophagus.** *Adult:* 2 mg/kg as slow IV injection over 3–5 min; laser tx must follow in 40–50 hr and again in 96–120 hr.
**ADV EFF** Abd pain, anemia, **bleeding,** chest pain, constipation, dyspnea, **GI perforation,** n/v, photosensitivity, **pleural effusion, respiratory toxicity**
**NC/PT** Monitor for pleural effusion, respiratory complications. Avoid contact w/drug. Protect pt from light exposure for 30 d after tx; photosensitivity may last up to 90 d. Pt should report difficulty breathing/swallowing, unusual bleeding.

DANGEROUS DRUG

## posaconazole (Noxafil)

**CLASS** Antifungal, azole
**PREG/CONT** High risk/NA

**IND & DOSE Px of invasive *Aspergillus, Candida* infections in immunosuppressed pts.** *Adult, child ≥13 yr:* 200 mg (5 mL) PO tid oral suspension; 300 mg PO bid DR tablet on day 1, then once a day. Or 300 mg IV bid on day 1, then 300 mg/d IV. **Tx of oropharyngeal candidiasis.** *Adult, child ≥13 yr:* 100 mg (2.5 mL) PO bid on day 1; then 100 mg/d PO for 13 d (oral suspension). For refractory infection, 400 mg (10 mL) PO bid; duration based on pt response.
**ADJUST DOSE** Hepatic impairment, severe renal impairment
**ADV EFF** Abd pain, anemia, constipation, cough, dizziness, dyspnea, electrolyte disturbances, epistaxis, fatigue, fever, headache, **hepatotoxicity,** insomnia, n/v/d, **prolonged QT,** rash
**INTERACTIONS** Calcium channel blockers, cimetidine, cyclosporine, digoxin, ergots, fosamprenavir, metoclopramide, midazolam, phenytoin, QT-prolonging drugs, quinidine, rifabutin, sirolimus, statins, tacrolimus, vincristine, vinblastine
**NC/PT** Culture before tx. Obtain baseline ECG; monitor LFTs. Check formulation, dose, and frequency; oral forms are not directly substitutable. Monitor drug regimen; many interactions possible. Shake bottle well before use. Give w/full meal or nutritional supplement. Maintain hydration, nutrition. Not for use in preg/breastfeeding. Pt should take safety precautions for CNS effects; report fever, urine/stool color changes.

DANGEROUS DRUG

## potassium acetate, potassium chloride (K-Lyte Cl), potassium gluconate (Klor-Con, K-Tab)

**CLASS** Electrolyte
**PREG/CONT** C/NA

**IND & DOSE Px of potassium deficiency.** *Adult:* 16–24 mEq/d PO. **Tx of potassium deficiency.** 40–100 mEq/d PO or IV. *Child:* 2–3 mEq/kg/d or 40 mEq/m²/d PO or IV; 2–6 mEq/kg/hr PO or IV for newborns.
**ADJUST DOSE** Elderly pts, renal impairment
**ADV EFF** Abd pain, hyperkalemia, n/v/d, tissue sloughing, venospasm
**INTERACTIONS** Potassium-sparing diuretics, salt substitutes using potassium
**NC/PT** Obtain baseline, periodic serial serum potassium level. Dilute in dextrose sol to 40–80 mEq/L; do not give undiluted. Monitor for cardiac arrhythmias during IV infusion.

Monitor injection site carefully. Wax tablet matrix may appear in stool. Pt should swallow tablet whole and not cut/crush/chew it; take w/food or after meals; avoid salt substitutes; report tingling in hands/feet, black tarry stools, pain at IV injection site.

**▶NEW DRUG**

## prabotulinumtoxinA-xvfs (Jeuveau)

**CLASS** Acetylcholine release inhibitor, neuromuscular transmission blocker

**PREG/CONT** Unkn/NA

**BBW** Risk of spread from injection area to produce sx consistent w/ botulinum toxin effects (hrs/wks after injection). Swallowing/breathing difficulties can be life-threatening. Reports of death.

**IND & DOSE Temporary improvement in appearance of glabellar lines associated w/corrugator and/ or procerus muscle activity.** *Adult:* 0.1 mL (4 units) IM in five sites for total dose of 20 units.

**ADV EFF** CV events, eyelid ptosis, headache, increased WBC, URI

**INTERACTIONS** Aminoglycosides, other drugs affecting neuromuscular transmission

**NC/PT** May cause eye dryness. Pt should report eye pain, eye irritation, photosensitivity, vision changes, unusual sx (including difficulty swallowing/speaking/breathing); avoid driving/potentially hazardous activities if loss of strength, muscle weakness, blurred vision, drooping eyelids occur.

## pralatrexate (Folotyn)

**CLASS** Antineoplastic, folate analog metabolic inhibitor

**PREG/CONT** High risk/NA

**IND & DOSE Tx of relapsed, refractory peripheral T-cell lymphoma.** *Adult:* 30 mg/m²/wk as IV push over 3–5 min for 6 wk in 7-wk cycle.

**ADJUST DOSE** Elderly pts, renal impairment

**ADV EFF Bone marrow suppression,** dehydration, dyspnea, fatigue, mucositis, n/v/d, night sweats, pain, rash, **serious to fatal dermatologic reactions,** TLS

**INTERACTIONS** NSAIDs, probenecid

**NC/PT** Monitor CBC/skin. Pt should also receive vitamin $B_{12}$ (1 mg IM q 8–10 wk) and folic acid (1–1.25 mg/d PO). Maintain hydration. Not for use in preg (contraceptives advised)/ breastfeeding. Provide skin care. Pt should avoid exposure to infection: report s&sx of infection, unusual bleeding, rash.

## pralidoxime chloride (Protopam Chloride)

**CLASS** Antidote

**PREG/CONT** C/NA

**IND & DOSE Antidote in poisoning due to organophosphate pesticides, chemicals w/anticholinesterase activity.** *Adult:* Atropine 2–4 mg IV. If cyanotic, 2–4 mg atropine IM while improving ventilation; repeat q 5–10 min until s&sx of atropine toxicity appear. Maintain atropinization for at least 48 hr. Give pralidoxime concomitantly: Initially, 1–2 g pralidoxime IV, preferably as 15–30 min infusion in 100 mL saline. After 1 hr, give second dose of 1–2 g IV if muscle weakness not relieved. Give additional doses cautiously q 10–12 hr. If IV route not feasible or pulmonary edema present, give IM or subcut. *Child ≤16 yr:* Loading dose, 20–50 mg/kg (max, 2,000 mg/dose) IV over 15–30 min, then continuous IV infusion of 10–20 mg/kg/hr. Or, 20–50 mg/kg (max, 2,000 mg/dose) IV over 15 30 min. Give second dose of 20–50 mg/kg in 1 hr if muscle weakness not relieved. May repeat dosing q 10–12 hr as needed. Or, for pt ≥40 kg, 1,800 mg IM/course of tx; <40 kg, 15 mg/kg IM q 15 min if needed, to total of three doses (45 mg/kg). **Adjunct to**

**atropine in poisoning by nerve agents w/anticholinesterase activity.** *Adult:* Give atropine, pralidoxime as soon as possible after exposure. Use autoinjectors, giving atropine first. Repeat both atropine, pralidoxime after 15 min. If sx after additional 15 min, repeat injections. If sx persist after third set of injections, seek medical help. **Tx of anticholinesterase overdose of myasthenia gravis drugs.** *Adult:* 1–2 g IV, then increments of 250 mg q 5 min.
**ADV EFF** Blurred vision, diplopia, dizziness, drowsiness, headache, pain at injection site, transient LFT increases
**NC/PT** For acute organophosphate poisoning, remove secretions, maintain patent airway, provide artificial ventilation as needed; then begin tx. After skin exposure to organophosphate poisoning, remove clothing, thoroughly wash hair/skin w/sodium bicarbonate or alcohol as soon as possible. Give by slow IV infusion. Have IV sodium thiopental or diazepam on hand if seizures occur. Pt should report pain at injection site, vision changes.

## pramipexole dihydrochloride (Mirapex)

**CLASS** Antiparkinsonian, dopamine receptor agonist
**PREG/CONT** Unkn/NA

**BBW** Use extreme caution in pts w/hx of hypotension, hallucinations, confusion, dyskinesias.
**IND & DOSE** **Tx of sx of Parkinson disease.** *Adult:* 0.125 mg PO tid for 1 wk; wk 2, 0.25 mg PO tid; wk 3, 0.5 mg PO tid; wk 4, 0.75 mg PO tid; wk 5, 1 mg PO tid; wk 6, 1.25 mg PO tid; wk 7, 1.5 mg PO tid. Once levels established, may use ER tablets for once-a-day dosing. **Tx of restless legs syndrome.** *Adult:* 0.125 mg/d PO 2–3 hr before bedtime. May increase q 4–7 d, if needed, to 0.25 mg/d; max, 0.5 mg/d.
**ADJUST DOSE** Renal impairment
**ADV EFF** Asthenia, confusion, constipation, dizziness, dyskinesia, extrapyramidal sx, fever, hallucinations, headache, impulsive behaviors, insomnia, orthostatic hypotension, psychotic-like behavior, retinal changes, somnolence
**INTERACTIONS** Cimetidine, diltiazem, dopamine antagonists, levodopa, quinidine, quinine, ranitidine, triamterene, verapamil
**NC/PT** Give w/extreme caution to pts w/hx of hypotension, hallucinations, confusion, dyskinesia. Taper gradually over at least 1 wk when stopping. Use caution in preg/breastfeeding. Pt should swallow ER tablet whole and not cut/crush/chew it; take safety precautions for CNS effects; report behavior changes, hallucinations, swelling, vision changes.

DANGEROUS DRUG

## pramlintide acetate

(Symlin)
**CLASS** Amylinomimetic, antidiabetic
**PREG/CONT** Low risk/NA

**BBW** Severe hypoglycemia associated w/combined use of insulin, pramlintide; usually seen within 3 hr of pramlintide injection. Monitor accordingly.
**IND & DOSE** **Adjunct tx in pts w/type 1, 2 diabetes who use mealtime insulin and have failed to achieve desired glucose control.** *Adult w/type 1 diabetes:* 15 mcg subcut before major meals; titrate at 15-mcg increments to maint of 30 or 60 mcg as tolerated. *Adult w/type 2 diabetes:* 60–120 mcg subcut immediately before major meals.
**ADV EFF** Cough, dizziness, **hypoglycemia,** injection-site reactions, n/v
**INTERACTIONS** Anticholinergics, oral drugs
**NC/PT** Doses of oral drugs, insulins will need reduction, usually by 50% based on pt response. Drug affects

gastric emptying; if rapid effect needed, give oral medication 1 hr before or 2 hr after pramlintide. Inject subcut more than 2 inches away from insulin injection site. Rotate sites. Do not mix in syringe w/insulin. Use caution in preg/breastfeeding. Store unopened vial in refrigerator; may store opened vial at room temp. Teach proper administration/disposal of needles/syringes. Pt should not take if not going to eat or share pen w/other pts; avoid alcohol; continue diet/exercise, other diabetes tx; monitor blood glucose level; report hypoglycemic reactions, injection-site pain/swelling.

**prasterone** (Intrarosa)
**CLASS** Steroid
**PREG/CONT** Unkn/NA

**IND & DOSE** **Tx of moderate to severe dyspareunia.** *Adult:* 6.5 mg/d as vaginal insert at bedtime.
**ADV EFF** Abnormal Pap smear, vaginal discharge
**NC/PT** Only for use in postmenopausal women. Do not use w/undiagnosed genital bleeding, hx of breast cancer. Not for use in preg/breastfeeding. Pt should insert into vagina daily at bedtime using supplied applicator.

**DANGEROUS DRUG**

**prasugrel** (Effient)
**CLASS** Platelet inhibitor
**PREG/CONT** Unkn/NA

**BBW** Risk of serious to fatal bleeding; do not use w/active bleeding or hx of TIA, stroke. Risk increased w/age >75 yr, weight <60 kg, bleeding tendency, warfarin/NSAID use. Do not use in likely candidates for CABG surgery; if pts taking drug need CABG, stop prasugrel at least 7 d before surgery. Suspect bleeding in pt who becomes hypotensive and has undergone invasive procedure. If possible, control bleeding w/o stopping prasugrel; stopping prematurely increases risk of thrombotic episodes.
**IND & DOSE** **To reduce risk of thrombotic CV events (including stent thrombosis) in pts w/acute coronary syndrome who are to be managed w/PCI.** *Adult:* 60 mg PO as single dose, then 10 mg/d PO w/o regard to food. Use 5 mg/d in pt <60 kg. Pt should also receive aspirin (75–325 mg/d).
**ADV EFF** **Bleeding,** fatigue, fever, headache, HTN, hyperlipidemia, **hypersensitivity reactions,** pain, rash, **risk of thrombotic episodes if stopped prematurely, thrombotic thrombocytopenic purpura**
**INTERACTIONS** NSAIDs
**NC/PT** Ensure pt also receives aspirin. Limit invasive procedures; monitor for bleeding. Stop drug 7 d before planned surgery. Protect from injury. Use caution in preg/breastfeeding. Do not stop prematurely; risk of rebound thrombotic events. Pt should wear medical ID; inform all health care providers about pramlintide use, increased risk of bleeding; report excessive bleeding, fever, purple skin patches; pink/brown urine, black or bloody stools, difficulty breathing.

**pravastatin sodium**
(Pravachol)
**CLASS** Antihyperlipidemic, statin
**PREG/CONT** High risk/NA

**IND & DOSE** **Adjunct to diet in tx of elevated total cholesterol, LDL cholesterol; px of MI in pts at risk for first MI; to slow progression of CAD in pts w/clinically evident CAD; to reduce risk of stroke, MI.** *Adult:* 40 mg/d PO at bedtime. Max, 80 mg/d. *Adult on immunosuppressants:* 10 mg/d PO; max, 20 mg/d. **Tx of heterozygous familial hypercholesterolemia as adjunct to diet/exercise:** *Child 14–18 yr:* 40 mg/d PO. *Child 8–13 yr:* 20 mg/d PO.
**ADJUST DOSE** Elderly pts; hepatic/renal impairment

**ADV EFF** Abd pain, blurred vision, cataracts, constipation, cramps, dizziness, flatulence, LFT elevations, n/v, **rhabdomyolysis**
**INTERACTIONS** Bile acid sequestrants, cyclosporine, digoxin, erythromycin, gemfibrozil, itraconazole, niacin, warfarin
**NC/PT** Ensure diet/exercise program for CAD. Not for use in preg (barrier contraceptives advised)/breastfeeding. Pt should take at bedtime, have periodic eye exams, report severe GI upset, urine/stool color changes, muscle pain.

## praziquantel (Biltricide)
**CLASS** Anthelmintic
**PREG/CONT** Low risk/NA

**IND & DOSE** **Tx of *Schistosoma* infections, liver fluke infections.** *Adult, child >4 yr:* Three doses of 20–25 mg/kg PO as one-day tx, w/4–6 hr between doses.
**ADV EFF** Abd pain, dizziness, fever, malaise, nausea, urticaria
**INTERACTIONS** Chloroquine, CP450 inducers, grapefruit juice
**NC/PT** Give w/food and water; GI upset common. Pt should swallow tablet whole and not chew it; avoid grapefruit juice. For child <6 yr, may crush tablet, mix w/food or liquid.

## prazosin hydrochloride (Minipress)
**CLASS** Alpha blocker, antihypertensive
**PREG/CONT** C/NA

**IND & DOSE** **Tx of HTN.** *Adult:* 1 mg PO bid–tid. Increase to total 20 mg/d in divided doses; range, 6–15 mg/d. If using w/other antihypertensives, reduce dose to 1–2 mg PO tid, titrate to control BP.
**ADV EFF** Abd pain, dizziness, drowsiness, dry mouth, headache, hypotension, lack of energy, nausea, paresthesia, weakness
**INTERACTIONS** Avanafil, beta blockers, sildenafil, tadalafil, vardenafil, verapamil
**NC/PT** First dose may cause syncope w/sudden loss of consciousness; limit first dose to 1 mg PO, give at bedtime. Use caution in breastfeeding. Pt should take safety precautions for CNS effects, use sugarless lozenges for dry mouth, report fainting.

## prednisoLONE, prednisoLONE sodium phosphate (Orapred ODT, Pred Forte, Pred Mild, Prelone)
**CLASS** Anti-inflammatory, corticosteroid
**PREG/CONT** C/NA

**IND & DOSE** **Mgt of inflammatory disorders; tx of hypercalcemia of cancer.** *Adult:* 5–60 mg/d PO based on condition, response. *Child:* 0.14–2 mg/kg/d PO in three–four divided doses. **Mgt of acute MS exacerbations.** *Adult:* 200 mg/d PO for 1 wk, then 80 mg q other day for 1 mo (sodium phosphate). **Mgt of nephrotic syndrome.** *Child:* 60 mg/m²/d PO in three divided doses for 4 wk (sodium phosphate). Then single doses for 4 wk. Or, 40 mg/m²/d PO. Mgt of inflammation of eyelid, conjunctiva, cornea, globe. *Adult, child:* 2 drops qid. For *Pred Mild/Forte,* sodium phosphate, 1–2 drops q hr during day, q 2 hr at night. W/favorable results, 1 drop q 4 hr, then 1 drop 3–4 ×/d to control sx.
**ADV EFF** Aggravation of infections, amenorrhea, **anaphylactic reactions,** edema, fluid retention, headache, hyperglycemia, hypotension, immunosuppression, impaired healing, increased appetite, **shock,** vertigo
**INTERACTIONS** Barbiturates, cyclosporine, estrogens, hormonal contraceptives, ketoconazole, neostigmine, phenytoin, pyridostigmine, rifampin, salicylates
**NC/PT** Individualize dose, depending on severity, response. Give daily dose before 9 a.m. to minimize adrenal

suppression. For maint, reduce initial dose in small increments at intervals until lowest satisfactory dose reached. If long-term tx needed, consider alternate-day tx w/short-acting corticosteroid. After long-term tx, withdraw slowly to prevent adrenal insufficiency. Monitor serum glucose level. Pt should avoid exposure to infection, bright light (eyes may be sensitive); learn proper eyedrop technique; report s&sx of infection, black tarry stools, difficulty breathing.

## predniSONE (Prednisone Intensol, Rayos)

**CLASS** Corticosteroid
**PREG/CONT** High risk/NA

**IND & DOSE** **Mgt of inflammatory disorders; tx of hypercalcemia of cancer; replacement tx w/adrenal insufficiency.** *Adult:* 5–60 mg/d PO titrated based on response. *Child:* 0.05–2 mg/kg/d PO or 4–5 mg/m$^2$/d PO in equal divided doses q 12 hr. **Mgt of acute MS exacerbations.** *Adult:* 200 mg/d PO for 1 wk, then 80 mg PO q other day for 1 mo.
**ADV EFF** Aggravation of infections, amenorrhea, **anaphylactic reactions,** edema, fluid retention, headache, hyperglycemia, hypotension, immunosuppression, impaired healing, increased appetite, **shock,** vertigo
**INTERACTIONS** Barbiturates, cyclosporine, estrogens, hormonal contraceptives, ketoconazole, neostigmine, phenytoin, pyridostigmine, rifampin, salicylates
**NC/PT** Individualize dose, depending on severity, response. Give daily dose before 9 a.m. to minimize adrenal suppression. For maint, reduce initial dose in small increments at intervals until lowest satisfactory dose reached. If long-term tx needed, consider alternate-day tx w/short-acting corticosteroid. After long-term tx, withdraw slowly to prevent adrenal insufficiency. Monitor serum glucose level. Pt should avoid exposure to infections, report s&sx of infection, worsening of condition.

## pregabalin (Lyrica)

**CLASS** Analgesic, antiepileptic, calcium channel modulator
**PREG/CONT** High risk/C-V

**IND & DOSE** **Mgt of neuropathic pain due to diabetic peripheral neuropathy.** *Adult:* 100 mg PO tid. Max, 300 mg/d. **Mgt of postherpetic neuralgia.** *Adult:* 75–150 mg PO bid or 50–100 mg PO tid; max, 600 mg/d. **Adjunct tx for partial-onset seizures.** *Adult, child ≥30 kg:* 150–600 mg/d PO divided into two–three doses. *Child <30 kg 1 mo–4 yr:* 14 mg/kg/d max PO divided into two–three doses; **Mgt of fibromyalgia.** *Adult:* 75–150 mg PO bid. Max, 450 mg/d. **Mgt of neuropathic pain associated w/spinal cord injuries.** *Adult:* 75 mg PO bid. Increase to 150 mg PO bid within 1 wk; may increase to 300 mg PO bid if insufficient relief.
**ADJUST DOSE** Renal impairment
**ADV EFF** **Angioedema,** confusion, constipation, dizziness, dry mouth, infection, neuropathy, peripheral edema, somnolence, **thrombocytopenia,** weight gain
**INTERACTIONS** Alcohol, CNS depressants, pioglitazone, rosiglitazone
**NC/PT** Taper when stopping. Not for use in preg (barrier contraceptives advised)/breastfeeding. Men should not father child during tx. Pt should take safety measures for CNS effects; avoid alcohol; report vision changes, weight gain, increased bleeding, thoughts of suicide.

**▶NEW DRUG**

## pretomanid tablets

**CLASS** Antituberculotic, nitroimidazole
**PREG/CONT** Unkn/NA

**IND & DOSE** **Tx of pulmonary extensively drug-resistant, tx-intolerant,**

**or nonresponsive multidrug-resistant TB, w/bedaquiline and linezolid.** *Adult:* 200 mg PO daily for 26 wk w/bedaquiline 400 mg PO daily for 2 wk followed by 200 mg 3 ×/wk for 24 wk and linezolid 1,200 mg PO daily for up to 26 wk. May give beyond 26 wk if needed. Give w/food.
**ADV EFF** Abd pain, acne, anemia, back pain, cough, diarrhea, dyspepsia, headache, hypoglycemia, **lactic acidosis, liver toxicity, myelosuppression,** n/v, **peripheral and optic neuropathy,** pruritus, **prolonged QT,** rash, weight loss
**INTERACTIONS** Organic anion transporter-3 substrates, strong/moderate CYP3A4 inducers
**NC/PT** Only given as combo regimen w/bedaquiline and linezolid. Regimen is not indicated for tx of latent or pulmonary infection due to *Mycobacterium tuberculosis,* drug-sensitive TB, or MDR-TB that is not tx-intolerant or nonresponsive to standard tx. Pt must take full course to maximize effectiveness of immediate tx and decrease likelihood of drug resistance/possible ineffectiveness of regimen or other antibacterial drugs in future. Pt should continue drug even if feeling better.

## primidone (Mysoline)
**CLASS** Antiepileptic
**PREG/CONT** D/NA

**BBW** Increased risk of suicidal ideation; monitor accordingly.
**IND & DOSE Control of tonic-clonic, psychomotor, focal epileptic seizures.** *Adult w/no previous tx:* Days 1–3, 100–125 mg PO at bedtime; days 4–6, 100–125 mg PO bid; days 7–9, 100–125 mg PO tid; day 10, maint, 250 mg tid. Max, 500 mg qid (2 g/d). *Adult on other epileptics:* 100–125 mg PO at bedtime. When primidone alone desired, do not complete transition in <2 wk. *Child <8 yr:* Days 1–3, 50 mg PO at bedtime; days 4–6, 50 mg PO bid; days 7–9, 100 mg PO bid; day 10, maint, 125–250 mg tid or 10–25 mg/kg/d in divided doses.
**ADV EFF** Anorexia, ataxia, fatigue, hyperirritability, megaloblastic anemia, nausea, rash
**INTERACTIONS** Acetazolamide, alcohol, carbamazepine, isoniazid, nicotinamide, phenytoins, succinimides
**NC/PT** Taper when stopping; evaluate for therapeutic serum level (5–12 mcg/mL). Monitor CBC, folic acid for megaloblastic anemia. Not for use in preg (barrier contraceptives advised)/breastfeeding. Pt should take safety measures for CNS effects; wear medical ID; avoid alcohol; report rash, fever, thoughts of suicide.

## probenecid (Probalan)
**CLASS** Antigout, uricosuric
**PREG/CONT** B/NA

**IND & DOSE Tx of hyperuricemia associated w/gout, gouty arthritis.** *Adult:* 0.25 g PO bid for 1 wk, then 0.5 g PO bid. Max, 2–3 g/d. **Adjuvant to tx w/penicillins, cephalosporins.** *Adult:* 2 g/d PO in divided doses. *Child 2–14 yr:* Initially, 25 mg/kg PO, then 40 mg/kg/d in four divided doses. Tx of gonorrhea. *Adult:* Single 1-g dose PO 30 min before penicillin. *Child <45 kg:* 23 mg/kg PO in one single dose 30 min before penicillin.
**ADJUST DOSE** Elderly pts, renal impairment
**ADV EFF Anaphylaxis,** anemia, anorexia, dizziness, n/v, rash, urinary frequency
**INTERACTIONS** Acyclovir, allopurinol, benzodiazepines, clofibrate, dapsone, methotrexate, NSAIDs, rifampin, sulfonamides, thiopental, zidovudine
**NC/PT** Check urine alkalinity; urates crystallize in acidic urine. Sodium bicarbonate, potassium citrate may be ordered to alkalinize urine. Pt should take w/meals, antacids; drink 2.5–3 L fluid/d; take safety precautions w/dizziness; report dark urine, painful urination, difficulty breathing.

DANGEROUS DRUG

## procarbazine hydrochloride (Matulane)

**CLASS** Antineoplastic
**PREG/CONT** High risk/NA

**IND & DOSE Part of MOPP regimen for tx of stage III, IV Hodgkin lymphoma.** *Adult:* 2–4 mg/kg/d PO for first wk, then 4–6 mg/kg/d PO. Maint, 1–2 mg/kg/d PO.
**ADJUST DOSE** Elderly pts, renal impairment
**ADV EFF Bone marrow suppression,** confusion, diarrhea, fever, hallucinations, **hepatotoxicity, hypertensive crisis, pneumonitis**
**INTERACTIONS** Alcohol, anticholinergics, antihistamines, MAOIs, oral anticoagulants, TCAs
**NC/PT** Monitor CBC, LFTs; do not give within 14 d of MAOIs. Not for use in preg (barrier contraceptives advised)/breastfeeding. Pt should follow prescription carefully; avoid exposure to infection, injury; report severe headache, unusual bleeding, s&sx of infection, difficulty breathing.

## prochlorperazine (Compro), prochlorperazine edisylate, prochlorperazine maleate (Procomp)

**CLASS** Antiemetic, antipsychotic, dopaminergic blocker, phenothiazine
**PREG/CONT** C/NA

**BBW** Increased risk of death if used to treat dementia-related psychosis in elderly pts; not approved for this use.
**IND & DOSE Mgt of manifestations of psychotic disorders.** *Adult:* 5–10 mg PO tid or qid. Range, 50–75 mg/d for mild/moderate disturbances, 100–150 mg/d PO for more severe disturbances. For immediate control of severely disturbed adults, 10–20 mg IM repeated q 2–4 hr (q hour for resistant cases). *Child 2–12 yr:* 2.5 mg PO or rectally bid–tid; max, 25 mg/d (6–12 yr), 20 mg/d (2–5 yr). *Child <12 yr:* 0.132 mg/kg by deep IM injection. Switch to oral as soon as possible (usually after one dose). **Tx of emesis.** *Adult:* 5–10 mg PO tid–qid; or 15 mg SR on arising; or 25 mg rectally bid; or 5–10 mg IM initially, then q 3–4 hr (max, 40 mg/d). *Child >2 yr:* 18.2–38.6 kg, 2.5 mg PO or rectally tid or 5 mg bid; max, 15 mg/d. 13.6–17.7 kg, 2.5 mg PO or rectally bid–tid; max, 10 mg/d. 9.1–13.2 kg, 2.5 mg PO or rectally daily–bid; max, 7.5 mg/d. *Child ≥2 yr, ≥9.1 kg:* 0.132 mg/kg IM (usually one dose). **Mgt of n/v related to surgery.** *Adult:* 5–10 mg IM 1–2 hr before anesthesia or periop and postop (may repeat once in 30 min); or 5–10 mg IV 15 min before anesthesia or periop and postop (may repeat once); or 20 mg/L isotonic sol added to IV infusion 15–30 min before anesthesia. **Tx of nonpsychotic anxiety.** *Adult:* 5 mg PO tid or qid; max, 20 mg/d for no ≤12 wk.
**ADV EFF** Akathisia, **aplastic anemia,** blurred vision, **bone marrow suppression, bronchospasm,** dizziness, drowsiness, dystonia, **HF, laryngospasm, NMS,** photosensitivity, pink to red-brown urine, pseudoparkinsonism, rash, **refractory arrhythmias,** tardive dyskinesia
**INTERACTIONS** Alcohol, anticholinergics, barbiturate anesthetics
**NC/PT** Monitor CBC, renal function; elderly pts may be more susceptible to adverse reactions. Maintain hydration. Avoid skin contact w/oral sol. Give IM injection deep into upper outer quadrant of buttock. Urine may be pink to red-brown. Pt should avoid sun exposure; take safety precautions for CNS effects; report unusual bleeding, swelling, fever, difficulty breathing.

**progesterone** (Crinone, Endometrin, Prometrium)
**CLASS** Hormone, progestin
**PREG/CONT** B (oral); X (injection)/NA

**BBW** Do not use for px of CV disease. Not effective for this use; may actually increase risk of CV disease. Increased risk of dementia; weigh risks. Increased risk of invasive breast cancer; monitor pt closely.
**IND & DOSE** **Tx of primary amenorrhea.** *Adult:* 5–10 mg/d IM for 6–8 consecutive d. Or, 400 mg PO in p.m. for 10 d. **Tx of secondary amenorrhea.** *Adult:* 4%–8% gel, 45–90 mg q other day; max, six doses. **Mgt of uterine bleeding.** *Adult:* 5–10 mg/d IM for six doses. If estrogen given, begin progesterone after 2 wk of estrogen tx. **Tx of endometrial hyperplasia.** *Adult:* 200 mg/d PO in p.m. for 12 d/28-day cycle w/daily conjugated estrogen. **Tx of infertility.** *Adult:* 90 mg vaginally daily in women needing progesterone supplementation; 90 mg vaginally bid for replacement. Continue for 10–12 wk into preg if it occurs. **Support for embryo implantation.** *Adult:* 100 mg vaginally 2–3 ×/d starting at oocyte retrieval, continuing for up to 10 wk.
**ADV EFF** Abd cramps, amenorrhea; breakthrough bleeding, spotting; breast tenderness; cervical erosion; change in menstrual flow, weight; constipation; dizziness; headache; **PE;** photosensitivity; rash; somnolence; **thromboembolic/thrombotic disease**
**INTERACTIONS** Grapefruit juice
**NC/PT** Obtain baseline, periodic (at least annual) hx, physical exam. Insert intrauterine system during or immediately after menstrual period. Give IM by deep injection. Stop at first sign of thromboembolic problems. Not for use in preg (contact prescriber if preg occurs)/breastfeeding. Pt should perform monthly breast self-exams; avoid grapefruit juice, sun exposure; stop if sudden vision loss, difficulty breathing, leg pain/swelling, chest pain.

**DANGEROUS DRUG**

**promethazine hydrochloride** (Phenadoz, Promethazine Plain, Promethegan)
**CLASS** Antiemetic, antihistamine, anti–motion sickness drug, dopaminergic blocker, phenothiazine, sedative-hypnotic
**PREG/CONT** C/NA

**BBW** Do not give to child <2 yr; risk of fatal respiratory depression. Use lowest effective dose, caution in child ≥2 yr. Give IM injection deep into muscle. Do not give subcut; tissue necrosis possible. Do not give intra-arterially; arteriospasm, limb gangrene possible. If IV route used, limit drug conc, rate of administration; ensure open IV line.
**IND & DOSE** **Relief of allergy s&sx.** *Adult:* 25 mg PO, rectally, preferably at bedtime. If needed, 12.5 mg PO before meals and at bedtime. Or, 25 mg IM or IV for serious reactions. May repeat within 2 hr if needed. *Child >2 yr:* 25 mg PO at bedtime or 6.25–12.5 mg tid. **Tx, px of motion sickness.** *Adult:* 25 mg PO bid 30–60 min before travel; repeat in 8–12 hr if needed. Then, 25 mg on rising and before evening meal. *Child >2 yr:* 12.5–25 mg PO, rectally bid. **Tx, px of n/v.** *Adult:* 25 mg PO; repeat doses of 12.5–25 mg as needed q 4–6 hr. Give rectally or parenterally if PO not tolerated. Or, 12.5–25 mg IM or IV; max, q 4–6 hr. *Child >2 yr:* 0.5 mg/lb body weight IM q 4–6 hr as needed. **Sedation, postop sedation, adjunctive use w/analgesics.** *Adult:* 25–50 mg PO, IM or IV. *Child >2 yr:* 12.5–25 mg PO rectally at bedtime. For postop sedation, 12.5–25 mg PO, IV or IM, rectally. **Preop use.** *Adult:* 50 mg PO night before surgery. *Child >2 yr:*

0.5 mg/lb body weight PO. **Obstetric sedation.** *Adult:* 50 mg IM or IV in early stages. When labor established, 25–75 mg w/reduced opioid dose. May repeat once or twice at 4-hr intervals. Max within 24 hr, 100 mg.
**ADV EFF** **Agranulocytosis,** confusion, dizziness, drowsiness, dysuria, epigastric distress, excitation, hypotension, **pancytopenia,** photosensitivity, poor coordination, thickened bronchial secretions, urinary frequency
**INTERACTIONS** Alcohol, anticholinergics, methohexital, phenobarbital anesthetic, thiopental
**NC/PT** Do not give subcut, deep IM. Maintain hydration. Pt should take safety precautions for CNS effects; avoid sun exposure; report unusual bleeding, rash, dark urine.

**DANGEROUS DRUG**

## propafenone hydrochloride (Rythmol SR)

**CLASS** Antiarrhythmic
**PREG/CONT** C/NA

**BBW** Arrange for periodic ECG to monitor effects on cardiac conduction; risk of serious proarrhythmias. Monitor pt response carefully, especially at start of tx; increase dosage at minimum of 3- to 4-day intervals.
**IND & DOSE** **Tx of documented life-threatening ventricular arrhythmias; tx of paroxysmal supraventricular tachycardia w/disabling s&sx in pts w/o structural heart disease.** *Adult:* 150 mg PO q 8 hr (450 mg/d). May increase at minimum of 3- to 4-day intervals to 225 mg PO q 8 hr (675 mg/d) to max 300 mg PO q 8 hr (900 mg/d). **To prolong time to recurrence of symptomatic atrial fibrillation in pts w/ structural heart disease.** *Adult:* 225 mg ER tablet PO q 12 hr; titrate at 5-day intervals to max 425 mg q 12 hr.
**ADJUST DOSE** Elderly pts; hepatic/ renal impairment
**ADV EFF** **Agranulocytosis**, arrhythmias, blurred vision, constipation, dizziness, headache, **cardiac arrest, coma,** fatigue, headache, **HF,** n/v, unusual taste
**INTERACTIONS** Beta blockers, cimetidine, cyclosporine, digoxin, quinidine, ritonavir, SSRIs, theophylline, warfarin
**NC/PT** Monitor ECG periodically. Not for use in preg/breastfeeding. Pt should swallow ER tablet whole and not cut/crush/chew it; take around the clock; use safety precautions for CNS effects; report difficulty breathing, fainting, palpitations.

## propantheline bromide (generic)

**CLASS** Anticholinergic, antispasmodic, parasympatholytic
**PREG/CONT** C/NA

**IND & DOSE** **Adjunct tx in peptic ulcer.** *Adult:* 7.5–15 mg PO 30 min before meals and at bedtime. *Child:* 1.5 mg/kg/d PO in divided doses tid–qid.
**ADJUST DOSE** Elderly pts; hepatic/ renal impairment
**ADV EFF** Blurred vision, decreased sweating, drowsiness, dry mouth, headache, n/v, urine retention
**INTERACTIONS** Antacids, anticholinergics, digoxin, phenothiazines
**NC/PT** Risk of heat prostration; maintain hydration. Not for use w/ severe glaucoma, GI obstruction, myasthenia gravis. Not for use in preg/breastfeeding. Pt should swallow ER tablet whole and not cut/crush/ chew it; take 30 min before meals and at bedtime; empty bladder before each dose; use sugarless lozenges for dry mouth; take safety precautions for CNS effects; report rash, eye pain.

**DANGEROUS DRUG**

## propofol (Diprivan)

**CLASS** Sedative/hypnotic
**PREG/CONT** B/NA

**IND & DOSE** **Induction of general anesthesia.** *Adult:* 2–2.5 mg/kg IV at 40 mg/10 sec. *Child 3–16 yr:*

2.5–3.5 mg/kg IV over 20–30 sec. **Induction of general anesthesia in neurosurgery.** *Adult:* 1–2 mg/kg IV at 20 mg/10 sec. **Induction of general anesthesia in cardiac surgery.** *Adult:* 0.5–1.5 mg/kg IV at 20 mg/10 sec. **Maintenance of general anesthesia.** *Adult:* 100–200 mcg/kg/min IV or 25–50 mg intermittent IV bolus, based on pt response. *Child 3–16 yr:* 125–150 mcg/kg/min IV, based on pt response. Monitored anesthesia care. *Adult:* 25–75 mcg/kg/min IV, based on pt response. **ICU sedation of intubated pts.** *Adult:* 5–50 mcg/kg/min IV as continuous infusion.
**ADJUST DOSE** Elderly, debilitated pts
**ADV EFF** Anxiety, **apnea,** chills, confusion, dry mouth, **hypoxemia,** injection-site reactions, **loss of responsiveness, MI, respiratory depression**
**INTERACTIONS** Benzodiazepines, opioid analgesics
**NC/PT** Monitor continuously. Perform frequent BP checks, oximetry; give oxygen; have emergency equipment on standby; ensure pt safety for CNS effects; taper after prolonged ICU use. Pt should be aware of sedation effects (do not drive; avoid important decisions/tasks requiring alertness); report difficulty breathing, chest pain, pain at injection site.

**DANGEROUS DRUG**

## propranolol hydrochloride (Hemangeol, Inderal, InnoPran XL)

**CLASS** Antianginal, antiarrhythmic, antihypertensive, beta blocker
**PREG/CONT** C/NA

**BBW** Do not stop abruptly after long-term tx (hypersensitivity to catecholamines possible, causing angina exacerbation, MI, ventricular arrhythmias). Taper gradually over 2 wk w/monitoring.
**IND & DOSE Tx of HTN.** *Adult:* 40 mg PO regular propranolol bid, or 80 mg (SR, ER) PO daily initially; range, 120–240 mg/d bid or tid or 120–160 mg (SR, ER) daily (max, 640 mg/d). **Tx of angina.** *Adult:* 80–320 mg/d PO divided bid, tid, or qid, or 80 mg (SR, ER) daily initially; usual dose, 160 mg/d (max, 320 mg/d). **Mgt of IHSS.** *Adult:* 20–40 mg PO tid or qid, or 80–160 mg PO (SR, ER) daily. **Post-MI.** *Adult:* 120 mg/d PO divided tid. After 1 mo, may titrate to 180–240 mg/d PO tid or qid (max, 240 mg/d). **Mgt of pheochromocytoma s&sx.** *Adult:* Preop, 60 mg/d PO for 3 d in divided doses; inoperable tumor, 30 mg/d in divided doses. **Px of migraine.** *Adult:* 80 mg/d PO (SR, ER) once or in divided doses; range, 160–240 mg/d. **Mgt of essential tremor.** *Adult:* 40 mg PO bid; maint, 120 mg/d (max, 320 mg/d). **Tx of arrhythmias.** *Adult:* 10–30 mg PO tid or qid, or 1–3 mg IV w/careful monitoring; max, 1 mg/min. May give second dose in 2 min, then do not repeat for 4 hr. **Tx of proliferating infantile hemangioma requiring systemic therapy.** *Child 5 wk–5 mo:* 0.6 mg/kg PO bid for 1 wk, then 1.1 mg/kg PO bid. After 2 wk, increase to maint 1.7 mg/kg PO bid; give doses at least 9 hr apart (*Hemangeol* sol only).
**ADV EFF** Arrhythmias, **bronchospasm,** constipation, decreased exercise tolerance/libido, fatigue, flatulence, gastric pain, serum glucose changes, **HF, laryngospasm,** n/v/d, **stroke**
**INTERACTIONS** Barbiturates, clonidine, epinephrine, ergots, ibuprofen, indomethacin, insulin, lidocaine, methimazole, naproxen, phenothiazines, piroxicam, prazosin, propylthiouracil, sulindac, theophyllines, thioridazine, verapamil
**NC/PT** Provide continuous cardiac, regular BP monitoring w/IV form. Change to oral form as soon as possible. Do not use sol for hemangioma in premature infants, infants <2 kg. Taper when stopping. Pt should take w/ food; take safety precautions for CNS effects; report difficulty breathing, swelling, numbness/tingling.

## propylthiouracil (PTU)
(generic)
**CLASS** Antithyroid drug
**PREG/CONT** High risk/NA

**BBW** Associated w/severe, possibly fatal, liver injury. Monitor carefully for liver adverse effects, especially during first 6 mo of tx. Do not use in child unless allergic to or intolerant of other tx; risk of liver toxicity higher in child. Drug of choice when antithyroid tx needed during or just before first trimester (fetal abnormalities are associated w/methimazole).
**IND & DOSE Tx of hyperthyroidism in pt who cannot tolerate methimazole and when radioactive iodine or surgery are not options.** *Adult:* 300 mg/d PO in divided doses q 8 hr, up to 400–900 mg/d in severe cases. Range, 100–150 mg/d in divided doses q 8 hr. *Child ≥6 intolerant to other tx:* 50 mg/d PO in divided doses q 8 hr. (Not drug of choice in child.)
**ADV EFF Agranulocytosis,** drowsiness, epigastric distress, fever, neuritis, n/v, paresthesia, rash, **severe liver injury,** vertigo
**INTERACTIONS** Cardiac glycosides, metoprolol, oral anticoagulants, propranolol, theophylline
**NC/PT** Monitor TSH, $T_3/T_4$. Prolonged tx will be needed. Alert surgeon that drug may increase risk of bleeding. Not for use in preg (but if antithyroid drug needed in first trimester, propylthiouracil is preferred). Pt should take around the clock; use safety precautions for CNS effects; report s&sx of infection, urine/stool color changes.

## protamine sulfate
(generic)
**CLASS** Heparin antagonist
**PREG/CONT** C/NA

**BBW** Keep emergency equipment on hand in case of anaphylactic reaction.
**IND & DOSE Tx of heparin, low-molecular-weight heparin overdose.** *Adult, child:* 1 mg IV neutralizes not <100 heparin units.
**ADV EFF Anaphylaxis,** hypotension, n/v, rash
**NC/PT** Monitor coagulation studies to adjust dose; screen for heparin rebound and response. Pt should report difficulty breathing, dizziness.

**DANGEROUS DRUG**

## protein C concentrate
(Ceprotin)
**CLASS** Anticoagulant, blood product
**PREG/CONT** C/NA

**IND & DOSE Replacement tx for pts w/severe congenital protein C deficiency.** *Adult, child:* 100–120 international units/kg by IV injection. Then 60–80 international units/kg IV q 6 hr for three more doses. Maint, 45–60 international units/kg IV q 6–12 hr.
**ADV EFF Anaphylactoid reaction, bleeding, hemothorax, hypotension,** light-headedness, pruritus, rash
**NC/PT** Risk of disease transmission w/blood products. Protect from light. Monitor for bleeding. Pt should report difficulty breathing, hives, rash, unusual bleeding.

## prothrombin complex concentrate (Kcentra)
**CLASS** Vitamin K anticoagulant reversal agent
**PREG/CONT** C/NA

**BBW** Risk of thromboembolic complications. Monitor closely; consider need to resume anticoagulant therapy when risks outweigh benefits.
**IND & DOSE Urgent reversal of acquired coagulation factor deficiency from warfarin overactivity w/major bleeding.** *Adult:* INR of 2–<4, 25 units/kg IV; max, 2,500 units. INR of 4–6, 35 units/kg IV; max, 3,500 units. INR

greater than 6, 50 units/kg IV; max, 5,000 units.
**ADV EFF** **Arterial/venous thrombotic events,** arthralgia, **blood-related infections,** DVT, headache, hypotension, n/v, **serious hypersensitivity reactions, stroke**
**NC/PT** Monitor INR during and after tx. Monitor for hypersensitivity reactions, sx of thrombotic events. Pt should know risks of receiving blood products. Risks in preg/breastfeeding unkn. Pt should report difficulty breathing, chest pain, acute leg pain, numbness/tingling, vision or speech changes, abnormal swelling.

## protriptyline hydrochloride (Vivactil)

**CLASS** TCA
**PREG/CONT** C/NA

**BBW** Limit drug access in depressed, potentially suicidal pts. Increased risk of suicidality in child, adolescent, young adult; monitor accordingly.
**IND & DOSE** **Relief of sx of depression.** *Adult:* 15–40 mg/d PO in three–four divided doses; max, 60 mg/d.
**ADJUST DOSE** Elderly pts
**ADV EFF** Anticholinergic effects, **bone marrow suppression,** constipation, dry mouth, extrapyramidal effects, **MI,** orthostatic hypotension, photosensitivity, rash, **stroke**
**INTERACTIONS** Alcohol, cimetidine, clonidine, fluoxetine, MAOIs, ranitidine, sympathomimetics, tramadol
**NC/PT** Do not stop suddenly. Monitor CBC periodically. Not for use in preg (contraceptives advised)/breastfeeding. Pt should avoid sun exposure; take safety precautions for CNS effects; use sugarless lozenges for dry mouth; report thoughts of suicide, excessive sedation.

**▶NEW DRUG**

## prucalopride succinate (Motegrity)

**CLASS** GI drug, selective serotonin type 4 receptor agonist
**PREG/CONT** Low risk/NA

**IND & DOSE** **Tx of chronic idiopathic constipation.** *Adult:* 2 mg PO daily. *Adult w/CrCl <30 mL/min:* 1 mg PO daily.
**ADV EFF** Abd pain, dizziness, fatigue, flatulence, headache, **hypersensitivity, intestinal perforation,** n/v, **suicidal ideation/behavior**
**INTERACTIONS** Strong CYP3A inducers/inhibitors
**NC/PT** Suicidal ideation/behavior has been reported in pts taking drug. Pt/caregivers should watch for unusual changes in mood/behavior, persistent worsening of depression sx, or emergence of suicidal thoughts/behavior. If sx occur, drug should be stopped immediately and prescriber contacted. Pt should take w/ or w/o food.

## pseudoephedrine hydrochloride, pseudoephedrine sulfate (Sudafed)

**CLASS** Nasal decongestant, sympathomimetic
**PREG/CONT** C/NA

**BBW** Administer cautiously to pts w/ CV disease, diabetes, hyperthyroidism, glaucoma, HTN, >65 yr; increased sensitivity to sympathetic amines possible in these pts.
**IND & DOSE** **Relief of nasal congestion.** *Adult, child >12 yr:* 60 mg PO q 4–6 hr (ER, 120 mg PO q 12 hr; CR, 240 mg/d PO); max, 240 mg/24 hr. *Child 6–12 yr:* 30 mg PO q 4–6 hr; max, 120 mg/24 hr. *Child 2–5 yr:* 15 mg PO (syrup) q 4–6 hr; max, 60 mg/24 hr.
**ADJUST DOSE** Elderly pts
**ADV EFF** Arrhythmias, anxiety, dizziness, drowsiness, fear, headache,

HTN, n/v, pallor, restlessness, **seizures,** tenseness, tremors
**INTERACTIONS** MAOIs, methyldopa, urine acidifiers/alkalinizers
**NC/PT** Avoid prolonged use. Underlying medical problems may be causing congestion. Pt should swallow ER tablet whole and not cut/crush/chew it; take safety precautions for CNS effects; report sweating, sleeplessness, chest pain.

## pyrantel pamoate (Pin-X, Reese's Pinworm)

**CLASS** Anthelmintic
**PREG/CONT** C/NA

**IND & DOSE** **Tx of enterobiasis, ascariasis.** *Adult, child >2 yr:* 11 mg/kg (5 mg/lb) PO as single oral dose. Max total dose, 1 g.
**ADJUST DOSE** Hepatic impairment
**ADV EFF** Abd cramps, anorexia, dizziness, drowsiness, headache, n/v/d
**INTERACTIONS** Piperazine, theophylline
**NC/PT** Culture before tx. Pt should shake suspension well; take w/fruit juice, milk; use strict hand washing, hygiene measures; launder undergarments, bed linens, nightclothes daily; disinfect toilet facilities daily, bathroom floors periodically; take safety precautions for CNS effects; report severe headache.

## pyrazinamide (generic)

**CLASS** Antituberculotic
**PREG/CONT** C/NA

**IND & DOSE** **Tx of active, drug-resistant TB.** *Adult, child:* 15–30 mg/kg/d PO; max, 2 g/d. Always use w/up to four other antituberculotics; give for first 2 mo of 6-mo tx program.
**ADV EFF** **Bone marrow suppression,** gouty arthritis, **hepatotoxicity,** n/v, photosensitivity, rash
**INTERACTIONS** Piperazine, theophylline
**NC/PT** Give only w/other antituberculotics. Monitor LFTs during tx. Pt should have regular medical follow-up, report unusual bleeding, urine/stool color changes, severe joint pain.

## pyridostigmine bromide (Mestinon, Regonol)

**CLASS** Antimyasthenic, cholinesterase inhibitor
**PREG/CONT** C/NA

**IND & DOSE** **Control of myasthenia gravis sx.** *Adult:* 600 mg PO over 24 hr; range, 60–1,500 mg. Or, 180–540 mg (ER) PO daily, bid. As supplement to oral dose preop, postop, during labor/myasthenic crisis, etc: Give 1/30 oral dose IM or very slow IV. May give 1 hr before second stage of labor completed. *Child:* 7 mg/kg/d PO divided into five or six doses (over 30 d); 5 mg/kg/d PO divided into five or six doses (≤29 d). **Neonates w/myasthenic mothers who have difficulty swallowing, sucking, breathing.** 0.05–0.15 mg/kg IM. Change to syrup as soon as possible. **Military w/threat of sarin nerve gas exposure.** *Adult:* 30 mg PO q 8 hr starting several hr before exposure; stop if exposure occurs. **Antidote for NMJ blocker.** Atropine sulfate 0.6–1.2 mg IV immediately before slow IV injection of pyridostigmine 0.1–0.25 mg/kg; 10–20 mg pyridostigmine usually suffices. Full recovery usually within 15 min; may take 30 min.
**ADV EFF** Abd cramps, **anaphylaxis,** bradycardia, **bronchospasm,** cardiac arrhythmias, dysphagia, increased respiratory secretions/lacrimation/salivation, **laryngospasm,** urinary frequency/incontinence
**INTERACTIONS** Corticosteroids, succinylcholine
**NC/PT** Have atropine on hand as antidote. Give IV slowly. Pt should swallow ER tablet whole and not cut/crush/chew it; report difficulty breathing, excessive sweating.

## QUEtiapine fumarate
(Seroquel)
**CLASS** Antipsychotic
**PREG/CONT** Moderate risk/NA

**BBW** Do not use in elderly pts w/ dementia-related psychosis; increased risk of CV mortality, including stroke, MI. Increased risk of suicidality in child, adolescent, young adult; monitor accordingly. Not approved for use in child.
**IND & DOSE Tx of schizophrenia.** *Adult:* 25 mg PO bid. Increase in increments of 25–50 mg bid–tid on days 2, 3. Range by day 4, 300–400 mg/d in two–three divided doses; max, 750 mg/d. Once stabilized, switch to ER, 300 mg/d PO in p.m.; range, 400–800 mg/d. *Child 13–17 yr:* Divided dose bid. Total dose: day 1, 50 mg PO; day 2, 100 mg; day 3, 200 mg; day 4, 300 mg; day 5, 400 mg. Range, 400–800 mg/d. **Tx of manic episodes of bipolar 1 disorder.** *Adult:* 100 mg/d PO divided bid on day 1; increase to 400 mg/d PO in bid divided doses by day 4, using 100-mg/d increments. Range, 400–800 mg/d in divided doses. ER: 300 mg/d PO on day 1; 600 mg on day 2; may adjust to 800 mg on day 3 if needed. *Child 10–17 yr:* 25 mg PO bid on day 1, 100 mg on day 2, 200 mg on day 3, 300 mg on day 4, 400 mg on day 5. Max, 600 mg/d. **Tx of depressive episodes of bipolar 1 disorder.** *Adult:* 50 mg (ER) PO on day 1, then 100 mg at bedtime on day 2; increase to desired dose of 300 mg/d by day 4. **Tx of major depressive disorder.** *Adult:* 50 mg (ER) PO at bedtime; on day 3, increase to 150 mg in evening. Range, 150–300 mg/d.
**ADJUST DOSE** Elderly, debilitated pts; hepatic impairment
**ADV EFF** Cataracts, dizziness, drowsiness, dry mouth, headache, hyperglycemia, **NMS,** orthostatic hypotension, **prolonged QT,** sweating, tardive dyskinesia
**INTERACTIONS** Alcohol, anticholinergics, antihypertensives, carbamazepine, CNS depressants, dopamine antagonists, glucocorticoids, levodopa, lorazepam, phenobarbital, phenytoin, QT-prolonging drugs, rifampin, thioridazine
**NC/PT** Monitor for hyperglycemia, leukopenia, neutropenia, agranulocytosis. Ensure hydration in elderly pts. Not for use in preg (barrier contraceptives advised)/breastfeeding. Pt should swallow ER tablet whole and not cut/crush/chew it; avoid alcohol; take safety precautions for CNS effects; report fever, unusual bleeding, rash, suicidal thoughts.

## quinapril hydrochloride
(Accupril)
**CLASS** ACE inhibitor, antihypertensive
**PREG/CONT** High risk/NA

**BBW** Should not be used during preg; can cause fetal injury or death. Advise barrier contraceptives.
**IND & DOSE Tx of HTN.** *Adult:* 10 or 20 mg/d PO; maint, 20–80 mg/d PO. **Adjunct tx of HF.** *Adult:* 5 mg PO bid; range, 10–20 mg PO bid.
**ADJUST DOSE** Elderly pts, renal impairment
**ADV EFF Angioedema,** cough, dizziness, headache, hyperkalemia, orthostatic hypotension, LFT changes, rash
**INTERACTIONS** ACE inhibitors, ARBs, lithium, potassium-sparing diuretics, renin inhibitors, tetracycline
**NC/PT** Alert surgeon to drug use; volume replacement may be needed after surgery. Maintain hydration. Not for use in preg (contraceptives advised)/breastfeeding. Pt should use care in situations that may lead to BP drop; take safety precautions w/ dizziness, hypotension; report fever, difficulty breathing, swelling of lips/ tongue, leg cramps.

DANGEROUS DRUG

## quiNIDine gluconate, quiNIDine sulfate

(generic)

**CLASS** Antiarrhythmic

**PREG/CONT** C/NA

**IND & DOSE** **Tx of atrial arrhythmias; paroxysmal, chronic ventricular tachycardia.** *Adult:* 400–600 mg (sulfate) PO q 2–3 hr until paroxysm terminated. *Child:* 30 mg/kg/24 hr PO in five equally divided doses. **Conversion of atrial fibrillation (AF).** *Adult:* 648 mg (gluconate) PO q 8 hr; may increase after three–four doses if needed. Or, 324 mg (gluconate) PO q 8 hr for 2 d, then 648 mg PO q 8 hr for 2 d. Or, 5–10 mg/kg (gluconate) IV. For ER, 300 mg (sulfate) PO q 8–12 hr; may increase cautiously if serum level in therapeutic range. For immediate-release, 400 mg (sulfate) PO q 6 hr; may increase after four–five doses if no conversion. **To reduce relapse into AF.** *Adult:* 324 mg (gluconate) PO q 8–12 hr. For ER, 300 mg (sulfate) PO q 8–12 hr. For immediate-release, 200 mg (sulfate) PO q 6 hr. **Tx of *Plasmodium falciparum* malaria.** *Adult:* 24 mg/kg gluconate IV in 250 mL normal saline infused over 4 hr; then 12 mg/kg IV infused over 4 hr q 8 hr for 7 d. Or, 10 mg/kg gluconate in 5 mL/kg IV as loading dose; then maint IV infusion of 20 mcg/kg/min. May switch to same oral dose of sulfate q 8 hr for 72 hr or until parasitemia decreased to ≤1%.

**ADJUST DOSE** Hepatic/renal impairment

**ADV EFF** **Bone marrow suppression, cardiac arrhythmias,** cinchonism, diarrhea, headache, **hepatic impairment,** light-headedness, nausea, rash, vision changes

**INTERACTIONS** Amiodarone, cimetidine, digoxin, grapefruit juice, hydantoins, NMJ blockers, oral anticoagulants, phenobarbital, rifampin, sodium bicarbonate, succinylcholine, sucralfate, TCAs, verapamil

**NC/PT** Give test dose of 200 mg PO or 200 mg IV for idiosyncratic reaction. Ensure pts w/atrial flutter, fibrillation digitalized before starting quinidine. Monitor for safe, effective serum level (2–6 mcg/mL). Pt should swallow ER tablet whole and not cut/crush/chew it; wear medical ID; take safety precautions for CNS effects; report vision disturbances, unusual bleeding, s&sx of infection.

## quinine sulfate

(Qualaquin)

**CLASS** Antimalarial, cinchonan

**PREG/CONT** C/NA

**BBW** Not for tx, px of nocturnal leg cramps; serious to life-threatening hematologic reactions possible. Chronic renal impairment has been reported. No evidence for therapeutic effectiveness for nocturnal leg cramps.

**IND & DOSE** **Tx of uncomplicated *Plasmodium falciparum* malaria.** *Adult:* 648 mg (two capsules) PO q 8 hr for 7 d.

**ADJUST DOSE** Renal impairment

**ADV EFF** Abd pain, **anaphylaxis,** anemia, blindness, blurred vision, cardiac arrhythmias, deafness, dizziness, headache, hearing impairment, hypoglycemia, n/v/d, **prolonged QT,** sweating, tinnitus, **thrombocytopenia including idiopathic thrombocytopenic purpura,** vertigo

**INTERACTIONS** CYP3A4 inducers/inhibitors, digoxin, NMJ blockers, QT-prolonging drugs, rifampin

**NC/PT** Monitor LFTs, renal function, blood glucose, CBC. Use caution in preg/breastfeeding. Pt should take safety precautions for CNS effects; report unusual bleeding, vision changes, difficulty breathing, palpitations, fainting.

## RABEprazole sodium
(AcipHex)
**CLASS** Proton pump inhibitor
**PREG/CONT** Unkn/NA

**IND & DOSE Tx of GERD.** *Adult, child ≥12 yr:* 20 mg/d PO for 4–8 wk; maint, 20 mg/d PO. *Child 1–11 yr:* 15 kg or more, 10 mg/d PO; <15 kg, 5 mg/d PO for up to 12 wk. **Healing of duodenal ulcer.** *Adult:* 20 mg PO daily for up to 4 wk. **Tx of pathological hypersecretory conditions.** *Adult:* 60 mg PO daily–bid. ***Helicobacter pylori* eradication.** *Adult:* 20 mg PO bid w/ amoxicillin 1,000 mg PO bid and clarithromycin 500 mg PO bid w/meals for 7 d.
**ADJUST DOSE** Hepatic impairment
**ADV EFF Acute interstitial nephritis,** asthenia, bone loss, CDAD, diarrhea, dizziness, dry mouth, headache, hypomagnesemia, n/v, pneumonia, URI sx, vitamin $B_{12}$ deficiency
**INTERACTIONS** Amoxicillin, atazanavir, azole antifungals, clarithromycin, cyclosporine, digoxin, methotrexate, rilpivirine, warfarin
**NC/PT** Contraindicated w/rilpivirine, clarithromycin, amoxicillin. Limit use in preg/breastfeeding. Pt should swallow tablet whole and not cut/crush/chew it; for sprinkle, sprinkle granules on room temp soft food or liquid. Pt should maintain other tx for condition; take safety precautions for CNS effects; maintain nutrition; report worsening of condition, severe diarrhea.

## radium Ra 223 dichloride (Xofigo)
**CLASS** Antineoplastic, radioactive particle–emitting agent
**PREG/CONT** High risk/NA

**IND & DOSE Tx of castration-resistant prostate cancer w/ symptomatic bone metastases and no known visceral metastatic disease.** *Adult:* 50 kBq (1.35 microcurie)/kg by slow IV injection (over 1 min) at 4-wk intervals for six injections.
**ADV EFF** Bone marrow suppression, n/v/d, peripheral edema; fractures/mortality when combined w/abiraterone plus prednisone/prednisolone
**NC/PT** Ensure proper dx, proper handling of drug. Monitor CBC; provide supportive measures. Use universal precautions w/body fluids. Pt should use gloves when handling body fluids; flush toilet several times; avoid preg (men should use barrier contraceptives during and for 6 mo after use)/breastfeeding; report extreme fatigue, bleeding, severe vomiting, diarrhea.

## ragweed pollen allergy extract (Ragwitek)
**CLASS** Allergen extract
**PREG/CONT** Unkn/NA

**BBW** Risk of severe life-threatening allergic reactions. Not for use in uncontrolled asthma, pts who may be unresponsive to epinephrine or inhaled bronchodilators. Observe pt for 30 min after initial dose; have emergency equipment on hand.
**IND & DOSE Immunotherapy for tx of ragweed pollen–induced allergic rhinitis w/ or w/o conjunctivitis confirmed by skin test.** *Adult 18–65 yr:* 1 tablet/d SL starting 12 wk before and continuing throughout season.
**ADV EFF** Cough, ear pruritus, mouth edema, oropharyngeal pain/pruritus, throat/tongue pruritus
**NC/PT** Ensure skin testing confirms allergy. Not for use w/uncontrolled asthma, hx of severe reactions, eosinophilic esophagitis. Begin 12 wk before expected ragweed season; continue throughout season. Tell pt to place tablet under tongue, allow it to stay until completely dissolved, and not to swallow for 1 min. Monitor pt for at least 30 min after first dose; have emergency equipment on hand. Stop tx in case of oral wounds or

inflammation; allow to heal completely before restarting. Use caution in preg/breastfeeding. Pt should report and stop tx w/oral inflammation or wounds; report difficulty breathing/ swallowing.

## raloxifene hydrochloride (Evista)

**CLASS** Selective estrogen receptor modulator
**PREG/CONT** X/NA

**BBW** Increased risk of DVT/PE; monitor accordingly. Increased risk of stroke, CV events in women w/documented CAD; weigh benefits/risks before use in these women.
**IND & DOSE** **Px/tx of osteoporosis in postmenopausal women; to reduce risk of invasive breast cancer in postmenopausal women w/osteoporosis and high risk of invasive breast cancer.** *Adult:* 60 mg/d PO.
**ADV EFF** Depression, dizziness, edema, flulike sx, hot flashes, lightheadedness, rash, vaginal bleeding, **VTE**
**INTERACTIONS** Cholestyramine, oral anticoagulants
**NC/PT** Obtain periodic CBC. Provide comfort measures for effects. Not for use in preg (contraceptives advised)/ breastfeeding. Pt should take safety precautions for CNS effects; report difficulty breathing, numbness/ tingling, pain/swelling in legs.

## raltegravir (Isentress)

**CLASS** Antiretroviral, integrase inhibitor
**PREG/CONT** C/NA

**IND & DOSE** **Tx of HIV-1 infection, w/other antiretrovirals.** *Adult and tx-naïve pts or pts w/viral suppression:* 400 mg PO bid or 1,200 mg (2 × 600 mg) film-coated tablets PO once/day. *Adults (tx-experienced):* 400-mg film-coated tablet PO bid. *Adults, w/rifampin:* 800 mg (2 × 400 mg)–(2 × 600 mg) film-coated tablets PO once/day or 300 mg PO chewable tablets bid. *Child 28–40 kg:* 200 mg PO chewable tablet bid. *Child at least 25 kg:* 400 mg PO film-coated tablet bid or 150 mg PO chewable tablet bid. *Child 4 wk and 3 kg or more:* 3–<4 kg, 25 mg PO bid; 4–<6 kg, 30 mg PO bid; 6–<8 kg, 40 mg PO bid; 8–<11 kg, 60 mg PO bid; 11–<14 kg, 75–80 mg PO bid; 14–<20 kg, 100 mg PO bid; 20–<25 kg, 150 mg PO bid. *Child 1–4 wk:* 2–<3 kg, 8 mg PO bid; 3–<4 kg, 10 mg PO bid; 4–<5 kg, 15 mg PO bid. *Child birth to 1 wk:* 2–<3 kg, 4 mg PO once/day; 3–<4 kg, 5 mg once/day; 4–<5 kg, 7 mg PO once/day. No data for preterm neonate dosing.
**ADV EFF** Diarrhea, dizziness, headache, fatigue, fever, insomnia, n/v, **rhabdomyolysis, serious to life-threatening skin reactions, including SJS**
**INTERACTIONS** Rifampin, St. John's wort
**NC/PT** Ensure pt taking other antivirals. Not for use in preg/breastfeeding. Calculate weight-based use of chewable tablets for child. Phenylalanine in chewable tablets; alert pts w/ phenylketonuria. Pt should not let prescription run out or stop temporarily (virus could become resistant to antivirals); take precautions to avoid spread (drug not a cure); avoid St. John's wort; report s&sx of infection, unexplained muscle pain/weakness, rash.

## ramelteon (Rozerem)

**CLASS** Melatonin receptor agonist, sedative-hypnotic
**PREG/CONT** C/NA

**IND & DOSE** **Tx of insomnia.** *Adult:* 8 mg PO within 30 min of bedtime.
**ADJUST DOSE** Hepatic impairment
**ADV EFF** Amenorrhea, **anaphylaxis, angioedema,** decreased testosterone, depression, diarrhea, galactorrhea, headache, insomnia, **suicidality**

**INTERACTIONS** Clarithromycin, fluconazole, fluvoxamine, itraconazole, ketoconazole, nefazodone, nelfinavir, ritonavir
**NC/PT** Not for use in preg/breastfeeding. Pt should take 30 min before bed; avoid activities after taking; plan on ≥8 hr sleep; report difficulty breathing, swelling, thoughts of suicide.

**ramipril** (Altace)
**CLASS** ACE inhibitor, antihypertensive
**PREG/CONT** High risk/NA

**BBW** Not for use in preg; risk of fetal harm. Advise contraceptives.
**IND & DOSE** **Tx of HTN.** *Adult:* 2.5 mg PO daily; range, 2.5–20 mg/d. **Tx of HF first few d post MI in stable pts.** *Adult:* 2.5 mg PO bid; if hypotensive, may use 1.25 mg PO bid; target dose, 5 mg PO bid. **To decrease risk of MI, stroke, death from CV disease in stable pts.** *Adult ≥55 yr:* 2.5 mg/d PO for 1 wk, then 5 mg/d PO for 3 wk; maint, 10 mg PO daily.
**ADJUST DOSE** Elderly pts, renal impairment
**ADV EFF** **Agranulocytosis, angioedema,** aphthous ulcers, **bone marrow suppression,** cough, dizziness, dysgeusia, gastric irritation, **HF, hyperkalemia,** light-headedness, proteinuria, rash, **SJS,** tachycardia
**INTERACTIONS** ACE inhibitors, ARBs, capsaicin, diuretics, lithium, NSAIDs, renin inhibitors
**NC/PT** Monitor renal function, BP, potassium. Stop diuretics 2–3 d before tx. Not for use in preg (barrier contraceptives advised)/breastfeeding. Alert surgeon of ramipril use; volume replacement may be needed postop. Pt should open capsules, sprinkle contents over small amount of applesauce or mix in applesauce/water (mixture is stable for 24 hr at room temp, 48 hr if refrigerated); take safety precautions for CNS effects; use caution in situations that could lead to fluid loss, decreased BP; maintain hydration; report unusual bleeding, swelling, rash.

**ramucirumab** (Cyramza)
**CLASS** Antineoplastic, endothelial growth factor receptor antagonist
**PREG/CONT** High risk/NA

**IND & DOSE** **Tx of advanced gastric or gastroesophageal junction adenocarcinoma as monotherapy or w/ paclitaxel, after other tx.** *Adult:* 8 mg/kg IV push or bolus q 2 wk as single agent or w/paclitaxel. **Tx of metastatic NSCLC, w/docetaxel, w/ disease progression w/platinum-based chemotherapy.** *Adult:* 10 mg/kg IV on day 1 of 21-day cycle, before docetaxel infusion. **Tx of colorectal cancer, w/Folfiri after prior tx.** *Adult:* 8 mg/kg IV q 2 wk before Folfiri. **Tx of hepatocellular carcinoma if alpha-fetoprotein ≥400 ng/mL after tx w/ sorafenib.** *Adult:* 8 mg/kg IV q 2 wk.
**ADV EFF** **Bleeding events,** fatigue, diarrhea, **GI perforation, hepatic impairment, HTN, impaired wound healing, infusion reactions, nephrotic syndrome, RPLS, thromboembolic events, thyroid dysfx**
**NC/PT** Monitor for infusion reactions, bleeding, clinical deterioration, HTN, thrombotic events, renal impairment; monitor LFTs. Withhold before surgery (impairs wound healing). Not for use in preg (contraceptives advised)/breastfeeding. Mark calendar w/tx days. Pt should report bleeding, severe GI pain, chest pain, difficulty breathing.

**ranibizumab** (Lucentis)
**CLASS** Monoclonal antibody, ophthal agent
**PREG/CONT** Moderate risk/NA

**IND & DOSE** **Tx of neovascular (wet) age-related macular degeneration; macular edema after retinal**

**vein occlusion.** 0.5 mg (0.05 mL) by intravitreal injection q 1–3 mo. **Tx of diabetic macular edema, diabetic retinopathy w/diabetic macular edema.** *Adult:* 0.3 mg by intravitreal injection once/mo. **Tx of myopic choroidal neovascularization.** *Adult:* 0.5 mg by intravitreal injection q 28 d for up to 3 mo.
**ADV EFF** Conjunctival hemorrhage, eye pain, hypersensitivity reactions, increased IOP, intraocular inflammation, ocular infection, retinal detachment, vision changes, vitreous floaters
**NC/PT** Monitor carefully for detached retina, increased IOP. Pt should be anesthetized before injection, receive antibiotic. Pt should report increased light sensitivity, vision changes, painful eye.

## raNITIdine hydrochloride (Zantac)
**CLASS** Gastric acid secretion inhibitor, histamine-2 antagonist
**PREG/CONT** B/NA

**IND & DOSE** **Tx of active duodenal ulcer.** *Adult:* 150 mg PO bid for 4–8 wk, or 300 mg PO once daily at bedtime, or 50 mg IM or IV q 6–8 hr *or* by intermittent IV infusion, diluted to 100 mL and infused over 15–20 min. Max, 400 mg/d; maint, 150 mg PO at bedtime. *Child 1 mo–16 yr:* 2–4 mg/kg PO bid for tx; once daily for maint. Max, 3,000 mg/d (tx), 1,500 mg/d (maint). Or, 2–4 mg/kg/d IV or IM q 6–8 hr; max, 50 mg q 6–8 hr. **Tx of active gastric ulcer.** *Adult:* 150 mg PO bid, or 50 mg IM or IV q 6–8 hr. **Tx of pathologic hypersecretory syndrome, GERD maint, esophagitis, benign gastric ulcer.** *Adult:* 150 mg PO bid; max, 6 g/d. **Tx of heartburn, acid indigestion.** *Adult:* 75 mg PO as needed.
**ADJUST DOSE** Elderly pts, renal impairment
**ADV EFF** Abd pain, bradycardia, **bone marrow suppression,** constipation, headache, n/v/d, pain at injection site, rash
**INTERACTIONS** Warfarin
**NC/PT** Give IM undiluted into large muscle; give oral drug w/meals and at bedtime. May continue antacids for pain relief. Pt should report unusual bleeding, s&sx of infection. Name confusion w/*Zantac* (ranitidine), *Zyrtec* (cetirizine), *Xanax* (alprazolam).

## ranolazine (Ranexa)
**CLASS** Antianginal, piperazineacetamide
**PREG/CONT** Low risk/NA

**IND & DOSE** **Tx of chronic angina.** *Adult:* 500 mg PO bid; max, 1,000 mg bid.
**ADJUST DOSE** Hepatic impairment (not recommended)
**ADV EFF** Constipation, dizziness, headache, nausea, **prolonged QT,** renal failure
**INTERACTIONS** Antipsychotics, digoxin, diltiazem, grapefruit juice, HIV protease inhibitors, ketoconazole, macrolide antibiotics, QT-prolonging drugs, rifampin, TCAs, verapamil
**NC/PT** Obtain baseline ECG, LFTs, renal function; monitor periodically. Continue other antianginals. Use caution in preg (contraceptives advised)/ breastfeeding. Pt should swallow tablet whole and not cut/crush/chew it; take safety measures w/dizziness; avoid grapefruit juice; use laxative for severe constipation; report fainting, palpitations.

## rasagiline (Azilect)
**CLASS** Antiparkinsonian, MAO type B inhibitor
**PREG/CONT** C/NA

**IND & DOSE** **Tx of s&sx of all stages of idiopathic Parkinson disease.** *Adult:* 1 mg/d PO as monotherapy; 0.5–1 mg/d PO w/levodopa.
**ADJUST DOSE** CYP1A2 inhibitors, hepatic impairment

**ADV EFF** Arthralgia, dizziness, dyspepsia, dry mouth, hallucinations, headache, hypotension, impulse control issues, **melanoma**, serotonin syndrome, vertigo
**INTERACTIONS** Cyclobenzaprine, CYP1A2 inhibitors (ciprofloxacin), dextromethorphan, MAOIs, meperidine, methadone, mirtazapine, SSRIs, St. John's wort, sympathomimetic amines, TCAs, tramadol, tyramine-rich food
**NC/PT** Obtain baseline LFTs, skin evaluation. Continue other Parkinson drugs. Use caution in preg/breastfeeding. Pt should avoid sun exposure, tyramine-rich foods, St. John's wort; take safety measures for CNS effects; tell all health care providers about prescribed/OTC drugs, herbs being used (drug reacts w/many other drugs); report skin changes, worsening of condition.

## rasburicase (Elitek)
**CLASS** Enzyme
**PREG/CONT** Moderate risk/NA

**BBW** Risk of anaphylaxis, hemolysis (in pts w/G6PD deficiency; screen before tx), methemoglobinemia, uric acid measurement alterations.
**IND & DOSE** **Mgt of plasma uric acid level in pts w/leukemia, lymphoma, solid tumor malignancies receiving anticancer tx expected to result in tumor lysis.** *Adult:* 0.2 mg/kg IV as single daily infusion over 30 min for 5 d. Start chemo 4–24 hr after first dose.
**ADV EFF** Abd pain, **anaphylaxis,** anxiety, constipation, fever, headache, **hemolysis,** methemoglobinemia, n/v/d
**NC/PT** Screen for G6PD deficiency. Monitor closely during infusion; stop immediately if hypersensitivity reactions. Monitor CBC. Blood drawn to monitor uric acid level must be collected in prechilled, heparinized vials and kept in ice-water bath; analysis must be done within 4 hr. Use caution in preg. Not for use in breastfeeding. Give analgesics for headache. Pt should report difficulty breathing, chest pain, rash.

**▶NEW DRUG**

## ravulizumab-cwvz
(Ultomiris)
**CLASS** Complement inhibitor, immunomodulator
**PREG/CONT** Unkn/NA

**BBW** Risk of life-threatening meningococcal infections/sepsis. Comply w/recommendation for meningococcal vaccination at least 2 wk before Ultomiris dose, unless risks of delay outweigh risk of meningococcal infection. Monitor for early sx of meningococcal infection. Drug only available through REMS program.
**IND & DOSE** **Tx of paroxysmal nocturnal hemoglobinuria.** *Adult ≥40 kg:* Weight-based loading dose IV followed in 2 wk by maint dosing scheduled q 8 wk. **Tx of atypical hemolytic uremic syndrome to inhibit complement-mediated thrombotic microangiopathy.** *Adult, child ≥1 mo ≥5 kg:* Weight-based loading dose followed in 2 wk by maint dosing q 4 or 8 wk (based on body weight).
**ADV EFF** Headache, HTN, n/v/d, pyrexia, URI
**NC/PT** See manufacturer's instruction for specific dosing. Risk of serious infections, including meningococcal infection, even post vaccination. Pt should carry Ultomiris Patient Safety Card at all times during tx and for at least 8 mo after final dose.

## raxibacumab (generic)
**CLASS** Monoclonal antibody
**PREG/CONT** B/NA

**IND & DOSE** **Tx/px of inhalational anthrax, w/antibacterial drugs.** *Adult, child >50 kg:* 40 mg/kg IV over 2 hr, 15 min. *Child* >40 kg: 40 mg/kg IV over 2 hr, 15 min. *Child 10–40 kg:*

60 mg/kg IV over 2 hr, 15 min. *Child ≤10 kg:* 80 mg/kg IV over 2 hr, 15 min.
**ADV EFF** Extremity pain, infusion reaction, pruritus, rash, somnolence
**NC/PT TEACH** Premedicate w/ diphenhydramine. Ensure use of antibacterials. Monitor for infusion reaction; slow, interrupt infusion as needed. Pt should report itching, difficulty breathing, rash.

## regorafenib (Stivarga)

**CLASS** Antineoplastic, kinase inhibitor
**PREG/CONT** High risk/NA

**BBW** Severe to fatal hepatotoxicity reported; monitor LFTs before, during tx.
**IND & DOSE Tx of metastatic colorectal cancer in pts previously treated w/other agents; tx of hepatocellular carcinoma if previously treated w/sorafenib; tx of advanced, unresectable GI stromal tumors if previously treated w/imatinib, sunitinib.** *Adult:* 160 mg/d PO for first 21 d of 28-d cycle. Give w/low-fat meal at same time of day. If dose decrease needed, 80 mg/d is lowest recommended dose.
**ADV EFF** Anorexia, **cardiac ischemia/infarction, dermatologic toxicity,** diarrhea, dysphonia, **GI perforation/fistula, hepatotoxicity, HTN,** mucositis, **RPLS,** weight loss, wound-healing complications
**INTERACTIONS** Grapefruit juice, St. John's wort, strong CYP3A4 inducers/inhibitors; avoid these combos
**NC/PT** Monitor LFTs. Decrease dose or stop drug if hepatotoxicity, acute worsening of infection, or severe skin reactions occur. Monitor for bleeding and problems w/wound healing. Not for use in preg/breastfeeding. Stop drug at least 24 hr before scheduled surgery. Pt should take daily w/low-fat meal at same time of day; report chest pain, severe GI pain, bleeding, urine/stool color changes.

**DANGEROUS DRUG**

## repaglinide (generic)

**CLASS** Antidiabetic, meglitinide
**PREG/CONT** C/NA

**IND & DOSE Adjunct to diet/exercise to lower blood glucose in pts w/ type 2 diabetes, as monotherapy or w/other antidiabetics.** *Adult:* 0.5–4 mg PO tid or qid 15–30 min (usually within 15 min) before meals; max, 16 mg/d.
**ADJUST DOSE** Hepatic/renal impairment
**ADV EFF** Diarrhea, headache, hypoglycemia, nausea, URI
**INTERACTIONS** Celery, coriander, dandelion root, fenugreek, garlic, gemfibrozil, ginseng, itraconazole, juniper berries
**NC/PT** Review complete diabetic teaching program. Pt should always take before meals (if meal is skipped or added, dose should be skipped or added appropriately); monitor serum glucose; continue diet/exercise program; report fever, unusual bleeding/bruising, frequent hypoglycemia.

## reslizumab (Cinqair)

**CLASS** Antiasthmatic, interleukin antagonist, monoclonal antibody
**PREG/CONT** High risk/NA

**BBW** Risk of anaphylaxis; pt must be monitored after infusion by professionals able to deal w/anaphylaxis.
**IND & DOSE Add-on maint tx of pts w/severe asthma w/eosinophilic phenotype.** *Adult:* 3 mg/kg IV over 20–50 min once q 4 wk.
**ADV EFF Anaphylaxis,** helminthic infections, **malignancy,** otopharyngeal pain
**NC/PT** Ensure proper dx. IV infusion only; not for push or bolus. Administer in setting prepared to deal w/anaphylactic reactions. Taper corticosteroids if appropriate; do not stop suddenly. Treat preexisting helminth infection

before use. Pt should avoid preg/ breastfeeding; mark calendar for infusion days; report difficulty breathing, edema, worsening of asthma sx.

## revefenacin (Yupelri)

**CLASS** Anticholinergic, long-acting

**PREG/CONT** Low risk/NA

**IND & DOSE** **Tx of COPD.** *Adult:* 175 mcg inhaled daily.
**ADV EFF** Back pain, cough, headache, hypersensitivity, narrow-angle glaucoma, nasopharyngitis, paradoxical bronchospasm, URI, urine retention
**INTERACTIONS** Anticholinergics, OATP1B1 and OAT1B3 inhibitors (may increase drug exposure)
**NC/PT** Drug for inhalation only. NOT indicated for acute sx. Discontinue if paradoxical bronchospasm. Avoid in hepatic impairment. Warn pt of possible worsening of narrow-angle glaucoma/urine retention. Discontinue if hypersensitivity reactions.

## ribavirin (Rebetol, Ribasphere, Virazole)

**CLASS** Antiviral

**PREG/CONT** High risk/NA

**BBW** Inhaled form not for use in adults; testicular lesions, birth defects possible. Monotherapy not effective for tx of chronic HCV; do not use alone for this indication. High risk of hemolytic anemia, which could lead to MI; do not use in significant, unstable CV disease. Monitor respiratory status frequently; pulmonary deterioration, death have occurred during, shortly after tx w/inhaled form. Risk of significant fetal defects; caution women to avoid preg during tx (barrier contraceptives advised). Male partners of preg women should not take drug.
**IND & DOSE** **Tx of hospitalized infant, child w/severe RSV infection of lower respiratory tract.** *Child:* Dilute aerosol powder to 20 mg/mL, deliver for 12–18 hr/d for at least 3 but not >7 d. **Tx of chronic HCV.** *Adult >75 kg:* Three 200-mg capsules PO in a.m., three 200-mg capsules PO in p.m. w/*Intron A* 3 million international units subcut 3 ×/wk, or w/Pegintron 180 mcg/wk subcut for 24–48 wk. *Adult ≤75 kg:* Two 200-mg capsules PO in a.m., three 200-mg capsules PO in p.m. w/*Intron A* 3 million international units subcut 3 ×/wk, or w/ Pegintron 180 mcg/wk subcut for 24–48 wk. *Child ≥3 yr:* 15 mg/kg/d PO in divided doses a.m. and p.m. Child 25–62 kg may use oral sol. Give w/ *Intron A* 3 million international units/ $m^2$ subcut 3 ×/wk.
**ADJUST DOSE** Anemia, renal impairment
**ADV EFF** Anemia, apnea, **cardiac arrest**, depression, deteriorating respiratory function, growth impairment in child, **hemolytic anemia**, nervousness, rash, **suicidality**
**INTERACTIONS** Antacids, nucleoside reverse transcriptase inhibitors
**NC/PT** Monitor CBC regularly. Review use/care of inhaler. Ensure pt on oral tx also taking other antivirals; not for monotherapy. Not for use in preg (barrier contraceptives advised)/ breastfeeding. Pt should report thoughts of suicide, chest pain, difficulty breathing.

## ribociclib (Kisqali)

**CLASS** Antineoplastic, kinase inhibitor

**PREG/CONT** High risk/NA

**IND & DOSE** **Combo tx w/aromatase inhibitor for HR-positive, HER2-negative advanced or metastatic breast cancer; w/fulvestrant for tx of postmenopausal women w/HR-positive, HER2-negative advanced or metastatic breast cancer as initial endocrine based therapy.** *Adult:* 600 mg/d PO for 21 consecutive d; then 7 d rest.

**ADV EFF** Alopecia, back pain, **bone marrow suppression,** constipation, headache, **hepatobiliary toxicity, ILD/ pneumonitis**, n/v/d, **prolonged QT**
**INTERACTIONS** CYP3A inducers/ inhibitors; avoid this combo. CYP3A substrates, QT-prolonging drugs
**NC/PT** Monitor LFTs, blood counts, QT interval before and q 2 wk during tx. Not for use in preg/breastfeeding. Pt may take w/ or w/o food once a day. Pt should report use of other drugs (many **INTERACTIONS** possible); cover head to prevent heat loss; report s&sx of infection, urine/stool color changes, severe n/v/d. Tx may need to be interrupted, dose reduced, or tx discontinued based on pt safety/ tolerability.

## rifabutin (Mycobutin)
**CLASS** Antibiotic
**PREG/CONT** B/NA

**IND & DOSE Px of disseminated *Mycobacterium avium* complex in pts w/advanced HIV infection.** *Adult:* 300 mg/d PO. *Child:* 5 mg/kg/d PO.
**ADV EFF** Abd pain, anorexia, CDAD, headache, nausea, neutropenia, rash, red to orange urine
**INTERACTIONS** Clarithromycin, delavirdine, indinavir, nelfinavir, oral contraceptives, ritonavir, saquinavir
**NC/PT** Negative TB test needed before starting tx. Not for use in preg (barrier contraceptives advised)/ breastfeeding. Urine, body fluids may turn red to orange, staining fabric, contact lenses. Pt should report diarrhea, difficulty breathing.

## rifAMPin (Rifadin)
**CLASS** Antibiotic, antituberculotic
**PREG/CONT** Unkn/NA

**IND & DOSE Tx of pulmonary TB.** *Adult:* 10 mg/kg/d PO or IV; max, 600 mg/d in single dose (w/other antituberculotics). *Child:* 10–20 mg/ kg/d PO or IV; max, 600 mg/d. **Tx of *Neisseria meningitidis* carriers to eliminate meningococci from nasopharynx.** *Adult:* 600 mg/d PO or IV for 4 consecutive d or 600 mg q 12 hr for 2 d. *Child >1 mo:* 10 mg/kg PO or IV q 12 hr for 2 d; max, 600 mg/dose. *Child <1 mo:* 5 mg/kg PO or IV q 12 hr for 2 d.
**ADJUST DOSE** Renal impairment
**ADV EFF Acute renal failure, bone marrow suppression,** discolored body fluids, dizziness, drowsiness, epigastric distress, fatigue, flulike sx, headache, heartburn, rash
**INTERACTIONS** Antiarrhythmics, benzodiazepine, buspirone, corticosteroids, cyclosporine, digoxin, doxycycline, fluoroquinolones, hormonal contraceptives, isoniazid, itraconazole, ketoconazole, methadone, metoprolol, nifedipine, oral anticoagulants, oral sulfonylureas, phenytoin, propranolol, quinidine, theophyllines, verapamil, zolpidem
**NC/PT** Monitor renal function, CBC, LFTs periodically. Ensure cultures and appropriate use of drug. Body fluids will turn reddish orange. Pt should take once/d on empty stomach 1 hr before or 2 hr after meals; take safety precautions for CNS effects; not wear soft contact lenses (may become permanently stained); report s&sx of infection, swelling, unusual bleeding/ bruising.

## rifamycin (Aemcolo)
**CLASS** Antibacterial
**PREG/CONT** Low risk/NA

**IND & DOSE Tx of travelers' diarrhea caused by noninvasive strains of *Escherichia coli.*** *Adult:* 388 mg PO bid for 3 d.
**ADV EFF** Constipation, headache, hypersensitivity
**NC/PT** Not recommended for diarrhea complicated by fever and/or bloody stool or due to pathogens other than noninvasive *E. coli.* Discontinue if diarrhea persists >48 hr or

worsens. Pt should take w/ or w/o food; swallow tablets whole w/glass of liquid; avoid alcohol.

## rifapentine (Priftin)

**CLASS** Antibiotic, antituberculotic
**PREG/CONT** Moderate risk/NA

**IND & DOSE** **Tx of active pulmonary TB.** *Adult, child ≥12 yr:* 600 mg PO twice wkly w/interval of at least 72 hr between doses. Continue for 2 mo, then 600 mg/wk PO for 4 mo w/other antituberculotics. **Tx of latent TB w/ isoniazid.** *Adult, child ≥12 yr:* 15 mg/kg/wk PO for 12 wk w/isoniazid; max, 900 mg/dose. *Child 2–11 yr:* >50 kg, 900 mg/wk PO; 32.1–50 kg, 750 mg/wk PO; 25.1–32 kg, 600 mg/wk PO; 14.1–25 kg, 450 mg/wk PO; 10–14 kg, 300 mg/wk PO.
**ADJUST DOSE** Elderly pts
**ADV EFF** Diarrhea, dizziness, headache, hematuria, **hepatotoxicity**, hyperuricemia, **hypersensitivity reactions**, proteinuria, pyuria, reddish body fluids
**INTERACTIONS** Antiarrhythmics, benzodiazepine, buspirone, corticosteroids, cyclosporine, digoxin, doxycycline, fluoroquinolones, hormonal contraceptives, isoniazid, itraconazole, ketoconazole, methadone, metoprolol, nifedipine, oral anticoagulants, oral sulfonylureas, phenytoin, propranolol, protease inhibitors, quinidine, theophyllines, verapamil, zolpidem
**NC/PT** Monitor LFTs. Always give w/ other antituberculotics. Body fluids will turn reddish orange. Not for use in preg (barrier contraceptives advised)/breastfeeding. Pt should mark calendar for tx days; take w/food (may crush tablets and add to semisolid food); not wear contact lenses (may become permanently stained); take safety precautions for CNS effects; report s&sx of infection, swelling, unusual bleeding/bruising, difficulty breathing.

## rifAXIMin (Xifaxan)

**CLASS** Antibiotic, antidiarrheal
**PREG/CONT** High risk/NA

**IND & DOSE** **Tx of traveler's diarrhea.** *Adult, child ≥12 yr:* 200 mg PO tid for 3 d. **To reduce recurrence of hepatic encephalopathy in pts w/ advanced liver disease.** *Adult:* 550 mg PO bid. **Tx of IBS w/diarrhea.** *Adult:* 550 mg PO tid for 14 d; may retreat up to two times w/recurrence.
**ADJUST DOSE** Hepatic impairment
**ADV EFF** CDAD, dizziness, fever, flatulence, headache, **hepatotoxicity**, nausea, **pseudomembranous colitis**, rash
**INTERACTIONS** P-gp inhibitors, warfarin
**NC/PT** Monitor LFTs w/long-term use. Do not use w/diarrhea complicated by fever, blood in stool. Not for use in preg/breastfeeding. Monitor INR closely if pt taking warfarin; dose adjustment may be needed. Pt should swallow tablet whole and not cut/crush/chew it; stop if diarrhea does not resolve or worsens in 48 hr; take safety precautions w/dizziness; report bloody diarrhea, urine/stool color changes, fever.

## rilonacept (Arcalyst)

**CLASS** Anti-inflammatory, interleukin blocker
**PREG/CONT** C/NA

**IND & DOSE** **Tx of cryopyrin-associated periodic syndromes, including familial cold autoinflammatory syndrome, Muckle-Wells syndrome.** *Adult:* Loading dose, 320 mg as two 160-mg (2-mL) subcut injections at different sites; then once-wkly subcut injections of 160 mg (2 mL). *Child 12–17 yr:* Loading dose, 4.4 mg/kg subcut; max, 320 mg. May give in divided doses if needed. Then once-wkly injections of 2.2 mg/kg; max, 160 mg.

**ADV EFF** Injection-site reactions, lipid changes, **serious infections,** URI
**INTERACTIONS** Live vaccines, TNF blockers
**NC/PT** Stop if infection occurs. Use caution in preg/breastfeeding. Teach proper administration/disposal of needles/syringes. Pt should rotate injection sites; report injection-site reactions, s&sx of infection.

## rilpivirine (Edurant)

**CLASS** Antiviral, nonnucleoside reverse transcriptase inhibitor (NNRTI)
**PREG/CONT** Low risk/NA

**IND & DOSE Combined w/other drugs for tx of HIV-1 infection in tx-naïve pts w/HIV-1 RNA of ≤100,000 copies/mL.** *Adult, child >12 yr:* 25 mg/d PO w/food, or 50 mg/d PO w/food if taken w/rifabutin. *Preg pt:* 25 mg/d PO w/food.
**ADV EFF** Body fat redistribution, depression, DRESS, headache, hypersensitivity reactions, immune reconstitution syndrome, insomnia, **prolonged QT,** rash, severe depressive disorder, **suicidality**
**INTERACTIONS** Antacids, CYP3A4 inducers/inhibitors, drugs that decrease stomach acid, other NNRTIs, QT-prolonging drugs, St. John's wort
**NC/PT** Monitor viral load, response carefully. Ensure pt taking other antivirals. Not for use in breastfeeding. Body fat may redistribute to back, breasts, middle of body. Check pt drug list carefully; drug interacts w/ many drugs. Pt should report all drugs, herbs, OTC products used; take once/d w/meal; take precautions to prevent spread (drug not a cure); continue to take other antivirals; report s&sx of infection, depression, thoughts of suicide, rash.

## riluzole (Exservan, Rilutek, Tiglutik)

**CLASS** ALS drug
**PREG/CONT** Unkn/NA

**IND & DOSE Tx of ALS.** *Adult:* 50 mg PO q 12 hr.
**ADV EFF** Abd pain, asthenia, anorexia, circumoral paresthesia, diarrhea, dizziness, **interstitial pneumonitis, liver injury, neutropenia,** somnolence, vertigo
**INTERACTIONS** Allopurinol, methyldopa, sulfasalazine, warfarin
**NC/PT** Monitor CBC, lung function, LFTs carefully. Protect from light. Use caution in preg/breastfeeding. Slows disease progress; not a cure. Pt should take on empty stomach 1 hr before or 2 hr after meal; use safety precautions w/dizziness; report s&sx of infection, difficulty breathing, urine/stool color changes.

## rimabotulinumtoxinB (Myobloc)

**CLASS** Neurotoxin
**PREG/CONT** Unkn/NA

**BBW** Drug not for tx of muscle spasticity; toxin may spread from injection area and cause s&sx of botulism (CNS alterations, trouble speaking and swallowing, loss of bladder control). Use only for approved indications.
**IND & DOSE Tx of cervical dystonia to reduce severity of abnormal head position and neck pain.** *Adult:* 2,500–5,000 units IM injected locally into affected muscles. **Tx chronic sialorrhea.** *Adult:* 1,500–3,500 units injected: 500–1,500 units in parotid gland and 250 units per submandibular gland; no more often than q 12 wk.
**ADV EFF Anaphylactic reactions,** dry mouth, dyspepsia, dysphagia, **spread of toxin that can lead to death**
**INTERACTIONS** Aminoglycosides, anticholinesterases, lincosamides, magnesium sulfate, NMJ blockers, polymyxin, quinidine, succinylcholine

**NC/PT** Store in refrigerator. Have epinephrine on hand in case of anaphylactic reactions. Do not inject in area of skin infection. Effects may not appear for 1–2 d; will persist for 3–4 mo. Not for use in preg/breastfeeding. Pt should report difficulty swallowing, breathing.

## rimantadine hydrochloride (Flumadine)

**CLASS** Antiviral
**PREG/CONT** C/NA

**IND & DOSE** **Px of illness caused by influenza A virus.** *Adult, child >10 yr:* 100 mg/d PO bid. *Child 1–9 yr:* 5 mg/kg/d PO; max, 150 mg/dose. **Tx of illness caused by influenza A virus.** *Adult, child >10 yr:* 100 mg/d PO bid as soon after exposure as possible, continuing for 7 d.
**ADJUST DOSE** Nursing home pts; hepatic/renal impairment
**ADV EFF** Ataxia, dizziness, dyspnea, **HF**, insomnia, light-headedness, mood changes, nausea
**INTERACTIONS** Acetaminophen, aspirin, cimetidine, intranasal influenza virus vaccine
**NC/PT** Pt should take full course of drug; take safety precautions for CNS effects; report swelling, severe mood changes.

## riociguat (Adempas)

**CLASS** Cyclase stimulator, pulmonary HTN drug
**PREG/CONT** High risk/NA

**BBW** Known teratogen. Serious to fatal birth defects; monthly negative preg test required. Available by limited access program for women.
**IND & DOSE** **Tx of thromboembolic pulmonary HTN, idiopathic pulmonary HTN.** *Adult:* 1.5–2.5 mg PO tid.
**ADJUST DOSE** Severe renal/hepatic impairment (not recommended); smokers
**ADJUST DOSE** Anemia, bleeding, constipation, dizziness, dyspepsia, headache, hypotension, n/v/d, **pulmonary edema**
**INTERACTIONS** Antacids; CYP inhibitors; nitrates; P-gp, phosphodiesterase inhibitors (contraindicated)
**NC/PT** Smokers may need higher doses. Monitor BP, respiratory status. Ensure negative preg test. Not for use w/ED drugs, nitrates. Pt should avoid preg (during and for 1 mo after use)/breastfeeding; monitor activity tolerance, respiratory sx; take safety precautions for CNS effects; report worsening of sx, bleeding, severe n/v, difficulty breathing.

▶**NEW DRUG**

## risankizumab-rzaa (Skyrizi)

**CLASS** Immunomodulator, interleukin-23 receptor antagonist
**PREG/CONTROLLED** Unkn/NA

**IND & DOSE** **Tx of moderate to severe plaque psoriasis in pts who are candidates for systemic tx or phototherapy.** *Adult:* 150 mg (two 75-mg injections) subcut at wk 0, 4, then q 12 wk.
**ADV EFF** Fatigue, headache, infections, injection-site reactions, tinea infections, TB
**INTERACTIONS** Live vaccines
**NC/PT** Evaluate for TB before giving drug; give all recommended immunizations. Pt/caregiver should give first self-injected dose under supervision of qualified health care professional and be trained in drug preparation/administration (choice of administration site, proper subcut injection technique/syringe disposal).

## risedronate sodium (Actonel, Atelvia)

**CLASS** Bisphosphonate
**PREG/CONT** Moderate risk/NA

**IND & DOSE** **Tx/px of postmenopausal osteoporosis.** *Adult:* 5 mg/d

PO taken in upright position w/6–8 oz water at least 30 min before or after other beverage, food; may switch to 35-mg tablet PO once/wk, or 75 mg PO on 2 consecutive d each mo (total, 2 tablets/mo), or one 150-mg tablet PO per mo. **Tx/px of glucocorticoid osteoporosis.** *Adult:* 5 mg/d PO. **Tx of Paget disease.** *Adult:* 30 mg/d PO for 2 mo taken in upright position w/6–8 oz water at least 30 min before or after other beverage, food; may retreat after at least 2-mo posttreatment period if indicated. **To increase bone mass in men w/osteoporosis.** *Adult:* 35 mg PO once/wk.

**ADJUST DOSE** Renal impairment

**ADV EFF** Anorexia, arthralgia, atypical femur fractures, diarrhea, dizziness, dyspepsia, **esophageal rupture,** headache, increased bone/muscle/joint pain, **osteonecrosis of jaw**

**INTERACTIONS** Aluminum, aspirin, calcium, magnesium

**NC/PT** Monitor serum calcium level. May increase risk of osteonecrosis of jaw; pts having invasive dental procedures should discuss risk. Not for use w/esophagus abnormalities, hypocalcemia. Not for use in breastfeeding. Not for use for longer than 3–5 yr. Give w/full glass of plain (not mineral) water at least 30 min before or after other beverage, food, medication. Have pt remain in upright position for at least 30 min to decrease GI effects. Pt should swallow DR tablet whole and not cut/crush/chew it; mark calendar if taking wkly; take supplemental calcium, vitamin D; report muscle twitching, difficulty swallowing, edema.

## risperiDONE (Perseris, Risperdal, Risperdal Consta)

**CLASS** Antipsychotic, benzisoxazole

**PREG/CONT** High risk/NA

**BBW** Not for use in elderly pts w/dementia; increased risk of CV mortality. Not approved for this use.

**IND & DOSE Tx of schizophrenia.** *Adult:* 1 mg PO bid or 2 mg PO once daily; target, 3 mg PO bid by third day. Range, 4–8 mg/d or 25 mg IM q 2 wk. Max, 50 mg IM q 2 wk. Delaying relapse time in long-term tx: 2–8 mg/d PO or 90–120 mg subcut/mo (*Perseris*). *Child 13–17 yr:* 0.5 mg/d PO; target, 3 mg/d. **Tx of bipolar I disorder.** *Adult:* 25–50 mg IM q 2 wk. **Tx of bipolar mania.** *Adult:* 2–3 mg/d PO; range, 1–6 mg/d. *Child 10–17 yr:* 0.5 mg/d PO; target, 2.5 mg/d. **Irritability associated w/autistic disorder.** *Child 5–17 yr:* 0.5 mg/d (20 kg or more), 0.25 mg/d PO (<20 kg). After at least 4 d, may increase to 1 mg/d (20 kg or more), 0.5 mg/d (<20 kg). Maintain dose for at least 14 d; then may increase in increments of 0.5 mg/d (20 kg or more), 0.25 mg/d (<20 kg) at 2-wk intervals.

**ADJUST DOSE** Elderly pts; hepatic/renal impairment

**ADV EFF** Agitation, **arrhythmias,** anxiety, aggression, bone marrow depression, cognitive/motor impairment, constipation, CV events, diabetes, dizziness, drowsiness, headache, hyperglycemia, hyperprolactinemia, insomnia, n/v, **NMS,** orthostatic hypotension, photosensitivity, **seizures,** tardive dyskinesia

**INTERACTIONS** Alcohol, carbamazepine, clonidine, levodopa

**NC/PT** If restarting tx, follow initial dose guidelines, using extreme care due to increased risk of severe adverse effects w/reexposure. Stop other antipsychotics before starting risperidone. Not for use in preg/breastfeeding. Pt should open blister units of orally disintegrating tablets individually (not push tablet through foil); use dry hands to remove tablet, immediately place on tongue but do not chew; mix oral sol in 3–4 oz water, coffee, orange juice, low-fat milk (not cola, tea); take safety precautions for CNS effects; avoid sun exposure; report s&sx of infection, palpitations, increased thirst/urination, chest pain. Name confusion between *Risperdal* (risperidone) and *Requip* (ropinirole).

**ritonavir** (Norvir)
**CLASS** Antiviral, protease inhibitor
**PREG/CONT** B/NA

**BBW** Potentially large increase in serum conc, risk of serious arrhythmias, seizures, fatal reactions w/alfuzosin, amiodarone, astemizole, bepridil, bupropion, clozapine, ergotamine, flecainide, meperidine, pimozide, piroxicam, propafenone, quinidine, rifabutin, terfenadine, voriconazole. Potentially large increase in serum conc of these sedatives/hypnotics: Alprazolam, clonazepam, diazepam, estazolam, flurazepam, midazolam, triazolam, zolpidem; extreme sedation, respiratory depression possible. Do not give ritonavir w/ any drugs listed above.
**IND & DOSE** **Tx of HIV infection, w/ other antiretrovirals.** *Adult:* 600 mg PO bid w/food. *Child:* 250 mg/m² PO bid. Increase by 50 mg/m² bid at 2- to 3-day intervals to max 400 mg/m² PO bid. Max, 600 mg bid.
**ADV EFF** Abd pain, anorexia, anxiety, asthenia, body fat redistribution, dizziness, dysuria, **hypersensitivity reactions,** n/v/d, pancreatitis, peripheral/circumoral paresthesia, prolonged PR
**INTERACTIONS** Grapefruit juice, QT-prolonging drugs, St. John's wort. See also *Black Box Warning* above.
**NC/PT** Carefully screen drug hx for potentially serious drug-drug interactions. Ensure use of other antivirals. Monitor LFTs, amylase, ECG. Not for use in breastfeeding. Pt should store capsules/oral sol in refrigerator; take w/food; avoid grapefruit juice, St. John's wort; use precautions to avoid spread (drug not a cure); report severe diarrhea, changes in drugs being taken, s&sx of infection, difficulty breathing. Name confusion between *Retrovir* (zidovudine) and ritonavir.

**DANGEROUS DRUG**

**riTUXimab** (Rituxan), **riTUXimab-abbs** (Truxima), **riTUXimab-pvvr** (Ruxience)
**CLASS** Antineoplastic, monoclonal antibody
**PREG/CONT** High risk/NA

**BBW** Fatal infusion reactions, severe cutaneous reactions, TLS possible. Risk of reactivation of HBV at drug initiation; screen for HBV before use.
**IND & DOSE** **Tx of non-Hodgkin lymphoma.** *Adult:* 375 mg/m² IV once wkly for four or eight doses. **To reduce s&sx of RA.** *Adult:* Two 1,000-mg IV infusions separated by 2 wk, w/methotrexate; after first two doses may not repeat sooner than q 16 wk. **Tx of chronic lymphocytic leukemia.** *Adult:* 375 mg/m² IV day before fludarabine/cyclophosphamide; then 500 mg/m² on day 1 of cycles 2–6 (q 28 d). **Tx of Wegener granulomatosis, microscopic polyangiitis.** *Adult, child ≥2 yr:* 375 mg/m² IV once wkly for 4 wk, w/glucocorticoids. **Tx of pemphigus vulgaris.** *Adult:* Two 1,000-mg IV infusions w/ glucocorticoids q 2 wk, then 500 mg IV at mo 12, then q 6 mo.
**ADV EFF** **Bowel obstruction,** bronchitis, cardiac arrhythmias, **HBV reactivation, infections,** infusion reactions, **PML, TLS,** URI
**INTERACTIONS** Live vaccines
**NC/PT** Premedicate w/acetaminophen, diphenhydramine to decrease fever, chills associated w/infusion. Protect from infection exposure. Monitor for HBV reactivation; stop if viral hepatitis occurs. Use caution in preg/breastfeeding. Pt should mark calendar of tx days; report severe abd pain, headache, s&sx of infection, urine/stool color changes.

## rivaroxaban (Xarelto)

**CLASS** Anticoagulant, factor Xa inhibitor

**PREG/CONT** C/NA

**BBW** Risk of epidural, spinal hematomas w/related neuro impairment, possible paralysis if used in pts receiving neuraxial anesthesia or undergoing spinal puncture. Carefully consider benefits/risks of neuraxial intervention in pts who are or will be anticoagulated. If rivaroxaban used, monitor frequently for neuro impairment; be prepared for rapid tx if necessary. Stopping drug increases risk of thromboembolic events; if stopped for any reason other than pathological bleeding, start another anticoagulant.

**IND & DOSE Px of DVT, which may lead to PE in pts undergoing knee/hip replacement.** *Adult:* 10 mg/d PO. Start within 6–10 hr of surgery; continue for 12 d after knee replacement, 35 d after hip replacement, continuously for atrial fibrillation (AF). **To reduce risk of stroke in pts w/nonvalvular AF; to reduce risk of recurrent DVT, PE.** *Adult: CrCl >50 mL/min:* 20 mg/d PO w/evening meal; *CrCl ≤50 mL/min:* 15 mg/d PO w/evening meal. **Tx of DVT, which may lead to PE in pts w/knee/hip replacement surgery.** *Adult:* Initially, 15 mg PO bid w/food for 21 d, then 20 mg/d PO for long-term tx. **To reduce risk of DVT and/or PE recurrence after 6 mo of anticoagulation.** *Adult:* 10 mg/d PO w/ or w/o food. **Px of venous thromboembolism in pts acutely ill and not at high risk for bleeding.** *Adult:* 10 mg/d PO w/ or w/o food for 31–39 d (including hospital stay and post discharge). **Px of CV events in pts w/CAD or peripheral artery disease.** *Adult:* 2.5 mg PO bid w/ or w/o food and w/aspirin daily.

**ADJUST DOSE** Renal/hepatic impairment

**ADV EFF Bleeding,** dysuria, elevated liver enzymes, **hemorrhage,** rash, rebound thrombotic events

**INTERACTIONS** Anticoagulants, aspirin, carbamazepine, clarithromycin, clopidogrel, erythromycin, ketoconazole, NSAIDs, phenytoin, platelet inhibitors, rifampin, ritonavir, St. John's wort, warfarin

**NC/PT** Not for use w/prosthetic heart valves or w/triple positive antiphospholipid syndrome. Monitor for bleeding. Do not stop abruptly (increased risk of thrombotic events). Taper when stopping; consider use of another anticoagulant. Not for use in preg (contraceptives advised)/breastfeeding. Pt should report all prescribed/OTC drugs, herbs being taken; take precautions to prevent injury; ensure no lapse in taking drug; report stool color changes, unusual bleeding, dizziness, chest pain.

## rivastigmine tartrate (Exelon)

**CLASS** Alzheimer disease drug, cholinesterase inhibitor

**PREG/CONT** Unkn/NA

**IND & DOSE Tx of moderate dementia of Alzheimer type.** *Adult:* 1.5 mg PO bid w/food. Range, 6–12 mg/d; max, 12 mg/d. Transdermal patch: One 4.6-mg/24 hr patch once/d; after ≥4 wk, may increase to one 9.5-mg/24 hr patch. **Tx of moderate Parkinson dementia.** *Adult:* Initially, 1.5 mg PO bid; titrate to effective range (3–12 mg/d PO bid in divided doses). Transdermal patch: one 4.6-mg/24 hr patch once/d; after ≥4 wk, may increase to one 9.5-mg/24 hr patch.

**ADV EFF** Abd pain, allergic dermatitis w/topical, anorexia, ataxia, bradycardia, confusion, fatigue, insomnia, n/v/d

**INTERACTIONS** Anticholinergics, beta blockers, metoclopramide, NSAIDs, other cholinesterase inhibitors, theophylline

**NC/PT** Establish baseline function before tx. Pt should take w/food; mix sol w/water, fruit juice, soda to improve compliance; apply patch to clean, dry skin (remove old patch before applying new one), rotate sites; take safety precautions for CNS effects; report severe GI effects, changes in neuro function, rash.

**rizatriptan** (Maxalt)
**CLASS** Antimigraine, serotonin selective agonist
**PREG/CONT** Unkn/NA

**IND & DOSE Tx of acute migraine attacks.** *Adult, child 6–17 yr:* 5 (<40 kg) or 10 mg (≥40 kg) PO at onset of headache; may repeat in 2 hr if needed. Max, 30 mg/d.
**ADJUST DOSE** Hepatic/renal impairment
**ADV EFF** Chest pain, dizziness, jaw pain, paresthesia, serotonin syndrome, somnolence, throat pressure, vertigo, weakness
**INTERACTIONS** Ergots, MAOIs, propranolol
**NC/PT** Do not give within 14 d of MAOIs. For acute attack only, not px or for cluster headaches. Monitor BP in pts w/known CAD. Not for use in preg/breastfeeding. Pt should place orally disintegrating tablet on tongue, then swallow; take safety measures for CNS effects; continue normal migraine relief measures; report chest pain, numbness/tingling.

**roflumilast** (Daliresp)
**CLASS** Phosphodiesterase-4 inhibitor
**PREG/CONT** High risk/NA

**IND & DOSE To reduce exacerbation risk in severe COPD.** *Adult:* Maint dose, 500 mcg/d PO w/ or w/o food. Starting at 250 mcg/d for 4 wk, then increasing to 500 mcg/d may decrease rate of tx discontinuation.
**ADJUST DOSE** Hepatic impairment
**ADV EFF** Bronchospasm, depression, diarrhea, dizziness, headache, insomnia, **suicidality,** weight loss
**INTERACTIONS** Carbamazepine, cimetidine, erythromycin, ethinyl estradiol, fluvoxamine, ketoconazole, phenobarbital, phenytoin, rifampin
**NC/PT** Not for acute bronchospasm. Monitor weight; if significant weight loss, stop drug. Not for use in preg (contraceptives advised)/breastfeeding. Pt should continue other COPD tx; report all drugs being taken, weight loss, thoughts of suicide, difficulty breathing.

**rolapitant** (Varubi)
**CLASS** Antiemetic, substance P/neurokinin 1 antagonist
**PREG/CONT** Low risk/NA

**IND & DOSE Combo px of delayed n/v associated w/emetogenic chemo.** *Adult:* 180 mg PO 1–2 hr before start of chemo, w/dexamethasone and 5-$HT_3$ receptor antagonist.
**ADV EFF** Anorexia, dizziness, hiccups, neutropenia
**INTERACTIONS** Pimozide, thioridazine (avoid use); CYP2D6 substrates, CYP3A4 inducers, digoxin, irinotecan, methotrexate, topotecan
**NC/PT** Premedicate w/dexamethasone and any 5-$HT_3$ receptor antagonist. Monitor drug regimen; many interactions possible. Monitor for infection. Pt should take safety precautions w/dizziness; avoid infection; report fever, syncope.

**romidepsin** (Istodax)
**CLASS** Antineoplastic, histone deacetylase inhibitor
**PREG/CONT** High risk/NA

**IND & DOSE Tx of pts w/cutaneous, peripheral T-cell lymphoma who have received at least one prior systemic tx.** *Adult:* 14 mg/$m^2$ IV over 4 hr on days 1, 8, 15 of 28-d cycle. Repeat q 28 d.
**ADJUST DOSE** Hepatic, severe renal impairment

**ADV EFF** Anemia, anorexia, **bone marrow suppression,** fatigue, **infections,** n/v/d, **prolonged QT, TLS**
**INTERACTIONS** CYP3A4 inducers/inhibitors, QT-prolonging drugs, warfarin
**NC/PT** Monitor CBC, LFTs, renal function. Obtain baseline, periodic ECG. Not for use in preg (contraceptives advised)/breastfeeding. Pt should mark calendar of tx days; avoid exposure to infection; report s&sx of infection, unusual bleeding/bruising.

## romiplostim (Nplate)

**CLASS** Thrombopoietin receptor agonist
**PREG/CONT** Moderate risk/NA

**IND & DOSE** **Tx of thrombocytopenia in pts w/chronic immune thrombocytopenic purpura if poor response to corticosteroids, immunoglobulins, or splenectomy.** *Adult, child ≥1 yr:* 1 mcg/kg/wk subcut; adjust in increments of 1 mcg/kg to achieve platelet count of $50 \times 10^9$. Max, 10 mcg/kg/wk. Not indicated for other types of thrombocytopenia.
**ADJUST DOSE** Hepatic, severe renal impairment
**ADV EFF** Abd pain, arthralgia, dizziness, dyspepsia, headache, insomnia, myalgia, pain, paresthesia, **progression to acute myelogenous leukemia, severe thrombocytopenia, thrombotic events**
**NC/PT** Pt must be enrolled in *Nplate NEXUS* program; drug must be given by health care provider enrolled in program who will do blood test for platelet count before injection. Monitor platelet count; dosage adjustment may be needed. Not for use in preg/breastfeeding. Not for home administration. Pt should take safety precautions w/dizziness; report difficulty breathing, numbness/tingling, leg pain.

**▶NEW DRUG**

## romosozumab-aqqg (Evenity)

**CLASS** Antiosteoporotic, sclerostin inhibitor
**PREG/CONT** Not indicated for women of reproductive potential/NA

**BBW** Risk of MI, stroke, CV death. Do not start if CV event in past yr; discontinue if CV event during tx.
**IND & DOSE** **Tx of osteoporosis in postmenopausal women at high risk for fracture or if intolerant to or have failed other osteoporosis tx.** *Adult:* 210 mg subcut once q mo for 12 mo.
**ADV EFF** Arthralgia, **atypical femoral fracture, CV events,** headache, **hypersensitivity, hypocalcemia, osteonecrosis of jaw**
**NC/PT** Limit duration to 12 monthly doses. If osteoporosis tx still warranted, consider continued tx w/antiresorptive. Pt should take calcium/vitamin D supplements daily to reduce hypocalcemia risk.

## rOPINIRole hydrochloride (Requip)

**CLASS** Antiparkinsonian, dopamine receptor agonist
**PREG/CONT** C/NA

**IND & DOSE** **Tx of idiopathic Parkinson disease.** *Adult:* 0.25 mg PO tid (1st wk); 0.5 mg PO tid (2nd wk); 0.75 mg PO tid (3rd wk); 1 mg PO tid (4th wk). May increase by 1.5 mg/d at 1-wk intervals to 9 mg/d, then by up to 3 mg/d at 1-wk intervals to max 24 mg/d. ER tablets: 2 mg/d PO. After 1–2 wk, may increase by 2 mg/d. Titrate w/wkly increases of 2 mg/d to max 24 mg/d. If used w/levodopa, decrease levodopa gradually; average reduction, 31% w/immediate-release ropinirole, 34% w/ER form. **Tx of restless legs syndrome.** *Adult:* 0.25 mg/d PO 1–3 hr before bed. After 2 d, increase to 0.5 mg/d PO; after 1 wk, to

1 mg/d PO. wk 3, increase to 1.5 mg/d; wk 4, 2 mg/d; wk 5, 2.5 mg/d; wk 6, 3 mg/d; wk 7, 4 mg/d PO.
**ADJUST DOSE** Elderly pts
**ADV EFF** Constipation, dizziness, hallucinations, hyperkinesia, hypokinesia, insomnia, nausea, orthostatic hypotension, psychotic behavior, somnolence, sudden onset of sleep, syncope, vision changes
**INTERACTIONS** Alcohol, ciprofloxacin, estrogens, levodopa, warfarin
**NC/PT** Withdraw gradually over 1 wk if stopping. Monitor orthostatic BP. Pt should swallow ER tablet whole and not cut/crush/chew it; take w/food; use safety precautions for CNS effects; change position slowly; report black tarry stools, hallucinations, falling asleep during daily activities. Name confusion between *Requip* (ropinirole) and *Risperdal* (risperidone).

## rosiglitazone (Avandia)
**CLASS** Antidiabetic, thiazolidinedione
**PREG/CONT** Unkn/NA

**BBW** Increased risk of HF, MI. Do not use in pts w/known heart disease, symptomatic HF; monitor accordingly.
**IND & DOSE As adjunct to diet/exercise to improve glycemic control in pts w/type 2 diabetes.** *Adult:* 4 mg PO daily; max, 8 mg/d.
**ADJUST DOSE** Hepatic impairment
**ADV EFF** Anemia, bone fractures, **CV events,** fluid retention, headache, **HF,** hypoglycemia, macular edema, **MI,** UTI, weight gain
**INTERACTIONS** CYP2C8 inducers/inhibitors, insulin
**NC/PT** Not for use w/established HF or in type 1 diabetes/ketoacidosis. Not for use in preg/breastfeeding. Monitor weight; check for s&sx of HF. Ensure full diabetic teaching. Pt should continue diet/exercise program; report weight gain of ≥3 lb/d, chest pain, swelling.

## rosuvastatin calcium
(Crestor, Ezallor)
**CLASS** Antihyperlipidemic, statin
**PREG/CONT** High risk/NA

**IND & DOSE Tx of hypercholesterolemia, mixed dyslipidemia, primary dysbetalipoproteinemia, hypertriglyceridemia; primary px of CAD; atherosclerosis.** *Adult:* 5–40 mg/d PO; 10 mg/d PO if combined w/other lipid-lowering drugs; 5 mg/d PO if combined w/cyclosporine. **Tx of heterozygous familial hypercholesterolemia.** *Child 10–17 yr:* 5–20 mg/d PO. *Child 8–<10 yr (girls must be at least 1 yr postmenarchal):* 5–10 mg/d PO. **Tx of homozygous familial hypercholesterolemia.** *Adult:* 20 mg/d PO. *Child 7–17 yr:* 20 mg/d PO.
**ADJUST DOSE** Asian pts, renal impairment
**ADV EFF** Diarrhea, dizziness, flulike sx, headache, ILD, **liver failure, myopathy,** nausea, pharyngitis, **rhabdomyolysis,** rhinitis
**INTERACTIONS** Antacids, cyclosporine, gemfibrozil, lopinavir/ritonavir, warfarin
**NC/PT** Risk of increased adverse effects in Asian pts; initiate tx w/5 mg/d PO and adjust based on lipid levels, adverse effects. Obtain baseline lipid profile. Not for use in preg (barrier contraceptives advised)/breastfeeding. Pt should take at bedtime; have regular blood tests; continue diet/exercise program; take antacids at least 2 hr after rosuvastatin; report muscle pain w/fever, unusual bleeding/bruising.

## rotigotine (Neupro)
**CLASS** Antiparkinsonian, dopamine agonist
**PREG/CONT** Moderate risk/NA

**IND & DOSE Tx of s&sx of Parkinson disease.** *Adult:* 2 mg/24 hr transdermal patch; range, 2–8 mg/24 hr patch. **Tx of moderate to severe restless**

**legs syndrome.** *Adult:* 1 mg/24 hr transdermal patch; max, 3 mg/24 hr transdermal patch.
**ADV EFF** Anorexia, application-site reactions, dizziness, dyskinesia, edema, hallucinations, headache, hyperpyrexia, hypotension, insomnia, **melanoma,** n/v, orthostatic hypotension, **severe allergic reaction**
**INTERACTIONS** Antipsychotics, dopamine antagonists, metoclopramide
**NC/PT** Apply to clean, dry skin; press firmly for 30 sec. Rotate application sites; remove old patch before applying new one. Taper after long-term use. Remove patch before MRI. Not for use in preg; use caution in breastfeeding. Pt should not open patch until ready to apply; remove old patch before applying new one; rotate application sites; not stop use suddenly; take safety precautions for CNS effects; report application-site reactions, skin reactions, difficulty breathing, fever, changes in behavior, dizziness.

## rucaparib (Rubraca)

**CLASS** ADP-ribose polymerase inhibitor, antineoplastic
**PREG/CONT** High risk/NA

**IND & DOSE** **Tx of deletions BRC4 mutation–associated advanced ovarian, fallopian tube, or primary peritoneal cancer after ≥two chemos; tx of recurrent epithelial ovarian, fallopian tube, or primary peritoneal cancer in pts who have been treated w/platinum-based chemo.** *Adult:* 600 mg PO bid. Continue until progression or unacceptable toxicity.
**ADV EFF** Abd pain, **acute myeloid leukemia,** anorexia, fatigue, **myelodysplastic syndrome,** n/v/d, photosensitivity, thrombocytopenia
**NC/PT** Ensure proper dx. Ensure pt is not preg; contraceptive use recommended during and for 6 mo after tx (fetal toxicity can occur). Not for use in breastfeeding. Take w/o regard to food, approx q 12 hr. Pt should avoid sun exposure; report extreme fatigue/weakness, abnormal bruising/bleeding, severe n/v.

## rufinamide (Banzel)

**CLASS** Antiepileptic, sodium channel blocker
**PREG/CONT** Unkn/NA

**IND & DOSE** **Adjunct tx of seizures associated w/Lennox-Gastaut syndrome.** *Adult:* 400–800 mg/d PO in two equally divided doses; target, 3,200 mg/d PO in two equally divided doses. *Child ≥1 yr:* 10 mg/kg/d PO in two equally divided doses; target, 45 mg/kg/d or 3,200 mg/d.
**ADJUST DOSE** Hepatic/renal impairment
**ADV EFF** Ataxia, coordination disturbances, dizziness, fatigue, headache, nausea, **seizures, severe hypersensitivity reactions,** somnolence, **suicidality**
**INTERACTIONS** CYP450 inducers, hormonal contraceptives, valproate
**NC/PT** Withdraw gradually; do not stop abruptly. Stable for 90 d. Women taking drug during preg should enroll in North American Antiepileptic Drug Preg Registry. Pt should take w/food; swallow tablet whole and not cut/crush/chew it; store suspension upright; measure using medical measuring device; take safety precautions for CNS effects; report difficulty breathing, rash, thoughts of suicide, mood changes.

## ruxolitinib (Jakafi)

**CLASS** Kinase inhibitor
**PREG/CONT** High risk/NA

**IND & DOSE** **Tx of intermediate, high-risk myelofibrosis.** *Adult:* 5–20 mg PO bid. Dosage based on platelet count. **Tx of polycythemia vera after inadequate response to hydroxyurea.** *Adult:* 10 mg PO bid. **Tx of steroid-refractory acute GVHD.** *Adult, child ≥12 yr:* 5 mg PO daily.
**ADJUST DOSE** Hepatic/renal impairment

**ADV EFF** Anemia, **bone marrow suppression,** bruising, dizziness, headache, **serious infections,** skin cancer, thrombocytopenia
**INTERACTIONS** CYP450 inhibitors, fluconazole
**NC/PT** Monitor CBC q 2–4 wk. Stop drug after 6 mo if no spleen reduction or sx improvement. Not for use in preg/breastfeeding. Monitor for infection. Pt should take safety precautions w/dizziness; report s&sx of infection, unusual bleeding.

## sacrosidase (Sucraid)

**CLASS** Enzyme
**PREG/CONT** C/NA

**IND & DOSE Oral replacement of genetically determined sucrase deficiency.** *Adult, child >15 kg:* 2 mL PO or 44 drops/meal or snack PO. *Adult, child ≤15 kg:* 1 mL or 22 drops/meal or snack PO.
**ADV EFF** Abd pain, constipation, dehydration, headache
**NC/PT** Do not use in known allergy to yeast. Must dilute w/60–120 mL water, milk, infant formula before giving. Do not dilute/consume w/fruit juice. Refrigerate bottle; discard 4 wk after opening. Give cold or at room temp. Pt should report difficulty breathing, swelling of tongue/face.

## safinamide (Xadago)

**CLASS** Antiparkinsonian, MAO type B inhibitor
**PREG/CONT** High risk/NA

**IND & DOSE Adjunct tx to levodopa/carbidopa in pts w/Parkinson disease having "off" episodes.** *Adult:* 50 mg/d PO; may increase to 100 mg after 2 wk.
**ADJUST DOSE** Hepatic impairment
**ADV EFF** Dyskinesia, falling asleep during ADLs, hallucinations, impulse control issues, serotonin syndrome
**INTERACTIONS** Dextromethorphan, MAOIs, opioids, SSRIs, serotonergic drugs, sympathomimetics, tyramine
**NC/PT** Monitor for HTN, serotonin syndrome, psychotic behaviors; withdrawal s&sx possible when discontinuing, w/high fever/confusion. Pt should report other drugs being used (many reactions possible); continue levodopa/carbidopa; avoid preg (contraceptives advised)/breastfeeding; take safety precautions w/CNS effects; report changes in behavior, unintentional muscle movements, falling asleep during ADLs.

## saliva substitute (Entertainer's Secret, Moi-Stir, MouthKote, Salivart)

**CLASS** Saliva substitute
**PREG/CONT** Unkn/NA

**IND & DOSE Mgt of dry mouth, throat in xerostomia, hyposalivation.** *Adult:* Spray for ½ second or apply to oral mucosa.
**ADV EFF** Excessive electrolyte absorption
**NC/PT** Monitor pt while eating; swallowing may be impaired and additional tx needed. Pt should swish around in mouth after application; report difficulty swallowing, headache, leg cramps.

## salmeterol xinafoate (Serevent Diskus)

**CLASS** Antiasthmatic, long-acting beta selective agonist
**PREG/CONT** High risk/NA

**BBW** Ensure drug not used for acute asthma or w/worsening/deteriorating asthma; risk of death. Increased risk of asthma-related hospitalization when used in child, adolescent. When long-acting sympathomimetic, inhaled corticosteroid needed, fixed-dose comb strongly recommended. Do not use for asthma unless combined w/long-term asthma-control medication; risk of death. Use only as additional tx in pts not controlled by other medications.

**IND & DOSE Maint tx for asthma, bronchospasm.** *Adult, child ≥4 yr:* 1 inhalation (50 mcg) bid at 12-hr intervals w/ inhaled corticosteroid. **Px of exercise-induced asthma.** *Adult, child ≥4 yr:* 1 inhalation 30 min or more before exertion. **Long-term maint of bronchospasm w/COPD.** *Adult:* 1 inhalation (50 mcg) bid at 12-hr intervals.
**ADV EFF Asthma-related deaths** (risk higher in black pts), **bronchospasm, cough,** headache, pain, palpitations, tachycardia, tremors
**INTERACTIONS** Beta blockers, diuretics, hypersensitivity if severe milk allergy, MAOIs, protease inhibitors, strong P450 3A4 inhibitors (contraindicated), TCAs
**NC/PT** Arrange for periodic evaluation of respiratory condition. Not for tx of acute asthma attack. Must be used w/an inhaled corticosteroid. Review proper use of *Diskus*. Pt should never take drug alone for tx of asthma; take safety precautions w/tremors; report irregular heartbeat, difficulty breathing, worsening of asthma.

## salsalate (generic)

**CLASS** Analgesic, NSAID, salicylate
**PREG/CONT** High risk/NA

**BBW** Increased risk of GI bleeding, CV events; monitor accordingly.
**IND & DOSE Relief of pain, sx of inflammatory conditions.** *Adult:* 3,000 mg/d PO in divided doses.
**ADV EFF Acute salicylate toxicity, anaphylactoid reactions to anaphylactic shock, bone marrow suppression, bronchospasm,** constipation, **CV collapse,** dizziness, dyspepsia, GI pain, insomnia, **renal/respiratory failure**
**INTERACTIONS** Alcohol, antacids, carbonic anhydrase inhibitors, corticosteroids, insulin, probenecid, spironolactone, sulfonylureas, urine alkalinizers, valproic acid
**NC/PT** Do not give to pt w/chickenpox. Use caution in preg/breastfeeding. Pt should take w/full glass of water (w/food if GI upset); continue other measures for relief of pain/inflammation; report rapid, difficult breathing, ringing in ears.

## sapropterin dihydrochloride (Kuvan)

**CLASS** Coenzyme factor, phenylalanine reducer
**PREG/CONT** Moderate risk/NA

**IND & DOSE W/diet to reduce blood phenylalanine level in hyperphenylalaninemia caused by tetrahydrobiopterin-responsive phenylketonuria.** *Pt ≥7 yr:* 10–20 mg/kg/d based on blood phenylalanine level. *Pt 1 mo–6 yr:* 10 mg/kg/d PO.
**ADV EFF** Abd pain, **GI mucosal inflammation,** headache, hyperactivity, **hypersensitivity,** hypophenylalaninemia, n/v/d, pharyngolaryngeal pain
**NC/PT** Do not use w/levodopa, ED drugs, drugs that inhibit folate metabolism. Must use w/phenylalanine dietary restrictions. Protect from moisture; do not use if outdated. Monitor phenylalanine level; adjust dose as needed. Pt should swallow tablets whole or dissolve in water/apple juice and drink within 15 min; report severe headache, anorexia, fever.

## saquinavir mesylate (Invirase)

**CLASS** Antiviral, protease inhibitor
**PREG/CONT** Unkn/NA

**IND & DOSE Tx of HIV infection, w/ritonavir and other antivirals.** *Adult, child >16 yr:* 1,000 mg PO bid w/ritonavir 100 mg bid given together within 2 hr after meal, or if tx-naïve, first 7 d 500 mg bid w/ritonavir 100 mg bid together within 2 hr after meal.
**ADJUST DOSE** Hepatic impairment
**ADV EFF Anaphylaxis,** asthenia, diabetes mellitus, diarrhea, dizziness, dyslipidemia, dyspepsia, fatigue, fat

redistribution, GI pain, headache, hemophilia, **hypersensitivity,** n/v, pneumonia, **prolonged PR/QT**
**INTERACTIONS** Antiarrhythmics, carbamazepine, clarithromycin, delavirdine, dexamethasone, ergots, grapefruit juice, indinavir, ketoconazole, midazolam, nelfinavir, nevirapine, phenobarbital, phenytoin, QT-prolonging drugs, rifabutin, rifampin, ritonavir, sildenafil, statins, triazolam, St. John's wort
**NC/PT** Store at room temp; use by expiration date. Carefully evaluate drug hx; many potentially DANGEROUS DRUG interactions. Drug contains lactose monohydrate. Give within 2 hr after full meal, always w/ritonavir. Monitor for opportunistic infections. Health care provider should register preg pt in Antiretroviral Preg Registry. Not for use in breastfeeding. Pt should take precautions to prevent spread (drug not a cure); avoid grapefruit juice, St. John's wort; take safety precautions w/dizziness; report severe headache, urine/stool color changes. Name confusion between saquinavir and *Sinequan*.

## sarecycline (Seysara)
**CLASS** Antibiotic, tetracycline
**PREG/CONT** High risk/NA

**IND & DOSE** **Tx of inflammatory lesions of nonnodular moderate to severe acne vulgaris in pts ≥9 yr.** *85–136 kg:* 150 mg PO/d; *55–84 kg:* 100 mg PO/d; *33–54 kg:* 60 mg PO/d.
**ADV EFF** Bone growth inhibition, CDAD, intercranial HTN, **light-headedness/dizziness/vertigo, nausea, photosensitivity,** teeth discoloration/enamel hypoplasia
**INTERACTIONS** Antacids/iron preparations (impair absorption); anticoagulants (decrease anticoagulant dosage as appropriate); penicillin/oral retinoids (avoid coadministration); P-glycoprotein substrates
**NC/PT** Not recommended for child <9 yr or preg pt. Pt should not ingest food 4 hr before and 2 hr after taking drug; avoid dairy products/antacids/multivitamins for 4 hr after taking drug; seek medical attention for watery/bloody stools, headache, blurred vision; avoid UV light (increased burn risk).

## sargramostim (Leukine)
**CLASS** Colony-stimulating factor
**PREG/CONT** High risk/NA

**IND & DOSE** **Myeloid reconstitution after autologous, allogenic bone marrow transplantation.** *Adult:* 250 mcg/m$^2$/d for 21 d as 2-hr IV infusion starting 2–4 hr after autologous bone marrow infusion and not less than 24 hr after last dose of chemo, radiation. Do not give until postmarrow infusion ANC <500 cells/mm$^3$. Continue until ANC greater than 1,500 cells/mm$^3$ for 3 consecutive d. **Bone marrow transplantation failure, engraftment delay.** *Adult:* 250 mcg/m$^2$/d for 14 d as 2-hr IV infusion; may repeat after 7 d off tx if no engraftment. If still no engraftment, may give third dose of 500 mcg/m$^2$/d for 14 d after another 7 d off tx. **Neutrophil recovery after chemo in AML.** *Adult:* 250 mcg/m$^2$/d IV over 4 hr starting about day 11 or 4 d after chemo induction. **Mobilization of peripheral blood progenitor cells (PBPCs).** *Adult:* 250 mcg/m$^2$/d IV over 24 hr or subcut once daily; continue throughout harvesting. **Post-PBPC transplant.** *Adult:* 250 mcg/m$^2$/d IV over 24 hr or subcut once daily starting immediately after PBPC infusion; continue until ANC greater than 1,500 cells/mm$^3$ for 3 consecutive d. **Tx of delayed neutrophil recovery or graft failure after bone marrow transplant.** *Adult, child ≥2 yr:* 250 mcg/m$^2$/d for 14 d as 2-hr IV infusion. **Tx after myelosuppressive radiation.** *Adult, child >40 kg:* 7 mcg/kg subcut daily. *Child 15–40 kg:* 10 mcg/kg subcut daily. *Child <15 kg:* 12 mcg/kg subcut daily.

**ADV EFF** Alopecia, bone pain, diarrhea, effusions, fever, **hemorrhage, hypersensitivity,** n/v/d, supraventricular arrhythmias
**INTERACTIONS** Corticosteroids, lithium
**NC/PT** Give no less than 24 hr after cytotoxic chemo and within 2–4 hr of bone marrow infusion. Store in refrigerator; do not freeze/shake. Not for use in preg (barrier contraceptives advised). Use powder within 6 hr of mixing. If using powder, use each vial for one dose; do not reenter vial. Discard unused drug. Infuse over 2 hr. Do not use in-line membrane filter or mix w/other drugs or in other diluent. Monitor CBC, body weight, hydration status. Pt should cover head at temp extremes (hair loss possible); avoid exposure to infection; report fever, s&sx of infection, difficulty breathing, bleeding.

## sarilumab (Kevzara)

**CLASS** Antirheumatic, interleukin antagonist
**PREG/CONT** High risk/NA

**BBW** Risk of serious to fatal infections; if infection occurs, stop drug until controlled. TB has been reported; closely monitor for s&sx of infection.
**IND & DOSE Tx of adults w/ moderately to severely active RA after inadequate response to DMARDs.** *Adult:* 200 mg subcut q 2 wk; may combine w/other DMARDs.
**ADJUST DOSE** Neutropenia
**ADV EFF Bone marrow suppression, GI perforation,** injection-site rash, hypersensitivity reactions, hepatic impairment, **serious infections**
**INTERACTIONS** Vaccines; avoid combo
**NC/PT** Continuously monitor for s&sx of infection; monitor blood count. Pt should mark calendar for injection days; learn proper preparation/injection techniques, disposal of needles/syringes; avoid preg/breastfeeding; report severe or persistent GI pain, difficulty breathing, rash, unusual bleeding, fatigue, fever or s&sx of infection.

**DANGEROUS DRUG**

## sAXagliptin (Onglyza)

**CLASS** Antidiabetic, DPP-4 inhibitor
**PREG/CONT** Unkn/NA

**IND & DOSE As adjunct to diet/exercise to improve glycemic control in type 2 diabetics.** *Adult:* 2.5–5 mg/d PO w/o regard to meals.
**ADJUST DOSE** Renal impairment
**ADV EFF** Headache, HF, hypoglycemia, hypersensitivity reactions, **pancreatitis,** peripheral edema, serious to debilitating arthralgia, URI, UTI
**INTERACTIONS** Strong CYP3A4/5 inhibitors
**NC/PT** Not for use in type 1 diabetes, ketoacidosis. Reduce dose if given w/ strong CYP3A4/5 inhibitors. Monitor blood glucose, $HbA_{1c}$, renal function before, periodically during tx. Ensure thorough diabetic teaching program. Pt may be switched to insulin during times of stress. Pt should continue diet/exercise program, other prescribed diabetes drugs; report all other prescribed/OTC drugs, herbs being taken (dose adjustment may be needed), edema, uncontrolled glucose levels, severe headache, s&sx of infection, joint pain, rash, difficulty breathing.

## scopolamine hydrobromide (Transderm-Scop)

**CLASS** Anticholinergic, antiemetic, anti–motion sickness drug, antiparkinsonian, belladonna alkaloid, parasympatholytic
**PREG/CONT** Low risk/NA

**IND & DOSE Tx of motion sickness.** *Adult:* Apply 1 transdermal system to postauricular skin at least 4 hr before

antiemetic effect needed or in evening before scheduled surgery; delivers scopolamine 1 mg over 3 d. May replace system q 3 d. **Obstetric amnesia, preoperative sedation.** *Adult:* 0.32–0.65 mg subcut or IM. May give IV after dilution in sterile water for injection. May repeat up to qid. *Child:* General guidelines, 0.006 mg/kg subcut, IM or IV; max, 0.3 mg. *3 yr–6 yr:* 0.2–0.3 mg IM or IV. *6 mo–3 yr:* 0.1–0.15 mg IM or IV. **Sedation, tranquilization.** *Adult:* 0.6 mg subcut or IM tid–qid. **Antiemetic.** *Adult:* 0.6–1 mg subcut. *Child:* 0.006 mg/kg subcut. **Refraction.** *Adult:* Instill 1–2 drops into eye(s) 1 hr before refracting. **Uveitis.** *Adult:* Instill 1–2 drops into eye(s) up to qid.
**ADJUST DOSE** Elderly pts
**ADV EFF** **Anaphylaxis,** blurred vision, constipation, decreased sweating, dizziness, drowsiness, dry mouth, nasal congestion, photophobia, pupil dilation, urinary hesitancy, urine retention
**INTERACTIONS** Alcohol, antidepressants, antihistamines, haloperidol, phenothiazines
**NC/PT** Ensure adequate hydration. Provide temp control to prevent hyperpyrexia. Avoid use in preg pt w/ severe preeclampsia due to risk of eclamptic seizures. W/transdermal system, have pt wash hands thoroughly after handling patch, dispose of patch properly to avoid contact w/child, pets, remove old patch before applying new one, do not cut patch. Pt should empty bladder before each dose; avoid alcohol, hot environments; use laxative for constipation; take safety precautions for CNS effects; report severe dry mouth, difficulty breathing.

## sebelipase (Kanuma)
**CLASS** Hydrolytic lysosomal cholesteryl ester
**PREG/CONT** Mild risk/NA

**IND & DOSE** **Tx of lysosomal acid lipase deficiency.** *Adult, child:* 1 mg/kg IV over at least 2 hr once q other wk. *Child ≤6 mo w/rapidly progressive deficiency:* 1–3 mg/kg IV once a wk.
**ADV EFF** Anemia, asthenia, constipation, cough, fever, headache, **hypersensitivity reactions,** nasopharyngitis, n/v/d, rash
**NC/PT** Increased risk of hypersensitivity reaction w/known egg or egg-product allergies. Monitor for hypersensitivity reactions, slow infusion, consider pretreatment w/antipyretics, antihistamines. Pt should report difficulty breathing, chest pain, rash.

## secnidazole (Solosec)
**CLASS** Antimicrobial
**PREG/CONT** Unkn/NA

**IND & DOSE** **Tx of bacterial vaginosis in adult women.** *Adult:* 2-g packet of granules taken once.
**ADV EFF** Abd pain, dysgeusia, headache, n/v/d, vulvovaginal candidiasis
**NC/PT** Use only for infections strongly suspected to be caused by bacteria. Monitor for vulvovaginal candidiasis; tx w/antifungal may be needed. Carcinogenic; not meant for prolonged use. Pt should sprinkle contents on applesauce, yogurt, or pudding (drug not meant to be dissolved in liquids) and consume entire mixture in 30 min w/o crunching/chewing granules (pt may take glass of water afterward); avoid breastfeeding; report vaginal itching/discharge, worsening of infection.

**DANGEROUS DRUG**

## secobarbital sodium (Seconal Sodium)
**CLASS** Antiepileptic, barbiturate, sedative-hypnotic
**PREG/CONT** D/C-II

**IND & DOSE** **Intermittent use as sedative-hypnotic.** *Adult:* 100 mg PO at bedtime for up to 2 wk. **Preop sedation.** *Adult:* 200–300 mg PO 1–2 hr before surgery. *Child:* 2–6 mg/kg PO

1–2 hr before surgery; max, 100 mg/dose.
**ADJUST DOSE** Elderly, debilitated pts; hepatic/renal impairment
**ADV EFF** **Anaphylaxis, angioedema,** agitation, anxiety, apnea, ataxia, bradycardia, confusion, constipation, dizziness, epigastric pain, hallucinations, hyperkinesia, hypotension, hypoventilation, insomnia, **laryngospasm,** n/v/d, psychiatric disturbances, respiratory depression, sleep disorders, **SJS,** somnolence, syncope
**INTERACTIONS** Alcohol, anticoagulants, antihistamines, corticosteroids, doxycycline, estrogens, hormonal contraceptives, hypnotics, metoprolol, metronidazole, oxyphenbutazone, phenylbutazone, propranolol, quinidine, sedatives, theophylline, verapamil
**NC/PT** Monitor blood levels, watch for anaphylaxis, angioedema w/above interacting drugs. Not for use in preg (barrier contraceptives advised)/breastfeeding. Barbiturates may produce irritability, excitability, inappropriate tearfulness, aggression in child; stay w/child who receives preop sedation. Taper gradually after repeated use. Pt should avoid alcohol; take safety precautions; report difficulty breathing, swelling, rash.

## **secretin** (ChiRhoStim)
**CLASS** Diagnostic agent
**PREG/CONT** Unkn/NA

**IND & DOSE** **To stimulate pancreatic secretions to aid in dx of pancreatic exocrine dysfx, gastric secretions to aid in dx of gastrinoma.** *Adult:* 0.2–0.4 mcg/kg IV over 1 min.
**ADV EFF** Abd pain, **allergic reactions,** flushing, n/v
**INTERACTIONS** Anticholinergics, $H_2$-receptor antagonists, proton pump inhibitors (PPIs); discontinue anticholinergics at least five half-lives, $H_2$-receptor antagonists at least 2 d, and PPIs before administration
**NC/PT** Monitor carefully during infusion for allergic reaction; have emergency equipment on hand. Do not use w/acute pancreatitis. Pt should report severe abd pain, difficulty breathing.

## **secukinumab** (Cosentyx)
**CLASS** Interleukin antagonist
**PREG/CONT** Moderate risk/NA

**IND & DOSE** **Tx of moderate to severe plaque psoriasis in pts who are candidates for systemic therapy or phototherapy.** *Adult:* 300 mg subcut at wk 0, 1, 2, 3, and 4 followed by 300 mg subcut q 4 wk; 150 mg subcut may be acceptable in some pts. **Tx of active psoriatic arthritis, active ankylosing spondylitis.** *Adult:* 150 mg subcut at wk 0, 1, 2, 3, and 4 and q 4 wk thereafter.
**ADV EFF** Cold sx, Crohn disease exacerbation, diarrhea, hypersensitivity reactions, **infections,** TB activation, URI
**INTERACTIONS** Live vaccines
**NC/PT** Test for TB before tx. Monitor pts w/Crohn disease. Use caution in preg/breastfeeding. Do not inject within 2 inches of navel. Pt should refrigerate drug and learn proper use/disposal of *Sensoready Pen,* subcut administration, rotation of injection sites; report difficulty breathing, swelling, chest tightness, rash, fainting, s&sx of infection.

## **selegiline hydrochloride** (Emsam, Zelapar)
**CLASS** Antidepressant, antiparkinsonian, MAO type B inhibitor
**PREG/CONT** High risk/NA

**BBW** Increased risk of suicidality in child, adolescent, young adult; monitor accordingly. *Emsam* is contraindicated in child <12 yr; risk of hypertensive crisis.
**IND & DOSE** **Mgt of pts w/Parkinson disease whose response to levodopa/carbidopa has decreased.** *Adult:*

10 mg/d PO in divided doses of 5 mg each at breakfast, lunch. After 2–3 d, attempt to reduce levodopa/carbidopa dose; reductions of 10%–30% typical. For orally disintegrating tablet, 1.25 mg/d PO in a.m. before breakfast. May increase after 6 wk to 2.5 mg/d; max, 10 mg/d. **Tx of major depressive disorder.** *Adult, child>12 yr:* One patch *(Emsam)* daily to dry, intact skin on upper torso, upper thigh, or outer surface of upper arm. Start w/6-mg/24 hr system; increase to max 12 mg/24 hr if needed, tolerated.
**ADJUST DOSE** Elderly pts
**ADV EFF** Abd pain, **asthma,** confusion, dizziness, dyskinesia, falling asleep during daily activities, fever, hallucinations, headache, HTN, loss of impulse control, light-headedness, local reactions to dermal patch, melanoma risk, n/v, **serotonin syndrome,** vivid dreams
**INTERACTIONS** Carbamazepine, fluoxetine, meperidine, methadone, opioid analgesics, oxcarbazepine, TCAs, tramadol, tyramine-rich foods
**NC/PT** Not for use in breastfeeding. Pt should place oral tablet on top of tongue, avoid food, beverage for 5 min; apply dermal patch to dry, intact skin on upper torso, upper thigh, or outer upper arm, replace q 24 hr (remove old patch before applying new one); continue other parkinsonians; take safety precautions for CNS effects; report all drugs being used (dose adjustments may be needed); report confusion, fainting, thoughts of suicide.

## selexipag (Uptravi)

**CLASS** Prostacyclin receptor agonist
**PREG/CONT** Low risk/NA

**IND & DOSE** **Tx of pulmonary arterial HTN.** *Adult:* Initially, 200 mcg PO bid; increase at wkly intervals to 1,600 mcg PO bid.
**ADJUST DOSE** Hepatic impairment, moderate CYP2C8 inhibitors
**ADV EFF** Extremity/jaw pain, flushing, headache, n/v/d, **pulmonary edema**
**INTERACTIONS** Strong/moderate CYP2C8 inhibitors; avoid combo
**NC/PT** Ensure proper dx. Not for use w/severe hepatic impairment or breastfeeding. Adjust dose based on pt response. Pt should monitor activity level and breathing; report difficulty breathing, severe n/v/d.

**▶NEW DRUG**

## selinexor (Xpovio)

**CLASS** Antineoplastic, nuclear export inhibitor
**PREG/CONT** High risk/ NA

**IND & DOSE** **Tx of relapsed/refractory multiple myeloma, w/dexamethasone, in pts w/at least four prior tx and whose disease is refractory to at least two proteasome inhibitors, at least two immunomodulatory agents, and an anti-CD38 monoclonal antibody.** *Adult:* 80 mg PO w/dexamethasone 20 mg PO on days 1 and 3 of each wk until disease progression or unacceptable toxicity.
**ADV EFF** Anemia, dyspnea, fatigue, **GI toxicity, hyponatremia, infections, neurotoxicity, neutropenia, thrombocytopenia,** weight loss
**NC/PT** Monitor CBC, standard blood chemistry, and body weight at baseline/during tx, more frequently first 2 mo of tx. Provide px concomitant tx w/5-$HT_3$ antagonist and/or other antinausea agents before/during tx. Consider IV hydration for pt w/dehydration risk. Pt should swallow tablet whole w/water, not break/chew/crush/divide; maintain adequate fluid/caloric intake during tx.

DANGEROUS DRUG

## semaglutide (Ozempic, Rybelsus)

**CLASS** Antidiabetic, glucagon-like peptide 1 (GLP-1) receptor agonist

**PREG/CONT** Moderate risk/NA

**BBW** Drug causes thyroid C-cell tumors in rodents; it is unknown if drug causes thyroid C-cell tumors, including medullary thyroid carcinoma (MTC), in humans as the human relevance of semaglutide-induced rodent thyroid C-cell tumors has not been determined. Contraindicated in pts w/personal, family history of MTC or in pts w/multiple endocrine neoplasia syndrome type 2 (MEN 2). Counsel pts about MTC risk and thyroid tumors sx.

**IND & DOSE** **Adjunct to diet/exercise to improve glycemic control in pts w/type 2 diabetes mellitus (DM); to reduce risk of major CV events in pts w/type 2 DM and established CV disease.** *Adult: Ozempic:* Initially, 0.25 mg subcut q wk. After 4 wk, increase to 0.5 mg subcut q wk. If, after at least 4 wk, additional glycemic control needed, increase to 1 mg subcut q wk. *Rybelsus:* Initially, 3 mg PO daily for 30 d; then increase to 7 mg PO daily. Max, 14 mg PO daily if needed.

**ADV EFF** Abd pain, **acute kidney injury**, constipation, **diabetic retinopathy, hypersensitivity, hypoglycemia,** n/v/d, pancreatitis

**NC/PT** Contraindicated in MEN 2. Not recommended as first-line therapy. Has not been studied in pts w/history of pancreatitis. Not indicated for pts w/type 1 diabetes mellitus or in diabetic ketoacidosis. Give *Ozempic* in abdomen, thigh, or upper arm on same day of wk w/ or w/o meals. Give *Rybelsus* at least 30 min before food/other drugs w/no more than 4 oz of plain water; have pt swallow whole. Discontinue in women at least 2 mo before planned preg. Pt should immediately report severe abd pain, vision changes, hypersensitivity s&sx; avoid fluid depletion (risk of dehydration); never share pen w/others (risk of infection transmission).

## sertraline hydrochloride (Zoloft)

**CLASS** Antidepressant, SSRI

**PREG/CONT** High risk/NA

**BBW** Increased risk of suicidality in child, adolescent, young adult; monitor accordingly.

**IND & DOSE** **Tx of major depressive disorder, OCD.** *Adult:* 50 mg PO once daily, a.m. or p.m.; may increase to max 200 mg/d. *Child 13–17 yr:* For OCD, 50 mg/d PO; max, 200 mg/d. *Child 6–12 yr:* For OCD, 25 mg/d PO; max, 200 mg/d. **Tx of panic disorder, PTSD.** *Adult:* 25–50 mg/d PO, up to max 200 mg/d. **Tx of PMDD.** *Adult:* 50 mg/d PO daily or just during luteal phase of menstrual cycle. Range, 50–150 mg/d. **Tx of social anxiety disorder.** *Adult:* 25 mg/d PO; range, 50–200 mg/d.

**ADJUST DOSE** Hepatic/renal impairment

**ADV EFF** Anxiety, diarrhea, dizziness, drowsiness, dry mouth, fatigue, headache, insomnia, nausea, nervousness, painful menstruation, rhinitis, serotonin syndrome, **suicidality,** vision changes

**INTERACTIONS** Cimetidine, MAOIs, pimozide, St. John's wort

**NC/PT** Do not give within 14 d of MAOIs. Dilute oral concentrate in 4 oz water, ginger ale, lemon-lime soda, lemonade, orange juice only; give immediately after diluting. Risk of congenital heart defects; not for use in preg (barrier contraceptives advised). May take up to 4–6 wk to see depression improvement. Pt should take safety precautions for CNS effects; avoid St. John's wort; report difficulty breathing, thoughts of suicide.

## sevelamer hydrochloride (Renagel), sevelamer carbonate (Renvela)

**CLASS** Calcium-phosphate binder
**PREG/CONT** Low risk/NA

**IND & DOSE To reduce serum phosphorus level in hemodialysis pts w/ESRD.** *Adult:* 1–4 tablets PO w/ each meal based on serum phosphorus level; may increase by 1 tablet/ meal to achieve desired serum phosphorus level (*Renagel*). Or, 800 mg PO tid w/meals (*Renvela*); modify based on phosphorus level.
**ADV EFF** Bowel obstruction/ perforation, cough, diarrhea, dyspepsia, fecal impaction, headache, hypotension, thrombosis, vomiting
**NC/PT** Do not use w/ hypophosphatemia or bowel obstruction. May decrease fat-soluble vitamins and folic acid serum levels in preg women; supplementation may be needed. Pt should take other oral drugs at least 1 hr before or 3 hr after sevelamer; have blood tests regularly to monitor phosphorus level, report chest pain, difficulty breathing, severe abd pain.

## sildenafil citrate (Revatio, Viagra)

**CLASS** ED drug, phosphodiesterase-5 inhibitor
**PREG/CONT** B/NA

**IND & DOSE Tx of ED.** *Adult:* 50 mg PO 1 hr before anticipated sexual activity; range, 25–100 mg PO. May take 30 min–4 hr before sexual activity. Limit use to once/d (*Viagra*). **Tx of pulmonary arterial HTN.** *Adult:* 20 mg PO tid at least 4–6 hr apart w/o regard to food (*Revatio*), or 2.5–10 mg by IV bolus tid (*Revatio*).
**ADJUST DOSE** Elderly pts; hepatic/ renal impairment
**ADV EFF** Dyspepsia, flushing, headache, hearing/vision loss, hypotension, insomnia, priapism, rhinitis
**INTERACTIONS** Alcohol, alpha adrenergic blockers, amlodipine, cimetidine, erythromycin, grapefruit juice, itraconazole, ketoconazole, nitrates, protease inhibitors, ritonavir, saquinavir
**NC/PT** Ensure proper dx before tx. *Revatio* contraindicated in child 1–17 yr; deaths have been reported. Reserve IV use for pts unable to take orally. *Viagra* ineffective in absence of sexual stimulation. Pt should take appropriate measures to prevent STDs; report difficult urination, sudden hearing/ vision loss, erection lasting longer than 4 hr.

## silodosin (Rapaflo)

**CLASS** Alpha blocker, BPH drug
**PREG/CONT** B/NA

**IND & DOSE Tx of s&sx of BPH.** *Adult:* 8 mg/d PO w/meal.
**ADJUST DOSE** Hepatic/renal impairment
**ADV EFF** Abnormal/retrograde ejaculation, dizziness, headache, liver impairment, orthostatic hypotension, rash
**INTERACTIONS** Clarithromycin, cyclosporine, ED drugs, itraconazole, ketoconazole, other alpha blockers, nitrates, ritonavir
**NC/PT** Rule out prostate cancer before tx. Pt undergoing cataract surgery at risk for intraop floppy iris syndrome; alert surgeon about drug use. Pt should take safety precautions w/ dizziness, orthostatic hypotension; use caution when combined w/nitrates, ED drugs, antihypertensives; report urine/ stool color changes, worsening of sx.

## siltuximab (Sylvant)

**CLASS** Interleukin-6 antagonist
**PREG/CONT** Moderate risk/NA

**IND & DOSE Tx of multicentric Castleman disease in pts HIV-negative**

**and herpesvirus-negative.** *Adult:* 11 mg/kg IV over 1 hr q 3 wk.
**ADV EFF GI perforation, infection, infusion reaction**, rash, **severe hypersensitivity reactions**, URI
**INTERACTIONS** Live vaccines
**NC/PT** Ensure proper dx. Do not give to pt w/infections. Monitor for infection during tx; provide tx. Do not give drug until infection resolves. Have emergency equipment on hand during infusion. Pt should report s&sx of infection, difficulty breathing, severe abd pain; avoid breastfeeding during tx and for 3 mo after final dose.

## simeprevir (Olysio)
**CLASS** Hepatitis C drug, protease inhibitor
**PREG/CONT** High risk/NA

**BBW** Cases of HBV reactivation resulting in fulminant hepatitis, hepatic failure, and death have been noted in pts w/HCV and HBV.
**IND & DOSE Tx of chronic HCV genotype 1 or 4, w/other antiretrovirals.** *Adult:* 150 mg/d PO w/food; combined w/peginterferon alfa and ribavirin for 12 wk, then peginterferon alfa and ribavirin for 24–36 wk. May combine w/ sofosbuvir in genotype 1 for 12- to 24-wk course.
**ADJUST DOSE** Hepatic impairment (contraindicated)
**ADV EFF Bradycardia, liver failure,** nausea, photosensitivity, rash
**INTERACTIONS** Amiodarone (may cause bradycardia), CYP3A inducers/ inhibitors, warfarin
**NC/PT** Ensure concurrent use of peginterferon alfa and ribavirin or sofosbuvir; not for monotherapy. Monitor HR. Monitor INR closely if pt taking warfarin. Negative preg test required monthly; pt should avoid preg or fathering a child (two forms of contraception advised). Not for use in breastfeeding. Pt should swallow capsule whole and not cut/crush/chew it; avoid sun exposure; use precautions to avoid spread of disease; report rash, itching, severe nausea, urine/ stool color changes.

## simethicone (Flatulex, Gas-X, Phazyme)
**CLASS** Antiflatulent
**PREG/CONT** C/NA

**IND & DOSE Relief of sx of excess gas in digestive tract.** *Adult:* 40–360 mg PO as needed after meals, at bedtime; max, 500 mg/d. *Child 2–12 yr, >11 kg:* 40 mg PO as needed after meals, at bedtime. *Child <2 yr:* 20 mg PO as needed after meals, at bedtime; max, 240 mg/d.
**ADV EFF** Constipation, diarrhea, flatulence
**NC/PT** Pt should shake drops thoroughly before each use; add drops to 30 mL cool water, infant formula, other liquid to ease administration to infants; let strips dissolve on tongue; chew chewable tablets thoroughly before swallowing; report extreme abd pain, vomiting.

## simvastatin (Zocor)
**CLASS** Antihyperlipidemic, statin
**PREG/CONT** High risk/NA

**IND & DOSE Tx of hyperlipidemia; px of coronary events.** *Adult:* 10–20 mg PO, up to 40 mg, daily in evening. Range, 5–40 mg/d; max, 40 mg/d. **Tx of familial hypercholesterolemia; to reduce elevated triglycerides (TG) in hypertriglyceridemia and TG and VLDL-C in primary dysbetalipoproteinemia.** *Adult:* 40 mg/d PO in evening. *Child 10–17 yr:* 10 mg/d PO in evening; range, 10–40 mg/d. Do not progress to 80 mg/d; increased risk of rhabdomyolysis.
**ADJUST DOSE** Renal impairment; hepatic impairment (contraindicated)
**ADV EFF** Abd pain, **acute renal failure**, cramps, flatulence, headache, **liver failure**, n/v/d, **rhabdomyolysis/ myopathy**

**INTERACTIONS Strong CYP3A4 inhibitors, cyclosporine, danazol, gemfibrozil; contraindicated w/ these drugs.** Amiodarone, amlodipine, digoxin, diltiazem, dronedarone, fibrates, grapefruit juice, hepatotoxic drugs, lomitapide, niacin, ranolazine, verapamil, warfarin
**NC/PT** Not for use w/strong CYP3A4 inhibitors, gemfibrozil, cyclosporine, danazol. Monitor LFTs. Avoid 80-mg dose because of increased risk of muscle injury, rhabdomyolysis; if pt already stable on 80 mg, monitor closely. Not for use in preg (barrier contraceptives advised)/breastfeeding. Pt should continue diet; take in p.m.; have blood tests regularly; avoid grapefruit juice; report urine/stool color changes, muscle pain/soreness.

▶ **NEW DRUG**

## siponimod (Mayzent)
**CLASS** MS drug, sphingosine 1-phosphate receptor modulator
**PREG/CONT** High risk/NA

**IND & DOSE Tx of relapsing forms of MS w/CYP2C9 genotype *1/*1, *1/*2, or *2/*2.** *Adult:* Initially, 0.25 mg PO daily (days 1, 2), then 0.5 mg PO daily (day 3), 0.75 mg PO daily (day 4), 1.25 mg PO daily (day 5). On day 6, begin 2 mg PO daily as maint dose. **Tx of relapsing forms of MS w/CYP2C9 genotype *1/*3 or *2/*3.** *Adult:* Initially, 0.25 mg PO daily (days 1, 2), 0.5 mg PO daily (day 3), 0.75 mg PO daily (day 4). On day 5, begin 1 mg PO daily as maint dose.
**ADV EFF AV conduction delays, bradycardia,** headache, **HTN, infections, liver injury, respiratory decline**
**INTERACTIONS** CYP2C9/CYP3A4 inducers/inhibitors, live vaccines
**NC/PT** Before initiation, obtain genotype determination, CBC, LFTs, indicated vaccination, ophthalmic/cardiac evaluation. Initial drug titration decreases risk of CV adverse effects. Not indicated for pts w/CYP2C9*3/*3 genotype, MI, angina, stroke, TIA or HF requiring hospitalization in last 6 mo, **CLASS** III/IV HF, Mobitz type II second-degree, third-degree AV block, sick sinus syndrome if no functional pacemaker.

## sipuleucel-T (Provenge)
**CLASS** Cellular immunotherapy
**PREG/CONT** NA/NA

**IND & DOSE Tx of asymptomatic, minimally symptomatic metastatic castrate-resistant prostate cancer.** *Adult:* 50 million autologous CD54+ cells activated w/PAP-GM-CSF suspended in 250 mL lactated Ringer injection IV.
**ADV EFF Acute infusion reactions,** back pain, chills, fatigue, fever, headache, joint ache, nausea
**INTERACTIONS** Immunosuppressants
**NC/PT** Autologous use only. Leukapheresis will be done 3 d before infusion. Ensure pt identity. Premedicate w/oral acetaminophen and antihistamine. Risk of acute infusion reactions; closely monitor pt during infusion. Universal precautions required. Pt should report difficulty breathing, s&sx of infection.

## sirolimus (Rapamune)
**CLASS** Immunosuppressant
**PREG/CONT** High risk/NA

**BBW** Risk of increased susceptibility to infection; graft loss, hepatic artery thrombosis w/liver transplant; bronchial anastomotic dehiscence in lung transplants.
**IND & DOSE Px for organ rejection in renal transplant.** *Adult, child ≥13 yr:* ≥40 kg: Loading dose of 6 mg PO as soon after transplant as possible, then 2 mg/d PO. <40 kg: Loading dose of 3 mg/$m^2$, then 1 mg/$m^2$/d PO. **Tx of pts w/lymphangioleiomyomatosis.** *Adult:* 2 mg/d PO; titrate to achieve trough concentrations of 5–15 ng/mL.
**ADJUST DOSE** Hepatic impairment

**ADV EFF** Abd pain, **anaphylaxis,** anemia, **angioedema,** arthralgia, delayed wound healing, edema, fever, headache, HTN, **ILD,** lipid profile changes, pain, pneumonitis, skin cancer, thrombocytopenia
**INTERACTIONS** CYP3A4 inducers/inhibitors, grapefruit juice, live vaccines
**NC/PT** Always use w/adrenal corticosteroids, cyclosporine. Monitor pulmonary/renal function, LFTs. Not for use in preg (contraceptives advised)/breastfeeding. Risk of male infertility. Pt should avoid grapefruit juice, sun exposure; report difficulty breathing, swelling.

**DANGEROUS DRUG**

## SITagliptin phosphate
(Januvia)
**CLASS** Antidiabetic, DPP-4 inhibitor
**PREG/CONT** Unkn/NA

**IND & DOSE As adjunct to diet/exercise to improve glycemic control in type 2 diabetics.** *Adult:* 100 mg/d PO.
**ADJUST DOSE** Renal impairment
**ADV EFF** Headache, **hypersensitivity reactions,** hypoglycemia, **pancreatitis, renal failure, severe to disabling arthralgia, SJS,** URI, UTI
**INTERACTIONS** Atazanavir, celery, clarithromycin, coriander, dandelion root, fenugreek, garlic, ginseng, indinavir, itraconazole, juniper berries, ketoconazole, nefazodone, nelfinavir, ritonavir, saquinavir, telithromycin
**NC/PT** Not for use in type 1 diabetics, ketoacidosis. Monitor for s&sx of HF (other DPP-4 inhibitors have been shown to increase risk). Monitor blood glucose, $HbA_{1c}$, renal function, pancreatic enzymes before, periodically during tx. Ensure thorough diabetic teaching program. May switch pt to insulin during times of stress. Health care provider should report prenatal Januvia exposure to the Preg Registry. Pt should continue diet/exercise program, other prescribed diabetes drugs; report all other prescribed/OTC drugs, herbs being take, difficulty breathing, rash, joint pain.

## sodium bicarbonate
(generic)
**CLASS** Antacid, electrolyte; systemic, urine alkalinizer
**PREG/CONT** C/NA

**IND & DOSE Urine alkalinization.** *Adult:* 3,900 mg PO, then 1,300–2,600 mg PO q 4 hr. *Child:* 84–840 mg/kg/d PO. **Antacid.** *Adult:* 300 mg–2 g PO daily–qid usually 1–3 hr after meals, at bedtime. **Adjunct to advanced CV life support during CPR.** *Adult:* Inject IV either 300–500 mL of 5% sol or 200–300 mEq of 7.5% or 8.4% sol as rapidly as possible. Base further doses on subsequent blood gas values. Or, 1 mEq/kg dose, then repeat 0.5 mEq/kg q 10 min. *Child ≥2 yr:* 1–2 mEq/kg (1 mL/kg 8.4% sol) by slow IV. *Child <2 yr:* 4.2% sol; max, 8 mEq/kg/d IV. **Severe metabolic acidosis.** *Adult, child:* Dose depends on blood carbon dioxide content, pH, pt's clinical condition. Usually, 90–180 mEq/L IV during first hr, then adjust PRN. **Less urgent metabolic acidosis.** *Adult, adolescent:* 5 mEq/kg as 4–8 hr IV infusion.
**ADJUST DOSE** Elderly pts, renal impairment
**ADV EFF** Local irritation, tissue necrosis at injection site, systemic alkalosis
**INTERACTIONS** Amphetamines, anorexiants, doxycycline, ephedrine, flecainide, lithium, methotrexate, quinidine, pseudoephedrine, salicylates, sulfonylureas, sympathomimetics, tetracyclines
**NC/PT** Monitor ABGs. Calculate base deficit when giving parenteral sodium bicarbonate. Adjust dose based on response. Give slowly. Do not attempt complete correction within first 24 hr; increased risk of systemic alkalosis. Monitor cardiac rhythm,

potassium level. Pt should chew tablets thoroughly before swallowing, follow w/full glass of water; avoid oral drug within 1–2 hr of other oral drugs; report pain at injection site, headache, tremors.

## sodium ferric gluconate complex (Ferrlecit)

**CLASS** Iron product
**PREG/CONT** B/NA

**IND & DOSE Tx of iron deficiency in pts undergoing long-term hemodialysis who are on erythropoietin.** *Adult:* Test dose: 2 mL diluted in 50 mL normal saline injection IV over 60 min. *Adult:* 10 mL diluted in 100 mL normal saline injection IV over 60 min. *Child ≥6 yr:* 0.12 mL/kg diluted in 25 mL normal saline by IV infusion over 1 hr for each dialysis session.
**ADV EFF** Cramps, dizziness, dyspnea, flushing, hypotension, **hypersensitivity reactions,** injection-site reactions, **iron overload,** n/v/d, pain
**NC/PT** Monitor iron level, BP. Most pts will initially need eight doses given at sequential dialysis sessions, then periodic use based on hematocrit. Do not mix w/other drugs in sol. Have emergency equipment on hand for hypersensitivity reactions. Use caution in preg/breastfeeding. Pt should take safety precautions for CNS effects; report difficulty breathing, pain at injection site.

## sodium fluoride (Fluoritab, Flura, Karigel, Pharmaflur)

**CLASS** Mineral
**PREG/CONT** C/NA

**IND & DOSE Px of dental caries.** *Adult:* 10 mL rinse once daily or wkly; swish around teeth, spit out. Or, apply thin ribbon to toothbrush or mouth tray for 1 min; brush, rinse, spit out. *Child:* Fluoride in drinking water >0.6 ppm: No tx. Fluoride in drinking water 0.3–0.6 ppm: 6–16 yr, 0.5 mg/d PO; 3–6 yr, 0.25 mg/d PO. Fluoride in drinking water <0.3 ppm: 6–16 yr, 1 mg/d PO; 3–6 yr, 0.5 mg/d PO; 6 mo–3 yr, 0.25 mg/d PO. *Child 6–12 yr:* 10 mL/d rinse; have pt swish around teeth for 1 min, spit out. Or, 4–6 drops gel on applicator. Have pt put applicator over teeth, bite down for 6 min, spit out excess gel.
**ADV EFF** Eczema, gastric distress, headache, rash, teeth staining, weakness
**INTERACTIONS** Dairy products
**NC/PT** Do not give within 1 hr of milk, dairy products. Pt may chew tablets, swallow whole, or add to drinking water, juice. Pt should brush, floss teeth before using rinse, then spit out fluid (should not swallow fluid, cream, gel, rinse); have regular dental exams; report increased salivation, diarrhea, seizures, teeth mottling.

## sodium oxybate (Xyrem)

**CLASS** Anticataplectic, CNS depressant
**PREG/CONT** Unkn/C-III

**BBW** Counsel pt that drug, also called GHB, is known for abuse. Pt will be asked to view educational program, agree to safety measures to ensure only pt has drug access, and agree to return for follow-up at least q 3 mo. Severe respiratory depression, coma, death possible. Available only through restricted access program.
**IND & DOSE Tx of excessive daytime sleepiness, cataplexy in pts w/narcolepsy.** *Adult:* 4.5 g/d PO divided into two equal doses of 2.25 g. Give at bedtime and again 2½–4 hr later. May increase no more often than q 1–2 wk to max 9 g/d in increments of 1.5 g/d (0.75 g/dose). Range, 6–9 g daily.
**ADJUST DOSE** Hepatic impairment
**ADV EFF CNS depression,** confusion, dizziness, dyspepsia, flulike sx, headache, n/v/d, pharyngitis, **respiratory depression, sleep walking,** somnolence, suicidality, URI

**INTERACTIONS** Alcohol, CNS depressants
**NC/PT** Dilute each dose w/60 mL water in child-resistant dosing cup. Give first dose of day when pt still in bed; should stay in bed after taking. Give second dose 2½–4 hr later, w/pt sitting up in bed. After second dose, pt should lie in bed. Not for use in preg (contraceptives advised); appears in human milk. Monitor elderly pts for impaired motor/cognitive function. Pt should take safety precautions for CNS effects; avoid eating for at least 2 hr before bed; keep drug secure; avoid alcohol, CNS depressants; report difficulty breathing, confusion, suicidal thoughts.

## sodium polystyrene sulfonate (Kalexate, Kionex, SPS)

**CLASS** Potassium-removing resin
**PREG/CONT** C/NA

**IND & DOSE** **Tx of hyperkalemia.** *Adult:* 15–60 g/d PO best given as 15 g daily–qid. May give powder as suspension w/water, syrup (20–100 mL). May introduce into stomach via NG tube. Or, 30–50 g by enema q 6 hr, retained for 30–60 min or as long as possible. *Child:* Give lower doses, using exchange ratio of 1 mEq potassium/g resin as basis for calculation.
**ADV EFF** Anorexia, constipation, gastric irritation, hypokalemia, n/v
**INTERACTIONS** Antacids
**NC/PT** Give resin through plastic stomach tube, or mixed w/diet appropriate for renal failure. Give powder form in oral suspension w/syrup base to increase palatability. Give enema after cleansing enema; help pt retain for at least 30 min. Monitor serum electrolytes; correct imbalances. If severe constipation, stop drug until function returns; do not use sorbitol, magnesium-containing laxatives. Pt should report confusion, constipation, irregular heartbeat.

## sodium zirconium cyclosilicate (Lokelma)

**CLASS** Antidote, potassium binder
**PREG/CONT** Low risk/NA

**IND & DOSE** **Tx of hyperkalemia.** *Adult:* Initially, 10 g PO 3 × a day for up to 48 hr. Maint, 10 g PO daily; adjust as needed to obtain desired serum potassium.
**ADV EFF** Edema, GI motility problems
**INTERACTIONS** Drugs w/pH-dependent solubility; administer at least 2 hr before or after
**NC/PT** Avoid in pts w/severe GI motility problems (severe constipation, bowel obstruction/impaction, including abnormal postop bowel motility disorders); may be ineffective and worsen GI conditions. Some pts may need to lower dietary sodium. Pt should drink full dose.

## sofosbuvir (Sovaldi)

**CLASS** Hepatitis C drug, nucleoside analog inhibitor
**PREG/CONT** Unkn/NA

**BBW** Risk of HBV reactivation resulting in fulminant hepatitis, hepatic failure, and death in pts w/HCV and HBV. Test all pts for HBV before therapy.
**IND & DOSE** **Tx of HCV (genotype 1, 2, 3, or 4) w/o cirrhosis or w/cirrhosis w/other antivirals.** *Adult:* 400 mg/d PO w/peginterferon and ribavirin for 12 wk (genotype 1 or 4); w/ribavirin for 12 wk (genotype 2) or 24 wk (genotype 3). **Tx chronic HCV (genotype 2 or 3) w/o cirrhosis or w/compensated cirrhosis w/other antivirals.** *Child ≥3 yr ≥35 kg:* 400 mg/d PO w/ribavirin for 12 wk (genotype 2) or 24 wk (genotype 3). *Child ≥3 yr 17–35 kg:* 200 mg/d PO w/ribavirin for 12 wk (genotype 2) or 24 wk (genotype 3). *Child ≥3 yr <17 kg:* 150 mg/d PO w/ ribavirin for 12 wk (genotype 2) or 24 wk (genotype 3).

**ADJUST DOSE** HCV/HIV coinfection, pts w/hepatocellular carcinoma awaiting liver transplant
**ADV EFF** Anemia, bradycardia, fatigue, headache, insomnia, nausea
**INTERACTIONS** Amiodarone, rifampin, St. John's wort
**NC/PT** Ensure proper dx. Monthly negative preg test required (use of barrier contraceptives advised for men and women during and for 6 mo after use). Drug is not a cure. Pt should eat small meals for nausea; take analgesic for headache; avoid St. John's wort; consult prescriber before stopping drug; take precautions to avoid spread of disease; report severe headache, urine/stool color changes.

## solifenacin succinate
(VESIcare)
**CLASS** Muscarinic receptor antagonist, urinary antispasmodic
**PREG/CONT** C/NA

**IND & DOSE Tx of overactive bladder.** *Adult:* 5–10 mg/d PO swallowed whole w/water.
**ADJUST DOSE** Moderate to severe hepatic impairment, severe renal impairment
**ADV EFF** Constipation, dizziness, dry eyes, dry mouth, **prolonged QT,** tachycardia, urine retention
**INTERACTIONS** CYP3A4 inhibitors, ketoconazole, potassium chloride, QT-prolonging drugs
**NC/PT** Arrange tx for underlying cause. Not for use in breastfeeding. Pt should empty bladder before each dose if urine retention an issue; swallow tablet whole and not cut/crush/chew it; use sugarless lozenges for dry mouth, laxatives for constipation; take safety precautions w/dizziness; report inability to void, fever, blurred vision.

## somatropin (Genotropin, Humatrope, Norditropin Flexpro, Nutropin, Nutropin AQ NuSpin, Omnitrope, Saizen, Serostim, Zomacton, Zorbtive)
**CLASS** Hormone
**PREG/CONT** C; B (*Genotropin, Omnitrope, Saizen, Serostim, Zorbtive*)/NA

**IND & DOSE (Adult) Tx of GH deficiency; replacement of endogenous GH in adults w/GHD w/multiple hormone deficiencies** (*Genotropin, Humatrope, HumatroPen, Norditropin, Nutropin, Nutropin AQ, Omnitrope, Saizen*). *Genotropin, Omnitrope,* 0.04–0.08 mg/kg/wk subcut divided into seven daily injections. *Humatrope, HumatroPen,* 0.006–0.0125 mg/kg/d subcut. *Nutropin, Nutropin AQ,* usual, 0.006 mg/kg/d subcut; max, 0.0125 mg/kg/d (over 35 yr), 0.025 mg/kg/d (<35 yr). *Norditropin,* 0.004–0.016 mg/kg/d subcut. *Saizen,* up to 0.005 mg/kg/d subcut; may increase up to 0.01 mg/kg/d after 4 wk. *Zomacton,* up to 0.1 mg subcut 3 ×/wk. **Tx of AIDS-wasting or cachexia.** *Serostim,* >55 kg: 6 mg/d subcut; 45–55 kg: 5 mg/d subcut; 35–45 kg: 4 mg/d subcut; <35 kg: 0.1 mg/kg/d subcut. **Tx of short bowel syndrome in pts receiving specialized nutritional support** (*Zorbtive*). 0.1 mg/kg/d subcut for 4 wk; max, 8 mg/d.
**IND & DOSE (Child) Tx of growth failure related to renal dysfx.** 0.35 mg/kg/wk subcut divided into daily doses (*Nutropin, Nutropin AQ*). **Tx of girls w/Turner syndrome.** 0.33 mg/kg/wk divided into six–seven subcut injections (*Genotropin*). Or, up to 0.375 mg/kg/wk subcut divided into equal doses 6–7 ×/wk (*Humatrope, HumatroPen*). Or, up to 0.067 mg/kg/d subcut (*Norditropin*). Or, up to 0.375 mg/kg/wk subcut divided into equal doses (*Nutropin, Nutropin AQ*). **Long-term tx of growth failure due to Prader-Willi syndrome.** 0.24 mg/kg/wk

subcut divided into daily doses (*Genotropin, Norditropin Flexpro*). **Small for gestational age.** 0.48 mg/kg/wk (*Genotropin*). **Tx of short stature, growth failure in short stature homeobox (SHOX)-containing gene deficiency.** 0.35 mg/kg/wk subcut (*Humatrope, HumatroPen*). **Tx of short stature in Noonan syndrome.** Up to 0.066 mg/kg/d subcut (*Norditropin*). **Long-term tx of idiopathic short stature when epiphyses not closed and diagnostic evaluation excludes other causes treatable by other means.** 0.47 mg/kg/wk subcut divided into six–seven doses (*Genotropin*). Or, 0.18–0.3 mg/kg/wk subcut or IM given in divided doses 3 time/wk (*Humatrope, HumatroPen*). Or, 0.3 mg/kg/wk subcut in divided daily doses (*Nutropin, Nutropin AQ*). **Long-term tx of growth failure due to lack of adequate endogenous GH secretion.** 0.18–0.3 mg/kg/wk subcut divided into doses 6–7 ×/wk (*Humatrope, HumatroPen*). Or, 0.3 mg/kg/wk subcut in divided daily doses (*Nutropin, Nutropin AQ*). Or, 0.16–0.24 mg/kg/wk subcut divided into daily doses (*Genotropin*). Or, 0.16–0.24 mg/kg/wk subcut divided into daily doses (*Omnitrope*). Or, 0.06 mg/kg subcut, IM 3 ×/wk (*Saizen*). Or, 0.024–0.034 mg/kg subcut, 6–7 ×/wk (*Norditropin*). Or, up to 0.1 mg/kg subcut 3 ×/wk (*Zomacton*). **Tx of short stature w/no catch-up growth by 2–4 yr.** 0.35 mg/kg/wk subcut injection divided into equal daily doses (*Humatrope, HumatroPen*), 0.024–0.034 mg/kg subcut 6–7 ×/wk (*Norditropin*).
**ADV EFF** Development of GH antibodies, headache, hypothyroidism, insulin resistance, **leukemia, neoplasms,** pain, pain at injection site
**INTERACTIONS** CYP450 inducers/inhibitors
**NC/PT** Arrange tests for glucose tolerance, thyroid function, growth hormone antibodies; tx as indicated. Ensure cancer screening during tx. Rotate injection sites. Teach proper administration/disposal of needles/syringes. Pt should have frequent blood tests; report increased thirst/voiding, fatigue, cold intolerance.

## sonidegib (Odomzo)

**CLASS** Antineoplastic, hedgehog pathway inhibitor
**PREG/CONT** High risk/NA

**BBW** Can cause embryo-fetal death, birth defects. Advise contraceptives for women. Advise males of risk through semen and need for condom use during and for at least 8 mo after tx ends.
**IND & DOSE Tx of locally advanced basal cell carcinoma recurring after surgery or radiation or if pt not candidate for surgery/radiation.** *Adult:* 200 mg/d PO at least 1 hr before or 2 hr after meal.
**ADV EFF** Abd pain, alopecia, anorexia, fatigue, headache, myalgia, n/v/d, premature fusion of epiphyses, rash, skeletal pain, weight loss
**INTERACTIONS** CYP3A inducers/inhibitors
**NC/PT** Obtain serum CK/creatinine levels before/periodically during tx, and as clinically indicated. Rule out preg before use (contraceptives advised). Men should use condoms during and for 8 mo after tx. Not for use in breastfeeding. Pt cannot donate blood during and for 20 mo after last dose. Pt should take on empty stomach 1 hr before or 2 hr after meals; try small, frequent meals; report severe musculoskeletal pain, weight loss.

**DANGEROUS DRUG**

## sorafenib tosylate (Nexavar)

**CLASS** Antineoplastic, kinase inhibitor
**PREG/CONT** D/NA

**IND & DOSE Tx of advanced renal cell, hepatocellular carcinoma, differentiated thyroid carcinoma**

**refractory to other tx.** *Adult:* 400 mg PO bid on empty stomach.
**ADV EFF** Alopecia, fatigue, **GI perforation, hand-foot syndrome, hemorrhage, hepatitis,** HTN, **MI,** n/v/d, **prolonged QT,** skin reactions, weight loss, wound-healing complications
**INTERACTIONS** CYP3A4 inducers, grapefruit juice, QT-prolonging drugs
**NC/PT** Obtain baseline, periodic ECG; monitor BP regularly. Not for use in preg (contraceptives advised)/ breastfeeding. Pt should take on empty stomach; avoid grapefruit juice; cover head at temp extremes (hair loss possible); report headache, rash, nonhealing wounds, bleeding.

## sotalol hydrochloride
(Betapace, Betapace AF, Sorine, Sotylize)
**CLASS** Antiarrhythmic, beta blocker
**PREG/CONT** B/NA

**BBW** Do not give for ventricular arrhythmias unless pt unresponsive to other antiarrhythmics and has life-threatening ventricular arrhythmia. Monitor response carefully; proarrhythmic effect can be pronounced. Do not initiate tx if baseline QT interval >450 msec. If QT interval increases to ≥500 msec during tx, reduce dose, extend infusion time, or stop drug.
**IND & DOSE Tx of life-threatening ventricular arrhythmias** (*Betapace*); **maint of sinus rhythm after atrial fibrillation (AF) conversion** (*Betapace AF, Sotylize*). *Adult:* 80 mg PO bid. Adjust gradually, q 3 d, until appropriate response; may need 240–320 mg/d PO; up to 120 mg bid PO (*Betapace AF, Sotylize*). Or, 75 mg IV over 5 hr bid; may increase in increments of 75 mg/d q 3 d. Range, 225–300 mg once or twice a day for ventricular arrhythmias; 112.5 mg once or twice a day IV for AF if oral not possible. Converting between oral, IV doses: 80 mg oral–75 mg IV; 120 mg oral–112.5 mg IV; 160 mg oral–150 mg IV. *Child >2 yr w/normal renal function:* 30 mg/m$^2$ tid PO. Max, 60 mg/m$^2$ tid.
**ADJUST DOSE** Elderly pts, renal impairment
**ADV EFF Bronchospasm,** cardiac arrhythmias, constipation, decreased exercise tolerance/libido, ED, flatulence, gastric pain, **HF, laryngospasm,** n/v/d, **pulmonary edema, QT prolongation, stroke**
**INTERACTIONS** Antacids, aspirin, bismuth subsalicylate, clonidine, hormonal contraceptives, insulin, magnesium salicylate, NSAIDs, prazosin, QT-prolonging drugs, sulfinpyrazone
**NC/PT** Monitor QT interval. Switch from IV to oral as soon as possible. Do not stop abruptly; withdraw gradually. Not for use in breastfeeding. Pt should take on empty stomach; take safety precautions w/dizziness; report difficulty breathing, confusion, edema, chest pain.

## spironolactone
(Aldactone, CaroSpir)
**CLASS** Aldosterone antagonist, potassium-sparing diuretic
**PREG/CONT** High risk/NA

**BBW** Drug a tumorigen, w/chronic toxicity in rats; avoid unnecessary use.
**IND & DOSE Dx of hyperaldosteronism.** *Adult:* Long test, 400 mg/d PO for 3–4 wk; correction of hypokalemia, HTN presumptive evidence of primary hyperaldosteronism. Short test, 400 mg/d PO for 4 d. If serum potassium increases but decreases when drug stopped, presumptive dx can be made. **Tx of edema.** *Adult:* 100 mg/d PO; range, 25–200 mg/d. Or, 75 mg/d PO (*CaroSpir*). **Tx of HTN.** *Adult:* 50–100 mg/d PO for at least 2 wk. Or, 20–75 mg/d PO (*CaroSpir*). **Tx of hypokalemia.** *Adult:* 25–100 mg/d PO. **Tx of hyperaldosteronism.** *Adult:* 100–400 mg/d PO in preparation for surgery. **Tx of severe HF.** *Adult:* 25–50 mg/d PO if potassium ≤5 mEq/L, creatinine ≤2.5 mg/dL; 20 mg/d PO (*CaroSpir*).

**ADV EFF** Cramping, diarrhea, dizziness, drowsiness, gynecomastia, headache, hirsutism, hyperkalemia, voice deepening
**INTERACTIONS** ACE inhibitors, anticoagulants, antihypertensives, ARBs, corticosteroids, ganglionic blockers, heparin, licorice, potassium-rich diet, salicylates
**NC/PT** Monitor electrolytes periodically. Not for use in preg/breastfeeding. Pt should avoid potassium-rich foods, excessive licorice intake; take safety precautions w/dizziness; weigh self daily, report change of ≥3 lb/d; report swelling, muscle cramps/weakness.

## stavudine (d4T) (Zerit)
**CLASS** Antiviral, nucleoside reverse transcriptase inhibitor
**PREG/CONT** C/NA

**BBW** Monitor closely for pancreatitis during tx; fatal, nonfatal pancreatitis has occurred. Monitor LFTs; lactic acidosis, severe hepatomegaly possible.
**IND & DOSE** **Tx of HIV-1 infection w/other antivirals.** *Adult, child >13 d:* ≥60 kg, 40 mg PO q 12 hr; 30–<60 kg, 30 mg PO q 12 hr; <30 kg, 1 mg/kg/dose PO q 12 hr. *Child birth–13 d:* 0.5 mg/kg/dose PO q 12 hr.
**ADJUST DOSE** Renal impairment
**ADV EFF** Agranulocytopenia, asthenia, dizziness, fever, GI pain, headache, **hepatomegaly w/steatosis, lactic acidosis,** n/v/d, **pancreatitis,** paresthesia
**INTERACTIONS** Didanosine, doxorubicin, ribavirin, zidovudine
**NC/PT** Monitor LFTs, pancreatic function, neuro status before, q 2 wk during tx. Always give w/other antivirals. Not for use in preg (barrier contraceptives advised)/breastfeeding. Pt should take precautions to prevent spread (drug not a cure); avoid infections; take safety precautions for CNS effects; report numbness/tingling, severe headache, difficulty breathing.

▶ **NEW DRUG**

## stiripentol (Diacomit)
**CLASS** Anticonvulsant
**PREG/CONT** Unkn/NA

**IND & DOSE** **Tx of seizures associated w/Dravet syndrome in pts taking clobazam.** *Adult, child ≥2 yr:* 50 mg/kg/d PO in two or three divided doses. Max, 3,000 mg/d.
**ADV EFF** **Neutropenia,** somnolence, **suicidal ideation/behavior, thrombocytopenia,** weight loss, **withdrawal**
**INTERACTIONS** Suspension powder contains phenylalanine; CYP1A2, CYP2B6, CYP3A4, P-gp, BCRP substrates
**NC/PT** If adverse reactions, consider lower clobazam dose; reduce dose or discontinue gradually. Pt should swallow capsules whole w/glass of water during meal; not break or open capsules; mix powder for suspension in glass of water and take immediately during meal; enroll in preg exposure registry if preg.

## streptomycin sulfate (generic)
**CLASS** Antibiotic
**PREG/CONT** D/NA

**BBW** Risk of severe neurotoxic, nephrotoxic reactions; monitor closely. Do not use w/other neurotoxic, nephrotoxic drugs.
**IND & DOSE** **Tx of subacute bacterial endocarditis, resistant TB.** *Adult:* 15 mg/kg/d IM, or 25–30 mg/kg IM 2 or 3 ×/wk. *Child:* 20–40 mg/ kg/d IM or 25–30 mg/kg/IM 2 or 3 ×/wk. **Tx of tularemia.** *Adult:* 1–2 g/d IM for 7–14 d. **Tx of plaque.** *Adult:* 2 g/d IM in two divided doses for at least 10 d.
**ADJUST DOSE** Renal impairment
**ADV EFF** Dizziness, hearing loss, injection-site reactions, **renal toxicity, respiratory paralysis,** ringing in ears
**INTERACTIONS** Diuretics
**NC/PT** Monitor renal function, hearing regularly. Monitor injection sites.

Teach appropriate administration/disposal of needles/syringes. Ensure pt w/TB is also receiving other drugs. Not for use in preg (barrier contraceptives advised)/breastfeeding. Pt should take safety precautions for CNS effects; report difficulty breathing, dizziness, edema, hearing changes.

**streptozocin** (Zanosar)
**CLASS** Alkylating drug, antineoplastic
**PREG/CONT** D/NA

**BBW** Monitor for renal/hepatic toxicity. Special drug handling required.
**IND & DOSE** **Tx of metastatic islet cell carcinoma of pancreas.** *Adult:* 500 mg/m$^2$ IV for 5 consecutive d q 6 wk; or 1,000 mg/m$^2$ IV once/wk for 2 wk, then increase to 1,500 mg/m$^2$ IV each wk.
**ADJUST DOSE** Renal impairment
**ADV EFF** **Bone marrow suppression,** dizziness, drowsiness, glucose intolerance, n/v/d, **severe to fatal renal toxicity**
**INTERACTIONS** Doxorubicin
**NC/PT** Monitor LFTs, renal function closely. Handle drug as biohazard. Monitor CBC to determine dose. Give antiemetics for n/v. Not for use in preg/breastfeeding. Pt should avoid exposure to infection; maintain nutrition; report unusual bleeding/bruising, increased thirst, swelling.

**succimer** (Chemet)
**CLASS** Antidote, chelate
**PREG/CONT** C/NA

**IND & DOSE** **Tx of lead poisoning in child w/blood level >45 mcg/dL.** *Child:* 10 mg/kg or 350 mg/m$^2$ PO q 8 hr for 5 d; reduce to 10 mg/kg or 350 mg/m$^2$ PO q 12 hr for 2 wk (tx runs for 19 d).
**ADV EFF** Back pain, dizziness, drowsiness, flank pain, headache, n/v, rash, urination difficulties
**INTERACTIONS** EDTA
**NC/PT** Monitor serum lead level, transaminase levels before, q 2 wk during tx. Continue tx for full 19 d. Have pt swallow capsule whole; if unable to swallow capsule, open and sprinkle contents on soft food or give by spoon followed by fruit drink. Pt should maintain hydration; report difficulty breathing, tremors.

**sucralfate** (Carafate)
**CLASS** Antiulcer drug
**PREG/CONT** B/NA

**IND & DOSE** **Tx, maint of duodenal, esophageal ulcers.** *Adult:* 1 g PO qid on empty stomach for 4–8 wk; maint, 1 g PO bid.
**ADV EFF** Constipation, dizziness, dry mouth, gastric discomfort, rash, vertigo
**INTERACTIONS** Antacids, ciprofloxacin, digoxin, ketoconazole, levothyroxine, penicillamine, phenytoin, quinidine, tetracycline, theophylline, warfarin
**NC/PT** Pt should take on empty stomach, 1 hr before or 2 hr after meals, and at bedtime; avoid antacids within 30 min of sucralfate; take safety precautions for CNS effects; use laxative for constipation; report severe gastric pain.

DANGEROUS DRUG

**sufentanil** (Dsuvia), **sufentanil citrate** (generic)
**CLASS** General anesthetic, opioid agonist analgesic
**PREG/CONT** Moderate risk /C-II

**BBW** *Dsuvia:* Accidental exposure/ingestion, especially in child, can result in respiratory depression, death. Available only through REMS Program. Should only be administered by health care provider in certified medical setting. Serious, life-threatening, or fatal respiratory depression may occur. Monitor closely, especially during initiation. Risk of opioid addiction, abuse, misuse. Assess risk before prescribing; monitor regularly for these behaviors. Use w/CYP3A4 inhibitors (or discontinuation of CYP3A4 inducers) can result in fatal sufentanil overdose. Use of opioids w/ benzodiazepines or other CNS depressants, including alcohol, may result in profound sedation, respiratory depression, coma, death. Reserve concomitant prescribing for pts for whom alternative tx options are inadequate; limit dosage/duration to minimum required; observe pt for respiratory depression/sedation s&sx.

**BBW** *Sufenta:* Accidental exposure, especially in child, can result in respiratory depression/death. Risk of opioid addiction, abuse, misuse. Use w/ CYP3A4 inhibitors, benzodiazepines, other CNS depressants can result in overdose/death. Only available via restricted program to be administered by health care provider in certified medical center.

**IND & DOSE** **Adjunct to general anesthesia.** *Adult:* Initially, 1–2 mcg/kg IV. Maint, 10–25 mcg; max, 1 mcg/kg/hr of expected surgical time. **Anesthesia.** *Adult:* Initially, 8–30 mcg/kg IV; supplement w/doses of 0.5–10 mcg/kg IV. Max, 30 mcg/kg for procedure. Give w/oxygen, skeletal muscle relaxant. *Child 2–12 yr:* Initially, 10–25 mcg/kg IV; supplement w/doses of 25–50 mcg IV. Give w/oxygen, skeletal muscle relaxant. **Epidural analgesia.** *Adult:* 10–15 mcg via epidural administration w/10 mL bupivacaine 0.125%. May repeat twice at 1-hr or longer intervals (total, three doses). **Tx of acute pain severe enough to require opioid analgesic and when alternative tx is inadequate, in supervised health care setting (*Dsuvia*).** *Adult:* 30 mcg SL prn w/at least 1 hr between doses; max, 12 tablets in 24 hr.

**ADV EFF** **Adrenal insufficiency (*Dsuvia*), arrhythmias, bradycardia, bronchospasm, cardiac arrest,** clamminess, confusion, constipation, dizziness, dry mouth, headache, floating feeling, **hypotension (*Dsuvia*), laryngospasm,** lethargy, lightheadedness, n/v, **respiratory depression (*Dsuvia*),** sedation, **serotonin syndrome (*Dsuvia*), shock,** tachycardia, urinary hesitancy, urine retention, vertigo

**INTERACTIONS** Barbiturates, beta blockers, calcium channel blockers, general anesthetics, grapefruit juice, hypnotics, opiate agonists, sedatives

**NC/PT** *Dsuvia:* Contraindicated if significant respiratory depression, acute or severe bronchial asthma, GI obstruction, hypersensitivity. Do not use for >72 hr. Pt should minimize talking and not eat or drink for 10 min after each dose. *Sufentanil citrate:* Protect vials from light. Provide opioid antagonist. Have equipment for assisted, controlled respiration on hand during parenteral administration. Give to breastfeeding women 4–6 hr before next feeding. Pt should avoid grapefruit juice; take safety precautions for CNS effects; report difficulty breathing, palpitations. Name confusion between sufentanil and fentanyl; use extreme caution.

---

## **sugammadex** (Bridion)

**CLASS** Modified gamma cyclodextrin, reversal agent

**PREG/CONT** Low risk/NA

**IND & DOSE** **Reversal of neuromuscular blockade induced by rocuronium/vecuronium in adults undergoing surgery.** *Adult:* For rocuronium/vecuronium: 4 mg/kg IV as a single bolus, based on twitch response; 2 mg/kg if response is faster. Rocuronium only: 16 mg/kg IV as a single bolus if there is need to reverse blockade within 3 min after single dose of rocuronium.

**ADJUST DOSE** Severe renal impairment

**ADV EFF** **Bradycardia,** extremity pain, headache, hypotension, n/v/d, pain

**INTERACTIONS** Hormonal contraceptives, toremifene
**NC/PT** Monitor cardiac/respiratory function. Pt should be on ventilator support. Use of anticholinergic for bradycardia is recommended. Twitch response should determine success and dosing. Pt should use second method of contraception (hormonal contraceptives may be ineffective) and continue for 7 d post drug administration.

## sulfADIAZINE (generic)

**CLASS** Sulfonamide antibiotic
**PREG/CONT** C; d (labor & delivery)/NA

**IND & DOSE** **Tx of acute infections caused by susceptible bacteria strains.** *Adult:* 2–4 g PO, then 2–4 g/d PO in three–six divided doses. *Child >2 mo:* 75 mg/kg PO, then 150 mg/kg/d PO in four–six divided doses; max 6 g/d **Tx of toxoplasmosis.** *Adult:* 1–1.5 g PO qid w/pyrimethamine for 3–4 wk. *Child >2 mo:* 100–200 mg/kg/d PO w/pyrimethamine for 3–4 wk. **Suppressive, maint tx in HIV pts.** *Adult:* 0.5–1 g PO q 6 hr w/oral pyrimethamine, leucovorin. *Infant, child:* 85–120 mg/kg/d PO in two–four divided doses w/oral pyrimethamine, leucovorin. *Adolescent:* 0.5–1 g PO q 6 hr w/oral pyrimethamine, leucovorin. **Px of recurrent attacks of rheumatic fever.** *Adult:* >30 kg, 1 g/d PO; <30 kg, 0.5 g/d PO.
**ADV EFF** Abd pain, crystalluria, headache, hematuria, **hepatocellular necrosis,** n/v, photosensitivity, rash, **SJS**
**INTERACTIONS** Acetohexamide, chlorpropamide, cyclosporine, glyburide, glipizide, oral anticoagulants, phenytoin, tolbutamide, tolazamide
**NC/PT** Culture before tx. Pt should take on empty stomach 1 hr before or 2 hr after meals w/full glass of water; drink 8 glasses of water/d; avoid sun exposure; take safety precautions for CNS effects; report bloody urine, ringing in ears, difficulty breathing. Name confusion between sulfadiazine and *Silvadene* (silver sulfadiazine).

## sulfaSALAzine (Azulfidine)

**CLASS** Anti-inflammatory, antirheumatic, sulfonamide
**PREG/CONT** B/NA

**IND & DOSE** **Tx of ulcerative colitis; to prolong time between acute attacks.** *Adult:* 3–4 g/d PO in evenly divided doses. Maint, 2 g/d PO in evenly spaced doses (500 mg qid); max, 4 g/d. *Child ≥6 yr:* 40–60 mg/kg/24 hr PO in three–six divided doses. Maint, 30 mg/kg/24 hr PO in four equally divided doses; max, 2 g/d.
**ADV EFF** Abd pain, **agranulocytosis, aplastic anemia,** crystalluria, headache, hematuria, **hepatocellular necrosis,** n/v, paresthesia, photosensitivity, **SJS, thrombocytopenia**
**INTERACTIONS** Digoxin, folate
**NC/PT** Pt should take w/meals; swallow DR tablet whole and not cut/crush/chew it; drink 8 glasses of water/d; avoid sun exposure; take safety precautions for CNS effects; report difficulty breathing, bloody urine, rash.

## sulindac (generic)

**CLASS** NSAID
**PREG/CONT** High risk/NA

**BBW** Increased risk of CV events, GI bleeding; monitor accordingly. Contraindicated for periop pain in CABG surgery.
**IND & DOSE** **Tx of pain of RA, osteoarthritis, ankylosing spondylitis.** *Adult:* 150 mg PO bid. **Tx of acute painful shoulder, acute gouty arthritis.** *Adult:* 200 mg PO bid for 7–14 d (acute painful shoulder), 7 d (acute gouty arthritis).
**ADJUST DOSE** Hepatic/renal impairment
**ADV EFF** **Anaphylactoid reactions to fatal anaphylactic shock, bone**

**marrow suppression,** constipation, CV events, dizziness, drowsiness, dyspepsia, edema, fatigue, GI pain, headache, insomnia, **HF,** n/v, vision disturbances
**INTERACTIONS** Beta blockers, diuretics, lithium
**NC/PT** Not for use in preg/breastfeeding. Pt should take w/food, milk if GI upset; take safety precautions for CNS effects; report swelling, difficulty breathing, black tarry stools.

## SUMAtriptan succinate
(Imitrex, Onzetra Xsail, Zembrace)
**CLASS** Antimigraine drug, triptan
**PREG/CONT** C/NA

**IND & DOSE Tx of acute migraine attacks.** *Adult:* 25, 50, or 100 mg PO; may repeat in ≥2 hr. Max, 200 mg/d. Or, 6 mg subcut; may repeat in 1 hr. Max, 12 mg/24 hr. Or, 5, 10, or 20 mg into one nostril, or 10 mg divided into two doses (5 mg each), one in each nostril, repeated q 2 hr; max, 40 mg/24 hr. Or, 22 mg nasal powder via nosepiece in each nostril (each side delivers 11 mg [*Onzetra Xsail*]); max, 44 mg/d. Or, 3 mg subcut; max, 12 mg/d in separate doses at least 1 hr apart (*Zembrace*). **Tx of cluster headaches.** *Adult:* 6 mg subcut; may repeat in 1 hr. Max, 12 mg/24 hr.
**ADJUST DOSE** Hepatic impairment
**ADV EFF** Altered BP, arrhythmias, burning/tingling sensation, chest pain/pressure, dizziness, feeling of tightness, GI ischemic reactions, headache, injection-site reactions, **MI, serotonin syndrome, shock**
**INTERACTIONS** Ergots, MAOIs, St. John's wort
**NC/PT** For tx, not px, of acute migraines. May repeat dose in 2 hr if needed. Teach proper administration of each form; use of Xsail powdered nasal delivery device; disposal of needles/syringes for subcut use. Needle shield of prefilled syringe contains dry natural rubber, which may cause allergic reactions in latex-sensitive pt. Not for use in preg (barrier contraceptives advised)/breastfeeding. If breastfeeding, pt should wait 12 hr after tx. Pt should continue migraine comfort measures; take safety precautions for CNS effects; avoid St. John's wort; report chest pain, swelling, numbness/tingling.

**DANGEROUS DRUG**

## SUNItinib (Sutent)
**CLASS** Antineoplastic, kinase inhibitor
**PREG/CONT** High risk/NA

**BBW** Risk of serious to fatal hepatotoxicity; monitor LFTs closely.
**IND & DOSE Tx of GI stromal tumor, advanced renal cell carcinoma.** *Adult:* 50 mg/d PO for 4 wk, then 2 wk of rest. Repeat cycle. **Tx of progressive neuroendocrine cancerous pancreatic tumors.** 37.5 mg/d PO continuously. **Adjuvant tx of renal cell carcinoma in pts at high risk for recurrence post nephrectomy.** *Adult:* 50 mg/d PO for 4 wk, then 2 wk of rest, for total of nine cycles.
**ADJUST DOSE** Hepatic impairment, ESRD pts on hemodialysis
**ADV EFF** Abd pain, arthralgia, asthenia, anorexia, **cardiotoxicity,** constipation, cough, **dermatologic toxicity to SJS,** dyspnea, edema, fatigue, fever, **hemorrhage, hepatotoxicity, HTN,** hypoglycemia, mucositis, n/v/d, **prolonged QT,** proteinuria, skin color changes, **thyroid dysfx, thrombotic microangiopathy**
**INTERACTIONS** CYP3A4 inducers/inhibitors, grapefruit juice, QT-prolonging drugs
**NC/PT** Obtain baseline, periodic ECG, BP. Monitor LFTs, renal function. Not for use in preg (barrier contraceptives advised)/breastfeeding. Pt should mark calendar for tx days; take safety precaution for CNS effects; report unusual bleeding, palpitations, urine/stool color changes, rash, chest pain.

**suvorexant** (Belsomra)
**CLASS** Insomnia drug, orexin receptor antagonist
**PREG/CONT** C/NA

**IND & DOSE Tx of insomnia w/ difficulty w/sleep onset or maint.** *Adult:* 10 mg PO within 30 min of going to bed w/at least 7 hr til planned awakening; may increase to 20 mg/d.
**ADJUST DOSE** Hepatic impairment
**ADV EFF** Daytime somnolence, depression, respiratory impairment, sleep driving, sleep paralysis
**INTERACTIONS** CYP3A4 inducers/ inhibitors, digoxin
**NC/PT** Ensure timing of dose; allow 7 hr for sleep. Not for use in preg; use w/caution in breastfeeding. Pt should use safety precautions w/daytime somnolence, sleep driving, CNS effects; report cognitive impairment, difficulty breathing.

**tacrolimus** (Astagraf XL, Envarsus XR, Prograf, Protopic)
**CLASS** Immunosuppressant
**PREG/CONT** High risk/NA

**BBW** High risk of infection, lymphoma. Protect from infection; monitor closely. ER form not recommended for liver transplants; risk of death in female liver transplant pts.
**IND & DOSE Px of rejection after kidney transplant.** *Adult:* 0.2 mg/kg/d PO divided q 12 hr, or 0.03–0.05 mg/ kg/d as continuous IV infusion. Or, 0.1 mg/kg/d PO ER capsule preop, 0.15–0.2 mg/kg/d PO ER capsule postop; if using basiliximab, 0.15 mg/ kg/d PO ER capsule. Transferring from regular release to *Envarsus ER*, 80% of tacrolimus dose as once/d ER form. *Child who can swallow capsules intact:* 0.3 mg/kg PO daily after basiliximab, MMF and steroids (Astagraf XL). *Child:* 0.3 mg/kg/day PO dosed every 12 hours (Prograf). **Px of rejection after liver transplant.** *Adult:* 0.10–0.15 mg/kg/d PO divided q 12 hr; give initial dose no sooner than 6 hr after transplant. Or, 0.03–0.05 mg/kg/d as continuous IV infusion. *Child:* 0.15–0.20 mg/kg/d PO, or 0.03–0.05 mg/kg/d IV infusion. **Px of rejection after heart transplant.** *Adult:* 0.075 mg/kg/d PO or IV in two divided doses q 12 hr; give first dose no sooner than 6 hr after transplant. **Tx of atopic dermatitis.** *Adult:* Apply thin layer 0.03% or 0.1% ointment to affected area bid; rub in gently, completely. *Child 2–15 yr:* Apply thin layer 0.03% ointment bid.
**ADJUST DOSE** Hepatic/ renal impairment
**ADV EFF** Abd pain, **anaphylaxis,** constipation, diarrhea, fever, **GI perforation,** headache, **hepatotoxicity,** hyperglycemia, **infections, RPLS, prolonged QT,** renal impairment
**INTERACTIONS** Calcium channel blockers, carbamazepine, cimetidine, clarithromycin, cyclosporine (contraindicated), erythromycin, grapefruit juice, live vaccines, metoclopramide, nicardipine, phenobarbital, phenytoin, QT-prolonging drugs, rifamycins, sirolimus (contraindicated), statins, St. John's wort
**NC/PT** *Envarsus XR, Astagraf XL* not interchangeable w/any other forms. Check drug regimen; many interactions possible. Ensure concurrent use of corticosteroids in liver transplants; use w/mycophenolate or azathioprine in heart/kidney transplants. Monitor LFTs, serum tacrolimus, neuro status. Use IV route only if PO not possible; switch to PO as soon as possible. Not for use in preg/breastfeeding. Pt should avoid sun exposure (topical form), infection; avoid grapefruit juice, St. John's wort, live vaccines; report unusual bleeding, s&sx of infection, all drugs being taken, severe GI pain.

**tadalafil** (Adcirca, Alyq, Cialis)
**CLASS** Impotence drug, phosphodiesterase-5 inhibitor
**PREG/CONT** Low risk/NA

**IND & DOSE** **Tx of ED, BPH w/ED (*Cialis*).** *Adult:* 10 mg PO before anticipated sexual activity; range, 5–20 mg PO. Limit use to once/d. Or, 2.5–5 mg/d PO w/o regard to timing of sexual activity. **Tx of pulmonary arterial HTN (*Adcirca, Alyq*).** 40 mg/d PO.
**ADJUST DOSE** Hepatic/renal impairment; tx w/CYP3A4 inhibitors
**ADV EFF** Diarrhea, dizziness, dyspepsia, dry mouth, flulike sx, flushing, headache, **MI, priapism, SJS,** vision loss
**INTERACTIONS** Alcohol, alpha blockers, erythromycin, grapefruit juice, indinavir, itraconazole, ketoconazole, nitrates, rifampin, ritonavir; riociguat (contraindicated)
**NC/PT** Ensure proper dx. For pulmonary HTN, pt should monitor activity and limitations. For ED, does not protect against STDs, will not work in absence of sexual stimulation. Pt should not use w/nitrates, antihypertensives, grapefruit juice, alcohol; report vision changes, loss of vision, erection lasting >4 hr, sudden hearing loss.

**▶NEW DRUG**

**tafamidis** (Vyndamax), **tafamidis meglumine** (Vyndaqel)
**CLASS** Endocrine-metabolic agent, transthyretin stabilizer
**PREG/CONT** High risk based on animal studies/NA

**IND & DOSE** **Tx of cardiomyopathy of wild-type or hereditary transthyretin-mediated amyloidosis to reduce CV mortality/CV-related hospitalization.** *Adult:* 61 mg (tafamidis) or 80 mg (tafamidis meglumine) PO daily w/ or w/o food.
**INTERACTIONS** BCRP substrates
**NC/PT** Pts may voluntarily register in Transthyretin Amyloidosis Outcome Survey and provide information to assess disease progression, genotype/phenotype relationships, impact of interventions on disease progression. Advise preg pt of potential fetal risk and to avoid breastfeeding during tx.

**▶NEW DRUG**

**tagraxofusp-erzs** (Elzonris)
**CLASS** Antineoplastic, anti-CD123 agent
**PREG/CONT** High risk/NA

**BBW** Risk of capillary leak syndrome.
**IND & DOSE** **Tx of blastic plasmacytoid dendritic cell neoplasm.** *Adult, child ≥2 yr:* 12 mcg/kg IV once daily on days 1–5 of 21-d cycle. May extend to d 10 if dose delays. Continue until disease progression or unacceptable toxicity.
**ADV EFF** **Capillary leak syndrome,** edema, fatigue, **hepatotoxicity, hypersensitivity, hypoalbuminemia,** hypoglycemia, nausea, weight increase
**NC/PT** Before first dose, ensure serum albumin is ≥3.2 g/dL. Give $H_1$- and $H_2$-histamine antagonists, acetaminophen, and corticosteroid before each infusion. Administer in inpatient setting or in suitable outpatient ambulatory care setting equipped w/appropriate monitoring for pts w/hematopoietic malignancies. Observe pts for minimum of 4 hr after each infusion.

**talazoparib** (Talzenna)
**CLASS** Antineoplastic, poly polymerase inhibitor
**PREG/CONT** High risk/NA

**IND & DOSE** **Tx of adults w/deleterious germline BRCA-mutated HER2-negative locally advanced or metastatic breast cancer.** *Adult:* 1 mg

PO daily. Give 0.75 mg PO daily if renal impairment (CrCl 30–59 mL/min).
**ADV EFF** Alopecia, anemia, decreased appetite, diarrhea, fatigue, headache, neutropenia, thrombocytopenia, vomiting
**INTERACTIONS** P-gp/BCRP inhibitors; may increase adverse effects
**NC/PT** Monitor for myelodysplastic syndrome/acute myeloid leukemia and myelosuppression by checking Hgb, platelets, WBCs. Calcium decreases, glucose and liver enzymes increases possible. May reduce dosage if adverse effects, renal insufficiency. High risk of embryo-fetal toxicity (contraceptives advised during and for at least 7 mo post tx). Pt should swallow capsule whole; take w/ or w/o food; avoid breastfeeding until at least 1 mo after final dose.

## talc (Sclerosol, Steritalc)
**CLASS** Sclerosing drug
**PREG/CONT** B/NA

**IND & DOSE To decrease recurrence of malignant pleural effusion.** *Adult:* 5 g in 50–100 mL sodium chloride injection injected into chest tube after pleural fluid drained; clamp chest tube, have pt change positions for 2 hr; unclamp chest tube, continue external suction.
**ADV EFF Acute pneumonitis,** dyspnea, hypotension, localized bleeding, **MI, RDS,** tachycardia
**NC/PT** Ensure proper chest tube placement, pt positioning, draining. Pt should report difficulty breathing, chest pain.

## taliglucerase alfa (Elelyso)
**CLASS** Enzyme
**PREG/CONT** Low risk/NA

**IND & DOSE Long-term enzyme replacement tx for adult, child w/type 1 Gaucher disease.** *Adult, child ≥4 yr:* 60 units/kg IV q other wk as 60- to 120-min infusion. If switching from imiglucerase, start at unit/kg dose used in last imiglucerase dose.
**ADV EFF Anaphylaxis,** arthralgia, back pain, headache, influenza, **infusion reaction,** pain, pharyngitis, throat infection, URI
**NC/PT** Give IV only. Monitor for infusion reactions; decrease infusion rate, consider use of antipyretics, antihistamines. Pt should mark calendar for infusion dates; report difficulty breathing, fever, chest/back pain, rash.

## talimogene laherparepvec (Imlygic)
**CLASS** Oncolytic viral therapy
**PREG/CONT** High risk/NA

**IND & DOSE Local tx of unresectable cutaneous, subcut, nodal lesions in melanoma recurrent after surgery.** *Adult:* Initially, up to 4 mL at concentration of $10^6$ plaque-forming units(pfu)/mL injected into lesions; subsequent doses up to 4 mL at concentration of $10^8$ pfu/mL.
**ADV EFF** Chills, fatigue, fever, flulike sx, herpetic infections, injection-site reaction, plasmacytoma at injection site
**NC/PT** Accidental drug exposure may lead to herpetic infection; should not be prepared or handled by immunocompromised or preg providers. Providers and pt contacts should avoid exposure to dressings or bodily fluids of pt receiving drug. Provide proper treatment to pt who develops herpetic infections. Monitor injection site; treat appropriately if infection, delayed healing occurs. Monitor pt for plasmacytoma at injection site. May cause airway obstruction if injection near major airway. Not for use in preg (contraceptives advised)/breastfeeding. Pt should keep injection sites covered; wear gloves when changing dressings; avoid touching or scratching injection sites; caution preg or immunocompromised contacts to avoid

dressings, bodily fluids, injection sites; report pain, s&sx of infection at injection site, continued fever.

**DANGEROUS DRUG**

## tamoxifen citrate

(Soltamox)

**CLASS** Antiestrogen, antineoplastic

**PREG/CONT** High risk/NA

**BBW** Alert women w/ductal carcinoma in situ (DCIS) and those at high risk for breast cancer of risks of serious to potentially fatal drug effects, including stroke, embolic events, uterine malignancies; discuss benefits/risks.

**IND & DOSE** **Tx of estrogen receptor–positive metastatic breast cancer.** *Adult:* 20–40 mg/d PO. Give doses of >20 mg/d in divided doses, a.m. and p.m. **To reduce breast cancer incidence in high-risk women; tx of DCIS; adjuvant tx w/early-stage estrogen receptor–positive breast cancer.** *Adult:* 20 mg/d PO.

**ADV EFF** Corneal changes, depression, dizziness, **DVT**, edema, hot flashes, n/v, **PE**, rash, **stroke,** vaginal bleeding

**INTERACTIONS** Bromocriptine, cytotoxic agents, grapefruit juice, oral anticoagulants

**NC/PT** Monitor CBC periodically. Not for use in preg (barrier contraceptives advised)/breastfeeding. Pt should have regular gynecologic exams; take safety precautions for CNS effects, report leg pain/swelling, chest pain, difficulty breathing.

## tamsulosin hydrochloride (Flomax)

**CLASS** Alpha-adrenergic blocker, BPH drug

**PREG/CONT** NA/NA

**IND & DOSE** **Tx of s&sx of BPH.** *Adult:* 0.4–0.8 mg PO daily 30 min after same meal each day.

**ADV EFF** Abnormal ejaculation, dizziness, headache, insomnia, intraop floppy iris syndrome, orthostatic hypotension, priapism, somnolence

**INTERACTIONS** Alpha-adrenergic antagonists, avanafil, cimetidine, saw palmetto, sildenafil, tadalafil, vardenafil

**NC/PT** Ensure accurate dx. Not for use in women. Alert surgeon; increased risk of intraop floppy iris syndrome w/cataract/glaucoma surgery. Monitor for prostate cancer. Pt should swallow capsule whole and not cut/crush/chew it; change position slowly to avoid dizziness; not take w/ED drugs; take safety precautions for CNS effects; avoid saw palmetto; report fainting, worsening of sx, prolonged erection. Name confusion between *Flomax* (tamsulosin) and *Fosamax* (alendronate).

## tapentadol (Nucynta, Nucynta ER)

**CLASS** Norepinephrine reuptake inhibitor, opioid receptor analgesic

**PREG/CONT** High risk/C-II

**BBW** Risk of abuse; limit use w/hx of addiction; FDA mandates a REMS. Risk of fatal respiratory depression, highest at start and w/dose changes; monitor accordingly. Accidental ingestion of ER form can cause fatal overdose in child; secure drug. Risk of fatally high tapentadol level w/alcohol; pt should avoid alcohol, all medications containing alcohol, and other CNS depressants.

**IND & DOSE** **Relief of moderate to severe pain.** *Adult:* 50–100 mg PO q 4–6 hr. **Mgt of moderate to severe chronic pain when round-the-clock opioid use needed** (ER form). *Adult:* 100–250 mg PO bid. Reduce initial dose to 50 mg in analgesic-naïve pt; max, 500 mg/d. **Relief of pain of diabetic peripheral neuropathy** (*Nucynta ER*). *Adult:* 50 mg PO bid.

**ADJUST DOSE** Elderly, debilitated pts; hepatic impairment
**ADV EFF** Dizziness, drowsiness, headache, n/v, respiratory depression, **serotonin syndrome, seizures,** withdrawal sx
**INTERACTIONS** Alcohol, CNS depressants, general anesthetics, hypnotics, MAOIs, opioids, phenothiazines, sedatives, St. John's wort, SSRIs, TCAs, triptans
**NC/PT** Assess pain before, periodically during tx. Withdraw gradually. Do not give within 14 d of MAOIs. Not for use w/severe asthma, respiratory depression, paralytic ileus. Not for use in preg/breastfeeding. Pt should avoid alcohol, St. John's wort; take safety precautions for CNS effects; report difficulty breathing, rash.

## tasimelteon (Hetlioz)
**CLASS** Melatonin receptor agonist
**PREG/CONT** High risk/NA

**IND & DOSE** **Tx of non-24 hr-sleep-wake disorder in totally blind pts.** *Adult:* 20 mg before bedtime at same time each night.
**ADJUST DOSE** Severe hepatic impairment, smokers
**ADV EFF** Elevated alanine aminotransferase, headache, nightmares, somnolence, URI, UTI
**INTERACTIONS** Fluvoxamine, ketoconazole, rifampin
**NC/PT** Monitor LFTs. Pt should swallow capsule whole and not cut/crush/chew it; avoid preg/breastfeeding; limit activities after taking drug; take safety measures w/somnolence; report changes in behavior, severe somnolence.

## tbo-filgrastim (Granix)
**CLASS** Leukocyte growth factor
**PREG/CONT** High risk/NA

**IND & DOSE** **To reduce duration of severe neutropenia w/nonmyeloid malignancies in pts receiving myelosuppressive anticancer drugs.** *Adult, child ≥1 mo:* 5 mcg/kg/d subcut, first dose no earlier than 24 hr after myelosuppressive chemo. Continue until neutrophil count has recovered to normal range.
**ADV EFF** **Acute respiratory distress syndrome,** allergic reactions, **alveolar hemorrhage, aortitis,** bone pain, capillary leak syndrome, leukocytosis, sickle cell crisis, **splenic rupture**
**NC/PT** Monitor CBC, respiratory function. Do not give within 24 hr before scheduled chemo; not recommended for use w/chemo, radiation. Stop if sickle cell crisis suspected. Not for use in preg/breastfeeding. Teach proper subcut injection technique, proper disposal of needles/syringes. Pt should report difficulty breathing, edema, rash.

## tedizolid (Sivextro)
**CLASS** Antibacterial, oxazolidinone
**PREG/CONT** Moderate risk/NA

**IND & DOSE** **Tx of acute skin/skin-structure infections caused by susceptible bacteria.** *Adult:* 200 mg/d PO, or IV infused over 1 hr for 6 d.
**ADV EFF** CDAD, dizziness, headache, n/v/d
**NC/PT** Perform culture/sensitivity to ensure proper use. Safety for use in neutropenia not known; consider other tx in pts w/neutropenia. Use w/caution in preg/breastfeeding. Pt should complete full course; use safety precautions w/dizziness; report diarrhea w/blood or mucus.

## teduglutide (Gattex)
**CLASS** Glucagon-like peptide-2
**PREG/CONT** B/NA

**IND & DOSE** **Tx of pts w/short bowel syndrome who are dependent on**

**parenteral support.** *Adult, child ≥1 yr:* 0.05 mg/kg subcut daily.
**ADJUST DOSE** Renal impairment
**ADV EFF** Abd pain/distention, **biliary and pancreatic disease, fluid overload,** headache, **intestinal obstruction, neoplastic growth,** n/v
**INTERACTIONS** Oral drugs
**NC/PT** Subcut use only. Single-use vial; discard within 3 hr of reconstitution. Ensure complete colonoscopy, polyp removal before tx and at least q 5 yr. Rotate injection sites. Monitor for fluid overload; support as needed. Oral drugs may not be absorbed; monitor pt, consider need for oral drug dosage adjustment. Monitor pancreatic function. Pt should learn preparation of subcut injection, disposal of needles/syringes; rotate injection sites; schedule periodic blood tests; report severe abd pain, chest pain, swelling in extremities, severe epigastric pain, difficulty swallowing.

## telavancin (Vibativ)
**CLASS** Antibiotic, lipoglycopeptide
**PREG/CONT** High risk/NA

**BBW** Fetal risk; women of childbearing age should have serum preg test before start of tx. Avoid use in preg; advise contraceptive use. Nephrotoxicity possible, not for use in severe renal impairment; balance risk in moderate impairment. Monitor renal function in all pts.
**IND & DOSE Tx of complicated skin/skin-structure infections caused by susceptible strains of gram-positive organisms. Tx of hospital-acquired and ventilator-assisted pneumonia caused by *Staphylococcus aureus* when other tx not suitable.** *Adult:* 10 mg/kg IV infused over 60 min once q 24 hr for 7–14 d.
**ADJUST DOSE** Renal impairment
**ADV EFF** Bleeding, CDAD, dizziness, foamy urine, **nephrotoxicity,** n/v, **prolonged QT,** red man syndrome (w/rapid infusion), taste disturbance
**INTERACTIONS** Heparin, nephrotoxic drugs, QT-prolonging drugs
**NC/PT** Culture before tx. Infuse over at least 60 min. Monitor clotting time, renal function periodically. Not for use in preg (contraceptives advised)/breastfeeding. Negative preg test needed before tx. Urine may become foamy. Pt should take safety precautions for CNS effects; report fever, unusual bleeding, irregular heartbeat.

## telithromycin (Ketek)
**CLASS** Ketolide antibiotic
**PREG/CONT** C/NA

**BBW** Contraindicated w/myasthenia gravis; life-threatening respiratory failure possible.
**IND & DOSE Tx of mild to moderately severe community-acquired pneumonia caused by susceptible strains.** *Adult:* 800 mg/d PO for 7–10 d.
**ADJUST DOSE** Renal impairment
**ADV EFF Anaphylaxis,** CDAD, diarrhea, dizziness, headache, **hepatic impairment,** n/v, **prolonged QT, pseudomembranous colitis,** superinfections, visual disturbances
**INTERACTIONS** Serious reactions w/atorvastatin, lovastatin, midazolam, pimozide, simvastatin; avoid these combos. Also, carbamazepine, digoxin, metoprolol, phenobarbital, phenytoin, QT-prolonging drugs, rifampin, theophylline
**NC/PT** Culture before tx. Monitor LFTs. Treat superinfections. Pt should swallow tablet whole and not cut/crush/chew it; take safety precautions w/dizziness; avoid quickly looking between distant and nearby objects (if visual difficulties); report bloody diarrhea, difficulty breathing, unusual bleeding.

**telmisartan** (Micardis)
**CLASS** Antihypertensive, ARB
**PREG/CONT** High risk/NA

**BBW** Rule out preg before tx. Suggest barrier contraceptives during tx; fetal injury, deaths have occurred.
**IND & DOSE Tx of HTN.** *Adult:* 40 mg/d PO. Range, 20–80 mg/d; max, 80 mg/d. **To reduce CV risk in high-risk pts unable to take ACE inhibitors.** *Adult:* 80 mg/d PO.
**ADJUST DOSE** Hepatic/renal impairment
**ADV EFF** Dermatitis, dizziness, flatulence, gastritis, headache, hyperkalemia, hypotension, light-headedness, palpitations, rash
**INTERACTIONS** ACE inhibitors, ARBs, digoxin, potassium-sparing diuretics, renin inhibitors
**NC/PT** Monitor renal function, LFTs, potassium level. Monitor BP carefully. Alert surgeon; volume replacement may be needed postop. Not for use in preg (contraceptives advised)/breastfeeding. Pt should take safety precautions for CNS effects; report fever, severe dizziness.

**telotristat etiprate** (Xermelo)
**CLASS** Antidiarrheal, tryptophan hydroxylase inhibitor
**PREG/CONT** Low risk/NA

**IND & DOSE Tx of carcinoid syndrome diarrhea w/somatostatin analog therapy.** *Adult:* 250 mg PO tid w/food.
**ADV EFF** Abd pain, constipation, decreased appetite, depression, fever, flatulence, headache, peripheral edema
**INTERACTIONS** CYP3A substrates
**NC/PT** Give w/somatostatin analog. Monitor for constipation/abd pain; discontinue if severe. Monitor breastfed babies for constipation. Pt should take w/food; monitor bowel function; report constipation/abd pain.

**temazepam** (Restoril)
**CLASS** Benzodiazepine, sedative-hypnotic
**PREG/CONT** High risk/C-IV

**BBW** Concomitant use of benzodiazepines and opioids may result in profound sedation, respiratory depression, coma, death. Taper dosage gradually after long-term use; risk of refractory seizures. Assess for s&sx of respiratory depression/sedation.
**IND & DOSE Short-term tx of insomnia.** *Adult:* 15–30 mg PO before bedtime for 7–10 d; 7.5 mg may be sufficient for some pts
**ADJUST DOSE** Elderly, debilitated pts
**ADV EFF Anaphylaxis, angioedema,** bradycardia, confusion, constipation, **CV collapse,** diarrhea, drowsiness, drug dependence, fatigue, hiccups, nervousness, tachycardia, urticaria
**INTERACTIONS** Alcohol, aminophylline, CNS depressants, dyphylline, theophylline
**NC/PT** Not for use in preg (contraceptives advised)/breastfeeding. Pt should take for no longer than 7–10 d; avoid alcohol; take safety precautions for CNS effects; report difficulty breathing, face/eye swelling, continued sleep disorders.

**DANGEROUS DRUG**

**temozolomide** (Temodar)
**CLASS** Alkylating agent, antineoplastic
**PREG/CONT** High risk/NA

**IND & DOSE Tx of refractory astrocytoma.** *Adult:* 150 mg/m$^2$/d PO or IV for 5 consecutive d for 28-d tx cycle. **Tx of glioblastoma multiforme.** *Adult:* 75 mg/m$^2$/d PO or IV for 42 d w/focal radiation therapy; then six cycles: Cycle 1, 150 mg/m$^2$/d PO, IV for 5 d then 23 d rest; cycles 2–6, 200 mg/m$^2$/d PO or IV for 5 d then 23 d rest.

**ADJUST DOSE** Elderly pts; hepatic/renal impairment
**ADV EFF** Alopecia, amnesia, **bone marrow suppression, cancer,** constipation, dizziness, headache, **hepatotoxicity,** insomnia, n/v/d, ***Pneumocystis jirovecii* pneumonia,** rash, **seizures**
**INTERACTIONS** Valproic acid
**NC/PT** Monitor LFTs. Monitor CBC before each dose; adjustment may be needed. Not for use in preg (contraceptives advised)/breastfeeding. Pt should take safety precautions for CNS effects; avoid exposure to infection; report unusual bleeding, difficulty breathing.

**DANGEROUS DRUG**

## temsirolimus (Torisel)

**CLASS** Antineoplastic, kinase inhibitor
**PREG/CONT** High risk/NA

**IND & DOSE** **Tx of advanced renal cell carcinoma.** *Adult:* 25 mg/wk IV infused over 30–60 min; give 30 min after giving prophylactic diphenhydramine 25–50 mg IV.
**ADJUST DOSE** Elderly pts, hepatic impairment
**ADV EFF** Abd pain, alopecia, body aches, **bowel perforation,** confusion, constipation, drowsiness, **hepatic impairment,** hyperglycemia, **hypersensitivity/infusion reactions, infections, interstitial pneumonitis, nephrotoxicity,** n/v/d, painful urination, proteinuria, rash, wound-healing problems
**INTERACTIONS** CYP3A4 inducers/inhibitors, grapefruit juice, live vaccines, St. John's wort; ramipril and/or amlodipine increase risk of angioedema
**NC/PT** Monitor LFTs, renal/respiratory function. Premedicate to decrease infusion reaction risk. Not for use in preg (barrier contraceptives advised)/breastfeeding. Pt should mark calendar of tx days; cover head at temp extremes (hair loss possible); take safety precautions for CNS effects; avoid St. John's wort, grapefruit juice; report difficulty breathing, severe abd pain, urine/stool color changes.

**DANGEROUS DRUG**

## tenecteplase (TNKase)

**CLASS** Thrombolytic enzyme
**PREG/CONT** C/NA

**BBW** Arrange to stop concurrent heparin, tenecteplase if serious bleeding occurs.
**IND & DOSE** **To reduce mortality associated w/acute MI.** *Adult:* Initiate tx as soon as possible after onset of acute MI. Give as IV bolus over 5 sec. Dose based on weight (max, 50 mg/dose): ≥90 kg, 50 mg; 80–89 kg, 45 mg; 70–79 kg, 40 mg; 60–69 kg, 35 mg; <60 kg, 30 mg.
**ADJUST DOSE** Elderly pts
**ADV EFF** **Bleeding,** cardiac arrhythmias, **MI,** rash, urticaria
**INTERACTIONS** Aminocaproic acid, anticoagulants, aspirin, clopidogrel, dipyridamole, heparin, ticlopidine
**NC/PT** Can only give IV under close supervision. Do not add other drugs to infusion sol. Stop current heparin tx. Apply pressure to all dressings. Avoid invasive procedures. Monitor coagulation studies; watch for s&sx of bleeding. Pt should report blood in urine, bleeding, chest pain, difficulty breathing.

## tenofovir alafenamide (Vemlidy), tenofovir disoproxil fumarate (Viread)

**CLASS** Antiviral, nucleoside reverse transcriptase inhibitor
**PREG/CONT** Low risk/NA

**BBW** Severe HBV exacerbation has occurred when anti–HBV tx stopped; monitor for several mo if drug discontinued.
**IND & DOSE** **Tx of HIV-1 infection, w/other antivirals.** *Adult, child ≥12 yr,*

≥35 kg: 300 mg/d PO. *Child 2–11 yr:* 8 mg/kg/d PO. **Tx of chronic HBV.** *Adult, child ≥12 yr, ≥35 kg:* 300 mg/d PO (tablet), or 8 mg/kg powder PO (powder) up to 300 mg/d (*Viread*). Or, for adults, 25 mg/d PO (*Vemlidy*).
**ADJUST DOSE** Renal impairment, severe hepatic impairment
**ADV EFF** Asthenia, body fat redistribution, headache, **lactic acidosis,** n/v/d, renal impairment, **severe hepatomegaly w/steatosis**
**INTERACTIONS** Atazanavir, didanosine, lopinavir, ritonavir
**NC/PT** Always give w/other antivirals. Test for HIV before using tenofovir alafenamide; should not be used alone in pts w/HIV infection. Monitor LFTs, renal function regularly; stop at first sign of lactic acidosis. Not for use in preg/breastfeeding. Body fat may redistribute to back, middle, chest. Pt should take precautions to avoid disease spread (drug not a cure); avoid exposure to infections; report urine/stool color changes, rapid respirations.

## terazosin hydrochloride (generic)
**CLASS** Alpha blocker, antihypertensive, BPH drug
**PREG/CONT** C/NA

**BBW** Give first dose just before bed to lessen likelihood of first-dose syncope due to orthostatic hypotension.
**IND & DOSE Tx of HTN.** *Adult:* 1 mg PO at bedtime. Slowly increase to achieve desired BP response. Usual range, 1–5 mg PO daily. **Tx of BPH.** *Adult:* 1 mg PO at bedtime. Increase to 2, 5, or 10 mg PO daily. May need 10 mg/d for 4–6 wk to assess benefit.
**ADV EFF Allergic anaphylaxis,** blurred vision, dizziness, drowsiness, dyspnea, headache, nasal congestion, n/v, orthostatic hypotension, palpitations, priapism, sinusitis
**INTERACTIONS** ED drugs, nitrates, other antihypertensives
**NC/PT** If not taken for several days, restart w/initial dose. Always start first dose at bedtime to lessen likelihood of syncope; have pt lie down if syncope occurs. Pt should take safety precautions for CNS effects; use caution w/ED drugs; report fainting, dizziness.

## terbinafine hydrochloride (Lamisil)
**CLASS** Allylamine, antifungal
**PREG/CONT** Unkn/NA

**BBW** Monitor regularly for s&sx of hepatic impairment; liver failure possible.
**IND & DOSE Tx of onychomycosis of fingernail, toenail.** *Adult:* 250 mg/d PO for 6 wk (fingernail), 12 wk (toenail). **Tx of tinea capitis.** *Adult:* 250 mg/d PO for 6 wk. *Child ≥4 yr:* >35 kg, 250 mg/d PO for 6 wk; 25–35 kg, 187.5 mg/d PO for 6 wk; <25 kg, 125 mg/d PO for 6 wk. **Tx of athlete's foot.** *Adult, child:* Apply topically between toes bid for 1 wk. **Tx of ring worm, jock itch.** *Adult, child:* Apply topically once daily for 1 wk.
**ADV EFF** Abd pain, dyspepsia, headache, **hepatic failure,** nausea, pruritus, rash
**INTERACTIONS** Cimetidine, cyclosporine, dextromethorphan, rifampin
**NC/PT** Culture before tx. Contraindicated w/chronic or active liver disease. Monitor LFTs before and regularly during tx. Not for use in preg/breastfeeding. Pt should sprinkle oral granules on spoonful of nonacidic food such as mashed potatoes, swallow entire spoonful w/o chewing; take analgesics for headache; report urine/stool color changes, unusual bleeding, rash. Name confusion w/*Lamisil* (terbinafine), *Lamictal* (lamotrigine), *Lamisil AF* (tolnaftate), *Lamisil AT* (terbinafine).

## terbutaline sulfate
(Brethine)
**CLASS** Antiasthmatic, beta selective agonist, bronchodilator, sympathomimetic
**PREG/CONT** B/NA

**BBW** Do not use injectable form in preg women for px, prolonged tx (beyond 48–72 hr) of preterm labor in hospital or outpt setting; risk of serious maternal heart problems, death.
**IND & DOSE Px, tx of bronchial asthma, reversible bronchospasm.** *Adult, child >15 yr:* 2.5–5 mg PO tid at 6-hr intervals during waking hours; max, 15 mg/d. Or, 0.25 mg subcut into lateral deltoid area. If no significant improvement in 15–30 min, give another 0.25-mg dose. Max, 0.5 mg/4 hr. *Child 12–15 yr:* 2.5 mg PO tid; max, 7.5 mg/24 hr.
**ADJUST DOSE** Elderly pts
**ADV EFF** Anxiety, apprehension, **bronchospasm,** cardiac arrhythmias, cough, fear, nausea, palpitations, **pulmonary edema, respiratory difficulties,** restlessness, sweating
**INTERACTIONS** Diuretics, halogenated hydrocarbons, MAOIs, sympathomimetics, TCAs, theophylline
**NC/PT** Due to similar packaging, terbutaline injection confused w/ *Methergine* injection (methylergonovine maleate); use extreme caution. Have beta blocker on hand for arrhythmias, respiratory distress. Pt should take safety precautions for CNS effects; report chest pain, difficulty breathing, irregular heartbeat, failure to respond to usual dose.

## teriflunomide (Aubagio)
**CLASS** MS drug, pyrimidine synthesis inhibitor
**PREG/CONT** High risk/NA

**BBW** Risk of severe hepatotoxicity; monitor LFTs before tx and at least monthly for 6 mo. Risk of major birth defects. Contraindicated in preg; contraceptives required.
**IND & DOSE Tx of relapsing MS.** *Adult:* 7 or 14 mg/d PO.
**ADJUST DOSE** Severe hepatic impairment
**ADV EFF** Alopecia, **BP changes,** flu-like sx, hyperkalemia, immunosuppression, infections, **neutropenia,** n/v, paresthesia, **peripheral neuropathy, renal failure, severe skin reactions**
**INTERACTIONS** Alosetron, cholestyramine, duloxetine, hormonal contraceptives, paclitaxel, pioglitazone, repaglinide, rosiglitazone, theophylline, tizanidine, warfarin
**NC/PT** Do not begin tx if acute infection; monitor for s&sx of infection, changes in potassium levels, BP changes, peripheral neuropathy, skin reactions. Monitor LFTs before, during tx. Not for use in preg (contraceptives required)/breastfeeding; advise pt of risk of fetal harm. Pt should take once daily; avoid exposure to infection; report urine/stool color changes, extreme fatigue, fever, infection, skin reactions, muscle cramping, numbness/tingling.

## teriparatide (Bonsity, Forteo)
**CLASS** Calcium regulator, parathyroid hormone
**PREG/CONT** Unkn/NA

**BBW** Increased risk of osteosarcoma in rats; do not use in pts w/increased risk of osteosarcoma (Paget disease, unexplained alkaline phosphatase elevations, open epiphyses, prior external beam, implant radiation involving skeleton). Not recommended for bone disease other than osteoporosis.
**IND & DOSE Tx of postmenopausal women w/osteoporosis, glucocorticoid-related osteoporosis, hypogonadal osteoporosis in men.** *Adult:* 20 mcg/d subcut in thigh or abd wall for no more than 2 yr.

**ADV EFF** Arthralgia, hypercalcemia, nausea, orthostatic hypotension, pain, urolithiasis
**INTERACTIONS** Digoxin
**NC/PT** Do not use in pts at risk for osteosarcoma; use for no more than 2 yr. Monitor serum calcium. Not for use in preg/breastfeeding. Teach proper administration/disposal of needles, delivery device. Pt should rotate injection sites; have blood tests to monitor calcium level; change positions slowly after injection; report constipation, muscle weakness.

## tesamorelin (Egrifta)
**CLASS** GHRF analog
**PREG/CONT** High risk/NA

**IND & DOSE** **To reduce excess abd fat in HIV-infected pts w/lipodystrophy related to antiviral use.** *Adult:* 2 mg/d subcut into abd skin.
**ADV EFF** **Acute illness,** arthralgia, **cancer,** edema, fluid retention, glucose intolerance, hypersensitivity reactions, injection-site reactions, **neoplasms**
**INTERACTIONS** Anticonvulsants, corticosteroids, cyclosporine, estrogen, progesterone, testosterone
**NC/PT** Monitor blood glucose. Arrange for cancer screening. Teach proper administration/disposal of needles/syringes. Not for use in preg/breastfeeding. Pt should rotate injection sites; report s&sx of infection, injection-site reaction, increased thirst.

## testosterone (Androderm, AndroGel, Aveed, Fortesta, Jatenzo, Natesto, Testim, Testopel, Vogelxo)
**CLASS** Androgen, hormone
**PREG/CONT** High risk/C-III

**BBW** Risk of toxic effects (enlarged genitalia, greater-than-normal bone age) in child exposed to pt using transdermal form (*AndroGel, Testim, Vogelxo*). Pt should wash hands after applying, cover treated area w/ clothing to reduce exposure. Risk of serious pulmonary oil microembolism, anaphylaxis (*Aveed*); observe pt for 30 min and be prepared for supportive tx. Risk of thrombotic events; monitor accordingly. Risk of HTN (*Jatenzo*).
**IND & DOSE** **Replacement tx in hypogonadism.** *Adult:* Initially, 237 mg PO daily and adjust to 158–396 mg PO bid (*Jatenzo*); or 50–400 mg (cypionate, enanthate) IM q 2–4 wk; or 750 mg (*Aveed*) IM, then 750 mg 4 wk later, then q 10 wk; or 150–450 mg (enanthate pellets) implanted subcut q 3–6 mo. Or, initially 4-mg/d system (patch) applied to nonscrotal skin; then 2 mg/d system (*Androderm*). Or, 50 mg/d *AndroGel, Testim, Vogelxo* (preferably in a.m.) applied to clean, dry, intact skin of shoulders, upper arms, or abdomen. Or, 4 actuations (40 mg) *Fortesta* applied to inner thighs in a.m. Or, 1 pump actuation (30 mg) Or, 4 actuations (50 mg) *AndroGel* 1.62%, *Vogelxo* once daily in a.m. to shoulders or upper arms. Or 11 mg (*Natesto*) intranasally tid (2 pumps, one in each nostril). **Tx of males w/delayed puberty.** *Adult:* 50–200 mg enanthate IM q 2–4 wk for 4–6 mo, or 150 mg pellets subcut q 3–6 mo. **Tx of carcinoma of breast, metastatic mammary cancer.** *Adult:* 200–400 mg IM enanthate q 2–4 wk.
**ADV EFF** Androgenic effects, chills, dizziness, fatigue, fluid retention, headache, **hepatocellular carcinoma,** hypoestrogenic effects, leukopenia, nasal reactions (*Natesto*), polycythemia, rash, **thrombotic events**
**INTERACTIONS** Anticoagulants, corticosteroids, grapefruit juice, insulin, metronidazole
**NC/PT** Obtain testosterone level before use; efficacy in age-related low testosterone has not been established. Monitor blood glucose, serum calcium, serum electrolytes, lipids, LFTs. Women using drug should avoid preg/breastfeeding. Review proper

administration of each delivery form; sprays not interchangeable. Pt should wash hands after administrating topical forms; mark calendar of tx days; remove old transdermal patch before applying new one; cover topical gel application sites if in contact w/child; avoid grapefruit juice; report swelling, urine/stool color changes, unusual bleeding/bruising, chest pain, difficult breathing.

## tetrabenazine (Xenazine)

**CLASS** Anti-chorea drug, vesicular monoamine transporter-2 inhibitor
**PREG/CONT** Moderate risk/NA

**BBW** Increased risk of depression, suicidality; monitor accordingly.
**IND & DOSE** **Tx of chorea associated w/Huntington disease.** *Adult:* 12.5 mg/d PO in a.m. After 1 wk, increase to 12.5 mg PO bid; max, 100 mg/d in divided doses.
**ADV EFF** Akathisia, anxiety, confusion, depression, fatigue, insomnia, nausea, Parkinson-like sx, **prolonged QT,** sedation, URI
**INTERACTIONS** Alcohol, antiarrhythmics, antipsychotics, dopamine agonists, fluoxetine, MAOIs, paroxetine, quinidine
**NC/PT** Obtain accurate depression evaluation before use. Obtain baseline of chorea sx. Do not give within 14 d of MAOIs. Avoid if hepatic impairment. Not for use in preg (contraceptives advised)/breastfeeding. Pt should take safety measures for CNS effects, avoid alcohol; report tremors, behavior changes, depression, thoughts of suicide.

## tetracycline hydrochloride (generic)

**CLASS** Antibiotic
**PREG/CONT** D/NA

**IND & DOSE** **Tx of infections caused by susceptible bacteria.** *Adult:* 1–2 g/d PO in two to four equal doses; max, 500 mg PO qid. *Child >8 yr:* 25–50 mg/kg/d PO in four equal doses. **Tx of brucellosis.** *Adult:* 500 mg PO qid for 3 wk w/1 g streptomycin IM bid first wk and daily second wk. **Tx of syphilis.** *Adult:* 30–40 g PO in divided doses over 10–15 d (*Sumycin*); 500 mg PO qid for 15–30 d (all others). **Tx of uncomplicated gonorrhea.** *Adult:* 500 mg PO q 6 hr for 7 d. **Tx of gonococcal urethritis.** *Adult:* 500 mg PO q 4–6 hr for 4–6 d. **Tx of uncomplicated urethral, endocervical, rectal infections w/*Chlamydia trachomatis*.** *Adult:* 500 mg PO qid for at least 7 d. **Tx of severe acne.** *Adult:* 1 g/d PO in divided doses; then 125–500 mg/d.
**ADV EFF** **Anaphylaxis; bone marrow suppression;** discoloring, inadequate calcification of primary teeth of fetus if used by preg women, of permanent teeth if used during dental development; **hepatic impairment;** phototoxic reactions; superinfections
**INTERACTIONS** Aluminum, bismuth, calcium salts; charcoal; dairy products; food; hormonal contraceptives; iron, magnesium salts; penicillins; urinary alkalinizers; zinc salts
**NC/PT** Culture before tx. Arrange tx of superinfections. Not for use in preg (hormonal contraceptives may be ineffective; barrier contraceptives advised). Pt should take on empty stomach 1 hr before or 2 hr after meals; not use outdated drugs; report rash, urine/stool color changes.

## tetrahydrozoline hydrochloride (Murine Plus, Opticlear, Tyzine, Visine)

**CLASS** Alpha agonist; decongestant; ophthal vasoconstrictor, mydriatic
**PREG/CONT** C/NA

**IND & DOSE** **Relief of nasal, nasopharyngeal mucosal congestion.** *Adult, child ≥6 yr:* 2–4 drops 0.1% sol in each nostril 3–4 ×/d; or 3–4 sprays

in each nostril q 4 hr as needed. Not more often than q 3 hr. *Child 2–6 yr:* 2–3 drops 0.05% sol in each nostril q 4–6 hr as needed Not more often than q 3 hr. **Temporary relief of eye redness, burning, irritation.** *Adult:* 1–2 drops into eye(s) up to qid.
**ADV EFF** Anxiety, **CV collapse w/ hypotension,** dizziness, drowsiness, headache, light-headedness, pallor, rebound congestion, restlessness, tenseness
**INTERACTIONS** Methyldopa, MAOIs, TCAs, urine acidifiers/alkalinizers
**NC/PT** Monitor BP in pt w/CAD. Review proper administration. Rebound congestion may occur when drug stopped. Pt should remove contact lenses before using drops; drink plenty of fluids; use humidifier for at least 72 hr; take safety precautions for CNS effects; report blurred vision, fainting.

## thalidomide (Thalomid)
**CLASS** Immunomodulator
**PREG/CONT** High risk/NA

**BBW** Associated w/severe birth defects. Women must have preg test, signed consent to use birth control to avoid preg during tx (STEPS program). Significant risk of VTEs when used in multiple myeloma w/dexamethasone; monitor accordingly.
**IND & DOSE Tx of erythema nodosum leprosum.** *Adult:* 100–300 mg/d PO at bedtime for at least 2 wk. Up to 400 mg/d for severe lesions. Taper in decrements of 50 mg q 2–4 wk. **Tx of newly diagnosed multiple myeloma.** *Adult:* 200 mg/d PO w/ dexamethasone.
**ADV EFF** Agitation, anorexia, anxiety, bradycardia, dizziness, dry skin, dyspnea, headache, nausea, **neutropenia,** orthostatic hypotension, **MI,** peripheral neuropathy, rash, **SJS,** somnolence, TLS
**INTERACTIONS** Alcohol, CNS depressants, dexamethasone (increased mortality), hormonal contraceptives
**NC/PT** Rule out preg; ensure pt has read, agreed to contraceptive use. Monitor BP, WBC count. Not for use in breastfeeding. Pt should take safety precautions for CNS effects; avoid exposure to infection; report chest pain, dizziness, rash, s&sx of infection.

## theophylline (Elixophyllin, Theo-24, Theochron)
**CLASS** Bronchodilator, xanthine
**PREG/CONT** C/NA

**IND & DOSE Sx relief or px of bronchial asthma, reversible bronchospasm.** *Note:* For dosages for specific populations, see manufacturer's details. *Adult, child >45 kg:* 300–600 mg/d PO, or 0.4 mg/kg/hr IV. *Child <45 kg:* Total dose in mg = [(0.2 × age in wk) + 5] × body wt in kg PO/d in four equal doses. Or, 0.7–0.8 mg/kg/hr IV (1–1.5 mg/kg/12 hr IV for neonate).
**ADV EFF** Anorexia, **death,** dizziness, headache, insomnia, irritability, **life-threatening ventricular arrhythmias,** n/v, restlessness, **seizures**
**INTERACTIONS** Barbiturates, benzodiazepines, beta blockers, charcoal, cigarette smoking, cimetidine, ciprofloxacin, erythromycin, halothane, hormonal contraceptives, NMJ blockers, ofloxacin, phenytoins, rifampin, ranitidine, St. John's wort, ticlopidine, thioamides, thyroid hormones
**NC/PT** Maintain serum level in therapeutic range (5–15 mcg/mL); adverse effects related to serum level. Do not add in sol w/other drugs. Not for use in preg (barrier contraceptives advised)/breastfeeding. Pt should take ER form on empty stomach 1 hr before or 2 hr after meals and not cut/crush/chew it; limit caffeine intake; avoid St. John's wort; report smoking changes (dose adjustment needed); take safety precautions for CNS effects; report irregular heartbeat, severe GI pain.

DANGEROUS DRUG

**thioguanine** (generic)
**CLASS** Antimetabolite, antineoplastic
**PREG/CONT** D/NA

**IND & DOSE Remission induction, consolidation, maint tx of acute nonlymphocytic leukemias.** *Adult, child ≥3 yr:* 2 mg/kg/d PO for 4 wk. If no clinical improvement, no toxic effects, increase to 3 mg/kg/d PO.
**ADV EFF** Anorexia, **bone marrow suppression, hepatotoxicity,** hyperuricemia, n/v, stomatitis, weakness
**NC/PT** Monitor CBC (dose adjustment may be needed), LFTs. Not for use in preg (contraceptives advised)/breastfeeding. Pt should drink 8–10 glasses of fluid/d; avoid exposure to infection; have regular blood tests; perform mouth care for mouth sores; report s&sx of infection, urine/stool color changes, swelling.

DANGEROUS DRUG

**thiotepa** (Tepadina)
**CLASS** Alkylating agent, antineoplastic
**PREG/CONT** High risk/NA

**IND & DOSE Tx of adenocarcinoma of breast, ovary.** *Adult:* 0.3–0.4 mg/kg IV at 1- to 4-wk intervals. Or, diluted in sterile water to conc of 10 mg/mL, then 0.6–0.8 mg/kg injected directly into tumor after local anesthetic injected through same needle. Maint, 0.6–0.8 mg/kg IV q 1–4 wk. Or, 0.6–0.8 mg/kg intracavity q 1–4 wk through same tube used to remove fluid from bladder. **Superficial papillary carcinoma of urinary bladder.** *Adult:* Dehydrate pt for 8–12 hr before tx. Instill 30–60 mg in 60 mL normal saline injection into bladder by catheter. Have pt retain for 2 hr. If pt unable to retain 60 mL, give in 30 mL. Repeat once/wk for 4 wk. **Control of intracavity effusions secondary to neoplasms of various serosal cavities.** *Adult:* 0.6–0.8 mg/kg infused directly into cavity using same tubing used to remove fluid from cavity.
**ADV EFF** Amenorrhea, **bone marrow suppression,** dizziness, fever, headache, n/v, skin reactions
**NC/PT** Monitor CBC; dose adjustment may be needed. IV sol should be clear w/out solutes. Not for use in preg/breastfeeding. Pt should mark calendar of tx days; avoid exposure to infections; take safety precautions w/ dizziness; report unusual bleeding, s&sx of infection, rash.

**thiothixene** (generic)
**CLASS** Antipsychotic, dopaminergic blocker, thioxanthene
**PREG/CONT** C/NA

**BBW** Increased risk of death if antipsychotics used to treat elderly pts w/ dementia-related psychosis; not approved for this use.
**IND & DOSE Mgt of schizophrenia.** *Adult, child >12 yr:* 2 mg PO tid (mild conditions), 5 mg bid (more severe conditions). Range, 20–30 mg/d; max, 60 mg/d.
**ADJUST DOSE** Elderly, debilitated pts
**ADV EFF Aplastic anemia, autonomic disturbances,** blurred vision, **bronchospasm,** drowsiness, dry mouth, extrapyramidal effects, gynecomastia, **HF, laryngospasm, nonthrombocytopenic purpura, pancytopenia,** photophobia, pink to red-brown urine, **refractory arrhythmias**
**INTERACTIONS** Alcohol, antihypertensives, carbamazepine
**NC/PT** Monitor renal function, CBC. Urine will turn pink to red-brown. Pt should avoid sun exposure; take safety precautions for CNS effects; maintain fluid intake; report s&sx of infection, unusual bleeding, difficulty breathing.

## thyroid, desiccated
(Armour Thyroid, Nature-Throid, Thyroid USP, Westhroid)
**CLASS** Thyroid hormone
**PREG/CONT** A/NA

**BBW** Do not use to treat obesity. Large doses in euthyroid pts may produce serious to life-threatening s&sx of toxicity.
**IND & DOSE Tx of hypothyroidism.** *Adult:* 30 mg/d PO, increased by 15 mg/d q 2–3 wk. Usual maint, 60–120 mg PO daily. *Child:* >12 yr, 90 mg/d PO; 6–12 yr, 60–90 mg/d PO; 1–5 yr, 45–60 mg/d PO; 6–12 mo, 30–45 mg/d PO; 0–6 mo, 7.5–30 mg/d PO.
**ADJUST DOSE** Elderly pts, long-standing heart disease
**ADV EFF Cardiac arrest,** hyperthyroidism, n/v/d, skin reactions
**INTERACTIONS** Antacids, cholestyramine, digoxin, theophylline, warfarin
**NC/PT** Monitor thyroid function to establish dose, then at least yearly. Pt should wear medical ID; report headache, palpitations, heat/cold intolerance.

## tiaGABine hydrochloride (Gabitril)
**CLASS** Antiepileptic
**PREG/CONT** High risk/NA

**BBW** Increased risk of suicidal ideation; monitor accordingly.
**IND & DOSE Adjunctive tx in partial seizures.** *Adult:* 4 mg/d PO for 1 wk; may increase by 4–8 mg/wk until desired response. Usual maint, 32–56 mg daily; max, 56 mg/d in two to four divided doses. *Child 12–18 yr:* 4 mg/d PO for 1 wk; may increase to 8 mg/d in two divided doses for 1 wk, then by 4–8 mg/wk. Max, 32 mg/d in two to four divided doses.
**ADV EFF** Asthenia, dizziness, GI upset, incontinence, eye changes, **potentially serious rash,** somnolence
**INTERACTIONS** Alcohol, carbamazepine, CNS depressants, phenobarbital, phenytoin, primidone, valproate
**NC/PT** Taper when stopping. Not for use in preg (contraceptives advised); use caution w/breastfeeding. Pt should not stop suddenly; take w/food; avoid alcohol, sleeping pills; wear medical ID; take safety precautions w/dizziness, vision changes; report rash, thoughts of suicide, vision changes.

## ticagrelor (Brilinta)
**CLASS** Antiplatelet
**PREG/CONT** Unkn/NA

**BBW** Significant to fatal bleeding possible; do not use w/active bleeding, CABG planned within 5 d, surgery. Maint aspirin doses above 100 mg reduce effectiveness; maintain aspirin dose at 75–100 mg/d.
**IND & DOSE To reduce rate of thrombotic CV events in pts w/acute coronary syndrome or hx of MI.** *Adult:* Loading dose, 180 mg PO; then 90 mg PO bid w/325 mg PO aspirin as loading dose, then aspirin dose of 75–100 mg/d PO for first year after event, then 60 mg/d PO maintenance.
**ADV EFF Bleeding,** dyspnea, **hepatotoxicity**
**INTERACTIONS** Potent CYP3A4 inducers (carbamazepine, dexamethasone, phenobarbital, phenytoin, rifampin), potent CYP3A4 inhibitors (atazanavir, clarithromycin, indinavir, itraconazole, ketoconazole, nefazodone, nelfinavir, ritonavir, saquinavir, telithromycin, voriconazole); avoid these combos. Digoxin, drugs affecting coagulation, lovastatin, simvastatin
**NC/PT** Continually monitor for s&sx of bleeding. Not for use w/hx of intracranial bleeding. Ensure concurrent use of 75–100 mg aspirin; do not stop drug except for pathological bleeding. Increased risk of CV events; if drug must be stopped, start another anticoagulant. Assess pt w/dyspnea for potential underlying cause. Not for use in preg (barrier contraceptive advised)/

breastfeeding. Pt should take drug exactly as prescribed w/prescribed dose of aspirin; not increase doses; not stop drug suddenly; report other drugs or herbs being used (many reactions possible; bleeding time may be prolonged), excessive bleeding, difficulty breathing, chest pain, numbness/tingling, urine/stool color changes.

## ticlopidine hydrochloride (generic)

**CLASS** Antiplatelet
**PREG/CONT** B/NA

**BBW** Monitor WBC count before, frequently while starting tx; if neutropenia present, stop drug immediately.
**IND & DOSE To reduce thrombotic stroke risk in pts who have experienced stroke precursors; px of acute stent thrombosis in coronary arteries.** *Adult:* 250 mg PO bid w/food.
**ADV EFF** Abd pain, **bleeding,** dizziness, **neutropenia,** n/v/d, pain, rash
**INTERACTIONS** Antacids, aspirin, cimetidine, digoxin, NSAIDs, theophylline
**NC/PT** Mark chart to alert all health care providers of use. Monitor WBC; watch for s&sx of bleeding. Pt should take w/meals; report unusual bleeding/bruising, s&sx of infection.

## tigecycline (Tygacil)

**CLASS** Glycylcycline antibiotic
**PREG/CONT** High risk/NA

**BBW** All-cause mortality higher in pts using tigecycline; reserve use for when no other tx is suitable.
**IND & DOSE Tx of complicated skin/skin-structure infections; community-acquired pneumonia; intra-abd infections caused by susceptible bacteria strains.** *Adult:* 100 mg IV, then 50 mg IV q 12 hr for 5–14 d; infuse over 30–60 min.
**ADJUST DOSE** Severe hepatic impairment
**ADV EFF Anaphylaxis,** CDAD, cough, **death,** dizziness, dyspnea, enamel hypoplasia, headache, **hepatic dysfx,** n/v/d, **pancreatitis,** photosensitivity, **pseudomembranous colitis,** superinfections
**INTERACTIONS** Oral contraceptives, warfarin
**NC/PT** Culture before tx. Limit use to serious need. Monitor LFTs, pancreatic function. Not for use in preg/breastfeeding. Risk of inhibition of bone growth if used in second and third trimesters, infancy, and childhood up to age 8 yr. Pt should avoid sun exposure; report bloody diarrhea, difficulty breathing, rash, pain at injection site.

## tildrakizumab-asmn (Ilumya)

**CLASS** Antipsoriatic agent; interleukin-23 inhibitor, monoclonal antibody
**PREG/CONT** Limited data/NA

**IND & DOSE Tx of adults w/ moderate to severe plaque psoriasis who are candidates for systemic tx or phototherapy.** *Adult:* 100 mg/mL subcut at wk 0, 4, and q 12 wk thereafter.
**ADV EFF** Diarrhea, **infections,** injection-site reactions, **hypersensitivity,** URI
**INTERACTIONS** Live vaccines; may increase infection risk
**NC/PT** Evaluate for TB before start of tx. Only administered by health care provider. Monitor for hypersensitivity (angioedema, urticaria), infections. Pt should have all age-appropriate immunizations, but avoid live vaccines.

## timolol maleate (Istalol, Timoptic)

**CLASS** Antiglaucoma, antihypertensive, beta blocker
**PREG/CONT** C/NA

**BBW** Do not stop abruptly after long-term tx (hypersensitivity to

catecholamines possible, causing angina exacerbation, MI, ventricular arrhythmias). Taper gradually over 2 wk w/monitoring.
**IND & DOSE Tx of HTN.** *Adult:* 10 mg bid PO; max, 60 mg/d in two divided doses. Usual range, 20–40 mg/d in two divided doses. **Px of reinfarction in MI.** 10 mg PO bid within 1–4 wk of infarction. **Px of migraine.** *Adult:* 10 mg PO bid; during maint, may give 20 mg/d as single dose. **To reduce IOP in chronic open-angle glaucoma.** 1 drop 0.25% sol bid into affected eye(s); adjust based on response to 1 drop 0.5% sol bid or 1 drop 0.25% sol daily. Or, 1 drop in affected eye(s) each morning (*Istalol*).
**ADV EFF** Arrhythmias, **bronchospasm,** constipation, decreased exercise tolerance, dizziness, ED, flatulence, gastric pain, **HF,** hyperglycemia, **laryngospasm,** n/v/d, ocular irritation w/eyedrops, **PE, stroke**
**INTERACTIONS** Antacids, aspirin, calcium, indomethacin
**NC/PT** Alert surgeon if surgery required. Do not stop abruptly; must be tapered. Teach proper eyedrop administration. Pt should take safety precautions w/dizziness; report difficulty breathing, swelling, numbness/tingling.

## Timothy grass pollen allergen extract (Grastek)

**CLASS** Allergen extract
**PREG/CONT** Low risk/NA

**BBW** Risk of severe, life-threatening allergic reactions. Not for use in uncontrolled asthma. Observe pt for 30 min after first dose; have emergency equipment on hand. Prescribe auto-injectable epinephrine; teach use.
**IND & DOSE Immunotherapy for tx of timothy grass pollen–induced allergic rhinitis w/ or w/o conjunctivitis confirmed by skin test in pts 5–65 yr.** *Adult, child ≥5 yr:* 1 tablet/d SL starting 12 wk before and continuing throughout season.
**ADV EFF** Cough, ear pruritus, mouth edema, oropharyngeal pain/pruritus, throat/tongue pruritus
**NC/PT** Ensure skin testing confirms allergy. Not for use in uncontrolled asthma, hx of severe reactions, eosinophilic esophagitis. Begin 12 wk before expected grass season and continue throughout season. First dose should be given under medical supervision; observe pt for at least 30 min and have emergency equipment on hand. Place tablet under tongue, allow to stay until completely dissolved; pt should not swallow for 1 min. Pt should also be prescribed auto-injectable epinephrine, taught its proper use, and instructed to seek medical help after using it. Stop tx if oral wounds/inflammation; allow to heal completely before restarting. Pt should report difficulty breathing/swallowing.

## tinidazole (Tindamax)

**CLASS** Antiprotozoal
**PREG/CONT** Unkn/NA

**BBW** Avoid use unless clearly needed; carcinogenic in lab animals.
**IND & DOSE Tx of trichomoniasis, giardiasis.** *Adult:* Single dose of 2 g PO w/food. *Child >3 yr:* For giardiasis, single dose of 50 mg/kg PO (up to 2 g) w/food. **Tx of amebiasis.** *Adult:* 2 g/d PO for 3 d w/food. *Child >3 yr:* 50 mg/kg/d PO (up to 2 g/d) for 3 d w/food. For giardiasis, **Tx of amebic liver abscess.** *Adult:* 2 g/d PO for 3–5 d w/food. *Child >3 yr:* 50 mg/kg/d PO (up to 2 g/d) for 3–5 d w/food. **Tx of bacterial vaginosis in nonpreg women.** *Adult:* 2 g/d PO for 2 d w/food or 1 g/d for 5 d w/food.
**ADV EFF** Anorexia, dizziness, drowsiness, metallic taste, neutropenia, **seizures, severe hypersensitivity reactions,** superinfections, weakness
**INTERACTIONS** Alcohol, cholestyramine, cimetidine, cyclosporine, disulfiram, 5-FU, ketoconazole, lithium, oral anticoagulants, oxytetracycline, phenytoin, tacrolimus

**NC/PT** Give w/food. Ensure proper hygiene, tx of superinfections. Urine may become very dark. Pt should take safety precautions w/dizziness; avoid alcohol during, for 3 d after tx; report vaginal itching, white patches in mouth, difficulty breathing, rash.

## tiopronin (Thiola, Thiola EC)

**CLASS** Thiol compound
**PREG/CONT** Low risk/NA

**IND & DOSE Px of cystine kidney stone formation in severe homozygous cystinuria.** *Adult:* 800 mg/d PO; increase to 1,000 mg/d in divided doses on empty stomach. *Child ≥20 kg:* 15 mg/kg/d PO on empty stomach; adjust based on urine cystine level.
**ADV EFF Hepatotoxicity,** nephrotoxicity, n/v/d, rash, skin/taste changes
**NC/PT** Monitor cystine at 1 mo, then q 3 mo. Monitor LFTs, renal function. Not for use in breastfeeding. Pt should drink fluids liberally (to 3 L/d); swallow EC tablets whole; report urine/stool color changes, rash.

## tiotropium bromide (Spiriva, Spiriva Respimat)

**CLASS** Anticholinergic, bronchodilator
**PREG/CONT** Unkn/NA

**IND & DOSE Long-term once-daily maint tx of bronchospasm associated w/COPD.** *Adult:* 2 inhalations/d of contents of one capsule (18 mcg) using *HandiHaler* device (*Spiriva, Spiriva Respimat*). **Long-term tx of asthma.** *Pts ≥6 yr:* 1.25 mcg/d as 2 inhalations once/d (*Spiriva Respimat*).
**ADV EFF** Abd pain, blurred vision, constipation, dry mouth, epistaxis, glaucoma, rash, urine retention
**INTERACTIONS** Anticholinergics
**NC/PT** Evaluate for glaucoma; stop drug if increased IOP. Not for use in acute attacks. Review proper use/care of *HandiHaler* device/*Respimat* inhaler. Pt should empty bladder before each dose; use sugarless lozenges for dry mouth; report eye pain, vision changes.

## tipranavir (Aptivus)

**CLASS** Antiviral, protease inhibitor
**PREG/CONT** C/NA

**BBW** Increased risk of hepatotoxicity in pts w/hepatitis; assess liver function before, periodically during tx. Giving w/ritonavir has caused nonfatal, fatal intracranial hemorrhage; monitor carefully.
**IND & DOSE Tx of HIV infection, w/other antiretrovirals.** *Adult:* 500 mg/d PO w/ritonavir 200 mg; w/food if tablets, w/ or w/o food if capsules or sol. *Child 2–18 yr:* 14 mg/kg w/ritonavir 6 mg/kg PO bid (375 mg/m² w/ritonavir 150 mg/m² PO bid). Max, 500 mg bid w/ritonavir 200 mg bid; w/food if tablets, w/ or w/o food if capsules or sol.
**ADV EFF** Abd pain, cough, depression, fever, flulike sx, headache, **hepatomegaly and steatosis**, hyperglycemia, n/v/d, **potentially fatal liver impairment,** redistribution of body fat, skin reactions
**INTERACTIONS** Amprenavir, atorvastatin, calcium channel blockers, cyclosporine, desipramine, didanosine, disulfiram, hormonal contraceptives, itraconazole, ketoconazole, lopinavir, meperidine, methadone, metronidazole, oral antidiabetics, saquinavir, sildenafil, sirolimus, SSRIs, St. John's wort, tacrolimus, tadalafil, vardenafil, voriconazole, warfarin. Contraindicated w/amiodarone, dihydroergotamine, ergotamine, flecainide, lovastatin, methylergonovine, midazolam, pimozide, propafenone, quinidine, rifampin, simvastatin, triazolam
**NC/PT** Not for use w/moderate or severe hepatic impairment, concurrent use of CYP3A inducers/CYP3A clearance–dependent drugs. Ensure

pt also taking ritonavir. Review drug hx before tx; multiple interactions possible. Serious complications possible. Monitor LFTs. Not for use in preg/breastfeeding. Pt should take w/ food; swallow capsule whole and not cut/crush/chew it; store capsules in refrigerator (do not refrigerate sol); not use after expiration date; use precautions to prevent spread (drug not a cure); avoid exposure to infection, St. John's wort; report general malaise, rash, urine/stool color changes, yellowing of skin/eyes.

## tirofiban hydrochloride

(Aggrastat)
**CLASS** Antiplatelet
**PREG/CONT** Low risk/NA

**IND & DOSE** **Tx of acute coronary syndromes, w/heparin; px of cardiac ischemic complications in PCI.** *Adult:* Initially, 25 mcg/kg IV within 5 min, then 0.15 mcg/kg/min IV for up to 18 hr.
**ADJUST DOSE** Renal impairment
**ADV EFF** **Bleeding,** bradycardia, dizziness, flushing, hypotension, syncope
**INTERACTIONS** Antiplatelets, aspirin, chamomile, don quai, feverfew, garlic, ginger, ginkgo, ginseng, grape seed extract, green leaf tea, heparin, horse chestnut seed, NSAIDs, turmeric, warfarin
**NC/PT** Obtain baseline, periodic CBC, PT, aPTT, active clotting time. Maintain aPTT between 50 and 70 sec, and active clotting time between 300 and 350 sec. Avoid noncompressible IV access sites to prevent excessive, uncontrollable bleeding. Not for use in breastfeeding. Pt should report light-headedness, palpitations, pain at injection site. Name confusion between *Aggrastat* (tirofiban) and argatroban.

**DANGEROUS DRUG**

## tisagenlecleucel

(Kymriah)
**CLASS** Antineoplastic, CD19-directed modified autologous T-cell immunotherapy
**PREG/CONT** High risk/NA

**BBW** Risk of cytokine release syndrome, severe to life-threatening neurotoxicities; do not give to pt w/ infections or inflammatory disorders. Monitor for neuro events; provide supportive tx. Available only through restricted access program.
**IND & DOSE** **Tx of pts ≤25 yr w/ B-cell precursor ALL refractory or in second relapse.** *Adult:* >50 kg: 0.1–2.5 × $10^8$ total CAR-positive viable T cells IV; ≤50 kg: 0.2–5 × $10^6$ CAR-positive viable T cells/kg IV. **Tx of relapsed or refractory diffuse large B-cell lymphoma.** *Adult:* 0.6–6 × $10^8$ CAR-positive viable T cells IV.
**ADV EFF** **Cytokine release syndrome,** decreased appetite, fatigue, fever, hypersensitivity reactions, hypogammaglobulinemia, **infections, secondary malignancies, serious neuro changes, prolonged cytopenia**
**NC/PT** Verify pt and dx before infusion. Premedicate w/acetaminophen, antihistamine. Ensure availability of tocilizumab before infusion. Monitor for hypersensitivity reactions, infection, bone marrow changes, CNS changes. Pt should expect frequent blood tests to evaluate toxicities; avoid driving or operating machinery during and for at least 8 wk after tx; avoid preg/breastfeeding; report fever, s&sx of infection, difficulty breathing, confusion, changes in thought processes, severe headache.

## tiZANidine (Zanaflex)

**CLASS** Alpha agonist, antispasmodic
**PREG/CONT** C/NA

**IND & DOSE** **Acute, intermittent mgt of increased muscle tone**

**associated w/spasticity.** *Adult:* Initially, 2 mg PO; can repeat at 6- to 8-hr intervals, up to three doses/24 hr. Increase by 2–4 mg/dose q 1–4 d; max, 36 mg/d.
**ADJUST DOSE** Hepatic/renal impairment
**ADV EFF** Asthenia, constipation, dizziness, drowsiness, dry mouth, hepatic injury, hypotension, sedation
**INTERACTIONS** Alcohol, baclofen, CNS depressants, hormonal contraceptives, other $alpha_2$-adrenergic agonists, QT-prolonging drugs
**NC/PT** Stop slowly to decrease risk of withdrawal, rebound CV effects. Continue all supportive measures for neuro damaged pt. Not for use in preg (hormonal contraceptives may be ineffective; barrier contraceptives advised). Pt should take around the clock for best results; use sugarless lozenges for dry mouth; avoid alcohol; take safety precautions for CNS effects; report vision changes, difficulty swallowing, fainting.

## tobramycin sulfate
(Aktob, Bethkis, Kitabis Pak, TOBI, Tobrex Ophthalmic)
**CLASS** Aminoglycoside antibiotic
**PREG/CONT** High risk (injection, inhalation); B (ophthal)/NA

**BBW** Injection may cause serious ototoxicity, nephrotoxicity, neurotoxicity. Monitor closely for changes in renal, CNS function.
**IND & DOSE Tx of serious infections caused by susceptible bacteria strains.** *Adult:* 3 mg/kg/d IM or IV in three equal doses q 8 hr; max, 5 mg/kg/d. *Child >1 wk:* 6–7.5 mg/kg/d IM or IV in three–four equally divided doses. *Premature infants, neonates ≤1 wk:* Up to 4 mg/kg/d IM or IV in two equal doses q 12 hr. **Mgt of cystic fibrosis pts w/*Pseudomonas aeruginosa*.** *Adult, child ≥6 yr:* 300 mg bid by nebulizer inhaled over 10–15 min. Give in 28-d cycles: 28 d on, 28 d rest. **Tx of superficial ocular infections due to susceptible organism strains.** *Adult, child ≥6 yr:* 1–2 drops into conjunctival sac of affected eye(s) q 4 hr, 2 drops/hr in severe infections. Or, ½ inch ribbon bid–tid.
**ADJUST DOSE** Elderly pts, renal impairment
**ADV EFF** Anorexia, bronchospasm w/inhalation, leukemoid reaction, palpitations, ototoxicity, **nephrotoxicity,** numbness/tingling, n/v/d, purpura, rash, superinfections, vestibular paralysis
**INTERACTIONS** Aminoglycosides, beta-lactam antibiotics, cephalosporins, NMJ blockers, penicillin, succinylcholine
**NC/PT** Culture before tx. Monitor hearing, renal function, serum concentration. Limit tx duration to 7–14 d to decrease toxic reactions. Do not mix in sol w/other drugs. Not for use in preg/breastfeeding (injection, inhaled). Review proper administration of eyedrops/nebulizer. Pt should mark calendar of tx days; store in refrigerator, protected from light; drink 8–10 glasses of fluid/d; take safety precautions for CNS effects; report hearing changes, dizziness, pain at injection site.

## tocilizumab (Actemra)
**CLASS** Antirheumatic, interleukin-6 receptor inhibitor
**PREG/CONT** High risk/NA

**BBW** Serious to life-threatening infections possible, including TB and bacterial, invasive fungal, viral, opportunistic infections. Perform TB test before tx. Interrupt tx if serious infection occurs; monitor for TB s&sx during tx.
**IND & DOSE Tx of moderately to severely active RA.** *Adult:* 4 mg/kg by IV infusion over 1 hr, then increase to 8 mg/kg based on clinical response; may repeat once q 4 wk; max,

800 mg/infusion. Or, *≥100 kg:* 162 mg subcut q wk. *<100 kg:* 162 mg subcut q other wk initially. **Tx of active systemic juvenile arthritis/Still disease (systemic idiopathic juvenile arthritis).** *Child ≥2 yr:* ≥30 kg, 8 mg/kg IV or 162 mg subcut q 2 wk; *<30 kg,* 12 mg/kg IV or 162 mg subcut q 2 wk. **Tx of giant cell arteritis.** *Adult:* 162 mg subcut q wk or q 2 wk, w/glucocorticoid taper. **Tx of pts 2 yr and over w/ severe chimeric antigen receptor cytokine release syndrome.** *≥30 kg:* 8 mg/kg IV over 60 min; *<30 kg:* 12 mg/kg IV over 60 min w/ or w/o corticosteroids. May give up to four total doses, if needed, q 8 hr. Max, 800 mg/infusion. **Tx of polyarticular juvenile idiopathic arthritis.** *Adult, child ≥2 yr:* ≥30 kg, 8 mg/kg IV q 4 wk or 162 mg subcut q 2 wks; <30 kg, 10 mg/kg IV q 4 wk or 162 mg subcut q 2 wk.
**ADV EFF** **Anaphylaxis,** dizziness, **GI perforation,** HTN, increased liver enzymes, nasopharyngitis, **potentially serious infections,** URI
**INTERACTIONS** Anti-CD20 monoclonal antibodies, cyclosporine, interleukin receptor antagonists, live vaccines, omeprazole, statins, TNF antagonists, warfarin
**NC/PT** Do not mix in sol w/other drugs. Do not start if low neutrophils (<2,000/mm³) or ALT or AST above 1.5 × ULN. Monitor CBC, LFTs, lipids carefully; dosage adjustment may be needed. Not for use in preg/breastfeeding. Pt should continue other drugs for arthritis; avoid live vaccines, exposure to infection; report s&sx of infection, difficulty breathing, easy bruising/bleeding.

## tofacitinib (Xeljanz, Xeljanz XR)

**CLASS** Antirheumatic, kinase inhibitor
**PREG/CONT** C/NA

**BBW** Risk of serious to fatal infections, including TB; test for TB before tx; do not give w/active infections. Risk of lymphoma, other malignancies. Epstein-Barr virus–associated posttransplant lymphoproliferative disorder when used in renal transplant. Risk of thrombosis in pts w/at least one CV risk factor.
**IND & DOSE** **Tx of adult w/moderately to severely active RA intolerant to other therapies; tx of adult w/active psoriatic arthritis w/o response or intolerant to methotrexate or other DMARDs.** *Adult:* 5 mg PO bid (*Xeljanz*) or 11 mg/d (*Xeljanz XR*). **Tx of ulcerative colitis.** *Adult:* 10 mg PO bid for at least 8 wk, then decrease to 5 mg if therapeutic benefit achieved (*Xeljanz*). Or, 22 mg PO daily for 16 wk, then decrease to 11 mg PO daily if therapeutic benefit achieved (*Xeljanz XR*).
**ADJUST DOSE** Hepatic/renal impairment
**ADV EFF** Diarrhea, **GI perforation,** headache, **lymphoma, malignancies, serious to fatal infections,** thrombosis, URI
**INTERACTIONS** Fluconazole, ketoconazole, rifampin, live vaccines
**NC/PT** Screen for TB, active infection before tx; monitor for s&sx of infection. Monitor for lymphoma/other malignancies. Not recommended for use w/other biologic DMARDs, azathioprine, cyclosporine. Not for use in preg/breastfeeding. Pt must swallow XR form whole and not cut/crush/chew it. Pt should take as directed; avoid exposure to infections; avoid vaccines; report severe GI pain, fever, s&sx of infection.

## TOLBUTamide (generic)

**CLASS** Antidiabetic, sulfonylurea
**PREG/CONT** C/NA

**BBW** Increased risk of CV mortality; monitor accordingly.
**IND & DOSE** **Adjunct to diet/exercise to control blood glucose in pts w/type 2 diabetes; w/insulin to**

**control blood glucose in select pts w/type 1 diabetes.** *Adult:* 1–2 g/d PO in a.m. before breakfast. Maint, 0.25–3 g/d PO; max, 3 g/d.
**ADJUST DOSE** Elderly pts
**ADV EFF** **Bone marrow suppression,** dizziness, fatigue, heartburn, hypoglycemia, rash, vertigo
**INTERACTIONS** Beta-adrenergic blockers, calcium channel blockers, chloramphenicol, corticosteroids, coumarins, estrogens, isoniazid, MAOIs, miconazole, nicotinic acid, oral contraceptives, phenothiazines, phenytoin, probenecid, salicylates, sulfonamides, sympathomimetics, thyroid products
**NC/PT** Review complete diabetic teaching program. Pt may be switched to insulin during high stress. Pt should take in a.m. w/breakfast (should not take if not eating that day); continue diet/exercise program; avoid exposure to infection; report uncontrolled blood glucose, dizziness.

## tolcapone (Tasmar)

**CLASS** Antiparkinsonian, COMT inhibitor
**PREG/CONT** C/NA

**BBW** Risk of potentially fatal acute fulminant liver failure. Monitor LFTs before, q 2 wk during tx; discontinue if s&sx of liver damage. Use for pts no longer responding to other therapies.
**IND & DOSE** **Adjunct w/levodopa/carbidopa in tx of s&sx of idiopathic Parkinson disease.** *Adult:* 100 mg PO tid; max, 600 mg.
**ADJUST DOSE** Hepatic/renal impairment
**ADV EFF** Confusion; constipation; disorientation; dry mouth; falling asleep during daily activities; **fulminant, possibly fatal liver failure;** hallucinations; hypotension; lightheadedness; n/v, rash, **renal toxicity,** somnolence, weakness
**INTERACTIONS** MAOIs
**NC/PT** Monitor LFTs before, q 2 wk during tx. Always give w/levodopa/carbidopa. Do not give within 14 d of MAOIs. Taper over 2 wk when stopping. Not for use in preg/breastfeeding. Pt should take w/meals; use sugarless lozenges for dry mouth; take safety precautions for CNS effects; use laxative for constipation; report urine/stool color changes, fever.

## tolmetin sodium (generic)

**CLASS** NSAID
**PREG/CONT** C (1st, 2nd trimesters); D (3rd trimester)/NA

**BBW** Increased risk of CV events, GI bleeding; monitor accordingly. Not for use for periop pain in CABG surgery.
**IND & DOSE** **Tx of acute flares; long-term mgt of RA, osteoarthritis.** *Adult:* 400 mg PO tid (1,200 mg/d) preferably including dose on arising and at bedtime. Maint, 600–1,800 mg/d in three–four divided doses for RA, 600–1,600 mg/d in three–four divided doses for osteoarthritis. **Tx of juvenile RA.** *Child ≥2 yr:* 20 mg/kg/d PO in three–four divided doses. Usual dose, 15–30 mg/kg/d; max, 30 mg/kg/d.
**ADV EFF** **Anaphylactoid reactions to fatal anaphylactic shock, bone marrow suppression, bronchospasm,** diarrhea, dizziness, dyspepsia, dysuria, GI pain, headache, HTN, insomnia, rash, somnolence, vision problems
**NC/PT** Pt should take w/milk if GI upset a problem; have periodic eye exams; take safety precautions for CNS effects; report s&sx of infection, difficulty breathing, unusual bleeding.

## tolterodine tartrate (Detrol)

**CLASS** Antimuscarinic
**PREG/CONT** C/NA

**IND & DOSE** **Tx of overactive bladder.** *Adult:* 1–2 mg PO bid. ER form, 2–4 mg/d PO.

**ADJUST DOSE** Hepatic/renal impairment
**ADV EFF** Blurred vision, constipation, dizziness, dry mouth, dyspepsia, n/v, vision changes, weight gain
**INTERACTIONS** CYP2D6, CYP3A4 inhibitors
**NC/PT** Pt should swallow capsule whole and not cut/crush/chew it; use sugarless lozenges for dry mouth; take laxative for constipation, safety precautions for CNS effects; report rash, difficulty breathing, palpitations.

**DANGEROUS DRUG**

## tolvaptan (Jynarque)

**CLASS** Vasopressin antagonist
**PREG/CONT** Unkn/NA

**BBW** May cause serious, potentially fatal liver injury. Acute liver failure requiring liver transplantation has been reported. Measure transaminases and bilirubin before start of treatment, at 2 wk and 4 wk after initiation, then monthly for first 18 mo, then q 3 mo thereafter. Is available only through REMS Program.
**IND & DOSE** **To slow kidney function decline in rapidly progressing autosomal dominant polycystic kidney disease.** *Adult:* Initially, 60 mg PO daily split as 45 mg and 15 mg 8 hr later; titration step: 90 mg PO daily split as 60 mg and 30 mg 8 hr later; target dose: 120 mg PO daily split as 90 mg and 30 mg 8 hr later.
**ADV EFF** **Hypernatremia, liver failure**, nocturia, pollakiuria, polydipsia, polyuria, thirst
**NC/PT** Concomitant use of strong CYP3A inhibitors is contraindicated; dose adjustment recommended if given w/moderate CYP3A inhibitors. Pt should drink water when thirsty to decrease risk of dehydration; stop drug for fatigue, anorexia, n/v, right upper abd discomfort/tenderness, fever, rash, pruritus, icterus, dark urine, jaundice; report known/suspected preg; avoid breastfeeding during tx.

## tolvaptan (Samsca)

**CLASS** Selective vasopressin receptor antagonist
**PREG/CONT** C/NA

**BBW** Initiate tx in hospital setting, w/ close supervision of sodium, volume. Not for use when rapid correction of hyponatremia needed; too-rapid correction of hyponatremia (eg, >12 mEq/L/24 hr) can cause osmotic demyelination, resulting in severe CNS adverse effects. Not for use for autosomal dominant polycystic kidney disease.
**IND & DOSE** **Tx of clinically significant hypervolemic, euvolemic hyponatremia.** *Adult:* 15 mg/d PO; may increase after at least 24 hr to max 60 mg/d.
**ADV EFF** Asthenia, constipation, dehydration, dry mouth, **hepatic injury**, hyperglycemia, polyuria, **serious liver toxicity**, thirst
**INTERACTIONS** CYP3A inducers/ inhibitors
**NC/PT** Do not use w/hypertonic saline sol. Limit tx duration to 30 d. If liver injury, discontinue. Monitor serum electrolytes. Not for use in emergency situation, preg/breastfeeding. Pt should report severe constipation, increasing thirst, fainting.

## topiramate (Qudexy XR, Topamax, Trokendi XR)

**CLASS** Antiepileptic, antimigraine
**PREG/CONT** High risk/NA

**BBW** Increased risk of suicidality; monitor accordingly. Reduce dose, stop, or substitute other antiepileptic gradually; stopping abruptly may precipitate status epilepticus.
**IND & DOSE** **Px of migraines:** *Adult, child ≥12 yr:* 25 mg PO in p.m. for 1 wk; wk 2, 25 mg PO bid a.m. and p.m.; wk 3, 25 mg PO in a.m., 50 mg PO in p.m.; wk 4, 50 mg PO a.m. and p.m. **Tx of**

**partial-onset and generalized seizure disorders.** *Adult, child ≥10 yr:* 25 mg PO bid, titrating to maint dose of 200 mg PO bid over 6 wk. wk 1, 25 mg bid; wk 2, 50 mg bid; wk 3, 75 mg bid; wk 4, 100 mg bid; wk 5, 150 mg bid; wk 6, 200 mg bid. Or ER form, 50 mg PO at bedtime, range 1–3 mg/kg for first wk; titrate at 1- to 2-wk intervals by 1- to 3-mg/kg increments to 5–9 mg/kg/d PO. Max dose: 400 mg/d. *Child 2–<10 yr:* 5–9 mg/kg/d PO in two divided doses. Start tx at nightly dose of 25 mg (or less, based on 1–3 mg/kg/d) for first wk. May titrate up by increments of 1–3 mg/kg/d (in two divided doses) at 1- to 2-wk intervals. ER form: 25 mg/d PO at bedtime. **Adjunct tx of Lennox-Gastaut syndrome.** *Adult:* 25 mg/d PO; titrate to 200 mg PO bid. ER form: 25–50 mg PO once daily; titrate to 200–400 mg/d. *Child ≥2 yr:* 1–3 mg/kg/d PO at bedtime; titrate to 5–9 mg/kg/d. ER form: 25 mg PO once daily at bedtime; titrate slowly to 5–9 mg/kg PO once daily.
**ADJUST DOSE** Hepatic/renal impairment
**ADV EFF** Ataxia, cognitive dysfx, dizziness, dysmenorrhea, dyspepsia, fatigue, metabolic acidosis, myopia, nausea, nystagmus, paresthesia, renal stones, somnolence, **suicidality**, URI, visual field defects
**INTERACTIONS** Alcohol, carbamazepine, carbonic anhydrase inhibitors, CNS depressants, hormonal contraceptives, phenytoin, valproic acid
**NC/PT** Taper if stopping. Not for use in preg (may make hormonal contraceptives ineffective; barrier contraceptives advised). Pt should not cut/crush/chew tablets (bitter taste); may swallow sprinkle capsule or XR forms whole or sprinkle contents on soft food, swallow immediately; should avoid alcohol; take safety precautions for CNS effects; report vision changes, flank pain, thoughts of suicide. Name confusion between *Topamax* and *Toprol-XL* (metoprolol).

**DANGEROUS DRUG**

## topotecan hydrochloride (Hycamtin)

**CLASS** Antineoplastic
**PREG/CONT** High risk/NA

**BBW** Monitor bone marrow carefully; do not give dose until bone marrow responsive.
**IND & DOSE Tx of metastatic ovarian cancer, small-cell lung cancer.** *Adult:* 1.5 mg/m²/d IV over 30 min for 5 d, starting on day 1 of 21-day course. Minimum four courses recommended. **Tx of persistent cervical cancer.** *Adult:* 0.75 mg/m² by IV infusion over 30 min on days 1, 2, 3 followed by cisplatin on day 1. Repeat q 21 d.
**ADJUST DOSE** Hepatic/renal impairment
**ADV EFF** Alopecia, **bone marrow suppression,** constipation, fever, infections, **interstitial pneumonitis,** n/v/d, pain
**INTERACTIONS** Cytotoxic drugs
**NC/PT** Monitor CBC; dose adjustment may be needed. Monitor for extravasation; stop immediately, manage tissue injury. Not for use in preg (barrier contraceptives advised)/breastfeeding. Pt should mark calendar of tx days; cover head at temp extremes (hair loss possible); avoid exposure to infection; take analgesics for pain; report difficulty breathing, unusual bleeding, s&sx of infection.

**DANGEROUS DRUG**

## toremifene citrate (Fareston)

**CLASS** Antineoplastic, estrogen receptor modulator
**PREG/CONT** D/NA

**BBW** Risk of prolonged QT. Obtain baseline, periodic ECG; avoid concurrent use of other QT-prolonging drugs.

**IND & DOSE Tx of advanced breast cancer in postmenopausal women.** *Adult:* 60 mg PO daily; continue until disease progression.
**ADV EFF** Depression, dizziness, headache, hepatotoxicity, hot flashes, n/v, **prolonged QT,** rash, uterine malignancy, vaginal discharge
**INTERACTIONS** Oral anticoagulants, other drugs that decrease calcium excretion, QT-prolonging drugs
**NC/PT** Obtain baseline ECG; monitor periodically during tx. Not for use in preg (barrier contraceptives advised)/ breastfeeding. Pt should take safety precautions w/dizziness; report palpitations, vision changes.

## torsemide (Demadex)

**CLASS** Loop diuretic, sulfonamide
**PREG/CONT** B/NA

**IND & DOSE Tx of edema associated w/HF.** *Adult:* 10–20 mg/d PO or IV; max, 200 mg/d. **Tx of edema associated w/chronic renal failure.** *Adult:* 20 mg/d PO or IV; max, 200 mg/d. **Tx of edema associated w/hepatic failure.** *Adult:* 5–10 mg/d PO or IV; max, 40 mg/d. **Tx of HTN.** *Adult:* 5 mg/d PO.
**ADV EFF** Anorexia, asterixis, dizziness, drowsiness, headache, hypokalemia, nocturia, n/v/d, orthostatic hypotension, ototoxicity, pain, phlebitis at injection site, polyuria
**INTERACTIONS** Aminoglycoside antibiotics, cisplatin, digoxin, ethacrynic acid, NSAIDs
**NC/PT** Monitor serum electrolytes. Pt should take early in day to prevent sleep disruption; weigh self daily, report changes of >3 lb/d; take safety precautions for CNS effects; report swelling, hearing loss, muscle cramps/weakness.

**DANGEROUS DRUG**

## tositumomab and iodine I-131 tositumomab

(Bexxar)
**CLASS** Antineoplastic, monoclonal antibody
**PREG/CONT** X/NA

**BBW** Risk of severe, prolonged cytopenia. Hypersensitivity reactions, including anaphylaxis, have occurred.
**IND & DOSE Tx of CD20-positive, follicular non-Hodgkin lymphoma.** *Adult:* 450 mg tositumomab IV in 50 mL normal saline over 60 min, 5 mCi I-131 w/35 mg tositumomab in 30 mL normal saline IV over 20 min; then repeat as therapeutic step, adjusting I-131 based on pt response.
**ADV EFF** Anorexia, asthenia, **cancer development,** fever, headache, hypothyroidism, n/v/d, **severe cytopenia**
**NC/PT** Radioactive; use special handling precautions. Rule out preg; not for use in preg (two types of contraceptives advised)/breastfeeding. Monitor CBC, renal function. Discuss limiting exposure to family; will take about 12 d to clear body. Pt should report s&sx of infection, unusual bleeding.

## trabectedin (Yondelis)

**CLASS** Alkylating agent, antineoplastic
**PREG/CONT** High risk/NA

**IND & DOSE Tx of pts w/unresectable metastatic liposarcoma/ leiomyosarcoma after anthracycline tx.** *Adult:* 1.5 mg/m$^2$ IV over 24 hr through central line q 3 wk.
**ADJUST DOSE** Hepatic impairment
**ADV EFF** Bone marrow suppression, capillary leak syndrome, **cardiomyopathy,** constipation, dyspnea, fatigue, **hepatotoxicity,** n/v/d, **neutropenic sepsis,** peripheral edema, **rhabdomyolysis**
**INTERACTIONS** Strong CYP3A inducers/inhibitors; avoid combo

**NC/PT** Monitor CBC, LFTs, creatinine levels carefully; dose based on response. Premedicate w/dexamethasone 30 min before each infusion. Not for use in preg (barrier contraceptives advised)/breastfeeding. Pt should avoid exposure to infections; mark calendar of tx days; report s&sx of infection, difficulty breathing, muscle pain, peripheral edema, urine/stool color changes.

DANGEROUS DRUG

**traMADol hydrochloride** (ConZip, Ultram)
**CLASS** Opioid analgesic
**PREG/CONT** High risk w/ prolonged use/NA

**BBW** REMS required due to risk of addiction, abuse. Risk of life-threatening respiratory depression w/accidental ingestion, especially in child. Risk of neonatal opioid withdrawal w/prolonged use. Risk of increased adverse effects if used w/other drugs affecting CYP450 isoenzymes, benzodiazepines, other CNS depressants.
**IND & DOSE Relief of moderate to moderately severe pain.** *Adult:* 50–100 mg PO q 4–6 hr; max, 400 mg/d. For chronic pain, 25 mg/d PO in a.m.; titrate in 25-mg increments q 3 d to 100 mg/d. Then, increase in 50-mg increments q 3 d to 200 mg/d. After titration, 50–100 mg q 4–6 hr PO; max, 400 mg/d. Or, 100-mg PO ER tablet once daily, titrated by 100-mg increments q 5 d; max, 300 mg/d. For orally disintegrating tablets, max, 200 mg/d PO.
**ADJUST DOSE** Elderly pts; hepatic/renal impairment
**ADV EFF Anaphylactoid reactions,** constipation, dizziness, headache, hypotension, n/v, sedation, **seizures, suicidality,** sweating, vertigo
**INTERACTIONS** Alcohol, carbamazepine, CNS depressants, MAOIs, SSRIs
**NC/PT** Control environment; use other measures to relieve pain. Limit use w/hx of addiction. Pt should swallow ER tablet whole and not cut/crush/chew it; take safety precautions for CNS effects; report thoughts of suicide, difficulty breathing.

**trametinib** (Mekinist)
**CLASS** Antineoplastic, kinase inhibitor
**PREG/CONT** High risk/NA

**IND & DOSE Tx of unresectable or metastatic melanoma w/BRAF V600E or V600K mutations, as monotherapy or w/dabrafenib; tx of metastatic NSCLC w/BRAF V600E; tx of advanced thyroid cancer w/ BRAF V600E and no locoregional tx options.** *Adult:* 2 mg/d PO 1 hr before or 2 hr after meal; may combine w/ dabrafenib 150 mg PO bid.
**ADJUST DOSE** Severe renal/hepatic impairment
**ADV EFF Cardiomyopathy,** diarrhea, **GI perforation, hemorrhage,** hyperglycemia, **ILD,** lymphedema, **malignancies,** ocular toxicities, **retinal pigment epithelial detachment, retinal vein occlusion, serious skin toxicity, VTE**
**NC/PT** Confirm presence of specific mutations before use. Ensure regular ophthal exams. Evaluate left ventricular ejection fraction before and q 2 mo during tx. Evaluate lung function; stop drug if sx of interstitial pneumonitis. Watch for rash, skin toxicity; stop drug if grade 2–4 rash does not improve w/3-wk interruption. Pt should take drug 1 hr before or 2 hr after meal; avoid preg/breastfeeding; know frequent testing and follow-up will be needed; be aware drug could impair fertility; report difficulty breathing, extreme fatigue, swelling of extremities, rash, vision changes.

**trandolapril** (Mavik)
**CLASS** ACE inhibitor, antihypertensive
**PREG/CONT** High risk/NA

**BBW** Rule out preg before tx; advise use of barrier contraceptives. Fetal

injury, death has occurred when used in second, third trimester.
**IND & DOSE** **Tx of HTN.** *Adult:* African-American pts: 2 mg/d PO. All other pts: 1 mg/d PO. Maint, 2–4 mg/d; max, 8 mg/d. **Tx of HF post-MI.** *Adult:* 1 mg/d PO; may start 3–5 d after MI. Adjust to target 4 mg/d.
**ADJUST DOSE** **Angioedema,** diarrhea, dizziness, headache, **hepatic failure, hypersensitivity reactions, MI,** renal impairment, tachycardia
**INTERACTIONS** ARBs, diuretics, lithium, potassium supplements, renin inhibitors
**NC/PT** Monitor LFTs. If pt on diuretic, stop diuretic 2–3 d before starting trandolapril; resume diuretic only if BP not controlled. If diuretic cannot be stopped, start at 0.5 mg PO daily; adjust upward as needed. Alert surgeon; volume replacement may be needed postop. Not for use in preg (barrier contraceptives advised)/breastfeeding. Pt should use care in situations that could lead to BP drop; take safety precautions for CNS effects; report difficulty breathing, swelling of lips/face, chest pain, urine/stool color changes.

## tranexamic acid

(Cyklokapron, Lysteda)
**CLASS** Antifibrinolytic
**PREG/CONT** B/NA

**IND & DOSE** **Tx of cyclic heavy menstrual bleeding.** *Adult:* 1,300 mg PO tid for max 5 d during monthly menstruation. **Short-term tx of hemophilia before and after tooth extraction.** *Adult:* 10 mg/kg IV w/replacement therapy before extraction, then 10 mg/kg IV 3–4 ×/d as needed for 2–8 d.
**ADJUST DOSE** Hepatic/renal impairment
**ADV EFF** Abd pain, **anaphylactic shock, anaphylactoid reactions,** arthralgia, back pain, fatigue, headache, n/v/d, **thromboembolic events,** visual disturbances
**INTERACTIONS** Hormonal contraceptives, TPAs
**NC/PT** Obtain baseline, periodic evaluation of bleeding. Not for use in preg (hormonal contraceptives may increase thromboembolic event risk; barrier contraceptives advised). Pt should report difficulty breathing, leg pain/swelling, severe headache, vision changes.

## tranylcypromine sulfate

(Parnate)
**CLASS** Antidepressant, MAOI
**PREG/CONT** Unkn/NA

**BBW** Limit amount available to suicidal pts. Not approved for child. Tyramine ingestion increases risk of hypertensive crisis; monitor BP. Allow for drug-free intervals.
**IND & DOSE** **Tx of major depressive disorder.** *Adult:* 30 mg/d PO in divided doses. If no improvement within 2–3 wk, increase in 10-mg/d increments q 1–3 wk. Max, 60 mg/d.
**ADJUST DOSE** Elderly pts
**ADV EFF** Abd pain, anorexia, blurred vision, confusion, constipation, dizziness, drowsiness, dry mouth, headache, hyperreflexia, **hypertensive crises,** hypomania, hypotension, insomnia, jitteriness, **liver toxicity,** n/v/d, orthostatic hypotension, photosensitivity, suicidal thoughts, twitching, vertigo
**INTERACTIONS** Alcohol, amphetamines, antidiabetics, beta blockers, bupropion, buspirone, general anesthetics, meperidine, SSRIs, sympathomimetics, TCAs, thiazides, tyramine-containing foods
**NC/PT** Have phentolamine, another alpha-adrenergic blocker on hand for hypertensive crisis. Monitor for s&sx of mania in pts w/bipolar disease. Do not use within 14 d of other MAOIs, within 10 d of buspirone, bupropion. Monitor LFTs, BP regularly. Pt should avoid diet high in tyramine-containing foods during, for 2 wk after tx; avoid alcohol, OTC appetite suppressants; take safety

precautions for CNS effects; change position slowly w/orthostatic hypotension; report rash, urine/stool color changes, thoughts of suicide.

DANGEROUS DRUG

**trastuzumab** (Herceptin), **trastuzumab-anns** (Kanjinti), **trastuzumab-dkst** (Ogivri), **trastuzumab-dttb** (Ontruzant), **trastuzumab-pkrb** (Herzuma), **trastuzumab-qyyp** (Trazimera)

**CLASS** Antineoplastic, monoclonal antibody (anti-HER2)

**PREG/CONT** High risk/NA

**BBW** Monitor pt during infusion; provide comfort measures, analgesics as appropriate for infusion reaction. Monitor cardiac status, especially if pt receiving chemo; do not give w/ anthracycline chemo. Have emergency equipment on hand for cardiotoxicity; cardiomyopathy possible. Monitor for possibly severe pulmonary toxicity, especially within 24 hours of infusion. Stop if s&sx of respiratory involvement. Embryotoxic; ensure pt is not preg before tx (advise use of contraceptive measures).

**IND & DOSE** **Tx of metastatic HER2 overexpressing breast cancer.** *Adult:* 4 mg/kg IV once by IV infusion over 90 min. Maint, 2 mg/kg/wk IV over at least 30 min as tolerated; max, 500 mg/dose. **Adjunct tx of HER2-overexpressing breast cancer.** *Adult:* After completion of doxorubicin, cyclophosphamide tx, give wkly for 52 wk. Initially, 4 mg/kg by IV infusion over 90 min; maint, 2 mg/kg/wk by IV infusion over 30 min. Or, initially, 8 mg/kg by IV infusion over 90 min; then 6 mg/kg by IV infusion over 30–90 min q 3 wk. During first 12 wk, give w/paclitaxel. **Tx of HER2-overexpressing metastatic gastric or gastroesophageal junction adenocancer.** *Adult:* 8 mg/kg IV over 90 min; then 6 mg/kg IV over 30–90 min q 3 wk until disease progression.

**ADV EFF** Abd pain, anemia, cardiomyopathy, chills, diarrhea, fever, headache, infections, injection-site reactions, leukopenia, **neutropenia,** paresthesia, **pulmonary toxicity, serious cardiotoxicity**

**NC/PT** Ensure HER2 testing before therapy. Do not mix w/other drug sols or add other drugs to IV line. Monitor cardiac status; have emergency equipment on hand. Monitor respiratory status, CBC. Pt should mark calendar of tx days; avoid exposure to infection; avoid preg (contraceptives advised)/breastfeeding (ensure 7-mo washout before breastfeeding); report chest pain, difficulty breathing, pain at injection site.

**traZODone hydrochloride** (generic)

**CLASS** Antidepressant

**PREG/CONT** C/NA

**BBW** Increased risk of suicidality; limit quantities in depressed, suicidal pts.

**IND & DOSE** **Tx of depression.** *Adult:* 150 mg/d PO in divided doses; max, 400 mg/d PO in divided doses. For severe depression, max, 600 mg/d PO.

**ADJUST DOSE** Elderly pts

**ADV EFF** Angle-closure glaucoma, blurred vision, constipation, dizziness, **NMS,** orthostatic hypotension, sedation, withdrawal syndrome

**INTERACTIONS** Alcohol, aspirin, CNS depressants, CYP3A4 inducers/ inhibitors, digoxin, MAOIs, NSAIDs, phenytoin, SSRIs, St. John's wort

**NC/PT** Do not give within 14 d of MAOIs. Taper when stopping; do not stop abruptly. Use caution in preg/ breastfeeding. Pt should take safety precautions for CNS effects; report fever, severe constipation, thoughts of suicide.

**treprostinil** (Orenitram, Remodulin, Tyvaso)
**CLASS** Endothelin receptor antagonist, vasodilator
**PREG/CONT** Unkn/NA

**IND & DOSE Tx of pulmonary arterial HTN.** *Adult:* 1.25 ng/kg/min subcut infusion. Increase rate in increments of no more than 1.25 ng/kg/min wkly for first 4 wk, then by 2.5 ng/kg/min wkly. Max, 40 ng/kg/min or 3 breaths (18 mcg), using *Tyvaso* Inhalation System, per tx session; 4 sessions/d, approx 4 hr apart during waking hours. Increase by additional 3 breaths/session at 1- to 2-wk intervals if needed, tolerated. Maint, 9 breaths (54 mcg)/session. For *Orenitram,* 0.125–0.25 mg PO bid–tid; titrate q 3–4 d as tolerated.
**ADJUST DOSE** Hepatic impairment
**ADV EFF** Edema, headache, infusion-site reaction, jaw pain, n/d, rash
**INTERACTIONS** Anticoagulants, antihypertensives, antiplatelets, diuretics, vasodilators
**NC/PT** See manufacturer's instructions if switching from epoprostenol (*Flolan*). Obtain baseline pulmonary status, exercise tolerance. Not for use in preg (barrier contraceptives advised). Taper slowly when stopping. Evaluate subcut infusion site wkly; give analgesics for headache. Teach proper care, use of continuous subcut infusion; if using inhalation, review proper use. Pt should swallow oral tablets whole w/food; continue usual tx procedures, report swelling, injection site pain/swelling, worsening of condition.

**DANGEROUS DRUG**

**tretinoin** (Atralin, Avita, Renova, Retin-A, Tretin-X)
**CLASS** Antineoplastic, retinoid
**PREG/CONT** High risk/NA

**BBW** Rule out preg before tx; arrange for preg test within 2 wk of starting tx. Advise use of two forms of contraception during tx, for 1 mo after tx ends. Should only be used under supervision of experienced practitioner or in institution experienced w/its use. Risk of rapid leukocytosis (40% of pts); notify physician immediately if this occurs. Stop drug, notify physician if LFTs over 5 × ULN, pulmonary infiltrates appear, or pt has difficulty breathing; serious side effects possible. Monitor for retinoic acid-APL syndrome (fever, dyspnea, acute respiratory distress, weight gain, pulmonary infiltrates, pleural/pericardial effusion, multiorgan failure); endotracheal intubation, mechanical ventilation may be needed.
**IND & DOSE To induce remission in acute promyelocytic leukemia (APL).** *Adult, child ≥1 yr:* 45 mg/m²/d PO in two evenly divided doses until complete remission; stop tx 30 d after complete remission obtained or after 90 d, whichever first. **Topical tx of acne vulgaris; mitigation of wrinkles; mottled hyperpigmentation.** *Adult, child ≥1 yr:* Apply once/d before bedtime. Cover entire affected area lightly, avoiding mucous membranes.
**ADV EFF** **Cardiac arrest,** dry skin, earache, fever, GI bleeding, headache, lipid changes, **MI,** n/v, **pseudotumor cerebri, rapid/evolving leukocytosis,** rash, sweating, visual disturbances
**INTERACTIONS** Hydroxyurea, keratolytic agents, ketoconazole, tetracyclines
**NC/PT** Monitor LFTs, lipids, vision. Not for use in preg (two forms of contraceptives, during and for 1 mo after tx, advised)/breastfeeding. Pt cannot donate blood during tx. Pt should not cut, crush oral capsule; have frequent blood tests; avoid products containing vitamin D; take safety precautions for CNS effects; use sugarless lozenges w/dry mouth; report severe/bloody diarrhea, difficulty breathing, thoughts of suicide.

**triamcinolone acetonide** (Kenalog), **triamcinolone hexacetonide** (Aristospan)
**CLASS** Corticosteroid
**PREG/CONT** C/NA

**IND & DOSE Hypercalcemia of cancer; mgt of various inflammatory disorders; tx of idiopathic thrombocytopenic purpura.** *Adult:* Individualize dose, depending on condition severity, pt response. Give daily dose before 9 a.m. to minimize adrenal suppression. If long-term tx needed, consider alternate-day tx. After long-term tx, withdraw slowly to avoid adrenal insufficiency. Range, 2.5–100 mg/d IM. *Child:* Individualize dose based on response, not formulae; monitor growth. **Maint, tx of bronchial asthma.** *Adult, child 6–12 yr:* 200 mcg inhalant released w/each actuation delivers about 100 mcg. Two inhalations tid–qid; max, 16 inhalations/d. **Tx of seasonal, perennial allergic rhinitis.** *Adult:* 2 sprays (220 mcg total dose) in each nostril daily; max, 4 sprays/d. *Child 6–12 yr:* 1 spray in each nostril once/d (100–110 mcg dose); max, 2 sprays/nostril/d. **Intra-articular relief of inflammatory conditions.** *Adult, child:* Acetonide, 2.5–15 mg intra-articular. Hexacetonide, 2–20 mg intra-articular; up to 0.5 mg/square inch of affected area intralesional. **Relief of inflammatory, pruritic s&sx of dermatoses.** *Adult, child:* Apply sparingly to affected area bid–qid. **Tx of oral lesions.** *Adult:* Press small dab (1/4 inch) to each lesion until thin film develops, 2–3 ×/d after meals.
**ADV EFF** Headache, increased appetite, immunosuppression, impaired wound healing, infections, menstrual changes, osteoporosis, sodium/fluid retention, vertigo, weight gain
**INTERACTIONS** Barbiturates, edrophonium, neostigmine, oral antidiabetics, phenytoin, pyridostigmine, rifampin, salicylates
**NC/PT** Not for acute asthmatic attack. Give in a.m. to mimic normal levels. Taper when stopping after long-term tx. Do not use occlusive dressings w/topical form. Review proper administration. Pt should avoid exposure to infection, joint overuse after intra-articular injection; keep topical forms away from eyes; report swelling, s&sx of infection, worsening of condition.

**triamcinolone acetonide, extended release** (Zilretta)
**CLASS** Corticosteroid
**PREG/CONT** Unkn/NA

**IND & DOSE Mgt of osteoarthritis pain of the knee.** *Adult:* 32 mg intra-articular injection once.
**ADV EFF** Contusions, cough, **hypersensitivity, joint infection/damage,** sinusitis
**NC/PT** Give only via intra-articular injection; serious neuro events have been reported after epidural or intrathecal administration.

**triamterene** (Dyrenium)
**CLASS** Potassium-sparing diuretic
**PREG/CONT** C/NA

**BBW** Risk of hyperkalemia (possibly fatal), more likely w/diabetics, elderly/severely ill pts; monitor potassium carefully.
**IND & DOSE Tx of edema associated w/systemic conditions.** *Adult:* 100 mg PO bid; max, 300 mg/d. **Tx of HTN.** *Adult:* 25 mg/d PO; usual dose, 50–100 mg/d.
**ADV EFF** Abd pain, anorexia, dizziness, drowsiness, dry mouth, **hyperkalemia,** n/v/d, rash, renal stones
**INTERACTIONS** Amantadine, lithium, potassium supplements

**NC/PT** Pt should take in a.m. to decrease sleep interruption, w/food if GI upset; weigh self regularly, report change of 3 lb/d; take safety precautions for CNS effects; avoid foods high in potassium; report swelling, difficulty breathing, flank pain, muscle cramps, tremors.

## triazolam (Halcion)

**CLASS** Benzodiazepine, sedative-hypnotic
**PREG/CONT** High risk/C-IV

**BBW** Concomitant use of benzodiazepines and opioids can result in sedation, respiratory depression, coma, death.
**IND & DOSE** **Tx of insomnia.** *Adult:* 0.125–0.25 mg PO before retiring. May increase to max 0.5 mg. Limit use to 7–10 d.
**ADJUST DOSE** Elderly, debilitated pts
**ADV EFF** **Anaphylaxis, angioedema,** bradycardia, confusion, constipation, **CV collapse,** diarrhea, drowsiness, drug dependence, fatigue, hiccups, nervousness, sleep-driving behaviors, tachycardia, urticaria
**INTERACTIONS** Alcohol, aminophylline, cimetidine, CNS depressants, disulfiram, dyphylline, grapefruit juice, hormonal contraceptives, itraconazole, ketoconazole, omeprazole, theophylline
**NC/PT** Taper gradually after long-term use. Monitor renal function, CBC periodically. Not for use in preg (barrier contraceptives advised)/breastfeeding. Pt should avoid grapefruit juice, alcohol; take safety precautions for CNS effects; report difficulty breathing, swelling of face/eyes, continued sleep disorders.

▶ **NEW DRUG**

## triclabendazole (Egaten)

**CLASS** Anthelmintic
**PREG/CONT** Unkn/NA

**IND & DOSE** **Tx of fascioliasis.** *Adult, child ≥6 yr:* 10 mg/kg PO q 12 hr w/food for two doses.
**ADV EFF** Abd pain, appetite decrease, diarrhea, headache, hyperhidrosis, musculoskeletal chest pain, n/v, pruritus, **prolonged QT,** urticaria
**INTERACTIONS** CYP2C19 substrates
**NC/PT** If dosage cannot be adjusted exactly, round upwards. Monitor QT w/ECG if risk of prolonged QT. Pt should swallow tablets whole or divide in half and take w/water, or crush and take w/applesauce.

## trientine hydrochloride (Clovique, Syprine)

**CLASS** Chelate
**PREG/CONT** C/NA

**IND & DOSE** **Tx of pts w/Wilson disease intolerant of penicillamine.** *Adult:* 750–1,250 mg/d PO in divided doses; max, 2 g/d. *Child:* 500–750 mg/d PO; max, 1,500 mg/d.
**ADV EFF** Abd pain, anorexia, epigastric pain, **hypersensitivity reactions,** iron deficiency, muscle spasm, myasthenia gravis, rash, rhabdomyolysis, SLE, weakness
**NC/PT** Pt should take on empty stomach 1 hr before, 2 hr after meals; swallow capsule whole and not cut/crush/chew it; monitor temp nightly for first mo of tx; space iron supplement at least 2 hr apart from trientine; report fever, muscle weakness/pain, difficulty breathing.

## trihexyphenidyl hydrochloride (generic)

**CLASS** Antiparkinsonian (anticholinergic type)
**PREG/CONT** C/NA

**BBW** Stop or decrease dosage if dry mouth interferes w/swallowing, speaking.
**IND & DOSE** **Adjunct in tx of parkinsonism.** *Adult:* 1 mg PO first day. Increase by 2-mg increments at 3- to 5-day intervals until total of 6–10 mg/d. Postencephalitic pts may need

12–15 mg/d. W/levodopa: Adjust based on response; usual, 3–6 mg/d PO. **Tx of drug-induced extrapyramidal sx.** *Adult:* 1 mg PO. May need to temporarily reduce tranquilizer dose to expedite control of extrapyramidal sx. Usual dose, 5–15 mg/d.
**ADJUST DOSE** Elderly pts
**ADV EFF** Blurred vision, confusion, constipation, decreased sweating, delusions, disorientation, dizziness, drowsiness, dry mouth, flushing, light-headedness, urine retention
**INTERACTIONS** Haloperidol, phenothiazines
**NC/PT** Pt should empty bladder before each dose; use caution in hot weather (decreased sweating can lead to heat stroke); use sugarless lozenges for dry mouth; take safety precautions for CNS effects; report eye pain, rash, rapid heartbeat, difficulty swallowing/speaking.

## trimethobenzamide hydrochloride (Tigan)
**CLASS** Antiemetic (anticholinergic)
**PREG/CONT** C/NA

**IND & DOSE** **Control of postop n/v, nausea associated w/gastroenteritis.** *Adult:* 300 mg PO tid–qid, or 200 mg IM tid–qid.
**ADJUST DOSE** Elderly pts
**ADV EFF** Blurred vision, dizziness, drowsiness, headache, hypotension, pain/swelling at injection site
**NC/PT** Ensure adequate hydration. Pt should avoid alcohol (sedation possible); take safety precautions for CNS effects; report unusual bleeding, visual disturbances, pain at injection site.

## trimethoprim (Primsol)
**CLASS** Antibiotic
**PREG/CONT** C/NA

**IND & DOSE** **Uncomplicated UTIs caused by susceptible bacteria strains.** *Adult, child ≥12 yr:* 100 mg PO q 12 hr or 200 mg PO q 24 hr for 10–14 d. **Tx of otitis media.** *Child <12 yr:* 10 mg/kg/d PO in divided doses q 12 hr for 10 d.
**ADJUST DOSE** Elderly pts, renal impairment
**ADV EFF** **Bone marrow suppression,** epigastric distress, exfoliative dermatitis, **hepatic impairment,** pruritus, rash
**INTERACTIONS** Phenytoin
**NC/PT** Culture before tx. Protect drug from light. Monitor CBC. Pt should take full course; avoid exposure to infection; report unusual bleeding, s&sx of infection, rash.

## trimipramine maleate (Surmontil)
**CLASS** TCA
**PREG/CONT** C/NA

**BBW** Limit access in depressed, potentially suicidal pts. Monitor for suicidal ideation, especially when beginning tx, changing doses. High risk of suicidality in child, adolescent, young adult.
**IND & DOSE** **Relief of sx of depression.** *Adult:* Inpts, 100 mg/d PO in divided doses. Gradually increase to 200 mg/d as needed; max, 250–300 mg/d. Outpts, 75 mg/d PO in divided doses. May increase to 150 mg/d; max, 200 mg/d. *Child ≥12 yr:* 50 mg/d PO w/gradual increases up to 100 mg/d.
**ADJUST DOSE** Elderly pts
**ADV EFF** Anticholinergic effects, **bone marrow suppression,** constipation, dry mouth, extrapyramidal effects, **MI,** orthostatic hypotension, photosensitivity, rash, **stroke**
**INTERACTIONS** Alcohol, cimetidine, clarithromycin, clonidine, fluoroquinolones, fluoxetine, MAOIs, ranitidine, sympathomimetics, tramadol
**NC/PT** Monitor CBC periodically. Not for use in preg (contraceptives advised). Pt should not stop suddenly; avoid sun exposure, alcohol; take safety

precautions for CNS effects; use sugarless lozenges for dry mouth; report thoughts of suicide, excessive sedation.

**DANGEROUS DRUG**

## triptorelin pamoate
(Trelstar)
**CLASS** Antineoplastic, LHRH analog
**PREG/CONT** High risk/NA

**IND & DOSE** **Palliative tx of advanced prostate cancer.** *Adult:* 3.75-mg depot injection IM once monthly into buttock, or 11.25-mg injection IM q 12 wk into buttock, or 22.5 mg IM q 24 wk into buttock.
**ADV EFF** **Anaphylaxis, angioedema,** bone pain, decreased erection, headache, **HF,** hot flashes, injection-site pain, insomnia, **prolonged QT,** sexual dysfx, urinary tract sx
**INTERACTIONS** Antipsychotics, metoclopramide, QT-prolonging drugs
**NC/PT** Monitor testosterone, PSA before, periodically during tx. Not for use in preg. Pt should mark calendar for injection days; use comfort measures for hot flashes/pain; report swelling, difficulty breathing, s&sx of infection at injection sites.

## trospium chloride
(generic)
**CLASS** Antimuscarinic, antispasmodic
**PREG/CONT** C/NA

**IND & DOSE** **Tx of s&sx of overactive bladder.** *Adult>75 yr:* 20 mg PO bid on empty stomach at least 1 hr before meals; monitor pt response and adjust down to 20 mg/d based on tolerance. *Adult<75 yr:* 20 mg PO bid on empty stomach, at least 1 hr before meals. Or, 60 mg ER tablet PO once/d.
**ADJUST DOSE** Renal impairment
**ADV EFF** Constipation, decreased sweating, dizziness, drowsiness, dry mouth, fatigue, headache, urine retention
**INTERACTIONS** Digoxin, metformin, morphine, other anticholinergics, procainamide, pancuronium, tenofovir, vancomycin
**NC/PT** Not for use in preg/breastfeeding. Pt should empty bladder before each dose; take on empty stomach 1 hr before, 2 hr after food; not cut/crush/chew ER tablet; use sugarless lozenges, mouth care for dry mouth; maintain hydration; use caution in hot environments (decreased sweating could lead to heat stroke); take safety precautions for CNS effects; report inability to urinate, fever.

## umeclidinium (Incruse Ellipta)
**CLASS** Anticholinergic, bronchodilator
**PREG/CONT** Unkn/NA

**IND & DOSE** **Long-term maint tx of airflow obstruction in COPD.** *Adult:* 62.5 mcg (1 oral inhalation)/d.
**ADV EFF** Allergic reactions, cough, narrow-angle glaucoma, **paradoxical bronchospasm,** URI, urine retention
**INTERACTIONS** Other anticholinergics; avoid combo
**NC/PT** Not for use in deteriorating COPD, acute bronchospasm. Not for use in pts w/hypersensitivity to milk proteins. Monitor closely w/known glaucoma, BPH, urine retention. Teach proper use of inhaler device. Pt should report sudden shortness of breath, vision problems, difficult/painful urination.

**▶NEW DRUG**

## upadacitinib (Rinvoq)
**CLASS** Antiarthritic, Janus kinase inhibitor
**PREG/CONT** High risk/NA

**BBW** Risk of serious infections leading to hospitalization/death, including TB, bacterial, fungal, viral, other opportunistic infections. Test for latent TB before dosing; if positive, treat TB

before starting Rinvoq. Monitor all pts for active TB during tx. Risk of lymphoma, other malignancies. Risk of thrombosis, including DVT, PE, arterial thrombosis.
**IND & DOSE Tx of moderate to severe RA in pts w/inadequate response to or intolerant of methotrexate, as monotherapy or w/ methotrexate or other nonbiologic DMARDS.** *Adult:* 15 mg PO once daily.
**ADV EFF** Cough, **GI perforation, infections, malignancy,** nausea, pyrexia, **thrombosis**
**INTERACTIONS** CYP3A4 inducers/ inhibitors, live vaccines
**NC/PT** Avoid initiation or interrupt tx if absolute lymphocyte count is <500 cells/mm$^3$, ANC is <1,000 cells/mm$^3$, or Hgb is <8 g/dL. Stop if acute infection. Do not use if severe hepatic impairment (Child-Pugh class C). Contraceptives advised during tx and for 4 wk after final dose. Pt should swallow tablets whole.

## uriden (Xuriden)
**CLASS** Pyrimidine analog
**PREG/CONT** Unkn/NA

**IND & DOSE Tx of hereditary orotic aciduria.** *Adult, child:* 60 mg/kg/d PO; may increase to 120 mg/kg/d if needed. Max, 8 g/d.
**ADV EFF** None reported
**NC/PT** Mix granules in applesauce, pudding, yogurt, milk, or baby formula; discard any granules left in packet. Administer as soon as mixed; pt should not chew granules. Tell pt blood tests will be taken regularly to monitor drug's effects.

## uridine triacetate (Vistogard, Xuriden)
**CLASS** Pyrimidine analog
**PREG/CONT** Unkn/NA

**IND & DOSE Emergency tx of 5-FU or capecitabine overdose or severe toxicity.** *Adult:* 10 g PO q 6 hr for 20 doses. *Child:* 6.2 g/m$^2$ PO q 6 hr for 20 doses; max, 10 g/dose. **Tx of hereditary orotic aciduria** (*Xuriden*). 60 mg/kg/d PO; may increase to 120 mg/kg/d.
**ADV EFF** N/v/d
**NC/PT** Mix packet w/3–4 oz soft food (applesauce, pudding, yogurt); give within 30 min. Do not allow pt to chew granules. Follow w/at least 4 oz water. If pt vomits within 2 hr, give complete dose again; give next dose at regular time. If a dose is missed, give as soon as possible and give next dose at regular time. May give via NG or gastrostomy tube. Tablet will not completely dissolve; do not crush or heat tablet. Pt should report vomiting, severe diarrhea.

## urofollitropin (Bravelle)
**CLASS** Fertility drug
**PREG/CONT** High risk/NA

**IND & DOSE Stimulation of ovulation.** *Adults who have received gonadotropin-releasing hormone agonist, antagonist suppression:* 150 units/d subcut or IM for first 5 d. Subsequent dosing should not exceed 75–150 units/adjustment. Max, 450 units/d. Tx beyond 12 d not recommended. If pt response appropriate, give HCG 5,000–10,000 units 1 d after last *Bravelle* dose. **Stimulation of follicle development.** *Adult:* 225 units/d subcut or IM for 5 d, then adjust dose q 2 d, not exceeding 75- to 150-unit increments; max, 450 units/d.
**ADV EFF** Congenital malformations, ectopic preg, multiple births, nausea, ovarian cyst, **ovarian hyperstimulation,** ovarian neoplasms, ovarian torsion, **pulmonary/vascular complications,** URI
**NC/PT** Ensure uterine health. Alert pt to risk of multiple births. Monitor regularly; monitor for thrombotic events. Teach proper administration/ disposal of needles/syringes. Pt should report abd/chest pain.

**ursodiol** (Actigall, URSO 250, Ursodiol, Urso Forte)
**CLASS** Gallstone-solubilizing drug
**PREG/CONT** B/NA

**IND & DOSE** **Gallstone solubilization.** *Adult:* 8–10 mg/kg/d PO in two–three divided doses. **Px of gallstones w/rapid weight loss.** *Adult:* 300 mg PO bid or 8–10 mg/kg/d PO in two–three divided doses. **Tx of biliary cirrhosis.** *Adult:* 13–15 mg/kg/d PO in two–four divided doses w/food.
**ADV EFF** Abd pain, cramps, diarrhea, epigastric distress, fatigue, headache, rash
**INTERACTIONS** Antacids, bile-acid sequestrants
**NC/PT** Drug not a cure; gallstones may recur. Schedule periodic oral cholecystograms or ultrasonograms to evaluate effectiveness at 6-mo intervals until resolution, then q 3 mo to monitor stone formation. Monitor LFTs periodically. Pt should avoid antacids; report yellowing of skin/eyes, gallstone attacks, bleeding.

**ustekinumab** (Stelara)
**CLASS** Monoclonal antibody
**PREG/CONT** Low risk/NA

**IND & DOSE** **Tx of pt w/moderate to severe plaque psoriasis if eligible for photo or systemic therapy.** *Adult, adolescent >12 yr:* >100 kg, 90 mg subcut, then 90 mg in 4 wk, then q 12 wk; 60–100 kg, 45 mg subcut, then 45 mg in 4 wk, then q 12 wk; <60 kg, 0.75 mg/kg subcut, then 0.75 mg/kg in 4 wk, then q 12 wk. **Tx of active psoriatic arthritis alone or w/ methotrexate.** *Adult:* Initially, 45 mg subcut, then 45 mg subcut 4 wk later, then 45 mg subcut q 12 wk. *Adult w/ coexisting moderate to severe plaque psoriasis weighing >100 kg:* 90 mg subcut, then 90 mg subcut 4 wk later, then 90 mg subcut q 12 wk. **Tx of moderate to severe active Crohn disease and ulcerative colitis.** *Adult:* >85 kg, 520 mg IV, then 90 mg subcut in 8 wk, then q 8 wk; >55–85 kg, 390 mg IV, then 90 mg subcut in 8 wk, then q 8 wk; <55 kg, 260 mg IV, then 90 mg subcut in 8 wk, then q 8 wk.
**ADV EFF** Fatigue, headache, **hypersensitivity reactions, malignancies, RPLS, serious infections, TB,** URI
**INTERACTIONS** Immunosuppressants, live vaccines, phototherapy
**NC/PT** Use caution in preg/breastfeeding. Ensure appropriate cancer screening. Pt should mark calendar of injection days, avoid live vaccines, report s&sx of infection, worsening of condition, difficulty breathing.

**valACYclovir hydrochloride** (Valtrex)
**CLASS** Antiviral
**PREG/CONT** Low risk/NA

**IND & DOSE** **Tx of herpes zoster.** *Adult:* 1 g PO tid for 7 d; most effective if started within 48 hr of sx onset (rash). **Tx of genital herpes.** *Adult:* 1 g PO bid for 7–10 d for initial episode. **Episodic tx of recurrent genital herpes.** *Adult:* 500 mg PO bid for 3 d, or 1 g/d for 5 d. **To suppress recurrent episodes of genital herpes.** *Adult:* 1 g/d PO; pts w/hx of <nine episodes in 1 yr may respond to 500 mg PO daily. **To suppress recurrent episodes of genital herpes in pts w/HIV.** 500 mg PO bid for 5–10 d. **To reduce risk of herpes zoster transmission.** *Adult:* 500 mg/d PO for source partner. For HIV-positive pts, 500 mg PO bid. **Tx of cold sores.** *Adult, child ≥12 yr:* 2 g PO bid for 1 day, 12 hr apart. **Tx of chickenpox.** *Child 2–18 yr:* 20 mg/kg PO tid for 5 d; max, 1 g tid.
**ADJUST DOSE** Renal impairment
**ADV EFF** Abd pain, **acute renal failure,** dizziness, headache, n/v/d, rash
**INTERACTIONS** Cimetidine, probenecid

**NC/PT** Begin tx within 48–72 hr of onset of shingles sx or within 24 hr of onset of chickenpox rash. Pt should take full course of tx; avoid contact w/ lesions; avoid intercourse when lesions present; take analgesics for headache; report severe diarrhea, worsening of condition. Name confusion between *Valtrex* (valacyclovir) and *Valcyte* (valganciclovir).

## valbenazine (Ingrezza)

**CLASS** Vesicular monoamine transporter-2 inhibitor
**PREG/CONT** High risk/NA

**IND & DOSE Tx of adults w/tardive dyskinesia.** *Adult:* 40 mg/d PO for 1 wk; then 80 mg/d PO.
**ADJUST DOSE** Hepatic impairment, severe renal impairment
**ADV EFF** Parkinsonism, **prolonged QT, somnolence**
**INTERACTIONS** MAOIs, QT-prolonging drugs, strong CYP3A4 inducers/inhibitors
**NC/PT** Obtain baseline ECG; monitor QT interval. Monitor LFTs, renal function. Pt should avoid preg (contraceptives advised)/breastfeeding (pt should not breastfeed for 5 d after final dose); take safety precautions w/somnolence effects; report fainting, palpitations, urine/stool color changes.

## valGANciclovir hydrochloride (Valcyte)

**CLASS** Antiviral
**PREG/CONT** High risk/NA

**BBW** Arrange for CBC before tx, at least wkly thereafter. Arrange for reduced dose if WBC/platelet counts fall. Toxicity includes granulocytopenia, anemia, thrombocytopenia. Advise pt drug has caused cancer, fetal damage, impairment of fertility in animals and that risk is possible in humans.
**IND & DOSE Tx of cytomegalovirus (CMV) infection.** *Adult:* 900 mg PO bid for 21 d; maint, 900 mg/d PO. **Px of CMV infection in high-risk kidney, pancreas-kidney, heart transplant.** *Adult:* 900 mg/d PO initiated within 10 d of transplant, continued for 100 d after transplant. **Px of CMV infection in high-risk kidney, heart transplant.** *Child 4 mo–16 yr:* Dose in mg = 7 × BSA × CrCl PO for 100 d (heart transplant), 200 d (kidney transplant). Max, 900 mg/d. May use oral sol, tablets.
**ADJUST DOSE** Renal impairment
**ADV EFF** Anemia, **bone marrow suppression,** confusion, dizziness, drowsiness, fertility impairment, fever, headache, insomnia, n/v/d, **renal failure,** tremor
**INTERACTIONS** Cytotoxic drugs, didanosine, mycophenolate, probenecid, zidovudine
**NC/PT** Cannot be substituted for ganciclovir capsules on one-to-one basis. Monitor CBC. Precautions needed for disposal of nucleoside analogs; consult pharmacy for proper disposal of unused tablets. Not for use in preg (men, women should use barrier contraceptives during, for 90 d after tx)/breastfeeding. Adults should use tablets, not solution. Avoid handling broken tablets. Pt should not cut/crush/chew tablets; drink 2–3 L water/d; have frequent blood tests, eye exams to evaluate progress; take safety precautions w/CNS effects; avoid exposure to infection; dispose of drug appropriately; report bruising/bleeding, s&sx of infection. Name confusion between *Valcyte* (valganciclovir) and *Valtrex* (valacyclovir).

## valproic acid (generic), divalproex sodium (Depakote, Depakote ER)

**CLASS** Antiepileptic
**PREG/CONT** High risk/NA

**BBW** Increased risk of suicidal ideation, suicidality; monitor accordingly. Arrange for frequent LFTs; stop drug

immediately w/suspected, apparent significant hepatic impairment. Continue LFTs to determine if hepatic impairment progresses despite discontinuation. Arrange counseling for women of childbearing age who wish to become preg; drug may be teratogenic. Not recommended for women of childbearing age; risk of neural tube defects, lower cognitive test scores in child when drug taken during preg compared to other anticonvulsants. Stop drug at any sign of pancreatitis; life-threatening pancreatitis has occurred.
**IND & DOSE** **Tx of simple, complex absence seizures.** *Adult:* 10–15 mg/kg/d PO, increasing at 1-wk intervals by 5–10 mg/kg/d until seizures controlled or side effects preclude further increases; max, 60 mg/kg/d PO. If total dose exceeds 250 mg/d, give in divided doses. *Child ≥10 yr:* 10–15 mg/kg/d PO. **Tx of acute mania, bipolar disorder.** *Adult:* 25 mg/kg/d PO. Increase rapidly to achieve lowest therapeutic dose. Max, 60 mg/kg/d PO (*Depakote ER* only). **Tx of bipolar mania:** *Adult:* 750 mg/d PO in divided doses; max, 60 mg/kg/d (*Depakote* only). **Px of migraine.** *Adult:* 250 mg PO bid; up to 1,000 mg/d has been used (*Depakote*); 500 mg/d ER tablet.
**ADV EFF** **Bleeding, bone marrow suppression,** depression, dizziness, **hepatic failure,** indigestion, **life-threatening pancreatitis,** n/v/d, rash
**INTERACTIONS** Alcohol, carbamazepine, charcoal, cimetidine, chlorpromazine, CNS depressants, diazepam, erythromycin, ethosuximide, felbamate, lamotrigine, phenobarbital, phenytoin, primidone, rifampin, salicylates, zidovudine
**NC/PT** Taper when stopping. Monitor CBC, LFTs, therapeutic serum level (usually 50–100 mcg/mL). Check drug regimen; many serious interactions possible, including DRESS/multiorgan hypersensitivity. Not for use in preg (barrier contraceptives advised); use caution w/breastfeeding. Pt should swallow tablet/capsule whole and not chew it; avoid alcohol, OTC sleeping pills; have frequent blood tests; wear medical ID; take safety precautions for CNS effects; avoid injury, exposure to infection; report bleeding, stool color changes, thoughts of suicide. Confusion between *Depakote DR* and *Depakote ER*. Dosage very different; serious adverse effects possible.

## valsartan (Diovan)

**CLASS** Antihypertensive, ARB
**PREG/CONT** High risk/NA

**BBW** Rule out preg before starting tx. Suggest barrier contraceptives during tx; fetal injury, deaths have occurred.
**IND & DOSE** **Tx of HTN.** *Adult:* 80 mg/d PO; range, 80–320 mg/d. *Child 6–16 yr:* 1.3 mg/kg/d PO (max, 40 mg). Target, 1.3–2.7 mg/kg/d PO (40–160 mg/d). **Tx of HF.** *Adult:* 40 mg PO bid; titrate to 80 mg and 160 mg bid, to highest dose tolerated by pt. Max, 320 mg/d. **Tx of post-MI left ventricular dysfx.** *Adult:* Start as early as 12 hr post-MI; 20 mg PO bid. May increase after 7 d to 40 mg PO bid. Titrate to 160 mg PO bid if tolerated.
**ADJUST DOSE** Hepatic/renal impairment
**ADV EFF** Abd pain, cough, dizziness, headache, hyperkalemia, hypotension, n/v/d, URI
**INTERACTIONS** ACE inhibitors, ARBs, lithium, NSAIDs, potassium-sparing diuretics, renin inhibitors
**NC/PT** Alert surgeon; volume replacement may be needed postop. Do not stop abruptly. Not for use in preg (barrier contraceptives advised)/breastfeeding. Pt should take safety precautions for CNS effects; use caution in situations that can lead to BP drop; report chills, preg.

## vancomycin hydrochloride (Firvanq, Vancocin)

**CLASS** Antibiotic
**PREG/CONT** C; low risk (oral)/NA

**BBW** Pt at risk for development of multiple drug-resistant organisms; ensure appropriate use.
**IND & DOSE** **Tx of severe to life-threatening infections caused by susceptible bacteria strains and unresponsive to other antibiotics.** *Adult:* 500 mg–2 g/d PO in three–four divided doses for 7–10 d. Or, 500 mg IV q 6 hr or 1 g IV q 12 hr. *Child:* 40 mg/kg/d PO in three–four divided doses for 7–10 d. Or, 10 mg/kg/dose IV q 6 hr. Max, 2 g/d. *Premature, full-term neonate:* Use w/caution because of incompletely developed renal function. Initially, 15 mg/kg IV, then 10 mg/kg q 12 hr in first wk of life, then q 8 hr up to age 1 mo. **Tx of pseudomembranous colitis due to *Clostridium difficile* or staphylococcal enterocolitis.** *Adult:* 500 mg–2 g/d PO in three–four divided doses for 7–10 d, or 125 mg PO tid–qid. *Child:* 40 mg/kg/d PO in four divided doses for 7–10 d. Max, 2 g/d.
**ADJUST DOSE** Elderly pts, renal failure
**ADV EFF** Fever, hypotension, nausea, **nephrotoxicity**, ototoxicity, paresthesia, "red man syndrome," superinfections, rash
**INTERACTIONS** Aminoglycosides, amphotericin B, atracurium, bacitracin, cisplatin, pancuronium, vecuronium
**NC/PT** Culture before tx. Monitor for red man syndrome during IV infusion. Monitor renal function. Monitor for safe serum level (conc of 60–80 mcg/mL toxic). Pt should take full course; perform hygiene measures to avoid possible infections of mouth, vagina; report ringing in ears, hearing loss, swelling.

## vardenafil hydrochloride (Levitra, Staxyn)

**CLASS** ED drug, phosphodiesterase type 5 inhibitor
**PREG/CONT** B/NA

**IND & DOSE** **Tx of ED.** *Adult:* 5–10 mg PO 1 hr before anticipated sexual activity; range, 5–20 mg PO. Limit use to once/d. *Staxyn* (oral disintegrating tablet) is not interchangeable w/*Viagra* tablet.
**ADJUST DOSE** Elderly pts, hepatic impairment
**ADV EFF** Abnormal ejaculation, angina, dyspnea, flushing, GERD, headache, hearing loss, hypotension, priapism, prolonged QT, rhinitis, vision changes/loss
**INTERACTIONS** Erythromycin, indinavir, itraconazole, ketoconazole nitrates, ritonavir (limit dose of these drugs to 2.5 mg/24 hr [72 hr w/ritonavir]); alpha blockers, nitrates
**NC/PT** Ensure dx. Do not use w/severe hepatic impairment, renal dialysis. Drug not effective w/o sexual stimulation; take 1 hr before sexual activity. Does not protect against STDs. Not for use in women. For oral disintegrating tablet: Place on tongue, allow to disintegrate; do not take w/water. Pt should avoid nitrates, alpha blocker antihypertensives; stop drug, immediately report loss of vision/hearing; report difficult urination, erection lasting longer than 4 hr, fainting.

## varenicline tartrate (Chantix)

**CLASS** Nicotine receptor antagonist, smoking deterrent
**PREG/CONT** High risk/NA

**IND & DOSE** **Aid to smoking cessation tx.** *Adult:* Pt should pick date to

stop smoking, begin tx 1 wk before that date. Or, pt can begin drug, quit smoking between d 8 and d 35 of tx. Days 1–3, 0.5 mg/d PO; days 4–7, 0.5 mg PO bid; day 8 to total of 12 wk, 1 mg PO bid.
**ADJUST DOSE** Severe renal impairment
**ADV EFF** Abd pain, abnormal dreams, constipation, depression, fatigue, flatulence, headache, hostility, insomnia, **MI,** nausea, neuropsychiatric events, rhinorrhea, **stroke, suicidality**
**INTERACTIONS** Cimetidine, nicotine transdermal systems
**NC/PT** Ensure comprehensive tx program. Not for use in preg/breastfeeding; Tx should last 12 wk; pt who successfully quits smoking in that time may benefit from another 12 wk to increase likelihood of long-term abstinence. Use caution w/known CAD. Pt should take after eating w/full glass of water; follow dosing protocol closely; if relapse occurs, discuss w/ prescribe; report failure to quit smoking, behavioral changes, thoughts of suicide, chest pain.

## vedolizumab (Entyvio)
**CLASS** Immunomodulator, integrin receptor antagonist
**PREG/CONT** Low risk/NA

**IND & DOSE Tx of ulcerative colitis, Crohn disease w/loss of response to TNF blockers, corticosteroids.** *Adult:* 300 mg IV over 30 min at 0, 2, and 6 wk, then q 8 wk.
**ADV EFF** Arthralgia, cough, **hypersensitivity reactions, infections,** pain, **RPLS,** URI
**NC/PT** Ensure proper dx, up-to-date immunizations before use. Stop if no evidence of benefit within 14 wk. Use w/caution in preg/breastfeeding. Pt should mark calendar for tx days; report s&sx of infection, fever, difficulty breathing, rash.

## velaglucerase (VPRIV)
**CLASS** Lysosomal enzyme
**PREG/CONT** Low risk/NA

**IND & DOSE Long-term replacement tx for type 1 Gaucher disease.** *Adult, child ≥4 yr:* 60 units/kg as 60-min IV infusion q other wk.
**ADV EFF** Abd pain, back pain, dizziness, headache, **hypersensitivity/infusion reactions,** joint pain, nausea, URI
**NC/PT** May use antihistamines, corticosteroids to alleviate infusion reactions. Consider slowing infusion or stopping tx if infusion reactions. Pt should mark calendar for infusion days; report difficulty breathing, pain at injection site.

## vemurafenib (Zelboraf)
**CLASS** Antineoplastic, kinase inhibitor
**PREG/CONT** High risk/NA

**IND & DOSE Tx of pts w/unresectable, metastatic melanoma w/BRAF V600E mutation as detected by approved BRAF test; tx of pts w/ Erdheim-Chester disease w/BRAF V600 mutation.** *Adult:* 960 mg PO bid approx 12 hr apart.
**ADV EFF** Alopecia, arthralgia, **cutaneous squamous cell carcinoma,** Dupuytren contracture/plantar fascial fibromatosis, fatigue, **hepatotoxicity,** nausea, **new malignant melanomas,** photosensitivity, pruritus, **prolonged QT, radiation sensitization, serious hypersensitivity reactions, serious ophthalmologic toxicity,** renal failure, **SJS,** skin papilloma
**INTERACTIONS** CYP substrates, QT-prolonging drugs, warfarin
**NC/PT** BRAF confirmation test required before use to ensure appropriate drug selection. Obtain baseline ECG; periodically monitor QT interval. Monitor skin, eye reactions. Not for use in preg/breastfeeding. Pt should cover head at temp extremes (hair

loss possible); avoid sun exposure; report rash, difficulty breathing, urine/stool color changes, vision changes.

## venetoclax (Venclexta)

**CLASS** Antineoplastic, BCL-2 inhibitor
**PREG/CONT** High risk/NA

**IND & DOSE Tx of chronic lymphocytic leukemia or small lymphocytic lymphoma; tx w/azacitidine or decitabine or cytarabine for acute myeloid leukemia in adults ≥75 yr or if unable to undergo induction chemo.** *Adult:* 20 mg/d PO for 7 d; increase wkly to 400 mg/d PO. See label for titration detail.
**ADV EFF** Anemia, **bone marrow suppression,** fatigue, n/v, URI
**INTERACTIONS** CYP3A inhibitors: contraindicated; CYP3A inducers, P-gp inhibitors/substrates, vaccines
**NC/PT** Provide px for TLS. Monitor blood counts; manage as needed. Pt should take w/meal; should not cut/crush/chew tablets; avoid preg/breastfeeding; report fever, unusual bleeding, extreme fatigue.

## venlafaxine hydrochloride (Effexor XR)

**CLASS** Antidepressant, anxiolytic
**PREG/CONT** High risk/NA

**BBW** Monitor pts for suicidal ideation, especially when starting tx, changing dose; high risk in child, adolescent, young adult. Not for use in child.
**IND & DOSE Tx of major depressive disorder.** *Adult:* Initially, 37.5–75 mg/d PO; target, 75 mg/d PO in two–three divided doses (or once/d, ER capsule). Increase at intervals of no less than 4 d up to 225 mg/d to achieve desired effect **Tx of generalized anxiety disorder.** *Adult:* 37.5–225 mg/d ER form PO. **Tx of panic disorder.** *Adult:* 37.5 mg/d PO for 7 d, then 75 mg/d for 7 d, then 75 mg/d wkly. Max, 225 mg/d (ER only). **Tx of social anxiety.** *Adult:* 75 mg/d PO; max, 75 mg/d.
**ADJUST DOSE** Hepatic/renal impairment
**ADV EFF** Abnormal ejaculation, activation of mania/hypomania, angle-closure glaucoma, asthenia, anorexia, bleeding, constipation, dizziness, dry mouth, headache, HTN, insomnia, nausea, nervousness, **serotonin syndrome,** somnolence, sweating, **suicidality**
**INTERACTIONS** Alcohol, MAOIs, serotonergic drugs, St. John's wort, trazodone
**NC/PT** To transfer to, from MAOI: Allow at least 14 d to elapse from stopping MAOI to starting venlafaxine; allow at least 7 d to elapse from stopping venlafaxine to starting MAOI. Not for use in preg/breastfeeding. Pt should swallow ER capsule whole and not cut/crush/chew it; take w/food; avoid alcohol, St. John's wort; take safety precautions for CNS effects; use sugarless lozenges w/dry mouth; report rash, thoughts of suicide.

**DANGEROUS DRUG**

## verapamil hydrochloride (Calan SR, Verelan, Verelan PM)

**CLASS** Antianginal, antihypertensive, calcium channel blocker
**PREG/CONT** Low risk/NA

**BBW** Monitor pt carefully during drug titration; dosage may be increased more rapidly w/hospitalized, monitored pts.
**IND & DOSE Tx of angina.** *Adult:* 80–120 mg PO tid. Maint, 240–480 mg/d. **Tx of arrhythmias.** *Adult:* 240–480 mg/d PO in divided doses. Or, 120–240 mg/d PO in a.m. ER capsules; max, 480 mg/d. Or, 120–180 mg/d PO in a.m. ER or SR tablets. Or, 5–10 mg

IV over 2 min; may repeat dose of 10 mg 30 min after first dose if initial response inadequate. In digitalized pts, 240–320 mg/d PO. *Child 1–15 yr:* 0.1–0.3 mg/kg IV over 2 min; max, 5 mg. Repeat dose 30 min after initial dose if response inadequate. Max for repeat dose, 10 mg. *Child ≤1 yr:* 0.1–0.2 mg/kg IV over 2 min. **Tx of HTN.** *Adult:* 40–80 mg PO tid; or 200–400 mg PO daily at bedtime (*Verelan PM*).
**ADJUST DOSE** Elderly pts, renal impairment
**ADV EFF** **Cardiac arrhythmias,** constipation, dizziness, edema, headache, HF, hypotension, nausea
**INTERACTIONS** Antihypertensives, beta blockers, calcium, carbamazepine, digoxin, flecainide, grapefruit juice, mammalian target of rapamycin (mTOR) inhibitors, prazosin, quinidine, rifampin, statins
**NC/PT** When pt stabilized, may switch to ER capsules (max, 480 mg/d), ER tablets (max, 240 mg q 12 hr), SR forms (max, 480 mg in a.m.). Protect IV sol from light. Monitor BP/cardiac rhythm closely. Not for use in breastfeeding. Pt should swallow ER, SR forms whole and not cut/crush/chew them; take safety precautions w/dizziness; avoid grapefruit juice; report swelling, difficulty breathing.

## verteporfin (Visudyne)
**CLASS** Ophthal drug
**PREG/CONT** High risk/NA

**IND & DOSE** **Tx of age-related macular degeneration, pathologic myopia, ocular histoplasmosis.** *Adult:* 6 mg/m² diluted in $D_5W$ to total 30 mL IV into free-flowing IV over 10 min at 3 mL/min using inline filter, syringe pump.
**ADJUST DOSE** Hepatic impairment
**ADV EFF** Dizziness, headache, injection-site reactions, malaise, photosensitivity, pruritus, rash, visual disturbances
**NC/PT** Stop infusion immediately if extravasation occurs. Laser light tx should begin within 15 min of starting IV; may repeat in 3 mo if needed. Avoid use in preg; not for use in breastfeeding. Protect pt from exposure to bright light for at least 5 d after tx. Pt should report vision changes, eye pain, injection-site pain/swelling.

**DANGEROUS DRUG**

## vestronidase alfa-vjbk
(Mepsevii)
**CLASS** Enzyme
**PREG/CONT** Unkn/NA

**BBW** Anaphylaxis has occurred, as early as first dose; observe pt during and for 60 min after infusion. Immediately discontinue infusion if anaphylaxis occurs.
**IND & DOSE** **Tx of mucopolysaccharidosis VII (Sly syndrome).** *Adult, child:* 4 mg/kg IV q 2 wk.
**ADV EFF** **Anaphylaxis,** diarrhea, **infusion-site extravasation**/swelling, peripheral swelling, pruritus, rash
**NC/PT** Premedicate w/nonsedating antihistamine w/ or w/o antipyretic 30–60 min before infusion. Infuse over approximately 4 hr. In first hr of infusion, infuse 2.5% of the total volume. After first hr, can increase rate to infuse remainder of the volume over 3 hr as tolerated.

## vigabatrin (Sabril, Vigadrone)
**CLASS** Antiepileptic, GABAase inhibitor
**PREG/CONT** High risk/NA

**BBW** Available only through restricted distribution program. Causes progressive, permanent, bilateral vision loss. Monitor vision; stopping drug may not stop vision loss. Increased risk of suicidality; monitor accordingly.
**IND & DOSE** **Adjunct tx of refractory complex seizures.** *Adult, child >60 kg:*

500 mg PO bid; increase slowly to max 1,500 mg PO bid. *Child–16 yr <60 kg:* Dose based on body weight; given in two divided doses. May increase dose in wkly intervals. **Tx of infantile spasms.** *Child:* 50 mg/kg/d PO in two divided doses; max, 150 mg/kg/d in two divided doses. May increase by 25–50 mg/kg/d q 3 d.
**ADJUST DOSE** Renal impairment
**ADV EFF** Abnormal coordination, anemia, arthralgia, confusion, edema, fatigue, nystagmus, **permanent vision loss,** somnolence, **suicidality,** tremor, weight gain
**NC/PT** Available only through limited access. Abnormal MRI signal changes have been reported in infants w/infantile spasms. Taper gradually to avoid withdrawal seizures. Monitor vision; permanent vision loss possible. For refractory complex seizures, give w/ other antiepileptics; for infantile spasms, use as monotherapy. Not for use in preg/breastfeeding. Pt should take precautions for CNS effects; report changes in vision, thoughts of suicide, extreme fatigue, weight gain.

## vilazodone hydrochloride (Viibryd)

**CLASS** SSRI
**PREG/CONT** High risk/NA

**BBW** High risk of suicidality in child, adolescent, young adult. Establish suicide precautions for severely depressed pts, limit quantity of drug dispensed. Vilazodone not approved for use in child.
**IND & DOSE Tx of major depressive disorder.** *Adult:* 10 mg/d PO for 7 d, then 20 mg/d PO for 7 d; maint, 40 mg/d PO.
**ADV EFF** Angle-closure glaucoma, bleeding, dizziness, dry mouth, insomnia, n/v/d, **NMS,** paresthesia, **seizures, serotonin syndrome, suicidality**
**INTERACTIONS** Alcohol, aspirin, diltiazem, ketoconazole, MAOIs, NSAIDs, serotonergic drugs, St. John's wort, warfarin
**NC/PT** Screen for bipolar disorder before use. Therapeutic effects may not occur for 4 wk. Taper when stopping. Not for use in preg/breastfeeding. Pt should take w/food in a.m.; avoid alcohol, NSAIDs, St. John's wort; take safety precautions for CNS effects; report seizures, thoughts of suicide.

**DANGEROUS DRUG**

## vinBLAStine sulfate (generic)

**CLASS** Antineoplastic, mitotic inhibitor
**PREG/CONT** High risk/NA

**BBW** Do not give IM, subcut due to severe local reaction, tissue necrosis. Fatal if given intrathecally; use extreme caution. Watch for irritation, infiltration; extravasation causes tissue damage, necrosis. If it occurs, stop injection immediately; give remainder of dose in another vein. Arrange for hyaluronidase injection into local area, after which apply moderate heat to disperse drug, minimize pain.
**IND & DOSE Palliative tx of lymphocytic/histiocytic lymphoma, generalized Hodgkin lymphoma (stages III, IV), mycosis fungoides, advanced testicular carcinoma, Kaposi sarcoma, Letterer-Siwe disease; tx of choriocarcinoma, breast cancer, Hodgkin lymphoma, advanced testicular germinal-cell cancers.** *Adult:* Initially, 3.7 mg/m$^2$ as single IV dose, followed at wkly intervals by increasing doses at 1.8-mg/m$^2$ increments; use these increments until max 18.5 mg/m$^2$ reached. When WBC count 3,000/mm$^3$, use dose one increment smaller for wkly maint. Do not give another dose until WBC count is 4,000/mm$^3$ even if 7 d have passed. *Child:* 2.5 mg/m$^2$ as single IV dose, followed at wkly intervals by increasing doses at 1.25-mg/m$^2$ increments. Max, 12.5 mg/m$^2$/dose.
**ADJUST DOSE** Hepatic impairment

**ADV EFF** Alopecia, anorexia, **bone marrow suppression,** cellulitis at injection site, headache, n/v/d, paresthesia, weakness
**INTERACTIONS** Erythromycin, grapefruit juice, phenytoins
**NC/PT** Do not give IM, subcut. Monitor CBC closely. Give antiemetic for severe n/v. Not for use in preg/breastfeeding. Pt should mark calendar of tx days; take safety precautions for CNS effects; cover head at temp extremes (hair loss possible); avoid exposure to infection, injury; avoid grapefruit juice; report pain at injection site, s&sx of infection, bleeding. Name confusion between vinblastine and vincristine.

DANGEROUS DRUG

## vinCRIStine sulfate

(Marqibo)
**CLASS** Antineoplastic, mitotic inhibitor
**PREG/CONT** High risk/NA

**BBW** Do not give IM, subcut due to severe local reaction, tissue necrosis. Fatal if given intrathecally; use extreme caution. Watch for irritation, infiltration; extravasation causes tissue damage, necrosis. If it occurs, stop injection immediately; give remainder of dose in another vein. Arrange for hyaluronidase injection into local area, after which apply moderate heat to disperse drug, minimize pain.
**IND & DOSE** **Tx of acute leukemia, Hodgkin lymphoma, non-Hodgkin lymphoma, rhabdomyosarcoma, neuroblastoma, Wilms tumor.** *Adult:* 1.4 mg/m² IV at wkly intervals. *Child >10 kg or BSA >1 m²:* 1–2 mg/m²/wk IV. Max, 2 mg/dose. *Child <10 kg or BSA <1 m²:* 0.05 mg/kg/wk IV. **Tx of adults w/Philadelphia chromosome–negative acute ALL who have relapsed after other tx.** *Adult:* 2.25 mg/m² IV over 1 hr q 7 d (*Marqibo*).
**ADJUST DOSE** Elderly pts, hepatic impairment
**ADV EFF** Alopecia, ataxia, constipation, cranial nerve manifestations, **death,** neuritic pain, paresthesia, photosensitivity, renal impairment, weight loss
**INTERACTIONS** Digoxin, grapefruit juice, L-asparaginase
**NC/PT** Do not give IM, subcut. Monitor renal function. Not for use in preg/breastfeeding. Pt should use laxative for constipation; take safety precautions for CNS effects; cover head at temp extremes (hair loss possible); avoid sun exposure; report pain at injection site, swelling, severe constipation. Name confusion between vinblastine and vincristine.

DANGEROUS DRUG

## vinorelbine tartrate

(Navelbine)
**CLASS** Antineoplastic, mitotic inhibitor
**PREG/CONT** High risk/NA

**BBW** Do not give IM, subcut due to severe local reaction, tissue necrosis. Fatal if given intrathecally; use extreme caution. Watch for irritation, infiltration; extravasation can cause tissue damage, necrosis. If it occurs, stop injection immediately; arrange for hyaluronidase injection into local area, after which apply moderate heat to disperse drug, minimize pain. Check CBC before each dose; severe granulocytosis possible. Adjust, delay dose as appropriate.
**IND & DOSE** **First-line tx of pts w/ unresectable advanced NSCLC, as monotherapy or w/cisplatin.** *Adult:* 30 mg/m²/wk as single IV injection as monotherapy; 25–30 mg/m²/wk as single IV injection w/cisplatin.
**ADJUST DOSE** Hepatic impairment
**ADV EFF** Alopecia, anorexia, constipation to bowel obstruction, headache, hepatic impairment, neurotoxicity, **severe bone marrow suppression,** paresthesia, **pulmonary toxicity,** vesiculation of GI tract
**INTERACTIONS** CYP3A4 inhibitors

**NC/PT** Check CBC before each dose; adjustment may be needed. Give antiemetic if needed. Institute bowel program; monitor for severe constipation. Monitor pulmonary function. Not for use in preg (contraceptives advised)/breastfeeding. Pt should mark calendar of tx days; cover head at temp extremes (hair loss possible); take safety precautions for CNS effects; avoid exposure to infection, injury; report pain at injection site, unusual bleeding, s&sx of infection, severe constipation, difficulty breathing.

## vismodegib (Erivedge)

**CLASS** Antineoplastic, hedgehog pathway inhibitor
**PREG/CONT** High risk/NA

**BBW** Risk of embryo-fetal death, severe birth defects; men, women advised to use barrier contraceptives.
**IND & DOSE Tx of pts w/metastatic or locally advanced basal cell carcinoma not candidates for surgery or radiation.** *Adult*: 150 mg/d PO.
**ADV EFF** Alopecia, anorexia, arthralgia, constipation, fatigue, muscle spasms, n/v/d
**NC/PT** Rule out preg before tx; advise men, women to use barrier contraceptives (due to risk of fetal toxicity). Not for use in breastfeeding; pt should not breastfeed during tx and for 24 mo after tx ends. Pt should take as directed; not donate blood during and for 24 mo after tx; do not donate semen during and for 3 mo after tx; cover head at temp extremes (hair loss possible); report weight loss, severe GI complaints.

## von Willebrand factor (recombinant) (Vonvendi)

**CLASS** Clotting factor
**PREG/CONT** Moderate risk/NA

**IND & DOSE Tx/control of bleeding episodes or periop mgt of bleeding in von Willebrand disease.** *Adult:* 40–80 international units/kg q 8–24 hr based on severity/location of bleeding. For elective surgery, give dose 12–24 hr before surgery to increase factor VIII level to at least 30 international units (IU)/dL (minor surgery) or 60 IU/dL (major surgery). For emergency surgery, base dose on baseline levels and weight 1 hr before surgery.
**ADV EFF Hypersensitivity reactions, thrombotic events,** von Willebrand antibody production, rash
**NC/PT** Not for use w/known allergy to mannitol, trehalose, sodium chloride, histidine, Tris, calcium chloride, polysorbate 80, hamster/mouse proteins. For each bleeding episode, administer w/approved factor VIII if factor VIII levels are below 40% or unkn. Use within 3 hr of reconstitution. Use caution in preg/breastfeeding. Teach proper administration/reconstitution, disposal of needles/syringes. Pt should wear medical ID; report difficulty breathing, chest pain, numbness/tingling, continued bleeding.

## vorapaxar (Zontivity)

**CLASS** Antiplatelet, protease-activated receptor-1 antagonist
**PREG/CONT** Low risk/NA

**BBW** Do not use w/hx of stroke, TIA, intracranial hemorrhage, active pathological bleeding. Increased risk of serious to fatal bleeding.
**IND & DOSE To reduce thrombotic CV events w/MI, peripheral arterial disease.** *Adult:* 2.08 mg (1 tablet)/d PO, w/aspirin and/or clopidogrel.
**ADV EFF Bleeding events**
**INTERACTIONS** Drugs affecting coagulation, strong CYP3A4 inducers/inhibitors
**NC/PT** Give daily, w/aspirin and/or clopidogrel. Use w/caution in preg; not for use in breastfeeding. Pt should alert surgeon/dentist about use; contact prescriber before stopping; report unusual bleeding.

**voriconazole** (Vfend)
**CLASS** Triazole antifungal
**PREG/CONT** High risk/NA

**IND & DOSE** **Tx of invasive aspergillosis, serious infections caused by susceptible fungi strains; candidemia in nonneutropenic pts w/disseminated skin infections and other deep tissue *Candida* infections; tx of scedosporiosis/fusariosis.** *Adult, child ≥15 yr and 12–14 yr if >50 kg:* Loading dose, 6 mg/kg IV q 12 hr for two doses, then 3–4 mg/kg IV q 12 hr or 200 mg PO q 12 hr. Switch to PO as soon as possible. *≥40 kg,* 200 mg PO q 12 hr; may increase to 300 mg PO q 12 hr if needed. *<40 kg,* 100 mg PO q 12 hr; may increase to 150 mg PO q 12 hr if needed. *Child 2–11 yr or 12–14 yr and <50 kg:* Loading dose, 9 mg/kg IV q 12 hr for two doses, then 8 mg/kg IV q 12 hr or 9 mg/kg PO q 12 hr (max, 350 mg q 12 hr). **Tx of esophageal candidiasis.** *Adult, child ≥15 yr and 12–14 if >50 kg:* 200 mg PO q 12 hr (100–150 mg PO q 12 hr if <40 kg) for 14 d or for at least 7 d after sx resolve. *Child 2–11 yr or 12–14 yr and <50 kg:* 4 mg/kg IV q 12 hr or 9 mg/kg PO q 12 hr (max, 350 mg q 12 hr).
**ADV EFF** **Anaphylactic reaction,** BP changes, dizziness, headache, **hepatotoxicity,** n/v/d, photosensitivity, **prolonged QT,** rash, **SJS,** visual disturbances
**INTERACTIONS** Benzodiazepine, calcium channel blockers, cyclosporine, omeprazole, oral anticoagulants, phenytoin, protease inhibitors, statins, St. John's wort, sulfonylureas, tacrolimus, vinblastine, vincristine, warfarin. Do not use w/carbamazepine, ergot alkaloids, mephobarbital, phenobarbital, pimozide, quinidine, rifabutin, rifampin, sirolimus
**NC/PT** Obtain baseline ECG, LFTs before, periodically during tx. Review drug list carefully; many interactions possible. Not for use in preg (contraceptives advised)/breastfeeding. Pt should take oral drug on empty stomach 1 hr before or 2 hr after meals; avoid sun exposure, St. John's wort; report all drugs/herbs being used, vision changes, urine/stool color changes, rash, difficulty breathing.

**DANGEROUS DRUG**
**vorinostat** (Zolinza)
**CLASS** Antineoplastic, histone deacetylase inhibitor
**PREG/CONT** D/NA

**BBW** Monitor for bleeding, excessive n/v, thromboembolic events.
**IND & DOSE** **Tx of cutaneous manifestations in cutaneous T-cell lymphoma.** *Adult:* 400 mg/d PO w/food; continue until disease progression or unacceptable toxicity.
**ADJUST DOSE** Hepatic impairment
**ADV EFF** Anorexia, dehydration, dizziness, **GI bleeding,** hyperglycemia, n/v/d, **thromboembolic events**
**INTERACTIONS** Warfarin
**NC/PT** Monitor CBC, electrolytes, serum blood glucose. Give antiemetics if needed. Encourage fluid intake of 2 L/d to prevent dehydration. Not for use in preg (barrier contraceptives advised)/breastfeeding. Pt should take safety precaution w/dizziness; use caution in hot environments; maintain hydration; report bloody diarrhea, numbness/tingling, chest pain, difficulty breathing.

**vortioxetine** (Trintellix)
**CLASS** Antidepressant, SSRI
**PREG/CONT** High risk/NA

**BBW** Increased risk of suicidality in child, adolescent, young adult, severely depressed pts. Limit quantity; monitor pt.
**IND & DOSE** **Tx of major depressive disorder.** *Adult:* 10 mg/d PO. Increase to 20 mg/d PO as tolerated.
**ADV EFF** Abnormal dreams, activation of mania, angle-closure glaucoma, constipation, dizziness, dry mouth,

hyponatremia, n/v/d, pruritus, **serotonin syndrome, suicidality**
**INTERACTIONS** Antihypertensives, aprepitant, aspirin, bupropion, carbamazepine, fluoxetine, linezolid, MAOIs, methylene blue (IV), NSAIDs, opioids, paroxetine, phenytoin, quinidine, rifampin, serotonergic drugs, SSRIs, St. John's wort
**NC/PT** Review drug regimen; many interactions possible. Monitor for hyponatremia, activation of mania. Not for use in preg/breastfeeding. Tapering when discontinuing is recommended. Pt should take in a.m.; avoid St. John's wort; take safety precautions for CNS effects; eat small, frequent meals for GI upset; report rash, mania, severe n/v, thoughts of suicide.

DANGEROUS DRUG

## warfarin sodium

(Coumadin, Jantoven)
**CLASS** Coumarin derivative, oral anticoagulant
**PREG/CONT** High risk/NA

**BBW** Evaluate pt regularly for s&sx of blood loss (petechiae, bleeding gums, bruises, dark stools, dark urine). Maintain INR of 2–3, 3–4.5 w/ mechanical prosthetic valves or recurrent systemic emboli; risk of serious to fatal bleeding.
**IND & DOSE** **Tx/px of PE, venous thrombosis; tx of thromboembolic complications of atrial fibrillation; px of systemic embolization after acute MI.** *Adult:* 2–5 mg/day PO or IV. Adjust according to PT response. Maint, 2–10 mg/day PO based on INR.
**ADJUST DOSE** Elderly pts
**ADV EFF** Alopecia, **calciphylaxis,** dermatitis, **hemorrhage,** n/v/d, priapism, red-orange urine
**INTERACTIONS** Acetaminophen, alcohol, allopurinol, amiodarone, androgens, angelica, azole antifungals, barbiturates, carbamazepine, cat's claw, cefazolin, cefotetan, cefoxitin, ceftriaxone, chamomile, chloramphenicol, cholestyramine, chondroitin, cimetidine, clofibrate, co-trimoxazole, danazol, disulfiram, erythromycin, famotidine, feverfew, fish oil, fluvastatin, garlic, ginkgo, glucagon, goldenseal, grape seed extract, green leaf tea, griseofulvin, horse chestnut seed, lovastatin, meclofenamate, mefenamic acid, methimazole, metronidazole, nalidixic acid, nizatidine, NSAIDs, phenytoin, propylthiouracil, psyllium, quinidine, quinine, quinolones, ranitidine, rifampin, simvastatin, sulfinpyrazone, thyroid drugs, turmeric, vitamins E, K
**NC/PT** Genetic testing can help determine reasonable dose. Decreased clearance w/CYP2C9*2, CYP2C9*3 variant alleles. Monitor blood clotting; target, INR of 2–3. IV use reserved for situations in which oral warfarin not feasible. Have vitamin K and/or prothrombin complex concentrate on hand for overdose. Check pt's drug regimen closely; many interactions possible. Carefully add/remove drugs from regimen; dose adjustment may be needed. Not for use in preg (contraceptives advised); use caution in breastfeeding. Urine may turn red-orange. Pt should not start or stop any drug, herb w/o consulting health care provider (dose adjustments may be needed); have regular blood tests; avoid injury; report bleeding/bruising.

## zafirlukast (Accolate)

**CLASS** Antiasthmatic, leukotriene receptor antagonist
**PREG/CONT** B/NA

**IND & DOSE** **Px, long-term tx of bronchial asthma.** *Adult, child ≥12 yr:* 20 mg PO bid on empty stomach 1 hr before or 2 hr after meals. *Child 5–11 yr:* 10 mg PO bid on empty stomach.
**ADV EFF** Headache, **Churg-Strauss syndrome,** dizziness, n/v/d
**INTERACTIONS** Calcium channel blockers, corticosteroids, cyclosporine, erythromycin, theophylline, warfarin
**NC/PT** Not for acute asthma attack. Pt should take on empty stomach q

day; consult health care provider before using OTC products; take safety precautions w/dizziness; report severe headache, fever, increased acute asthma attacks.

## zaleplon (Sonata)

**CLASS** Sedative-hypnotic (nonbenzodiazepine)
**PREG/CONT** Unkn/C-IV

**BBW** Risk of complex sleep behaviors (sleepwalking, sleep driving), which can lead to serious injuries, even death.
**IND & DOSE** **Short-term tx of insomnia.** *Adult:* 10 mg PO at bedtime. Pt must remain in bed for 4 hr after taking. Max, 20 mg/d.
**ADJUST DOSE** Elderly, debilitated pts; hepatic impairment
**ADV EFF** **Anaphylaxis, angioedema,** depression, dizziness, drowsiness, headache, short-term memory impairment, sleep disorders
**INTERACTIONS** Alcohol, CNS depressants, cimetidine, CYP3A4 inhibitors, rifampin
**NC/PT** Rule out medical causes for insomnia; institute sleep hygiene protocol. Pt will feel drug's effects for 4 hr; after 4 hr, pt may safely become active again. Pt should take dose immediately before bedtime; avoid alcohol, OTC sleeping aids; take safety precautions for CNS effects; report difficulty breathing, swelling, sleep-related behaviors.

## zanamivir (Relenza)

**CLASS** Antiviral, neuraminidase inhibitor
**PREG/CONT** C/NA

**IND & DOSE** **Tx of uncomplicated acute illness due to influenza virus.** *Adult, child ≥7 yr:* 2 inhalations (one 5-mg blister/inhalation administered w/*Diskhaler*, for total 10 mg) bid at 12-hr intervals for 5 d. Should start within 2 d of onset of flu sx; give two doses on first tx day, at least 2 hr apart; separate subsequent doses by 12 hr. **Px of influenza.** *Adult, child ≥5 yr:* Two inhalations (10 mg)/d for 28 d w/community outbreak, 10 d for household exposure.
**ADV EFF** Anorexia, **bronchospasm,** cough, diarrhea, dizziness, headache, nausea, **serious respiratory effects**
**NC/PT** Caution COPD, asthma pts of bronchospasm risk; pt should have fast-acting bronchodilator on hand. Review proper use of *Diskhaler* delivery system. Pt should take full course; if using bronchodilator, use before this drug; take safety precautions w/dizziness; report worsening of sx.

## ziconotide (Prialt)

**CLASS** Analgesic, N-type calcium channel blocker
**PREG/CONT** C/NA

**BBW** Severe neuropsychiatric reactions, neuro impairment; monitor pt closely. Do not use w/hx of psychosis.
**IND & DOSE** **Mgt of severe chronic pain in pts who need intrathecal tx.** *Adult:* 2.4 mcg/d by continuous intrathecal pump; may titrate to max 19.2 mcg/d (0.8 mcg/hr).
**ADV EFF** Confusion, dizziness, meningitis, nausea, **neuro impairment,** nystagmus, **psychotic behavior**
**NC/PT** Teach pt proper care of pump, injection site. Not for use in preg/breastfeeding. Pt should take safety precautions for CNS effects; report changes in mood/behavior, muscle pain/weakness, rash.

## zidovudine (Retrovir)

**CLASS** Antiviral, nucleoside reverse transcriptase inhibitor
**PREG/CONT** C/NA

**BBW** Monitor for hematologic toxicity, including neutropenia, severe anemia. Monitor LFTs; lactic acidosis w/severe hepatomegaly w/steatosis possible. Increased risk of symptomatic myopathy; monitor accordingly.

**IND & DOSE Tx of HIV, w/other antiretrovirals.** *Adult, child >12 yr:* 600 mg/d PO in divided doses as either 200 mg tid or 300 mg bid. Monitor hematologic indices q 2 wk. If significant anemia (Hgb <7.5 g/dL, reduction >25%) or granulocyte reduction >50% below baseline occurs, dose interruption necessary until evidence of bone marrow recovery. Or, 1 mg/kg 5–6 ×/d IV infused over 1 hr. *Child 6 wk–12 yr:* ≥30 kg, 600 mg/d PO in two–three divided doses. 9–<30 kg, 18 mg/kg/d PO in two–three divided doses. 4–<9 kg, 24 mg/kg/d PO in two–three divided doses. *Infant born to HIV-infected mother:* 2 mg/kg PO q 6 hr starting within 12 hr of birth to 6 wk of age, or 1.5 mg/kg IV over 30 min q 6 hr until able to take oral form. **Px of maternal-fetal transmission.** *Adult:* 100 mg PO 5 ×/d until start of labor.
**ADV EFF** Agranulocytosis, anorexia, asthenia, diarrhea, flulike sx, GI pain, headache, **hepatic decompensation, hypersensitivity reactions,** nausea, rash
**INTERACTIONS** Acyclovir, bone marrow suppressants, cyclosporine, cytotoxic drugs, ganciclovir, interferon alfa, methadone, nephrotoxic drugs, phenytoin, probenecid, ribavirin, St. John's wort, zidovudine
**NC/PT** Do not infuse IV w/blood product. Rubber stoppers contain latex. Not for use in breastfeeding. Pt should take drug around the clock; take precautions to prevent transmission (drug not a cure); avoid exposure to infection, St. John's wort; take w/ other antivirals; report s&sx of infection, rash, difficulty breathing, severe headache. Name confusion between *Retrovir* (zidovudine) and ritonavir.

## zileuton (Zyflo)
**CLASS** Antiasthmatic leukotriene synthesis inhibitor
**PREG/CONT** C/NA

**IND & DOSE Px, long-term tx of asthma.** *Adult, child ≥12 yr:* CR tablets, 1,200 mg (2 tablets) PO bid within 1 hr after a.m., p.m. meals for total daily dose of 2,400 mg. Tablets, 600 mg PO qid for total daily dose of 2,400 mg.
**ADJUST DOSE** Hepatic impairment
**ADV EFF** Diarrhea, dizziness, headache, **liver enzyme elevations,** neuropsychiatric events, pain, rash
**INTERACTIONS** Propranolol, theophylline, warfarin
**NC/PT** Not for acute asthma attack. Monitor LFTs, mood, behavior. Pt should take daily; take CR tablets on empty stomach 1 hr before or 2 hr after meals; swallow tablet whole and not cut/crush/chew it; take safety precaution for CNS effects; report acute asthma attacks, urine/stool color changes, rash.

## ziprasidone (Geodon)
**CLASS** Atypical antipsychotic, benzisoxazole
**PREG/CONT** High risk/NA

**BBW** Increased risk of death if used in elderly pts w/dementia-related psychosis. Do not use in these pts; not approved for this use.
**IND & DOSE Tx of schizophrenia.** *Adult:* Initially, 20 mg PO bid w/food; range, 20–100 mg PO bid. **Rapid control of agitated behavior.** *Adult:* 10–20 mg IM; may repeat 10-mg doses q 2 hr; may repeat 20-mg doses in 4 hr. Max, 40 mg/d. **Tx of bipolar mania.** *Adult:* 40 mg PO bid w/food. May increase to 60–80 mg PO bid w/food.
**ADV EFF Arrhythmias,** bone marrow suppression, cognitive/motor impairment, constipation, drowsiness, dyslipidemia, dyspepsia, fever, headache, hyperglycemia, hypotension, **NMS, prolonged QT, seizures, severe cutaneous reactions including SJS and DRESS,** somnolence, **suicidality,** tardive dyskinesia, weight gain
**INTERACTIONS** Antihypertensives, QT-prolonging drugs, St. John's wort
**NC/PT** Obtain baseline, periodic ECG; monitor serum glucose, weight. Use caution w/renal, hepatic impairment.

Not for use in preg (contraceptives advised)/breastfeeding. Pt should take safety precautions w/CNS effects; avoid St. John's wort; report palpitations, sx return.

## ziv-aflibercept (Zaltrap)

**CLASS** Antineoplastic, ligand binding factor
**PREG/CONT** High risk/NA

**BBW** Risk of hemorrhage; do not administer w/active bleeding. Risk of GI perforation, compromised wound healing. Stop at least 4 wk before elective surgery; do not start until all surgical wounds healed.
**IND & DOSE Tx of metastatic colorectal cancer resistant to oxaliplatin, w/5-FU, leucovorin, irinotecan.** *Adult:* 4 mg/kg IV over 1 hr q 2 wk.
**ADV EFF** Abd pain, anorexia, dehydration, diarrhea, dysphonia, epistaxis, fatigue, headache, hepatic impairment, **HTN, neutropenia, proteinuria, RPLS, thrombotic events**
**NC/PT** Not for use w/active bleeding; do not use within 4 wk of surgery. Monitor urine protein, BP, nutrition/hydration status; watch for s&sx of CV events. Not for use in preg (barrier contraceptives advised for men, women during and for 3 mo after tx)/breastfeeding. Pt should mark calendar for infusion dates; avoid exposure to infection; report chest pain, fever, s&sx of infection, difficulty breathing, numbness/tingling, severe diarrhea.

## zoledronic acid (Reclast, Zometa)

**CLASS** Bisphosphonate, calcium regulator
**PREG/CONT** High risk/NA

**IND & DOSE Tx of hypercalcemia of malignancy; bone metastases w/multiple myeloma.** *Adult:* 4 mg IV as single-dose infusion of not less than 15 min for hypercalcemia of malignancy w/albumin-corrected serum calcium of ≥12 mg/dL. May retreat w/4 mg IV if needed. Minimum of 7 d should elapse between doses w/careful monitoring of serum creatinine. Pts w/solid tumors should receive 4 mg IV q 3–4 wk to treat bone metastasis (*Zometa*). **Tx of Paget disease, postmenopausal osteoporosis, osteoporosis in men; px of new clinical fractures in pts w/low-trauma hip fractures; tx, px of glucocorticoid-induced osteoporosis; px of osteoporosis in postmenopausal women.** *Adult:* 5 mg IV infused via vented infusion line over at least 15 min. May consider retreatment as needed once q 2 yr for osteoporosis (*Reclast*).
**ADJUST DOSE** Renal impairment
**ADV EFF** Constipation; coughing; decreased phosphate, magnesium, potassium, calcium levels; dyspnea; femur fractures; fever; hypotension; infections; insomnia; **nephrotoxicity; osteonecrosis of jaw;** pain
**INTERACTIONS** Aminoglycosides, loop diuretics, nephrotoxic drugs
**NC/PT** Do not confuse *Reclast, Zometa;* dosage varies. Not for use in preg (contraceptives advised)/breastfeeding. Monitor renal function. Pt should have dental exam before tx; mark calendar of infusion dates; drink plenty of fluids; take supplemental vitamin D, calcium; avoid exposure to infection; report difficulty breathing, swelling, jaw pain.

## ZOLMitriptan (Zomig)

**CLASS** Antimigraine drug, triptan
**PREG/CONT** C/NA

**IND & DOSE Tx of acute migraine attacks.** *Adult:* 2.5 mg PO at onset of headache or w/beginning of aura; may repeat if headache persists after 2 hr. Max, 10 mg/24 hr. Or, 1 spray in nostril at onset of headache or beginning of aura; may repeat in 2 hr if needed. Max, 10 mg/24 hr (2 sprays).
**ADJUST DOSE** Hepatic impairment

**ADV EFF** BP changes, burning/pressure sensation, chest pain, dizziness, drowsiness, numbness, **prolonged QT,** vertigo, weakness
**INTERACTIONS** Cimetidine, ergots, hormonal contraceptives, MAOIs, QT-prolonging drugs, sibutramine
**NC/PT** For acute attack, not for px. Not for use in preg (may make hormonal contraceptives ineffective; barrier contraceptives advised)/breastfeeding. Pt should use right after removing from blister pack; not break/crush/chew tablet; place orally disintegrating tablet on tongue, let dissolve; use one spray only if using nasal spray (may repeat after 2 hours if needed); take safety precautions for CNS effects; report chest pain, swelling, palpitations.

## zolpidem tartrate
(Ambien, Ambien CR, Edluar, Zolpimist)
**CLASS** Sedative-hypnotic
**PREG/CONT** C/C-IV

**BBW** Risk of complex sleep behaviors (sleepwalking, sleep driving), which can cause serious injuries or death. Discontinue if these behaviors occur.
**IND & DOSE Short-term tx of insomnia.** *Adult:* Initially, 5 mg PO at bedtime (women), 10 mg PO at bedtime (men); max, 10 mg/d. ER tablets, 6.25 mg PO at bedtime (women), 6.25–12.5 mg/d PO (men). Oral spray, two–three sprays in mouth, over tongue at bedtime.
**ADJUST DOSE** Elderly pts, hepatic impairment
**ADV EFF Anaphylaxis, angioedema,** depression, dizziness, drowsiness, hangover, headache, next-day psychomotor impairment, severe injuries related to CNS effects, sleep behavior disorders, **suicidality,** suppression of REM sleep, vision disorders
**INTERACTIONS** Chlorpromazine, CNS depressants, imipramine, ketoconazole, rifampin
**NC/PT** Limit amount of drug given to depressed pts. Withdraw gradually after long-term use. Review proper administration of various forms. CR form should not be cut/crushed/chewed. Pt should have 7–8 hr of bedtime remaining. Not for use in preg/breastfeeding. Pt should take safety precautions for CNS effects; report difficulty breathing, abnormal sleep behaviors, swelling, thoughts of suicide.

## zonisamide (Zonegran)
**CLASS** Antiepileptic
**PREG/CONT** High risk/NA

**BBW** Increased risk of suicidal ideation, suicidality; monitor accordingly.
**IND & DOSE Adjuvant tx for partial seizures.** *Adult, child ≥16 yr:* 100 mg PO daily as single dose, not divided; may divide subsequent doses. May increase by 100 mg/d q 2 wk to achieve control. Max, 600 mg/d.
**ADJUST DOSE** Renal impairment
**ADV EFF** Anorexia, aplastic anemia, ataxia, cognitive/neuropsychiatric events, decrease in mental functioning, dizziness, DRESS, dry mouth, metabolic acidosis, nausea, renal calculi, **serious skin reactions to SJS, suicidality,** unusual taste
**INTERACTIONS** Carbamazepine, phenobarbital, phenytoin, primidone
**NC/PT** Withdraw gradually after long-term use. Monitor CBC. Pt should drink plenty of fluids; take safety precautions w/CNS effects; wear medical ID; report flank pain, urine/stool color changes, thoughts of suicide, rash, fever, swelling.

# Patient Safety and Medication Administration

## The rights of medication administration

In the clinical setting, the monumental task of ensuring medication safety can be managed by consistently using the rights of drug administration: right patient, right drug, right route, right dose, right time, right storage, right preparation, and right documentation/recording.

**Right patient: Check the patient's identification even if you think you know who the patient is.**

- Review the patient's diagnosis, and verify that the drug matches the diagnosis.
- Make sure all allergies have been checked before giving a drug.
- Ask patients specifically about OTC drugs, vitamin and mineral supplements, herbal remedies, and routine drugs that they may not think to mention.
- Review the patient's drug regimen to prevent potential interactions between the drug you are about to give and drugs the patient already takes.

**Right drug: Always review a drug order before administering the drug.**

- Do not assume that a computer system is always right. Always double-check.
- Make sure the drug name is correct. Ask for a brand name and a generic name; the chance of reading the name incorrectly is greatly reduced if both generic and brand names are used.
- Avoid taking verbal or telephone orders whenever possible. If you must, have a second person listen in to verify and clarify the order.
- Consider whether the drug makes sense for the patient's diagnosis.

**Right route: Review the available forms of a drug to make sure the drug can be given according to the order.**

- Check the routes available and the appropriateness of the route.
- Make sure the patient is able to take the drug by the route indicated.
- Do not use abbreviations for routes.

**Right dose: Make sure the dose about to be delivered is the dose the prescriber ordered.**

- There should always be a 0 to the left of a decimal point, and there should never be a 0 to the right of a decimal point. If you see an ordered dose that starts w/a decimal point, question it. And if a dose seems much too big, question that.
- Double-check drug calculations, even if a computer did the calculations.
- Check the measuring devices used for liquid drugs. Advise patients not to use kitchen teaspoons or tablespoons to measure drug doses.
- Do not cut tablets in half to get the correct dose without checking the warnings that come w/the drug.

**Right time**

- Ensure the timely delivery of the patient's drugs by scheduling dosing w/ other drugs, meals, or other consistent events to maintain the serum level.
- Teach patients the importance of timing critical drugs. As needed, make detailed medication schedules and prepare pill boxes.

**Right storage**

Some drugs require room temperature; others need to be frozen or chilled. Also, some may need to be kept out of sunlight.

**Right preparation**

Some tablets may be cut or crushed; others may not. Some parenteral medications may need to be reconstituted or diluted with specific solutions.

**Right documentation/recording: Document according to facility policy.**

- Include the drug name, dose, route, and time of administration.
- Note special circumstances, such as the patient having difficulty swallowing or the site of the injection.
- Include the patient's response to the drug and any special nursing interventions that were used.
- Remember, "if it isn't documented, it didn't happen." Accurate documentation provides continuity of care and helps prevent medication errors.

The bottom line in avoiding medication errors is simple: "If in doubt, check it out." A strange abbreviation, a drug or dosage that is new to you, and a confusing name are all examples that signal a need for follow-up. Look up the drug in your drug guide or call the prescriber or the pharmacy to double-check. Never give a drug until you have satisfied yourself that it is the right drug, given by the right route, at the right dose, at the right time, and to the right patient.

# Keeping patients safe

## Patient and family teaching

In today's world, patients are often left to manage on their own to administer most medications. Therefore, it is pertinent to work with patients/families to facilitate the safest medication regimen. Be sure to ask the patient/family what prescription, OTC, and herbal/dietary supplements the patient is taking, both on a regular basis and an "as needed" basis. If the patient/family are unsure, it may be helpful to obtain the list from their pharmacist or primary care provider. The patient/family are integral to safe medication administration and decreasing medication errors.

Medication errors present a constant risk, particularly for patients who take multiple drugs prescribed by multiple health care providers. Facilitating an organized medication regimen that the patient/family understand and embrace is key to preventing errors.

### Patient teaching to prevent medication errors

When being prescribed medications, patients should learn these key points to reduce the risk of medication errors.

- **Keep a list:** Keep a written and/or electronic list of all the drugs you take, including over-the-counter drugs, herbal products, and other supplements; carry this list w/you and show it to all your health care providers, including dentists and emergency personnel. If traveling in a different country, the brand name you are using may be used for a very different drug; it is important to know the generic name as well as the brand name. Refer to your list for safety.
- **Know the purpose of your drugs:** Make sure you know why you take each of your drugs.
- **Follow the directions:** Carefully read the label of each of your drugs, and follow the directions for taking it safely. Do not stop taking a drug without first consulting the prescriber. Make a calendar if you take drugs on alternating days. Using a weekly pillbox may also help ensure the medications are taken on the correct days.
- **Store carefully:** Always store drugs in a dry place safely out of the reach of children and pets and away from humidity and heat (the bathroom is a bad storage area). Make sure to keep all drugs in their original, labeled containers.
- **Speak up:** You, the patient, are the most important member of your health care team. *Never be afraid to ask questions* about your health or your treatments.

## Special populations

### *Keeping children safe*

Children present unique challenges related to medication errors. Advise the child's caregiver to take these steps to prevent medication errors:

- Keep a list of all medications you are giving your child, including prescription, over-the-counter, and herbal medications. Share this list w/any health care provider who cares for your child.
- Never use adult medications to treat a child.
- Read all labels before giving your child a drug. Check the ingredients and dosage to avoid overdose.
- Measure liquid medications using appropriate measuring devices.
- Call your health care provider immediately if your child seems to get worse or seems to be having trouble w/a drug.
- When in doubt, do not hesitate to ask questions. You are your child's best advocate.

### *Protecting elderly patients*

The elderly population is the most rapidly growing group in our country. Frequently, these patients have chronic diseases, are on multiple drugs, and have increasing health problems that can be a challenge to following a drug regimen. They are also more likely to suffer adverse reactions to drugs and drug combinations.

- Advise them to keep a medication list w/them to share w/all health care providers and to post a list somewhere in their home for easy access by emergency personnel.
- Prepare drug boxes for the week, draw up injectables (if stable) for the week, and provide daily reminders to take their medications.
- Be an advocate for elderly patients by asking questions, supplying information to providers, and helping elderly patients stay on top of their drug regimen and monitor their response.

### *Protecting women of childbearing age*

As a general rule, it is best to avoid taking any drugs while pregnant. In 2015, the FDA changed the regulation of medications from pregnancy categories to estimations of risk levels for pregnancy, fertility, and breastfeeding. All new medications approved by the FDA have risk levels assigned based on the current research. Other medications will have categories switched to risk levels as they are evaluated by the FDA. In this book, each medication will have either a pregnancy category OR a risk level based on the current FDA medication labels. The risk levels are "high," "moderate," or "low" based on the evidence OR "unknown" if there is lack of evidence.

- Advise women who may be pregnant to avoid High-Risk drugs (statins, hormones) that could cause serious harm to the fetus.
- Advise pregnant women to avoid all over-the-counter drugs and herbal therapies until they have checked w/the obstetrician for safety.
- Advise pregnant women to question all prescribed drugs and to check carefully to make sure that the drugs are safe for the fetus.
- Advise breastfeeding women to question the safety of prescribed drugs, over-the-counter drugs, or herbal therapies to make sure that the drugs or therapies will not adversely affect the baby.
- Encourage pregnant women to ask questions. Supply information and be an advocate for the fetus or newborn child.

# Avoiding dangerous abbreviations

Although abbreviations can save time, they also raise the risk of misinterpretation, which can lead to potentially disastrous consequences, especially when dealing w/drug administration. To help reduce the risk of being misunderstood, always take the time to write legibly and to spell out anything that could be misread. This caution extends to how you write numbers as well as drug names and other drug-related instructions. The Joint Commission is enforcing a growing list of abbreviations that should not be used in medical records to help alleviate this problem. It is important to be familiar w/the abbreviations used in your clinical area and to avoid the use of any other abbreviations.

## Common dangerous abbreviations

Try to avoid these common—and dangerous—abbreviations.

| *Abbreviation* | *Intended use* | *Potential misreading* | *Preferred use* |
|---|---|---|---|
| BT | bedtime | May be read as "bid" or twice daily | Spell out "bedtime." |
| cc | cubic centimeters | May be read as "u" or units | Use "milliliters," abbreviated as "mL" or "ml." |
| D/C | discharge or discontinue | May lead to premature discontinuation of drug therapy or premature discharge | Spell out "discharge" or "discontinue." |
| hs | at bedtime | May be read as "half-strength" | Spell out "at bedtime." |
| HS | half-strength | May be read as "at bedtime" | Spell out "half-strength." |
| IJ | injection | May be read as "IV" | Spell out "injection." |
| IN | intranasal | May be read as "IM" or "IV" | Spell out "intranasal" or use "NAS." |
| IU | international unit | May be read as "IV" or "10" | Spell out "international unit." |
| μg | microgram | May be read as "mg" | Use "mcg." |
| o.d. or O.D. | once daily | May be read as "right eye" | Spell out "once daily." |
| per os | by mouth | May be read as "left eye" | Use "PO" or spell out "orally." |

| | | | |
|---|---|---|---|
| q.d. or QD | daily | May be read as "qid" | Spell out "daily." |
| q1d | once daily | May be read as "qid" | Spell out "once daily." |
| qhs | every bedtime | May be read as "qhr" (every hour) | Spell out "nightly" or "at bedtime." |
| qn | every night | May be read as "qh" (every hour) | Spell out "nightly" or "at bedtime." |
| q.o.d. or QOD | every other day | May be read as "q.d." (daily) or "q.i.d." (four times daily) | Spell out "every other day." |
| SC, SQ | subcutaneous | May be read as "SL" (sublingual) or "5 every" | Spell out "subcutaneous" or use "subcut." |
| U or u | unit | May be read as "0" (100 instead of 10U) | Spell out "unit." |
| ×7d | for 7 days | May be read as "for seven doses" | Spell out "for 7 days." |
| ° | hour | May be read as a zero | Spell out "hour" or use "hr." |

## Reporting medication errors

Due to increases in the number of drugs available, the aging population, and more people taking many drugs, the possibilities for medication errors seem to be increasing. Institutions have adopted policies for reporting errors, but it is also important to submit information about errors to national/international programs. The FDA MedWatch Program provides a website (www.fda.gov/safety/medwatch-fda-safety-information-and-adverse-event-reporting-program) where the public may report adverse events regarding prescription medications, OTC medications, biologicals, and medical devices. The international institution Institute for Safe Medication Practices (ISMP; www.ismp.org/) provides a place for health care professionals to share potential or actual medications errors.

It is quite common that you may be involved in or witness a medication error. It is important to report the errors/adverse effects so that changes can be made to keep patients safer in the future. However, you may request to remain anonymous.

### What kind of errors should be reported?

Errors (or potential errors) to report include administration of the wrong drug or the wrong strength or dose of a drug, incorrect routes of administration, miscalculations, misuse of medical equipment, mistakes in prescribing or transcribing (misunderstanding of verbal orders), and errors resulting from sound-alike or look-alike names. In your report, you will be asked to include the following:

1. A description of the error or preventable adverse drug reaction. What went wrong?
2. Was this an actual medication accident or are you expressing concern about a potential error or writing about an error that was discovered before it reached the patient?
3. Patient outcome. Did the patient suffer any adverse effects?
4. Type of practice site where the event occurred
5. Generic and brand names of all products involved
6. Dosage form, concentration or strength, and so forth
7. If the error was based on a communication problem, is a sample of the order available? Are package label samples or pictures available if requested?
8. Your recommendations for error prevention.

The FDA and ISMP publish warnings and alerts based on clinician reports of medication errors. Their efforts have helped to increase recognition of the many types of errors, such as those involving sound-alike names, look-alike names and packaging, instructions on equipment and delivery devices, and others.

## Guidelines for safe disposal of medications

The White House Office of National Drug Control Policy, the Department of Health and Human Services, and the Environmental Protection Agency have established guidelines for the proper disposal of unused, unneeded, or expired medications to promote consumer safety, block access to them by potential abusers, and protect the water supply and the environment from possible contamination.

**Medical disposal guidelines**

***Disposing in trash***

- Take unused, unneeded, or expired medications out of their original containers.
- Mix the medication w/an undesirable substance, such as coffee grounds or used kitty litter, and place it in an impermeable, nondescript container, such as an empty can or a sealable storage bag. These steps help keep the medication from being diverted for illicit use or being accidentally ingested by children or animals.
- Place the closed container in your household trash. This is not the ideal way to dispose of a medication. Returning it to a drug take-back site is preferable, but if one is not available, follow these instructions.

***Disposing in toilet***

- Flush prescription drugs down the toilet only if the accompanying patient information specifically instructs you to do so.

***Disposing at a hospital or government-sponsored site***

- Return unused, unneeded, or expired prescription drugs to a pharmaceutical take-back location that offers safe disposal. Check w/your local hospital, health department, police department, or local government for a site near you.

# Appendices

Appendix A

# Alternative and complementary therapies

Many people use herbs and alternative therapies. Some of these products may contain ingredients that interact w/prescribed and OTC medications. Pt hx of alternative therapy use may explain unexpected reactions to some drugs. In the chart below, drugs that the substance interacts with are in **bold**.

| ***Substance*** | ***Reported uses, possible risks*** |
|---|---|
| acidophilus (probiotics) | *Oral:* px/tx of uncomplicated diarrhea; restoration of intestinal flora<br>RISK: **warfarin** |
| alfalfa | *Topical:* healing ointment, relief of arthritis pain<br>*Oral:* tx of arthritis, hot flashes; strength giving; to reduce cholesterol level<br>RISK: **warfarin, chlorpromazine, antidiabetics, hormonal contraceptives, hormone replacement** |
| allspice | *Topical:* anesthetic for teeth, gums; soothes sore joints, muscles<br>*Oral:* tx of indigestion, flatulence, diarrhea, fatigue<br>RISK: **antiplatelet drugs, anticoagulants** |
| aloe leaves | *Topical:* tx of burns, healing of wounds<br>*Oral:* tx of chronic constipation<br>RISK: hypokalemia; diabetic drugs, spontaneous abortion if used in third trimester; **digoxin** |
| androstenedione | *Oral, spray:* anabolic steroid to increase muscle mass/strength<br>RISK: CV disease, certain cancers; **estrogens** |
| angelica | *Oral:* "cure all" for gynecologic problems, headaches, backaches, appetite loss, GI spasms; increases circulation in periphery<br>RISK: **anticoagulants** |
| anise | *Oral:* relief of dry cough, tx of flatulence, bloating<br>RISK: **iron, contraceptives, estrogens, tamoxifen** |
| apple | *Oral:* blood glucose control, constipation, cancer, heart problems<br>RISK: **antidiabetics, fexofenadine** |
| arnica | *Topical:* relief of pain from muscle, soft-tissue injury<br>*Oral:* immune system stimulant; very toxic to child<br>RISK: **antihypertensives, anticoagulants, antiplatelet drugs** |

| *Substance* | *Reported uses, possible risks* |
|---|---|
| ashwagandha | *Oral:* to improve mental, physical functioning; general tonic; to protect cells during cancer chemo, radiation therapy<br>RISK: **anticoagulants, immunosuppressants, thyroid replacement, CNS depressants** |
| astragalus | *Oral:* to increase stamina, energy; to improve immune function, resistance to disease; tx of URI, common cold<br>RISK: **antihypertensives, cyclophosphamide, lithium, immunosuppressants** |
| barberry | *Oral:* antidiarrheal, antipyretic, cough suppressant<br>RISK: **antihypertensives, antiarrhythmics, cyclosporine;** spontaneous abortion if taken during preg |
| basil | *Oral:* analgesic, anti-inflammatory, hypoglycemic<br>RISK: **antidiabetics** |
| bayberry | *Topical:* to promote wound healing<br>*Oral:* stimulant, emetic, antidiarrheal<br>RISK: **antihypertensives** |
| bee pollen | *Oral:* to treat allergies, asthma, ED, prostatitis; suggested use to decrease cholesterol levels, premenstrual syndrome<br>RISK: **antidiabetics;** bee allergy |
| betel palm | *Oral:* mild stimulant, digestive aid<br>RISK: **MAOIs, beta blockers, digoxin, antiglaucoma drugs** |
| bilberry | *Oral:* tx of diabetes, diabetic retinopathy, CV problems, cataracts, night blindness; lowers cholesterol, triglycerides<br>RISK: **anticoagulants, alcohol, antidiabetics** |
| birch bark | *Topical:* tx of infected wounds, cuts; very toxic to child<br>*Oral:* as tea for relief of stomachache |
| blackberry | *Oral:* generalized healing; tx of diabetes<br>RISK: **antidiabetics** |
| black cohosh root | *Oral:* tx of PMS, menopausal disorders, RA. Contains estrogen-like components.<br>RISK: **hormone replacement, hormonal contraceptives, sedatives, antihypertensives, anesthetics, immunosuppressants, atorvastatin, cisplatin** |
| bromelain | *Oral:* tx of inflammation, sports injuries, URI, PMS; adjunct in cancer tx<br>RISK: n/v/d, menstrual disorders; **antibiotics, anticoagulants** |
| burdock | *Oral:* tx of diabetes; atropine-like adverse effects; uterine stimulant<br>RISK: **antidiabetics, anticoagulants** |

| *Substance* | *Reported uses, possible risks* |
|---|---|
| capsicum | *Topical*: external analgesic<br>*Oral:* tx of bowel disorders, chronic laryngitis, peripheral vascular disease<br>RISK: **warfarin, aspirin, ACE inhibitors, MAOIs, sedatives, cocaine** |
| catnip leaves | *Oral:* tx of bronchitis, diarrhea<br>RISK: **sedatives, lithium** |
| cat's claw | *Oral:* tx of allergies, arthritis; adjunct in tx of cancers, AIDS. Discourage use by transplant recipients, during preg/breastfeeding.<br>RISK: **oral anticoagulants, antihypertensives** |
| cayenne pepper | *Topical:* tx of burns, wounds; relief of toothache |
| celery | *Oral:* lowers blood glucose, acts as diuretic; may cause potassium depletion<br>RISK: **antidiabetics** |
| chamomile | *Topical:* tx of wounds, ulcers, conjunctivitis<br>*Oral:* tx of migraines, gastric cramps; relief of anxiety, inflammatory diseases. Contains coumarin; closely monitor pt taking anticoagulants.<br>RISK: **antidepressants;** ragweed allergies |
| chaste-tree berry | *Oral:* tx of PMS, menopausal problems; to stimulate lactation. Progesterone-like effects.<br>RISK: **hormone replacement, hormonal contraceptives** |
| chicken soup | *Oral:* breaks up respiratory secretions; bronchodilator; relieves anxiety |
| chicory | *Oral:* tx of digestive tract problems, gout; stimulates bile secretions |
| Chinese angelica (dong quai) | *Oral:* general tonic; tx of anemias, PMS, menopausal sx, antihypertensive, laxative. Use caution w/flu, hemorrhagic diseases.<br>RISK: **antihypertensives, vasodilators, anticoagulants, hormone replacement** |
| chondroitin | *Oral:* tx of osteoarthritis, related disorders (usually w/glucosamine)<br>RISK: **anticoagulants** |
| chong cao fungi | *Oral:* antioxidant; promotes stamina, sexual function |
| *Coleus forskohlii* | *Oral:* tx of asthma, HTN, eczema<br>RISK: **antihypertensives, antihistamines;** peptic ulcer |
| comfrey | *Topical:* tx of wounds, cuts, ulcers<br>*Oral:* gargle for tonsillitis<br>RISK: **eucalyptus;** monitor LFTs |

| *Substance* | *Reported uses, possible risks* |
|---|---|
| coriander | *Oral:* weight loss, lowers blood glucose<br>RISK: **antidiabetics** |
| creatine monohydrate | *Oral:* to enhance athletic performance<br>RISK: **insulin, caffeine** |
| dandelion root | *Oral:* tx of liver/kidney problems; decreases lactation (after delivery, w/weaning); lowers blood glucose<br>RISK: **antidiabetics, antihypertensives, quinolone antibiotics** |
| DHEA | *Oral:* slows aging, improves vigor ("Fountain of Youth"); androgenic side effects<br>RISK: **alprazolam, anastrozole, calcium channel blockers, exemestane, fulvestrant, antidiabetics** |
| di huang | *Oral:* tx of diabetes mellitus<br>RISK: **antidiabetics** |
| dried root bark of *Lycium chinense* Miller | *Oral:* lowers cholesterol, blood glucose<br>RISK: **antidiabetics** |
| echinacea (cone flower) | *Oral:* tx of colds, flu; stimulates immune system, attacks viruses; causes immunosuppression if used long term. May be hepatotoxic; discourage use for longer than 12 wk. Discourage use by pts w/SLE, TB, AIDS.<br>RISK: **hepatotoxic drugs, immunosuppressants, antifungals, caffeine** |
| elder bark and flowers | *Topical:* gargle for tonsillitis/pharyngitis<br>*Oral:* tx of fever, chills |
| ephedra | *Oral:* increases energy, relieves fatigue<br>RISK: serious complications, including death; increased risk of HTN, stroke, MI; **interacts w/many drugs; banned by FDA** |
| ergot | *Oral:* tx of migraine headaches, menstrual problems, hemorrhage<br>RISK: **antihypertensives, antidepressants** |
| eucalyptus | *Topical:* tx of wounds<br>*Oral:* decreases respiratory secretions; suppresses cough; very toxic in child<br>RISK: **comfrey** |
| evening primrose | *Oral:* tx of PMS, menopause, RA, diabetic neuropathy. Discourage use by pts w/epilepsy, schizophrenia.<br>RISK: **phenothiazines, antidepressants, anticoagulants** |
| false unicorn root | *Oral:* tx of menstrual/uterine problems. Not for use in preg/breastfeeding.<br>RISK: **lithium** |

| *Substance* | *Reported uses, possible risks* |
|---|---|
| fennel | *Oral:* tx of colic, gout, flatulence; enhances lactation<br>RISK: **ciprofloxacin, estrogens** |
| fenugreek | *Oral:* lowers cholesterol; reduces blood glucose; aids in healing<br>RISK: **antidiabetics, anticoagulants** |
| feverfew | *Oral:* tx of arthritis, fever, migraine. Not for use if surgery planned.<br>RISK: **anticoagulants** |
| fish oil | *Oral:* tx of coronary diseases, arthritis, colitis, depression, aggression, attention deficit disorder |
| garlic | *Oral:* tx of colds; diuretic; px of CAD; intestinal antiseptic; lowers blood glucose; anticoagulant effects; decreases BP; anemia<br>RISK: **antidiabetics, isoniazid, non-NRTIs, saquinavir, oral contraceptives** |
| ginger | *Oral:* tx of nausea, motion sickness, postop nausea (may increase risk of miscarriage)<br>RISK: **anticoagulants** |
| ginkgo | *Oral:* vascular dilation; increases blood flow to brain, improving cognitive function; tx of Alzheimer disease; antioxidant. Can inhibit blood clotting. Seizures reported w/ high doses.<br>RISK: **anticoagulants, aspirin, NSAIDs, phenytoin, carbamazepine, phenobarbital, TCAs, MAOIs, antidiabetics** |
| ginseng | *Oral:* aphrodisiac, mood elevator, tonic; antihypertensive; decreases cholesterol/blood glucose; adjunct in cancer chemo, radiation therapy. May cause irritability if used w/ caffeine. Inhibits clotting.<br>RISK: **anticoagulants, aspirin, NSAIDs, phenelzine, MAOIs, estrogens, corticosteroids, digoxin, antidiabetics** |
| glucosamine | *Oral:* tx of osteoarthritis, joint diseases; usually w/chondroitin<br>RISK: diabetic pts; **warfarin, some chemo agents** |
| goldenrod leaves | *Oral:* tx of renal disease, rheumatism, sore throat, eczema<br>RISK: **diuretics** |
| goldenseal | *Oral:* lowers blood glucose, aids healing; tx of bronchitis, colds, flulike sx, cystitis. May cause false-negative results in pts using drugs such as marijuana, cocaine. Large amounts may cause paralysis; overdose can cause death.<br>RISK: **anticoagulants, antihypertensives, acid blockers, barbiturates, sedatives, digoxin, cyclosporine** |

| *Substance* | *Reported uses, possible risks* |
|---|---|
| gotu kola | *Topical:* chronic venous insufficiency<br>RISK: **antidiabetics, cholesterol-lowering drugs, sedatives** |
| grape seed extract | *Oral:* tx of allergies, asthma; improves circulation; decreases platelet aggregation<br>RISK: **anticoagulants** |
| green tea leaf | *Oral:* antioxidant; to prevent cancer, CV disease; to increase cognitive function (caffeine effects)<br>RISK: **anticoagulants, milk** |
| guarana | *Oral:* decreases appetite; promotes weight loss; increases BP, risk of CV events<br>RISK: **amphetamines, cocaine, ephedrine** |
| guayusa | *Oral:* lowers blood glucose; promotes weight loss<br>RISK: **antihypertensives, iron, lithium** |
| hawthorn | *Oral:* tx of angina, arrhythmias, BP problems; decreases cholesterol<br>RISK: **digoxin, ACE inhibitors, CNS depressants** |
| hop | *Oral:* sedative; aids healing; alters blood glucose<br>RISK: **CNS depressants, antipsychotics** |
| horehound | *Oral:* expectorant; tx of respiratory problems, GI disorders<br>RISK: **antidiabetics, antihypertensives** |
| horse chestnut seed | *Oral:* tx of varicose veins, hemorrhoids, venous insufficiency<br>RISK: **anticoagulants** |
| hyssop | *Topical:* tx of cold sores, genital herpes, burns, wounds<br>*Oral:* tx of coughs, colds, indigestion, flatulence; toxic in child/pet<br>RISK: preg, pts w/seizures |
| jambolan | *Oral:* tx of diarrhea, dysentery; lowers blood glucose<br>RISK: **CNS depressants, java plum** |
| java plum | *Oral:* tx of diabetes mellitus<br>RISK: **antidiabetics** |
| jojoba | *Topical:* promotion of hair growth; relief of skin problems. Toxic if ingested. |
| juniper berries | *Oral:* increases appetite, aids digestion; diuretic; urinary tract disinfectant; lowers blood glucose<br>RISK: **antidiabetics;** preg |
| kava | *Oral:* tx of nervous anxiety, stress, restlessness; tranquilizer. Warn against use w/alprazolam; may cause coma. Advise against use w/Parkinson disease, hx of stroke. Risk of serious hepatotoxicity.<br>RISK: **St. John's wort, anxiolytics, alcohol** |

| *Substance* | *Reported uses, possible risks* |
|---|---|
| kudzu | *Oral:* reduces alcohol craving (undergoing research for use w/alcoholics)<br>RISK: **anticoagulants, aspirin, antidiabetics, CV drugs, estrogens** |
| lavender | *Topical:* astringent for minor cuts, burns; oil potentially poisonous<br>*Oral:* tx of insomnia, restlessness<br>RISK: **CNS depressants** |
| ledum tincture | *Topical:* tx of insect bites, puncture wounds; dissolves some blood clots, bruises |
| licorice | *Oral:* px of thirst; soothes coughs; treats "incurable" chronic fatigue syndrome; tx of duodenal ulcer. Acts like aldosterone. Blocks spironolactone effects. Can lead to digoxin toxicity because of aldosterone-lowering effects; advise extreme caution.<br>RISK: **thyroid drugs, antihypertensives, hormonal contraceptives;** renal/liver disease, HTN, CAD, preg, breastfeeding |
| ma huang | *Oral:* tx of colds, nasal congestion, asthma; contains ephedrine<br>RISK: **antihypertensives, antidiabetics, MAOIs, digoxin** |
| mandrake root | *Oral:* tx of fertility problems |
| marigold leaves and flowers | *Oral:* relief of muscle tension; increases wound healing<br>RISK: preg/breastfeeding |
| melatonin | *Oral:* relief of jet lag; tx of insomnia<br>RISK: **antihypertensives, benzodiazepines, beta blockers, methamphetamine** |
| milk thistle | *Oral:* tx of hepatitis, cirrhosis, fatty liver caused by alcohol/drug use<br>RISK: **drugs using CP450, CYP3A4, CYP2C9 systems** |
| milk vetch | *Oral:* improves resistance to disease; adjunct in cancer chemo, radiation therapy |
| mistletoe leaves | *Oral:* promotes weight loss; relief of diabetes s&sx<br>RISK: **antihypertensives, CNS depressants, immunosuppressants** |
| *Momordica charantia* (karela) | *Oral:* blocks intestinal absorption of glucose; lowers blood glucose; weight loss<br>RISK: **antidiabetics** |
| nettle | *Topical:* stimulation of hair growth, tx of bleeding<br>*Oral:* tx of rheumatism, allergic rhinitis; antispasmodic; expectorant<br>RISK: **diuretics, lithium, antidiabetics**; preg/breastfeeding |

| Substance | Reported uses, possible risks |
|---|---|
| nightshade leaves and roots | *Oral:* stimulates circulatory system; tx of eye disorders |
| octacosanol | *Oral:* tx of parkinsonism, enhancement of athletic performance<br>RISK: **carbidopa-levodopa;** preg/breastfeeding |
| parsley seeds and leaves | *Oral:* tx of jaundice, asthma, menstrual difficulties, urinary infections, conjunctivitis<br>RISK: **SSRIs, lithium, opioids, antihypertensives** |
| passionflower vine | *Oral:* sedative-hypnotic<br>RISK: **CNS depressants, MAOIs, alcohol, anticoagulants** |
| peppermint leaves | *Topical:* rubbed on forehead to relieve tension headaches<br>*Oral:* tx of nervousness, insomnia, dizziness, cramps, coughs<br>RISK: **cyclosporine, drugs metabolized by CYP450** |
| psyllium | *Oral:* tx of constipation; lowers cholesterol. Can cause severe gas, stomach pain. May interfere w/nutrient absorption.<br>RISK: **warfarin, digoxin, lithium, oral drugs, laxatives** |
| raspberry | *Oral:* healing of minor wounds; control/tx of diabetes, GI disorders, upper respiratory disorders<br>RISK: **antidiabetics; alcohol** |
| red clover | *Oral:* estrogen replacement in menopause; suppresses whooping cough; asthma<br>RISK: **anticoagulants, antiplatelet drugs, estrogens;** preg |
| red yeast rice | *Oral:* lowers cholesterol.<br>RISK: **cyclosporine, fibric acid, niacin, lovastatin, grapefruit juice** |
| rose hips | *Oral:* laxative; to boost immune system, prevent illness<br>RISK: **estrogens, iron, warfarin** |
| rosemary | *Topical:* relief of rheumatism, sprains, wounds, bruises, eczema<br>*Oral:* gastric stimulation; relief of flatulence, colic; stimulation of bile release<br>RISK: **alcohol** |
| rue extract | *Topical:* relief of pain associated w/sprains, groin pulls, whiplash<br>RISK: **antihypertensives, digoxin, warfarin** |
| saffron | *Oral:* tx of menstrual problems; abortifacient |
| sage | *Oral:* lowers BP, blood glucose<br>RISK: **antidiabetics, anticonvulsants, alcohol** |

| *Substance* | *Reported uses, possible risks* |
|---|---|
| SAM-e (adomet) | *Oral:* promotion of general well-being, health. May cause frequent GI complaints, headache<br>RISK: **antidepressants** |
| sarsaparilla | *Oral:* tx of skin disorders, rheumatism<br>RISK: **anticonvulsants** |
| sassafras | *Topical:* tx of local pain, skin eruptions<br>*Oral:* enhancement of athletic performance, "cure" for syphilis<br>RISK: Oil may be toxic to fetus, child, adult when ingested. **Interacts w/many drugs** |
| saw palmetto | *Oral:* tx of BPH<br>RISK: **estrogen-replacement, hormonal contraceptives, iron, finasteride, testosterone replacement** |
| schisandra | *Oral:* health tonic, liver protectant; adjunct in cancer chemo, radiation therapy<br>RISK: **drugs metabolized in liver;** preg (causes uterine stimulation) |
| squawvine | *Oral:* diuretic, tonic; aid in labor/delivery; tx of menstrual problems<br>RISK: **digoxin, alcohol** |
| St. John's wort | *Topical:* tx of puncture wounds, insect bites, crushed fingers/toes<br>*Oral:* tx of depression, PMS symptoms; antiviral. Discourage tyramine-containing foods; hypertensive crisis possible. Thrombocytopenia has occurred. Can increase light sensitivity; advise against taking w/drugs causing photo-sensitivity. Severe photosensitivity possible in light-skinned people.<br>RISK: **SSRIs, MAOIs, kava, digoxin, theophylline, AIDS antivirals, sympathomimetics, antineoplastics, hormonal contraceptives, serotogenic drugs** |
| sweet violet flowers | *Oral:* tx of respiratory disorders; emetic<br>RISK: **laxatives** |
| tarragon | *Oral:* weight loss; to prevent cancer; lowers blood glucose<br>RISK: **antidiabetics** |
| tea tree oil | *Topical:* antifungal, antibacterial; tx of burns, insect bites, irritated skin, acne; mouthwash |
| thyme | *Topical:* liniment, gargle; tx of wounds<br>*Oral:* antidiarrheal; relief of bronchitis/laryngitis. May increase light sensitivity; warn against using w/photosensitivity-causing drugs.<br>RISK: **MAOIs, SSRIs, anticoagulants, antiplatelets** |

| *Substance* | *Reported uses, possible risks* |
|---|---|
| turmeric | *Oral:* antioxidant, anti-inflammatory; tx of arthritis. May cause GI distress. Warn against use w/known biliary obstruction.<br>RISK: **oral anticoagulants, NSAIDs, immunosuppressants** |
| valerian | *Oral:* sedative-hypnotic; reduces anxiety, relaxes muscles. Can cause severe liver damage.<br>RISK: **barbiturates, alcohol, CNS depressants, benzodiazepines, antihistamines** |
| went rice | *Oral:* cholesterol/triglyceride-lowering effects. Warn against use in preg, liver disease, alcoholism, acute infection. |
| white willow bark | *Oral:* tx of fevers<br>RISK: **anticoagulants, NSAIDs, diuretics** |
| xuan shen | *Oral:* lowers blood glucose; slows HR; tx of HF<br>RISK: **antidiabetics** |
| yohimbe | *Oral:* tx of ED. Can affect BP; CNS stimulant. Has cardiac effects. Manic episodes have occurred in psychiatric pts.<br>RISK: **SSRIs, tyramine-containing foods, TCAs** |

Appendix B

# Topical drugs

Topical drugs are intended for surface use, not ingestion or injection. They may be very toxic if absorbed into the system, but they serve several purposes when used topically.
**PREG/CONT** Please refer to individual medication labels.
**ADV EFF** Burning, dermatitis, local irritation (common), stinging, toxic effects if absorbed systemically
**NC/PT** Apply sparingly to affected area as directed. Do not use w/open wounds, broken skin. Avoid contact w/eyes. Pt should report local irritation, allergic reaction, worsening of condition.

## *Acne, rosacea, melasma products*

**adapalene (Differin):** Not for use <12 yr. Avoid use on sunburned skin, w/other products, sun exposure. Apply thin film to affected area after washing q night at bedtime. Available as cream, gel; 0.1%, 0.3% conc.

**adapalene/benzyl peroxide (Epiduo):** For pt ≥9 yr. Avoid use on sunburned skin, w/other products, sun exposure. Apply thin film once a d to affected area on face and/or trunk after washing. Available as gel; 0.1%, 2.5% conc.

**alitretinoin (Panretin):** Tx of lesions of Kaposi sarcoma (1% gel). Apply as needed bid to cover lesions. Photosensitivity common. Inflammation, peeling, redness possible. Preg Category D.

**aminolevulinic acid hydrochloride (Ameluz):** Tx of mild to moderate actinic keratosis on face and scalp. Administered only by health care provider. Risk of eye injury, photosensitivity, bleeding, ophthalmic adverse reactions, mucous membrane irritation. Available as gel; 10%.

**azelaic acid (Azelex, Finacea):** Wash, dry skin. Massage thin layer into affected area bid. Wash hands thoroughly after applying. Improvement usually within 4 wk. Initial irritation usual; passes w/time.

**brimonidine (Mirvaso):** Tx of persistent facial erythema of rosacea in adult. Apply pea-size amount to forehead, chin, cheeks daily. Risk of vascular insufficiency, CV disease. Wash hands immediately after application; do not ingest.

**clindamycin (Clindesse, Cleocin, Evoclin): Tx of bacterial vaginitis (2% vaginal cream):** One applicatorful (100 mg) vaginally at any time of d. **Tx of acne vulgaris (1% foam):** Apply once daily to affected areas that have been washed, are fully dry.

**clindamycin/benzoyl peroxide (Acanya, BenzaClin, Duac, Onexton):** Tx of acne. Apply gel to affected areas bid. Wash area, pat dry before applying.

**clindamycin/tretinoin (Veltin, Ziana):** Tx of acne. Rub pea-size amount over entire face once daily at bedtime. Not for use in colitis. Avoid sun exposure.

**dapsone (Aczone Gel):** Tx of acne. Apply thin layer to affected areas bid. Methemoglobinemia has been reported. Closely follow Hgb, reticulocyte count in pts w/G6PD deficiencies.

**fluocinolone acetonide/hydroquinone/tretinoin (Tri-Luma):** Tx of melasma. Do not use in preg. Apply to depigmented area of melasma once each p.m. at least 30 min before bedtime after washing, patting dry; avoid occlusive dressings. Use sunscreen, protective clothing if outside (skin dryness, peeling possible).

**hydrogen peroxide (Eskata):** Tx of seborrheic keratoses. Given by health care provider; 40% solution.

**ingenol mebutate (Picato):** Tx of acne. Apply 0.015% gel once daily to face/scalp for 5 d. Apply 0.05% gel once daily to trunk/extremities for 2 d. Avoid periocular area, lips, mouth. Risk of hypersensitivity, ophthal reactions, herpes zoster.

**ivermectin (Soolantra):** Tx of rosacea. Apply 1% cream to affected areas daily. Not for oral, ophthal, intravaginal use.

**metroNIDAZOLE (MetroCream, MetroGel, MetroLotion, Noritate):** Tx of rosacea. Apply cream to affected area bid.

**oxymetazoline hydrochloride (Rhofade):** Tx of rosacea. Apply thin film to affected areas once daily. Tx of facial erythema associated w/rosacea (cream 1%). Apply pea-size amount daily in thin layer to entire face; wash hands after applying. Use caution w/known CV disease, angle-closure glaucoma.

**sodium sulfacetamide (Klaron):** Apply thin film to affected area bid. Wash affected area w/mild soap, water; pat dry. Avoid use in denuded, abraded areas.

**tazarotene (Avage, Fabior, Tazorac):** Tx of psoriasis. Avoid use in preg. Apply thin film once daily in p.m. Do not use w/irritants, products w/high alcohol content. Drying causes photosensitivity.

**tretinoin 0.025% cream (Avita):** Tx of acne. Apply thin layer once daily. Discomfort, peeling, redness possible first 2–4 wk. Worsened acne possible in first few wk.

**tretinoin 0.05% cream (Renova):** To remove fine wrinkles. Apply thin coat in p.m.

**tretinoin gel (Retin-A* Micro):** Tx of acne. Apply to cover once daily after washing. Inflammation exacerbation possible initially. Therapeutic effects usually seen in first 2 wk.

## *Analgesics*

**capsaicin (Axsain, Capsin, Capzasin, Icy Hot PM, No Pain-HP, Pain Doctor, Qutenza, Zostrix, Zostrix-HP):** Local pain relief for osteoarthritis, rheumatoid arthritis, neuralgias. Apply no more than tid–qid. Do not bandage tightly. Consult physician if condition worsens or persists after 14–28 d. **Qutenza:** Apply patch to relieve postherpetic neuralgia pain.

## *Antibiotics*

**ciprofloxacin (Cetraxal, Otiprio):** **Tx of child w/bilateral otitis media w/effusion undergoing tympanostomy tube placement:** 6 mg (0.1 mL) into each affected ear after middle ear suctioning. Risk of bacterial overgrowth.

**ciprofloxacin/dexamethasone (Ciprodex), ciprofloxacin/ hydrocortisone (Cipro-HC Otic Drops, Otiprio):** Apply to ears of child w/acute otitis media and tympanostomy tubes; apply to outer ear canal for acute otitis externa. Use bid for 7 d.

**mupirocin (Centany):** Tx of impetigo caused by susceptible strains. Apply small amt to affected area tid; may cover w/gauze dressing. Risk of superinfection.

**mupirocin calcium (Bactroban Nasal):** To eradicate nasal colonization of MRSA. Apply ½ of oint from single-use tubes between nostrils bid for 5 d. Risk of CDAD.

**neomycin/polymyxin B sulfates/ bacitracin zinc/hydrocortisone (Cortisporin):** Tx of corticosteroid-responsive dermatoses w/secondary infection. Apply thin film to affected area(s) 2–4 ×/d. Limit to 7 d or less.

**ozenoxacin (Xepi):** Tx of impetigo due to *Staphylococcus aureus* or *Streptococcus pyogenes* in adult, child ≥2 mo. Apply thin layer bid for 5 d.

**retapamulin (Altabax):** Tx of impetigo in pts ≥9 mo. Apply thin layer to affected area bid for 5 d.

## *Anti-diaper-rash drug*

**miconazole/zinc oxide/petrolatum (Vusion):** Culture for *Candida* before tx. Apply gently for 7 d; change diapers frequently, wash gently.

## *Antifungals*

**butenafine hydrochloride (Lotrimin Ultra, Mentax):** Tx of athlete's foot; tinea corporis, cruris; ringworm. Apply once/d for 4 wk.

**ciclopirox (Loprox, Penlac):** Tx of onychomycosis of fingernails, toenails in immunosuppressed pts. Apply directly to nails.

**clotrimazole (Cruex, Desenex, Lotrimin AF, Mycelex, Trivagizole):** Clean area; gently massage in up to bid for max 4 wk.

**econazole (Ecoza):** Apply daily or bid for 2–4 wk. Clean area before applying. Change socks at least once/d for athlete's foot.

**gentian violet (generic):** Apply locally up to bid. Do not apply to active lesions. Will stain skin, clothing.

**ketoconazole (Extina, Ketozole, Nizoral, Xolegel):** Tx of seborrheic dermatitis. Available as cream, foam, gel, shampoo. Use as shampoo daily.

**luliconazole (Luzu):** Tx of tinea cruris, tinea corporis, tinea pedis. Apply to affected area once a d for 1 wk, 2 wk for interdigital tinea pedis.

**naftifine hydrochloride (Naftin):** Tx of tinea cruris, tinea pedis, tinea corporis. Gently massage in bid for no more than 4 wk. Avoid occlusive dressings. Wash hands thoroughly after applying.

**oxiconazole (Oxistat):** Tx of tinea cruris, tinea pedis, tinea corporis. Apply q d to bid for max 1 mo.

**sertaconazole (Ertaczo):** Tx of interdigital tinea pedis. Apply between toes, to surrounding tissue bid for 4 wk.

**terbinafine (Lamisil):** Tx of onychomycosis of fingernails/toenails. Apply bid for 1–4 wk. Avoid occlusive dressings. Stop if local irritation.

**tolnaftate (Absorbine, Tinactin):** Tx of athlete's foot. Apply small amount bid for 2–3 wk; 4–6 wk if skin very thick. Clean, dry area before use. Change socks qid.

## *Antihistamine*

**azelastine hydrochloride (Astelin, Astepro, Dymista, Optivar):** 2 sprays/nostril bid. Do not use w/ alcohol, OTC antihistamines; dizziness, sedation possible.

## *Antipsoriatics*

**anthralin (Balnetar, Dritho-Cream HP, Fototar, Zithranol):** Apply daily; use protective dressings. Avoid contact w/eyes. May stain fabric, skin, hair, fingernails.

**betamethasone (Sernivo):** Apply to affected skin bid for up to 4 wk.

**calcipotriene (Dovonex, Sorilux):** Apply thin layer q d or bid. Monitor calcium w/extended use.

**calcipotriene/betamethasone (Enstilar, Taclonex):** Apply q d for 4 wk. Max, 100 g/wk. Avoid occlusive dressings. Limit to 30% of body area.

## *Antiseborrheic*

**selenium sulfide (Selsun Blue):** Massage 5–10 mL into scalp, leave on 2–3 min, rinse; repeat. May damage jewelry.

## *Antiseptics*

**benzalkonium chloride (Benza, Mycocide NS):** Mix in sol. Spray preop area; store instruments in sol (add antirust tablets). Rinse detergents, soaps from skin before use.

**chlorhexidine gluconate (BactoShield, Dyna-Hex, Exidine, Hibistat):** For surgical scrub, preop skin prep, wound cleansing. Scrub, leave on for 15 sec (3 min for surgical scrub), rinse.

**iodine (generic):** Wash area w/sol. Highly toxic. Avoid occlusive dressings. Stains skin, clothing.

**povidone iodine (ACU-Dyne, Betadine, Betagen, Iodex, Minidyne, Operand, Polydine):** Less irritating than iodine. May bandage area. May inactivate HIV.

**sodium hypochlorite (Dakin's solution):** Apply as antiseptic. Chemical burns possible.

## *Antivirals*

**acyclovir (Zovirax):** Apply 0.5-inch ribbon, rub in gently six times/d for 7 d.

**acyclovir/hydrocortisone (Xerese):** Tx of cold sores in pts ≥6 yr. Apply five times/d for 5 d.

**docosanol (Abreva):** Tx of oral, facial herpes simplex cold sores. Apply five times/d for 10 d. Do not overuse.

**imiquimod (Aldara):** Tx of external genital, perianal warts: Apply thin layer three times/wk at bedtime for up to 16 wk; remove w/soap, water after 6–10 hr. Tx of nonhyperkeratotic actinic keratosis on face, scalp in immunosuppressed pts: Apply before bed for 16 wk. Tx of superficial basal cell carcinoma in immunosuppressed pts: 10–40 mg applied to lesion five times/wk at bedtime for 6 wk.

**imiquimod (Zyclara):** Tx of nonhyperkeratotic, nonhypertrophic actinic keratoses on face, balding scalp: Apply daily at bedtime for 2 wk, then 2 wk of no tx. May repeat. Tx of genital, perianal warts in pts ≥12 yr: Apply daily.

**kunecatechins (sinecatechins) (Veregen):** External tx of genital, perianal warts in pts ≥18 yr. Apply to each wart tid for 16 wk. Do not cover tx area.

**penciclovir (Denavir):** Tx of cold sores on lips, face. Apply thin layer q 2 hr while awake for 4 d.

### *Burn tx*

**mafenide (Sulfamylon):** Apply to clean, dry, debrided wound q d or bid. Cover at all times w/drug. Monitor for infection, acidosis. Pretreat for pain.

**silver sulfadiazine (Silvadene, SSD Cream, Thermazene):** Apply q d to bid using 1/16-inch thickness. Dressings not necessary. Monitor for fungal infection.

### *Corticosteroids for inflammatory disorders*

**alclometasone dipropionate (generic):** 0.05% oint, cream

**beclomethasone (Beconase AQ, Qnasl):** Nasal spray for rhinitis

**betamethasone dipropionate:** 0.05% oint, cream, gel, lotion, aerosol

**betamethasone dipropionate augmented (Diprolene, Diprolene AF):** 0.05% oint, cream, lotion

**betamethasone valerate (Beta-Val, Luxiq, Valnac):** 0.1% oint, cream, lotion; 0.12% foam

**ciclesonide (Alvesco, Omnaris, Zetonna):** 80 or 160 mcg/actuation as nasal spray or for inhalation

**clobetasol propionate (Clobex, Cormax, Embeline, Olux):** 0.05% spray, oint, cream, foam, gel

**clocortolone pivalate (Cloderm):** 0.1% cream

**desonide (DesOwen, Verdeso):** 0.05% oint, lotion, cream, foam

**desoximetasone (Topicort):** 0.25% oint, cream

**dexamethasone (generic):** 0.05% cream, gel

**diflorasone diacetate (generic):** 0.1% cream

**fluocinolone acetate (Synalar):** 0.05% oint, cream; 0.01% sol

**fluocinonide (Fluonex, Lidex, Vanos):** 0.025% cream, oint; 0.01% cream; 0.05% cream, oint, gel, sol; 0.1% cream

**fluticasone fumarate (Veramyst):** 35 mcg/spray nasal spray

**fluticasone propionate (Cutivate):** 0.005% oint

**halcinonide (Halog):** 0.1% oint, cream

**halobetasol propionate (Ultravate):** 0.05% oint, cream

**hydrocortisone (Bactine Hydrocortisone, Cort-Dome, Dermolate, Dermtex HC, Cortizone-10, Hycort, Hytone, Tegrin-HC):** 0.25%, 0.5%, 1%, 2%, 2.5% cream, lotion, oint, sol

**hydrocortisone acetate (Anusol-HCL, Cortaid, Cortaid w/Aloe, Gynecort, Lanacort-5):** 0.5%, 1% cream, oint

**hydrocortisone buteprate (generic):** 0.1% cream

**hydrocortisone butyrate (Locoid):** 0.1% oint, cream

**hydrocortisone valerate (generic):** 0.2% oint, cream

**mometasone furoate (Asmanex Twisthaler, Elocon, Nasonex):** 220 mcg/actuation powder for oral inhalation; 0.1% oint, cream, lotion; 0.2% nasal spray

**prednicarbate (Dermatop):** 0.1% cream

**triamcinolone acetonide (Triderm):** 0.1% cream, lotion; 0.025% lotion

## *Eczema drug*

**crisabarole (Eucrisa):** Tx of mild to moderate eczema. Apply thin layer to affected area bid.

## *Emollients*

**dexpanthenol (generic):** To relieve itching, aids in healing skin irritation; q d to bid.

**urea (Aquacare; Gordon's Urea 40%; Nutraplus; Ureacin 10, 20):** Rub in bid–qid.

**vitamins A, D (generic):** To relieve minor burns, chafing, skin irritation; bid–qid for up to 7 d.

## *Estrogen*

**estradiol hemihydrate (Vagifem):** Tx of atrophic vaginitis. One tablet/d vaginally for 2 wk, then 1 tablet two times/wk. Taper over 3–6 mo.

## *Growth factor*

**becaplermin (Regranex):** Adjunct tx of diabetic foot ulcers. Must have adequate blood supply. Risk of cancer w/long-term use.

## *Hair removal product*

**eflornithine (Vaniqa):** For women only. Apply to unwanted facial hair bid for 24 wk; do not wash treated area for 4 hr.

## *Hemostatics*

**absorbable gelatin (Gelfoam):** Add 3–4 mL sterile saline to contents of jar; smear or press to cut surface. Assess for infection; do not use if area infected.

**absorbable fibrin sealant (TachoSil):** For CV surgery when usual techniques to control bleeding ineffective. Apply yellow side of patches directly to bleeding area. Do not use intravascularly or w/known hypersensitivity to human blood products, horse protein.

**human fibrin sealant (Artiss, Evicel, Tisseel):** Adjunct to decrease bleeding in vascular, liver surgery; to adhere autologous skin grafts for burns. Spray or drip onto tissue in short bursts to produce thin layer; may use second layer.

**human fibrin sealant (Raplixa):** Adjunct to decrease bleeding in small blood vessels in standard surgical techniques. Spray directly on site. Monitor for infection.

**microfibrillar collagen (Hemopad):** Apply dry directly to bleeding source. Monitor for infection. Remove any excess material once bleeding stopped.

**thrombin (Thrombinar, Thrombostat):** 100–1,000 units/mL. Prepare in sterile distilled water or isotonic saline. Mix freely w/blood on surface of injury; watch for allergic reactions.

**thrombin, recombinant (Recothrom):** Apply directly to bleeding site w/absorbable gelatin sponge; reserve for minor bleeds. Not for use w/hamster, snake protein allergies.

## *Immunomodulator*

**pimecrolimus (Elidel):** Tx of mild to moderate atopic dermatitis in nonimmunosuppressed pts >2 yr. Apply bid.

### *Keratolytics*

**podofilox (Condylox):** Apply to dry skin q 12 hr for 3 d.

**podophyllum resin (Podocon-25, Podofin):** Use minimum possible for wart removal; very toxic.

### *Local anesthetic*

**lidocaine/tetracaine (Synera):** Dermal analgesia for superficial venous access, dermatologic procedures. One patch to intact skin 20–30 min before procedure.

### *Lotions, solutions*

**Burow's solution aluminum acetate (Domeboro Powder):** Astringent wet dressing for inflammatory conditions, insect bites, athlete's foot, bruises. Dissolve packet, tablet in pint of water; apply q 15–30 min for 4–8 hr.

**calamine lotion (generic):** To relieve topical itching. Apply tid–qid.

**hamamelis water (A-E-R, Witch Hazel):** To relieve itching of vaginal infection, hemorrhoids; postepisiotomy, posthemorrhoidectomy care. Apply locally six times/d.

### *Nasal corticosteroid*

**fluticasone propionate (Flovent Diskus, Flovent HFA):** Px of asthma in pts >4 yr. Two sprays/nostril/d or 88–220 mcg bid using inhalation device, nasal inhalation.

### *Pediculicides, scabicides*

**benzyl alcohol (generic):** Tx of head lice in pts ≥6 mo. Apply 5% lotion to scalp, hair near scalp.

**crotamiton (Croton, Eurax):** Massage into skin of entire body; repeat in 24 hr. Bathe 48 hr after use. Change bed linens, clothing; wash in hot water, dry clean.

**ivermectin (Sklice):** Tx of head lice in pts ≥6 mo. Apply 0.5% lotion once to head for 10 min; no need for nit picking.

**lindane (generic):** Apply thin layer to entire body, leave on 8–12 hr, then wash thoroughly. For shampoo, 2 oz into dry hair, leave on 4 min, then rinse. Reapply in 7 d if needed.

**malathion (Ovide Lotion):** Apply to dry hair, leave on 8–12 hr, rinse. Repeat in 7–9 d. Contains flammable alcohol.

**permethrin (Elimite, Nix):** Thoroughly massage into skin, wash off after 8–14 hr. For shampoo, work into freshly washed, towel-dried hair, leave on 10 min, then rinse.

**spinosad (Natroba):** Tx of head lice in pts ≥4 yr. Apply to dry scalp, leave on 10 min, rinse. May repeat q 7 d.

Appendix C

# Ophthalmic drugs

Ophthal drugs are intended for direct administration into the conjunctiva of the eye.
**IND & DOSE** **Tx of glaucoma; to aid in dx of eye problems; tx of local ophthal infection, inflammation; to relieve s&sx of allergic reactions.** *Adult, child:* 1–2 drops to each eye bid–qid, or 0.25–0.5 inch oint to each eye.
**PREG/CONT** Please refer to individual medication labels.
**ADV EFF** Blurred vision (prolonged w/oint), burning, local irritation, stinging, tearing; headache
**NC/PT** **Sol, drops:** Wash hands thoroughly before giving; do not touch dropper to eye or other surface; have pt tilt head back or lie down and stare upward. Gently grasp lower eyelid; pull eyelid away from eyeball. Instill drop(s) into pouch formed by eyelid; release lid slowly. Have pt close eye, look downward. Apply gentle pressure to inside corner of eye for 3–5 min to retard drainage. Pt should not rub eyes, rinse eyedropper; avoid eyedrops that have changed color; separate administration by 5 min if more than one type of eyedrop used.
**Oint:** Wash hands thoroughly before giving; hold tube between hands for several min to warm; discard first cm of oint when opening tube for first time. Have pt tilt head back or lie down and stare upward. Gently pull out lower lid to form pouch; place 0.25–0.5 inch oint inside lower lid. Have pt close eyes for 1–2 min, roll eyeball in all directions. Remove excess oint from around eye. Separate administration by 10 min if using more than one kind of oint. Transient stinging, burning, blurred vision possible; pt should take appropriate safety measures. Sun sensitivity w/mydriatic agents (pupils will dilate); pt may need sunglasses. Pt should report severe eye discomfort, palpitations, nausea, headache.

**alcaftadine (Lastacaft):** Px of itching associated w/allergic conjunctivitis. 1 drop in each eye daily. Remove contacts. Not for tx of contact lens irritation.

**apraclonidine (Iopidine):** To control, prevent postop IOP elevation after argon-laser surgery; short-term adjunct tx in pts on max tolerated tx who need additional IOP reduction. Monitor for possible vasovagal attack. Do not give to pts w/clonidine allergy.

**azelastine hydrochloride (Optivar):** Tx of ocular itching associated w/allergic conjunctivitis in pts ≥3 yr. Antihistamine, mast cell stabilizer. 1 drop bid. Rapid onset, 8-hr duration.

**azithromycin (Azasite):** Tx of bacterial conjunctivitis in pts ≥1 yr. 1 drop bid 8–12 hr apart for 2 d, then once/d for 5 d.

**bepotastine besilate (Bepreve):** Tx of ocular itching from allergic rhinitis in pts ≥2 yr. Apply bid.

**besifloxacin (Besivance): Tx of pink eye:** 1 drop tid for 7 d (*Besivance*).

**bimatoprost (Latisse, Lumigan):** Tx of open-angle glaucoma, ocular hypertension: 1 drop daily in p.m. Tx of hypertrichosis of eyelashes: 1 drop each p.m.; iris darkening possible (*Latisse*).

**brimonidine tartrate (Alphagan P, Qoliana):** Tx of open-angle glaucoma, ocular hypertension. 1 drop tid. May stain contacts. Do not use w/MAOIs.

**brimonidine/brinzolamide (Simbrinza):** Tx of increased IOP. 1 drop in affected eye(s) tid.

**brimonidine/timolol (Combigan):** Tx of increased IOP. 1 drop q 12 hr. Do not wear contacts.

**brinzolamide (Azopt):** To decrease IOP in open-angle glaucoma. 1 drop tid; give 10 min apart from other drops.

**bromfenac (Bromsite, Prolensa):** Tx of postop inflammation, pain after cataract extraction. 1 drop bid starting 24 hr after surgery and for 2 wk; once/d w/*Bromday*.

**carbachol (Miostat):** Tx of glaucoma, miosis during surgery. 1–2 drops tid for glaucoma, one dose before surgery.

**carteolol hydrochloride (generic):** Tx of elevated IOP in open-angle glaucoma. 1 drop bid; monitor IOP closely.

**cetirizine (0.24%) (Zerviate):** Tx of ocular itching associated w/allergic conjunctivitis. 1 drop in each affected eye bid. Avoid touching eyelids/surrounding areas w/dropper tip.

**ciprofloxacin (Ciloxan): Tx of ocular infections, conjunctivitis:** Apply ¼-inch ribbon to eye sac tid for 2 d, then bid for 5 d, or 1–2 drops q 2 hr while awake for 2 d, then q 4 hr for 5 d.

**cyclopentolate (Ciclomydril, Cyclogyl, Pentolair):** Diagnostic procedures. Pts w/dark irises may need higher doses. Compress lacrimal sac for 2–3 min after giving.

**cycloSPORINE emulsion (Cequa, Restasis):** To increase tear production. 1 drop in each eye bid approx 12 hr apart. Remove contacts before use.

**dexamethasone intravitreal (Ozurdex):** Tx of macular edema after branch retinal artery, central retinal vein occlusion; tx of noninfectious uveitis of posterior segment of eye. Intravitreal injection. Monitor for infection, retinal detachment.

**diclofenac sodium (Voltaren):** Tx of photophobia in pts undergoing incisional refractive surgery; tx of postop ocular inflammation. 1 drop qid starting 24 hr after surgery and for 2 wk, or 1–2 drops within 1 hr of corneal surgery, then 1–2 drops 15 min after surgery, then qid for max 3 d.

**difluprednate (Durezol): Tx of postop ocular pain, inflammation:** 1 drop qid starting 24 after surgery and for 2 wk.

**dorzolamide (Trusopt):** Tx of increased IOP, open-angle glaucoma. 1 drop tid.

**dorzolamide/timolol (Cosopt):** To reduce IOP. 1 drop bid. Monitor for HF if absorbed systemically.

**emedastine (Emadine):** To relieve s&sx of allergic conjunctivitis in pts ≥3 yr. 1 drop q d to qid. Do not wear contacts. May cause headache, blurred vision.

**epinastine hydrochloride (Elestat):** Px of allergic conjunctivitis itching. 1 drop bid for entire time of exposure. Remove contacts.

**fluocinolone acetonide (Iluvien, Retisert):** Tx of chronic noninfectious uveitis of posterior segment of eye. 1 surgically implanted insert replaced after 30 mo if needed.

**fluorometholone (Flarex, FML):** Tx of inflammatory eye conditions. Stop if swelling; monitor IOP after 10 d.

**ganciclovir (Zirgan):** Tx of acute herpetic keratitis. 1 drop 5 ×/d until ulcer heals, then 1 drop tid for 7 d.

**gatifloxacin (Zymar, Zymaxid):** Tx of conjunctivitis caused by susceptible strains. 1 drop q 2 hr while awake up to 8 ×/d on days 1 and 2; then 1 drop q 4 hr while awake up to 4 ×/d for 5 d. Pt should not wear contact lenses; may cause blurred vision.

**homatropine (Homatropine HBr, Isopto-Homatropine):** Refraction; tx of inflammatory conditions, preop and postop when mydriasis needed. 5–10 min needed for refraction; dark irises may require bigger doses.

**ketorolac (Acular, Acuvail):** Tx of pain, inflammation after cataract surgery. 1 drop bid.

**ketotifen (Alaway):** Temporary relief of itching due to allergic conjunctivitis in pts ≥3 yr. 1 drop q 8–12 hr; remove contacts for 10 min.

**latanoprost (Xalatan):** Tx of open-angle glaucoma, ocular hypertension. Remove contacts before and for 15 min after drops. Allow 5 min between this and other drops.

**latanoprostene bunod (Vyzulta):** To reduce IOP in pt w/open-angle glaucoma or ocular HTN. 1 drop into eye/s q d in evening.

**levobunolol (AKBeta, Betagon):** Tx of bacterial conjunctivitis caused by susceptible strains. 1–2 drops q 2 hr while awake on days 1, 2; then q 4 hr while awake on days 3–7.

**levofloxacin (generic):** Tx of conjunctivitis caused by susceptible strains. 1 or 2 drops q 2 hr while awake up to 8 ×/d on days 1 and 2; then 1 drop q 4 hr while awake up to 4 ×/d for 3–7 d.

**lifitegrast (Xiidra):** Tx of s&sx of dry eye. 1 drop bid in each eye (dose 12 hr apart). Monitor for visual acuity changes.

**lodoxamide tromethamine (Alomide):** Tx of vernal conjunctivitis, keratitis in pts >2 yr. Do not wear contacts. Stop if stinging, burning persists.

**loteprednol etabonate (Alrex, Lotemax):** Tx of postop inflammation, ocular disease. 1–2 drops qid. Discard after 14 d. Prolonged use can cause eye nerve damage.

**loteprednol etabonate/tobramycin (Zylet):** Tx of ocular conditions w/risk of bacterial ocular infection. 1–2 drops q 4–6 hr for 24–48 hr.

**metipranolol (OptiPranolol):** Tx of chronic open-angle glaucoma, ocular hypertension. Vision changes possible; may need to use w/other drugs.

**mitoMYcin (Mitosol):** Adjunct to ab externo glaucoma surgery. Apply fully saturated sponges to tx area for 2 min. Topical only; biohazard disposal.

**moxifloxacin (Moxeza, Vigamox):** Tx of bacterial conjunctivitis caused by susceptible strains. *Moxeza* (pts ≥4 mo), 1 drop bid for 7 d. *Vigamox* (pts 1 ≥yr), 1 drop tid for 7 d. Do not wear contacts. Can cause blurred vision.

**natamycin (Natacyn):** Tx of fungal blepharitis, conjunctivitis, keratitis. 1–2 drops/d for 7 d.

**nedocromil sodium (Alocril):** Tx of allergic conjunctivitis itching. 1–2 drops bid through entire allergy season.

**neomycin/polymyxine B sulfates/ bacitracin zinc (Neosporin):** Tx of superficial eye bacterial infections. Apply oint q 3–4 hr for 7–10 d.

**netarsudil (Rhopressa):** Tx of glaucoma, ocular HTN. 1 drop into eye/s q d in evening.

**ocriplasmin (Jetrea):** Tx of symptomatic vitreomacular adhesion. 0.125 mg by intravitreal injection into affected eye as single dose. Potential for lens subluxation. Monitor vision.

**olopatadine hydrochloride (Pataday, Patanol, Pazeo):** Tx of allergic conjunctivitis itching in pts ≥3 yr. 1–2 drops q 6–8 hr. Not for use w/ contacts. Headache common.

**phenylephrine/ketorolac (Omidria):** Px of intraop miosis; pain reduction w/ cataract surgery. 4 mL in 500 mL ophthal irrigating solution, used as needed during surgery.

**pilocarpine (Adsorbocarpine, Piloptic, Pilostat):** Tx of chronic, acute glaucoma; mydriasis caused by drugs. 1–2 drops up to 6 ×/d.

**rimexolone (Vexol):** Tx of anterior uveitis; postop. Corticosteroid. Monitor for systemic absorption.

**sulfacetamide (Bleph-10):** Tx of ocular infections. 1–2 drops q 2–3 hr; gradually taper over 7–10 d.

**tafluprost (Zioptan):** Tx of elevated IOP in open-angle glaucoma/ocular hypertension. 1 drop in p.m.; permanent changes in eyelashes, iris color.

**timolol maleate (Timoptic, Timoptic XE):** Tx of increased IOP. 1 drop/d in a.m.

**travoprost (Travatan Z):** Tx of open-angle glaucoma, ocular hypertension. 1 drop each p.m.; iris darkening, eyelash growth common.

**trifluridine (Viroptic):** Tx of keratoconjunctivitis, recurrent epithelial keratitis due to herpes simplex 1, 2. Max, 9 drops/d in affected eye(s) no longer than 21 d.

**tropicamide (Mydriacyl, Tropicacyl, Tropicamide):** Refraction. 1–2 drops, repeat in 5 min. May repeat again in 30 min if needed.

**voretigene neparvovec (Luxturna):** Tx of vision loss due to biallelic *RPE65*-mediated inherited retinal disease. 0.3 mL injected subretinally in each eye on separate days but no fewer than 6 d apart. Systemic oral corticosteroids administered concomitantly.

Appendix D

# Laxatives

Many laxatives are available as OTC preparations and people may become dependent on them for GI movement. To limit long-term laxative use, it is best to optimize nutrition/physical activity and modify constipating medications. Laxatives for specific purposes are found in the drug monographs.
**IND & DOSE** Short-term relief of constipation; to prevent straining; to evacuate bowel for diagnostic procedures; to remove ingested poisons from lower GI tract; as adjunct in anthelmintic tx.
**PREG/CONT** Please refer to individual medication labels.
**ADV EFF** Abd cramps, cathartic dependence, dizziness, excessive bowel activity, perianal irritation, weakness
**NC/PT** Use as temporary measure. If taking orally, do not take within 1 hr of other drugs. Pt should swallow tablets whole; report sweating, flushing, muscle cramps, excessive thirst.

**bisacodyl (Bisa-Lax, Correctol, Dulcolax):** Stimulant. 5–15 mg PO; 2.5 g in water via enema. Onset, 6–12 hr; rapid. Tartrazine in *Dulcolax* tablets. May discolor urine. Not for child <6 yr.

**cascara:** Stimulant. 325 mg–6 g PO. Onset, 6–10 hr. Use caution if pt taking prescription drugs. May discolor urine. Not for children <18 yr.

**castor oil:** Stimulant. 15–60 mL PO. Onset, 2–6 hr. May be very vigorous; may cause abd cramping.

**docusate (Colace, Ex-Lax Stool Softener, Genasoft, Phillips' Liqui-Gels, Silace):** Detergent, softener. 50–300 mg PO. Onset, 12–72 hr. Gentle; beneficial w/painful anorectal conditions, dry or hard feces.

**glycerin (Fleet Babylax, Fleet Liquid Glycerin Suppository, Sani-Supp):** Hyperosmolar agent. Rectal suppository; 4 mL liquid by rectum (child rectal liquid). Onset, 15–60 min. Insert suppository high into rectum, retain 15 min. Insert liquid dispenser. Apply gentle, steady pressure until all liquid gone; then remove.

**lactulose (Cholac, Constilac, Enulose, Generlac):** Hyperosmolar agent. 15–30 mL PO. May also give rectally as enema. Onset, 24–48 hr. Also used for tx of portal system encephalopathy. More palatable if mixed w/fruit juice, milk, water.

**lubiprostone (Amitiza):** Chloride channel activator. 24 mcg PO bid w/ food, water. Onset, 1–2 hr. Also used for tx of women w/IBS w/constipation, chronic idiopathic constipation, opioid-induced constipation. Contains sorbitol; may cause nausea, diarrhea.

**magnesium citrate (Citrate of Magnesia):** Saline. 1 glassful PO. Onset, 0.5–3 hr. For child dose, reduce by half.

**magnesium (Milk of Magnesia, MOM, Phillip's MOM):** Saline. 30–60 mL PO at bedtime; 15–30 mL of conc PO. Onset, 0.5–3 hr. Take w/ liquids. Flavored forms available.

**magnesium sulfate (Epsom Salts):** Saline. 5–10 mL PO. Onset, 0.5–3 hr. Take mixed w/full glass of water. Child dose, reduce to 2.5–5 mL PO in ½ glass water.

**mineral oil (Kondremul):** Emollient. 5–45 mL PO. Onset, 6–8 hr. May decrease absorption of fat-soluble vitamins. Child ≥6 yr, reduce dose to 5–15 mL.

**polycarbophil (Equalactin, FiberCon, Konsyl Fiber):** Bulk. 1–2 tablets PO up to qid. Onset, 12–72 hr. Good w/IBS, diverticulitis. Swallow w/full glass of water to prevent sticking in esophagus, choking.

**polyethylene glycol (Glycolax, MiraLax):** Bulk. 17 g PO in 8 oz water daily for up to 2 wk. Onset, 48–72 hr. Do not use w/bowel obstruction. Diarrhea common.

**polyethylene glycolelectrolyte solutions w/multiple electrolytes (Colyte, GoLytely, Lax-Lyte, Moviprep, NuLytely, PEG 3350 and electrolytes, Plenvu, Trilyte):** Bulk/osmotic. 4 L oral sol PO before exam; however, different amounts may be needed per product labels. Onset, 1 hr. Used as bowel evacuant before exam/colonoscopy. Some sol require multiple doses. Do not use w/GI obstruction, megacolon.

**psyllium (Fiberall, Hydrocil Instant, Konsyl, Metamucil):** Bulk. 1 tsp or packet in water, juice 1–3 ×/d PO. Onset, 12–72 hr. Swallow w/full glass of water to prevent esophageal sticking, choking.

**senna (Agoral, Black Draught, Ex-Lax, Fletcher's Castoria, Senna-Gen, Senokot):** Stimulant. 1–8 tablets/d PO at bedtime; suppository/syrup, 10–30 mL PO. Onset, 6–10 hr. May cause abd cramps, discomfort.

**sodium picosulfate, magnesium oxide, anhydrous citric acid (Prepopik):** Bowel cleansing before colonoscopy. Reconstitute w/cold water, swallow immediately, follow w/clear liquids; repeat. Risk of fluid/electrolyte abnormalities.

Appendix E

# Combination products by therapeutic class

## *ALZHEIMER'S DISEASE DRUG*

### ▶ memantine and donepezil

Namzaric

**ER capsules:** 14 mg memantine, 10 mg donepezil; 28 mg memantine, 10 mg donepezil
**Usual adult dose:** 1 capsule/d PO in p.m. Pt should not cut/crush/chew capsule; can be opened and sprinkled on applesauce.

## *AMPHETAMINE*

### ▶ dextroamphetamine and amphetamine

CONTROLLED SUBSTANCE C-II
Adderall XR

**ER capsules:** 1.25 mg (5-mg capsule), 1.875 (7.5-mg tablet), 2.5 mg (10-mg capsule), 3.125 (12.5-mg tablet), 3.75 mg (15-mg capsule), 5 mg (20-mg capsule), 6.25 mg (25-mg capsule), 7.5 mg (30-mg capsule) of each component
**Usual adult, child dose:** 10–30 mg/d. **BBW** High risk of abuse; use caution. Decrease dose for renal impairment.

## *ANALGESICS*

### ▶ acetaminophen and codeine

CONTROLLED SUBSTANCE C-III
Tylenol with Codeine

**Elixir:** 12 mg codeine, 120 mg acetaminophen/5 mL
**Tablets:** No. 2: 15 mg codeine, 300 mg acetaminophen. No. 3: 30 mg codeine, 300 mg acetaminophen. No. 4: 60 mg codeine, 300 mg acetaminophen
**Usual adult dose:** 1 or 2 tablets PO q 4–6 hr as needed, or 15 mL q 4–6 hr.

### ▶ articaine hydrochloride and epinephrine

Orabloc, Ultacan

**Injection sol:** 4% (40 mg/mL) articaine hydrochloride, 1:200,000 (0.009 mg/mL) epinephrine; 4% (40 mg/mL) articaine hydrochloride, 1:100,000 (0.018 mg/mL) epinephrine
**Usual adult dose, child 4–16 yr:** 0.5–5 mL injected; max, 7 mg/kg.

### ▶ aspirin and codeine

CONTROLLED SUBSTANCE C-III
Empirin with Codeine

**Tablets:** No. 3: 30 mg codeine, 325 mg aspirin. No. 4: 60 mg codeine, 325 mg aspirin
**Usual adult dose:** 1 or 2 tablets PO q 4–6 hr as needed.

### ▶ aspirin and omeprazole

Yosprala

**DR tablets:** 81 mg DR aspirin/40 mg omeprazole. 325 mg DR aspirin/40 mg omeprazole
**Usual adult dose:** Used for px of CV events in pts at risk for gastric ulcers. 1 tablet/d PO 60 min before a meal; pt should not cut, crush, or chew.

### ▶ codeine, aspirin, caffeine, and butalbital

CONTROLLED SUBSTANCE C-III
Fiorinal with Codeine

**Capsules:** 30 mg codeine, 325 mg aspirin, 40 mg caffeine, 50 mg butabarbital
**Usual adult dose:** 1 or 2 capsules PO q 4 hr as needed for pain, up to 6/d. **BBW** Risk of death in children after tonsil/adenoid removal, many cases in children who are rapid metabolizers; not approved for this use. Risk of neonatal opioid withdrawal syndrome w/prolonged use during preg.

### ▶ diclofenac sodium and misoprostol

PREG CATEGORY X
Arthrotec

**Tablets:** '50': 50 mg diclofenac, 200 mcg misoprostol. '75': 75 mg diclofenac, 200 mcg misoprostol
**Usual adult dose:** *Osteoarthritis:* Arthrotec 50, PO tid. Arthrotec 50 or 75, PO bid. *Rheumatoid arthritis:* Arthrotec 50, PO tid or qid; Arthrotec 50 or 75, PO bid. **BBW** Misoprostol is abortifacient. Not for use in preg; negative preg test required.

### ▶ famotidine and ibuprofen

Duexis

**Tablets:** 26.6 mg famotidine, 800 mg ibuprofen
**Usual adult dose:** 1 tablet PO daily for arthritis pain. **BBW** NSAIDs increase risk of CV thrombotic events/GI adverse events that could be fatal. Contraindicated in pts undergoing CABG surgery.

### ▶ HYDROcodone bitartrate and acetaminophen

CONTROLLED SUBSTANCE C-II
Norco

**Elixir:** 2.5 mg hydrocodone, 167 mg acetaminophen/5 mL
**Tablets:** 2.5 mg hydrocodone, 500 mg acetaminophen; 5 mg hydrocodone, 500 mg acetaminophen; 5, 7.5, 10 mg hydrocodone, 400 mg acetaminophen; 7.5 mg hydrocodone, 500 mg acetaminophen; 7.5 mg hydrocodone, 650 mg acetaminophen; 10 mg hydrocodone, 650 mg acetaminophen
**Norco tablets:** 5 mg hydrocodone, 325 mg acetaminophen; 7.5 mg hydrocodone, 325 mg acetaminophen; 10 mg hydrocodone, 325 mg acetaminophen
**Usual adult dose:** Check brand-name products to determine specific dose combinations available. One or two tablets, capsules PO q 4–6 hr, up to 8/d. **BBW** Risk of potentially severe hepatotoxicity.

### ▶ HYDROcodone and ibuprofen

CONTROLLED SUBSTANCE C-II
Reprexain, Vicoprofen

**Tablets:** 2.5 mg hydrocodone, 200 mg ibuprofen; 7.5 mg hydrocodone, 200 mg ibuprofen; 10 mg hydrocodone, 200 mg ibuprofen

**Usual adult dose:** 1 tablet PO q 4–6 hr as needed.

### ▶ methylsalicylate and menthol
Salonpas

**Dermal patch:** 10% methylsalicylate, 3% menthol
**Usual adult dose:** Apply 1 patch to clean, dry affected area; leave on for 8–12 hr. Remove patch, apply another as needed. To relieve pain from sprains, bruises, strains, backache.

### ▶ naproxen and esomeprazole
Vimovo

**DR tablets:** 375 mg naproxen, 20 mg esomeprazole; 500 mg naproxen, 20 mg esomeprazole
**Usual adult dose:** 1 tablet PO bid. Not recommended in moderate to severe renal insufficiency, severe hepatic insufficiency; reduce w/mild to moderate hepatic insufficiency. **BBW** Risk of GI adverse events, CV events. Not for periop pain w/CABG.

### ▶ oxyCODONE and acetaminophen
CONTROLLED SUBSTANCE C-II
Percocet, Roxicet, Xartemis XR

**Tablets:** 2.25, 4.5, 5 mg oxycodone, 325 mg acetaminophen
**ER tablets:** 7.5 mg oxycodone, 325 mg acetaminophen
**Usual adult dose:** 1 or 2 tablets PO q 4–6 hr as needed; 2 tablets q 12 hr for ER form. **BBW** Risk of addiction, serious respiratory depression, fatal outcomes in child; hepatotoxicity; neonatal withdrawal if used in preg; increased adverse effects w/CNS depressants. Use caution.

### ▶ oxyCODONE and aspirin
CONTROLLED SUBSTANCE C-II
Percodan, Roxiprin

**Tablets:** 4.5 mg oxycodone, 325 mg aspirin
**Usual adult dose:** 1 or 2 tablets PO q 6 hr as needed. **BBW** Risk of addiction, serious respiratory depression, fatal outcomes in child; hepatotoxicity; neonatal withdrawal if used in preg; increased adverse effects w/ CNS depressants

### ▶ oxyCODONE and ibuprofen
CONTROLLED SUBSTANCE C-II
Generic

**Tablets:** 5 mg oxycodone, 400 mg ibuprofen
**Usual adult dose:** 1 tablet PO q 6 hr as needed for moderate to severe pain. Max, 4 tablets/24 hr for no more than 7 d.

### ▶ tramadol hydrochloride and acetaminophen
Ultracet

**Tablets:** 37.5 mg tramadol, 325 mg acetaminophen
**Usual adult dose:** 2 tablets PO q 4–6 hr as needed; max, 8 tablets/d. Reduce in elderly/renally impaired pts. **BBW** Risk of addiction/misuse, hepatotoxicity; do not exceed 4,000 mg acetaminophen/d. Risk of life-threatening respiratory depression, especially in children post tonsillectomy and/or adenoidectomy. Risk of neonatal opioid withdrawal syndrome w/prolonged use during preg.

### ANTIACNE DRUGS

**▶ ethinyl estradiol and norethindrone**
Estrostep Fe

**Tablets:** 1 mg norethindrone, 20 mcg ethinyl estradiol; 1 mg norethindrone, 30 mcg ethinyl estradiol; 1 mg norethindrone, 35 mcg ethinyl estradiol
**Usual adult dose:** 1 tablet PO each d (21 tablets have active ingredients; 7 are inert).

**▶ norgestimate and ethinyl estradiol**
Ortho Tri-Cyclen

**Tablets:** 0.18 mg norgestimate, 35 mcg ethinyl estradiol (7 tablets); 0.215 mg norgestimate, 35 mcg ethinyl estradiol (7 tablets); 0.25 mg norgestimate, 35 mcg ethinyl estradiol (7 tablets)
**Usual adult dose:** For women >15 yr, 1 tablet/d PO. Birth control agent used cyclically (21 tablets have active ingredients, 7 are inert). Approved for acne only if contraception is desired. **BBW** Contraindicated in women >35 yr who smoke; increased risk of CV events.

### ANTIANXIETY DRUGS

**▶ chlordiazepoxide hydrochloride and clidinium bromide**
Librax

**Capsules:** 5 mg chlordiazepoxide hydrochloride, 2.5 mg clidinium bromide
**Usual adult dose:** 1–2 capsules PO 3–4 ×/d before meals and at bedtime to control emotional/somatic factors in GI disorders and as adjunct in tx of peptic ulcer, IBS, acute enterocolitis. Risk of profound sedation, respiratory depression, coma, death w/concomitant opioid use.

### ANTIBACTERIALS

**▶ amoxicillin and clavulanic acid**
Augmentin, Augmentin ES-600, Augmentin XR

**Tablets:** '250': 250 mg amoxicillin, 125 mg clavulanic acid; '500': 500 mg amoxicillin, 125 mg clavulanic acid; '875': 875 mg amoxicillin, 125 mg clavulanic acid
**Powder for oral suspension:** '125': 125 mg amoxicillin, 31.25 mg clavulanic acid; '250': 250 mg amoxicillin, 62.5 mg clavulanic acid; '400': 400 mg amoxicillin, 57 mg clavulanic acid. **Sol** (*Augmentin ES-600*): 600 mg amoxicillin, 42.9 mg clavulanic acid/5 mL
**Chewable tablets:** '125': 125 mg amoxicillin, 31.25 mg clavulanic acid; '200': 200 mg amoxicillin, 28.5 mg clavulanic acid; '400': 400 mg amoxicillin, 57 mg clavulanic acid
**XR tablets:** 1,000 mg amoxicillin, 62.5 mg clavulanic acid
**Usual adult dose:** One 250-mg tablet or one 500-mg tablet PO q 8 hr. For severe infections, 875-mg tablet PO q 12 hr. W/difficulty swallowing, substitute 125-mg/5 mL or 250-mg/5 mL for 500-mg tablet, or 200-mg/5 mL or 400-mg/5 mL for 875-mg tablet.
**Usual child dose:** <40 kg, 20–40 mg amoxicillin/kg/d PO in divided doses q 8 hr (dose based on amoxicillin content) or q 12 hr; 90 mg/kg/d PO oral sol divided q 12 hr (*Augmentin ES-600*).

**▶ cefTAZidime and avibactam**
Avycaz

**Powder for injection:** 2 g ceftazidime, 0.5 g avibactam

**Usual adult dose:** 2.5 g IV q 8 hr over 2 hr for 5–14 d depending on infection. Tx of complicated UTI, intra-abd infections, hospital-acquired/ventilator-associated bacterial pneumonia.

## ▶ ceftolozane and tazobactam
Zerbaxa

**Powder for injection:** 1 g ceftolozane, 0.5 g tazobactam; reconstitute w/0.9% Sodium Chloride
**Usual adult dose:** 1.5 g (1 g ceftolozane, 0.5 g tazobactam) IV q 8 hr over 1 hr. Tx of complicated UTI/intra-abd infections, hospital-acquired/ventilator-associated bacterial pneumonia. Decrease dose in renal impairment; CDAD common.

## ▶ co-trimoxazole (TMP-SMZ)
Bactrim, Bactrim DS, Septra, Septra DS, Sulfatrim Pediatric

**Tablets:** 80 mg trimethoprim (TMP), 400 mg sulfamethoxazole (SMZ); 160 mg TMP, 800 mg SMZ
**Oral suspension:** 40 mg TMP, 200 mg SMZ/5 mL
**Usual adult dose:** *UTIs, shigellosis, acute otitis media:* 160 mg TMP/800 mg SMZ PO q 12 hr. Up to 14 d (UTI) or 5 d (shigellosis). *Acute exacerbations of chronic bronchitis:* 160 mg TMP/800 mg SMZ PO q 12 hr for 14 d. Pneumocystis jiroveci *pneumonitis:* 20 mg/kg TMP/100 mg/kg SMZ q 24 hr PO in divided doses q 6 hr for 14 d. *Traveler's diarrhea:* 160 mg TMP/800 mg SMZ PO q 12 hr for 5 d.
**Usual child dose:** *UTIs, shigellosis, acute otitis media:* 8 mg/kg/d TMP/40 mg/kg/d SMZ PO in two divided doses q 12 hr. For 10–14 d (UTIs, acute otitis media), 5 d (shigellosis). *Pneumocystis jiroveci pneumonitis:* 20 mg/kg TMP/100 mg/kg SMZ q 24 hr PO in divided doses q 6 hr for 14 d.

## ▶ erythromycin and sulfisoxazole
Generic

**Granules for oral suspension:** Erythromycin ethylsuccinate (equivalent of 200 mg erythromycin activity) and 600 mg sulfisoxazole/5 mL when reconstituted according to manufacturer's directions
**Usual child dose:** *Otitis media:* 50 mg/kg/d erythromycin and 150 mg/kg/d sulfisoxazole PO in divided doses qid for 10 d. Give without regard to meals. Refrigerate after reconstitution; use within 14 d.

## ▶ imipenem and cilastatin
Primaxin

**Powder for injection (IV):** 250 mg imipenem, 250 mg cilastatin; 500 mg imipenem, 500 mg cilastatin
**Powder for injection (IM):** 500 mg imipenem, 500 mg cilastatin. Follow manufacturer's instructions for reconstituting, diluting drug. Give each 250- to 500-mg dose by IV infusion over 20–30 min; infuse each 1-g dose over 40–60 min. Give 500–750 mg IM q 12 hr. Max, 1,500 mg/d.
**Usual adult dose:** Dose recommendations based on imipenem. Initially based on type, severity of infection; later on illness severity, degree of susceptibility of pathogens, and age, weight, CrCl. For adults w/normal renal function, 250 mg–1 g IV q 6–8 hr. Max, 50 mg/kg/d or 4 g/d, whichever less. Adjust in renal impairment.

## ▶ imipenem, cilastatin sodium, and relebactam
Recarbrio

**Vials:** 500 mg imipenem, 500 mg cilastatin sodium, 250 mg relebactam

**Usual adult dose:** 1.25 g IV over 30 min q 6 hr for 4–14 d. Adjust for renal impairment.

### ▶ omeprazole magnesium, amoxicillin, and rifabutin
Talicia

**DR capsules:** 10 mg omeprazole, 250 gm amoxicillin, 12.5 mg rifabutin
**Usual adult dose:** 4 capsules q 8 hr w/food for 14 d. Tx of *Helicobacter pylori* infection. Swallow capsules whole. Do not crush/chew or take w/ alcohol.

### ▶ piperacillin sodium and tazobactam sodium
Zosyn

**Powder for injection:** 2 g piperacillin, 0.25 g tazobactam; 3 g piperacillin, 0.375 g tazobactam; 4 g piperacillin, 0.5 g tazobactam
**Usual adult dose:** 12 g/1.5 g IV as 3.375 g q 6 hr over 30 min. Recommended for appendicitis; peritonitis; postpartum endometritis, PID; community-acquired pneumonia; nosocomial pneumonia if agent responsive in sensitivity testing. Adjust in renal impairment.

### ▶ rifAMPin, isoniazid, pyrazinamide
Rifater

**Tablets:** 120 mg rifampin, 50 mg isoniazid, 300 mg pyrazinamide
**Usual dose (≥16 yr):** Give single daily dose either 1 hr before or 2 hr after meal w/full glass of water. Pts ≤44 kg: 4 tablets; 45–54 kg: 5 tablets; ≥55 kg: 6 tablets. **BBW** Risk of fatal hepatitis w/isoniazid.

### ▶ quinupristin and dalfopristin
Synercid

Streptogramin antibiotics available only in combination
**Sol for IV use:** 500-mg/10-mL vial (150 mg quinupristin, 350 mg dalfopristin).
**Pts >16 yr:** *Complicated skin infections due to Staphylococcus aureus, Streptococcus pyogenes*: 7.5 mg/kg IV q 12 hr for 7 d. *Tx of life-threatening, susceptible infections associated w/ VREF*: 7.5 mg/kg IV q 8 hr. Dangerous when used w/QT-prolonging drugs.

### ▶ sulbactam and ampicillin
Unasyn

**Powder for injection:** 1.5-g vial (1 g ampicillin, 0.5 g sulbactam); 3-g vial (2 g ampicillin, 1 g sulbactam)
**Usual adult dose:** 0.5–1 g sulbactam w/1–2 g ampicillin IM or IV q 6–8 hr. **Usual child dose:** ≥40 kg, adult dose; max, 4 g/d. <40 kg, 300 mg/kg/d IV in divided doses q 6 hr.

## *ANTI–CORONARY ARTERY DISEASE DRUG*

### ▶ amLODIPine besylate and atorvastatin calcium
Caduet

**Tablets:** 2.5 mg amlodipine w/10, 20, 40 mg atorvastatin; 5 mg amlodipine w/10, 20, 40, 80 mg atorvastatin; 10 mg amlodipine w/10, 20, 40, 80 mg atorvastatin
**Usual adult dose:** 1 tablet PO daily in p.m. Adjust using individual products, then switch to appropriate combination product.

## ANTIDEPRESSANTS

### ▶ chlordiazepoxide and amitriptyline

CONTROLLED SUBSTANCE C-IV
Generic

**Tablets:** 5 mg chlordiazepoxide, 12.5 mg amitriptyline; 10 mg chlordiazepoxide, 25 mg amitriptyline
**Usual adult dose:** 10 mg chlordiazepoxide w/25 mg amitriptyline PO tid–qid up to six times/d. For pts intolerant of higher doses, 5 mg chlordiazepoxide w/12.5 mg amitriptyline PO tid–qid.

### ▶ OLANZapine and FLUoxetine

Symbyax

**Capsules:** 6 mg olanzapine, 25 mg fluoxetine; 6 mg olanzapine, 50 mg fluoxetine; 12 mg olanzapine, 25 mg fluoxetine; 12 mg olanzapine, 50 mg fluoxetine
**Usual adult dose:** 1 capsule PO daily in p.m. **BBW** Risk of suicidality; increased mortality in elderly pts w/dementia-related psychoses (not approved for that use). Monitor pt closely.

### ▶ perphenazine and amitriptyline

Generic

**Tablets:** 2 mg perphenazine, 10 mg amitriptyline; 2 mg perphenazine, 25 mg amitriptyline; 4 mg perphenazine, 10 mg amitriptyline; 4 mg perphenazine, 25 mg amitriptyline; 4 mg perphenazine, 50 mg amitriptyline
**Usual adult dose:** 2–4 mg perphenazine w/10–50 mg amitriptyline PO tid–qid.

## ANTIDIABETICS

### ▶ alogliptin and metFORMIN

Kazano

**Tablets:** 12.5 mg alogliptin, 500 mg metformin; 12.5 mg alogliptin, 1,000 mg metformin
**Usual adult dose:** Base on pt response, PO bid w/food; max, 25 mg alogliptin, 2,000 mg metformin/d. **BBW** Risk of lactic acidosis; monitor pt closely and stop drug, hospitalize pt.

### ▶ alogliptin and pioglitazone

Oseni

**Tablets:** 12.5 mg alogliptin, 15 mg pioglitazone; 12.5 mg alogliptin, 30 mg pioglitazone; 12.5 mg alogliptin, 45 mg pioglitazone; 25 mg alogliptin, 15 mg pioglitazone; 25 mg alogliptin, 30 mg pioglitazone; 25 mg alogliptin, 45 mg pioglitazone
**Usual adult dose:** Base on pt response, PO once daily. Max, 25 mg alogliptin, 45 mg pioglitazone. Limit w/HF, renal impairment. **BBW** Risk of HF; not for use w/known HF. Monitor pt closely.

### ▶ canagliflozin and metFORMIN

Invokamet, Invokamet XR

**Tablets:** 50 mg canagliflozin, 500 mg metformin; 50 mg canagliflozin, 1,000 mg metformin; 150 mg canagliflozin, 500 mg metformin; 150 mg canagliflozin, 1,000 mg metformin
**ER tablets:** 50 mg canagliflozin, 500 mg ER metformin; 50 mg canagliflozin, 1,000 mg ER metformin; 150 mg canagliflozin, 500 mg ER

metformin; 150 mg canagliflozin, 1,000 mg ER metformin
**Usual adult dose:** Base on pt response. PO bid w/meals. Max, 300 mg canagliflozin, 3,000 mg metformin/d. Reduce dose w/renal impairment. **BBW** Risk of lactic acidosis; monitor pt closely and stop drug, hospitalize pt. Risk of lower limb amputation in pts w/type II diabetes w/CV disease or at risk for CV disease.

### ▶ dapagliflozin and metFORMIN
Xigduo XR

**Tablets:** 5 mg dapagliflozin, 500 mg metformin; 5 mg dapagliflozin, 1,000 mg metformin; 10 mg dapagliflozin, 500 mg metformin; 10 mg dapagliflozin, 1,000 mg metformin
**Usual adult dose:** Base on pt response. PO once daily in a.m. w/ food. Max, 10 mg dapagliflozin, 2,000 mg metformin/d. Not for use w/severe renal impairment. **BBW** Risk of lactic acidosis; monitor pt closely and stop drug, hospitalize pt.

### ▶ dapagliflozin and sAXagliptin
Qtern

**Tablets:** 10 mg dapagliflozin, 5 mg saxagliptin
**Usual adult dose:** 1 tablet PO daily in a.m. w/ or w/o food. Withhold dose if GFR <60 mL/min/1.73 $m^2$.

### ▶ dapagliflozin, sAXagliptin, and metFORMIN
Qternmet

**Tablets:** 2.5 mg dapagliflozin, 2.5 mg saxagliptin, 1,000 mg metformin; 5 mg dapagliflozin, 2.5 mg saxagliptin, 1,000 mg metformin; 5 mg dapagliflozin, 5 mg saxagliptin, 1,000 mg metformin; 10 mg dapagliflozin, 5 mg saxagliptin, 1,000 mg metformin
**Usual adult dose:** 1 tablet PO daily in a.m. w/food. **BBW** Risk of lactic acidosis; monitor closely; stop drug, hospitalize pt.

### ▶ empagliflozin and linagliptin
Glyxambi

**Tablets:** 10 mg empagliflozin, 5 mg linagliptin; 25 mg empagliflozin, 5 mg linagliptin
**Usual adult dose:** 10 mg empagliflozin/5 mg linagliptin/d in a.m.; may increase if needed. Not for use w/severe renal impairment. Monitor pt for lactic acidosis, urosepsis, severe to disabling arthralgia.

### ▶ empagliflozin and metFORMIN
Synjardy, Synjardy XR

**Tablets:** 5 mg empagliflozin, 500 mg metformin; 5 mg empagliflozin, 1 g metformin; 12.5 mg empagliflozin, 500 mg metformin; 12.5 mg empagliflozin, 1 g metformin
**ER tablets:** 5 mg empagliflozin, 1,000 mg ER metformin; 10 mg empagliflozin, 1,000 mg ER metformin; 12.5 mg empagliflozin, 1,000 mg ER metformin; 25 mg empagliflozin, 1,000 mg ER metformin
**Usual adult dose:** 5 mg empagliflozin, 500 mg metformin; max daily dose, 25 mg empagliflozin, 2,000 mg metformin. May increase if needed. Not for use w/severe renal impairment. Monitor for lactic acidosis, urosepsis, severe to disabling arthralgia. **BBW** Risk of lactic acidosis; monitor pt closely and stop drug, hospitalize pt.

### ▶ ertugliflozin and metFORMIN
Segluromet

**Tablets:** 2.5 mg ertugliflozin, 500 mg metformin; 2.5 mg ertugliflozin, 1 g metformin; 5.5 mg ertugliflozin, 500 mg metformin; 7.5 mg ertugliflozin, 1 g metformin
**Usual adult dose:** Individualize based on current regimen. 7.5 mg ertugliflozin, 1 g metformin max bid dose. Assess renal function before starting; not recommended if GFR <60 mL/min/1.73 m$^2$. May need to stop before iodinated contrast imaging. **BBW** Risk of lactic acidosis; monitor closely; stop drug, hospitalize pt.

### ▶ ertugliflozin and SITagliptin
Steglujan

**Tablets:** 5 mg ertugliflozin, 100 mg sitagliptin; 15 mg ertugliflozin, 100 mg sitagliptin
**Usual adult dose:** 5 mg ertugliflozin/100 mg sitagliptin PO once daily. Assess renal function before starting; not recommended if GFR <60 mL/min/1.73 m$^2$.

### ▶ glipiZIDE and metFORMIN
Generic

**Tablets:** 2.5 mg glipizide, 250 mg metformin; 2.5 mg glipizide, 500 mg metformin; 5 mg glipizide, 500 mg metformin
**Usual adult dose:** Individualize doses. Max dose, 20 mg glipizide/ 2,000 mg metformin; give w/meals. Risk of hypoglycemia, lactic acidosis. Risk of lactic acidosis increases w/renal insufficiency. Stop before iodinated contrast imaging.

### ▶ glyBURIDE and metFORMIN
Generic

**Tablets:** 1.25 mg glyburide, 250 mg metformin; 2.5 mg glyburide, 500 mg metformin; 5 mg glyburide, 500 mg metformin
**Usual adult dose:** 1 tablet/d PO w/ meal, usually in a.m. **BBW** Risk of lactic acidosis; monitor pt closely and stop drug, hospitalize pt.

### ▶ insulin degludec and insulin aspart
Ryzodeg

**Solution:** 70 units insulin degludec, 30 units insulin aspart
**Usual adult dose:** Dose based on pt needs, blood glucose. Use w/*FlexTouch Pen*. For subcut injection only; not for IM, IV, or insulin pump. Do not mix or dilute. Not for use w/ diabetic ketoacidosis.

### ▶ insulin glargine and lixisenatide
Soliqua

**Solution in single-use pen:** 100 units insulin glargine/33 mcg lixisenatide
**Usual adult dose:** 15 units (15 units insulin glargine/33 mcg lixisenatide) subcut once/d within 1 hr of first meal of d; max dose, 60 units (60 units insulin glargine/20 mcg lixisenatide). Subcut injection only; not for IM, IV, or insulin pump. Do not mix or dilute.

### ▶ linagliptin and metFORMIN
Jentadueto, Jentadueto XR

**Tablets:** 2.5 mg linagliptin, 500 mg metformin; 2.5 mg linagliptin,

850 mg metformin; 2.5 mg linagliptin, 1,000 mg metformin
**ER tablets:** 2.5 mg linagliptin, 1,000 mg ER metformin; 5 mg linagliptin, 1,000 mg ER metformin
**Usual adult dose:** Base on current use of each drug, PO bid w/meals. Monitor pt for severe to disabling arthralgia or s&sx of HF. **BBW** Risk of lactic acidosis; monitor pt closely and stop drug, hospitalize pt.

### ▶ pioglitazone and glimepiride
Duetact

**Tablets:** 30 mg pioglitazone w/2 or 4 mg glimepiride
**Usual adult dose:** 1 tablet/d PO w/ first meal of d. **BBW** Risk of HF; not for use w/known HF. Monitor pt closely.

### ▶ pioglitazone and metFORMIN
ActoPlus Met

**Tablets:** 15 mg pioglitazone, 500 mg metformin; 15 mg pioglitazone, 850 mg metformin
**ER tablets:** 5 mg pioglitazone, 1,000 mg metformin; 30 mg pioglitazone, 1,000 mg metformin
**Usual adult dose:** 1 tablet PO once/d or bid w/meals; ER tablets, once/d. **BBW** Risk of lactic acidosis; monitor pt closely and stop drug, hospitalize pt. Risk of HF; not for use w/known HF. Monitor pt closely.

### ▶ rosiglitazone and glimepiride
Generic

**Tablets:** 4 mg rosiglitazone, 1 mg glimepiride; 4 mg rosiglitazone, 2 mg glimepiride; 4 mg rosiglitazone, 4 mg glimepiride; 8 mg rosiglitazone, 2 mg glimepiride; 8 mg rosiglitazone, 4 mg glimepiride
**Usual adult dose:** 4 mg rosiglitazone w/1 or 2 mg glimepiride PO once/d w/first meal of d. **BBW** Risk of HF; not for use w/known HF. Monitor pt closely.

### ▶ rosiglitazone and metFORMIN
Generic

**Tablets:** 1 mg rosiglitazone, 500 mg metformin; 2 mg rosiglitazone, 500 mg metformin; 2 mg rosiglitazone, 1 g metformin; 4 mg rosiglitazone, 500 mg metformin; 4 mg rosiglitazone, 1 g metformin
**Usual adult dose:** 4 mg rosiglitazone w/500 mg metformin PO once/d or in divided doses. **BBW** Risk of lactic acidosis; monitor pt closely and stop drug, hospitalize pt. Risk of HF; not for use w/known HF. Monitor pt closely.

### ▶ sAXagliptin and metFORMIN
Kombiglyze XR

**ER tablets:** 5 mg saxagliptin, 500 mg ER metformin; 5 mg saxagliptin, 1,000 mg ER metformin; 2.5 mg saxagliptin, 1,000 mg ER metformin
**Usual adult dose:** 1 tablet PO daily. Do not cut, crush, or allow pt to chew tablets. **BBW** Risk of lactic acidosis; monitor pt closely and stop drug, hospitalize pt.

### ▶ SITagliptin and metFORMIN
Janumet, Janumet XR

**Tablets:** 50 mg sitagliptin, 500 or 1,000 mg metformin
**ER tablets:** 50 mg sitagliptin, 500 mg or 1 g ER metformin; 100 mg sitagliptin, 1 g ER metformin
**Usual adult dose:** 1 tablet PO bid w/meals; max, 100 mg sitagliptin,

2,000 mg metformin/d. Risk of severe to disabling arthralgia or s&sx of HF. **BBW** Risk of lactic acidosis; monitor pt closely and stop drug, hospitalize pt.

## *ANTIDIARRHEAL*

### ▶ diphenoxylate hydrochloride and atropine sulfate

CONTROLLED SUBSTANCE C-V
Lomotil

**Tablets:** 2.5 mg diphenoxylate hydrochloride, 0.025 mg atropine sulfate
**Liquid:** 2.5 mg diphenoxylate hydrochloride, 0.025 mg atropine sulfate/5 mL
**Usual adult dose:** 5 mg PO qid.
**Usual child dose (use only liquid in child 2–12 yr):** 0.3–0.4 mg/kg PO daily in four divided doses.

## *ANTIDOTES*

### ▶ atropine and pralidoxime chloride

DuoDote

**Autoinjector:** atropine 2.1 mg/07 mL; 600 mg pralidoxime chloride/2 mL
**Usual adult dose, child >41 kg:** 1 injection IM in midlateral thigh if mild symptoms; 2 additional IM injections rapidly if severe symptoms for tx of poisoning by organophosphorus nerve agents/insecticides.

## *ANTIGLAUCOMA DRUG*

### ▶ netarsudil and latanoprost

Rocklatan

**Ophthal sol:** 0.2 mg/mL netarsudil (0.02%), 0.05 mg/mL latanoprost (0.005%)
**Usual adult dose:** 1 drop in affected eye(s) daily in evening for tx of elevated IOP in open-angle glaucoma.

## *ANTIHYPERTENSIVES*

### ▶ aliskiren and hydroCHLOROthiazide

Tekturna HCT

**Tablets:** 150 mg aliskiren, 12.5 mg hydrochlorothiazide; 150 mg aliskiren, 25 mg hydrochlorothiazide; 300 mg aliskiren, 12.5 mg hydrochlorothiazide; 300 mg aliskiren, 25 mg hydrochlorothiazide
**Usual adult dose:** 1 tablet/d PO. **BBW** Risk of birth defects/fetal death; avoid use in preg.

### ▶ amLODIPine and benazepril

Lotrel

**Capsules:** 2.5 mg amlodipine, 10 mg benazepril; 5 mg amlodipine, 10 mg benazepril; 5 mg amlodipine, 20 mg benazepril; 5 mg amlodipine, 40 mg benazepril; 10 mg amlodipine, 20 mg benazepril; 10 mg amlodipine, 40 mg benazepril
**Usual adult dose:** 1 tablet/d PO in a.m. **BBW** Risk of birth defects/fetal death; avoid use in preg.

### ▶ amLODIPine and celecoxib

Consensi

**Tablets:** 2.5 mg amlodipine, 200 mg celecoxib; 5 mg amlodipine, 200 mg celecoxib; 10 mg amlodipine, 200 mg celecoxib
**Usual adult dose:** 1 tablet/d PO. **BBW** NSAIDs increase risk of CV thrombotic events and GI adverse effects that can be fatal. Contraindicated w/CABG surgery.

**▶ amLODIPine and olmesartan**
Azor

**Tablets:** 5 mg amlodipine, 20 mg olmesartan; 10 mg amlodipine, 20 mg olmesartan; 5 mg amlodipine, 40 mg olmesartan; 10 mg amlodipine, 40 mg olmesartan
**Usual adult dose:** 1 tablet/d PO.
**BBW** Risk of birth defects/fetal death; avoid use in preg.

**▶ amLODIPine and perindopril**
Prestalia

**Capsules:** 2.5 mg amlodipine, 3.5 mg perindopril; 5 mg amlodipine, 7 mg perindopril; 10 mg amlodipine, 14 mg perindopril
**Usual adult dose:** Initially, 2.5 mg amlodipine/3.5 mg perindopril PO each d; adjust based on pt response.
**BBW** Risk of birth defects/fetal death; avoid use in preg.

**▶ amLODIPine and valsartan**
Exforge

**Tablets:** 5 mg amlodipine, 160 mg valsartan; 5 mg amlodipine, 320 mg valsartan; 10 mg amlodipine, 160 mg valsartan; 10 mg amlodipine, 320 mg valsartan
**Usual adult dose:** 1 tablet/d PO.
**BBW** Risk of birth defects/fetal death; avoid use in preg.

**▶ amLODIPine, valsartan, and hydroCHLOROthiazide**
Exforge HCT

**Tablets:** 5 mg amlodipine, 160 mg valsartan, 12.5 mg hydrochlorothiazide; 10 mg amlodipine, 160 mg valsartan, 12.5 mg hydrochlorothiazide; 5 mg amlodipine, 160 mg valsartan, 25 mg hydrochlorothiazide; 10 mg amlodipine, 320 mg valsartan, 25 mg hydrochlorothiazide
**Usual adult dose:** 1 tablet/d PO.
**BBW** Risk of birth defects/fetal death; avoid use in preg.

**▶ atenolol and chlorthalidone**
Tenoretic

**Tablets:** 50 mg atenolol, 25 mg chlorthalidone; 100 mg atenolol, 25 mg chlorthalidone
**Usual adult dose:** 1 tablet/d PO in a.m.

**▶ azilsartan and chlorthalidone**
Edarbyclor

**Tablets:** 40 mg azilsartan, 12.5 mg chlorthalidone; 40 mg azilsartan, 25 mg chlorthalidone
**Usual adult dose:** 1 tablet/d PO. Not for use in preg, renal failure. Monitor potassium level. **BBW** Risk of birth defects/fetal death; avoid use in preg.

**▶ bisoprolol and hydroCHLOROthiazide**
Ziac

**Tablets:** 2.5 mg bisoprolol, 6.25 mg hydrochlorothiazide; 5 mg bisoprolol, 6.25 mg hydrochlorothiazide; 10 mg bisoprolol, 6.25 mg hydrochlorothiazide
**Usual adult dose:** 1 tablet/d PO in a.m. Initially, 2.5/6.25-mg tablet/d PO. May need 2–3 wk for optimal antihypertensive effect.

**▶ candesartan and hydroCHLOROthiazide**
Atacand HCT

**Tablets:** 16 mg candesartan, 12.5 mg hydrochlorothiazide; 32 mg

candesartan, 12.5 mg hydrochlorothiazide
**Usual adult dose:** 1 tablet/d PO in a.m. **BBW** Risk of birth defects/fetal death; avoid use in preg.

### ▶ chlorthalidone and cloNIDine
Clorpres

**Tablets:** 15 mg chlorthalidone, 0.1 mg clonidine hydrochloride; 15 mg chlorthalidone, 0.2 mg clonidine hydrochloride; 15 mg chlorthalidone, 0.3 mg clonidine hydrochloride
**Usual adult dose:** 1 or 2 tablets/d PO in a.m.; may give once/d or bid.

### ▶ enalapril and hydroCHLOROthiazide
Vaseretic

**Tablets:** 5 mg enalapril maleate, 12.5 mg hydrochlorothiazide; 10 mg enalapril maleate, 25 mg hydrochlorothiazide
**Usual adult dose:** 1 or 2 tablets/d PO in a.m. **BBW** Risk of birth defects/fetal death; avoid use in preg.

### ▶ fosinopril and hydroCHLOROthiazide
Generic

**Tablets:** 10 mg fosinopril, 12.5 mg hydrochlorothiazide; 20 mg fosinopril, 12.5 mg hydrochlorothiazide
**Usual adult dose:** 1 tablet/d PO in a.m. **BBW** Risk of birth defects/fetal death; avoid use in preg.

### ▶ hydroCHLOROthiazide and benazepril
Lotensin HCT

**Tablets:** 6.25 mg hydrochlorothiazide, 5 mg benazepril; 12.5 mg hydrochlorothiazide, 10 mg benazepril; 12.5 mg hydrochlorothiazide, 20 mg benazepril; 25 mg hydrochlorothiazide, 20 mg benazepril
**Usual adult dose:** 1 tablet/d PO in a.m. **BBW** Risk of birth defects/fetal death; avoid use in preg.

### ▶ hydroCHLOROthiazide and captopril
Generic

**Tablets:** 15 mg hydrochlorothiazide, 25 mg captopril; 15 mg hydrochlorothiazide, 50 mg captopril; 25 mg hydrochlorothiazide, 25 mg captopril; 25 mg hydrochlorothiazide, 50 mg captopril
**Usual adult dose:** 1 or 2 tablets/d PO 1 hr before or 2 hr after meals. **BBW** Risk of birth defects/fetal death; avoid use in preg.

### ▶ hydroCHLOROthiazide and propranolol
Generic

**Tablets:** 25 mg hydrochlorothiazide, 40 mg propranolol; 25 mg hydrochlorothiazide, 80 mg propranolol
**Usual adult dose:** 1 or 2 tablets PO bid.

### ▶ irbesartan and hydroCHLOROthiazide
Avalide

**Tablets:** 150 mg irbesartan, 12.5 mg hydrochlorothiazide; 300 mg irbesartan, 12.5 mg hydrochlorothiazide; 300 mg irbesartan, 25 mg hydrochlorothiazide
**Usual adult dose:** 1 or 2 tablets/d PO. **BBW** Risk of birth defects/fetal death; avoid use in preg.

### ▶ lisinopril and hydroCHLOROthiazide
Zestoretic

**Tablets:** 10 mg lisinopril, 12.5 mg hydrochlorothiazide; 20 mg lisinopril, 12.5 mg hydrochlorothiazide; 20 mg lisinopril, 25 mg hydrochlorothiazide
**Usual adult dose:** 1 tablet/d PO in a.m. **BBW** Risk of birth defects/fetal death; avoid use in preg.

### ▶ losartan and hydroCHLOROthiazide
Hyzaar

**Tablets:** 50 mg losartan, 12.5 mg hydrochlorothiazide; 100 mg losartan, 12.5 mg hydrochlorothiazide; 100 mg losartan, 25 mg hydrochlorothiazide
**Usual adult dose:** 1 tablet/d PO in a.m. Also used to reduce stroke incidence in hypertensive pts w/left ventricular hypertrophy (not effective for this use in black pts). **BBW** Risk of birth defects/fetal death; avoid use in preg.

### ▶ metoprolol and hydroCHLOROthiazide
Dutoprol, Lopressor HCT

**Tablets:** 50 mg metoprolol, 25 mg hydrochlorothiazide; 100 mg metoprolol, 25 mg hydrochlorothiazide; 100 mg metoprolol, 50 mg hydrochlorothiazide
**ER tablets:** 25 mg metoprolol, 12.5 mg hydrochlorothiazide; 50 mg metoprolol, 12.5 mg hydrochlorothiazide, 100 mg metoprolol, 12.5 mg hydrochlorothiazide
**Usual adult dose:** 1 tablet/d PO. Pt should not cut, crush, or chew ER form (*Dutoprol*). **BBW** Risk of cardiac ischemia, angina, MI w/sudden cessation; taper drug. Alert pt to not stop drug.

### ▶ moexipril and hydroCHLOROthiazide
Generic

**Tablets:** 7.5 mg moexipril, 12.5 mg hydrochlorothiazide; 15 mg moexipril, 25 mg hydrochlorothiazide
**Usual adult dose:** 1 or 2 tablets/d PO 1 hr before or 2 hr after meal. **BBW** Risk of birth defects/fetal death; avoid use in preg.

### ▶ nadolol and bendroflumethiazide
Corzide

**Tablets:** 40 mg nadolol, 5 mg bendroflumethiazide; 80 mg nadolol, 5 mg bendroflumethiazide
**Usual adult dose:** 1 tablet/d PO in a.m.

### ▶ nebivolol and valsartan
Byvalson

**Tablets:** 5 mg nebivolol/80 mg valsartan
**Usual adult dose:** 1 tablet/d PO. Do not give w/bradycardia, heart block, HF, severe hepatic impairment. **BBW** Fetal toxicity; not for use in preg.

### ▶ olmesartan, amLODIPine, and hydroCHLOROthiazide
Tribenzor

**Tablets:** 40 mg olmesartan, 10 mg amlodipine, 25 mg hydrochlorothiazide
**Usual adult dose:** 1 tablet/d PO. **BBW** Risk of birth defects/fetal death; avoid use in preg.

**▶ olmesartan medoxomil and hydrochlorothiazide**
Benicar HCT

**Tablets:** 20 mg olmesartan, 12.5 mg hydrochlorothiazide; 40 mg olmesartan, 12.5 mg hydrochlorothiazide; 40 mg olmesartan, 25 mg hydrochlorothiazide
**Usual adult dose:** 1 tablet/d PO in a.m. **BBW** Risk of birth defects/fetal death; avoid use in preg.

**▶ quinapril and hydroCHLOROthiazide**
Accuretic

**Tablets:** 10 mg quinapril, 12.5 mg hydrochlorothiazide; 20 mg quinapril, 12.5 mg hydrochlorothiazide
**Usual adult dose:** 1 tablet/d PO in a.m. **BBW** Risk of birth defects/fetal death; avoid use in preg.

**▶ telmisartan and amLODIPine**
Twynsta

**Tablets:** 40 mg telmisartan, 5 mg amlodipine; 40 mg telmisartan, 10 mg amlodipine; 80 mg telmisartan, 5 mg amlodipine; 80 mg telmisartan, 10 mg amlodipine
**Usual adult dose:** 1 tablet/d PO. **BBW** Risk of birth defects/fetal death; avoid use in preg.

**▶ telmisartan and hydroCHLOROthiazide**
Micardis HCT

**Tablets:** 40 mg telmisartan, 12.5 mg hydrochlorothiazide; 80 mg telmisartan, 12.5 mg hydrochlorothiazide; 80 mg telmisartan, 25 mg hydrochlorothiazide
**Usual adult dose:** 1 tablet/d PO; max, 160 mg telmisartan and 25 mg hydrochlorothiazide/d. **BBW** Risk of birth defects/fetal death; avoid use in preg.

**▶ trandolapril and verapamil**
Tarka

**Tablets:** 1 mg trandolapril, 240 mg verapamil; 2 mg trandolapril, 180 mg verapamil; 2 mg trandolapril, 240 mg verapamil; 4 mg trandolapril, 240 mg verapamil
**Usual adult dose:** 1 tablet/d PO w/ food. Pt should not cut, crush, or chew tablet. **BBW** Risk of birth defects/fetal death; avoid use in preg.

**▶ valsartan and hydroCHLOROthiazide**
Diovan HCT

**Tablets:** 80 mg valsartan, 12.5 mg hydrochlorothiazide; 160 mg valsartan, 12.5 mg hydrochlorothiazide; 160 mg valsartan, 25 mg hydrochlorothiazide; 320 mg valsartan, 12.5 mg hydrochlorothiazide; 320 mg valsartan, 25 mg hydrochlorothiazide
**Usual adult dose:** 1 tablet/d PO. **BBW** Risk of birth defects/fetal death; avoid use in preg.

## *ANTIMALARIAL*

**▶ atovaquone and proguanil**
Malarone

**Tablets:** 250 mg atovaquone, 100 mg proguanil; *child:* 62.5 mg atovaquone, 25 mg proguanil
**Usual adult dose:** *Malaria px:* 1 tablet PO once daily w/food or milky drink 1 or 2 d before entering malaria-endemic area; continue through stay and 7 d after return. Do not use for px if severe renal impairment. *Malaria tx:*

4 tablets PO daily for 3 d. Base child dose on body weight.

## *ANTIMIGRAINE DRUGS*

### ▶ acetaminophen, aspirin, and caffeine
Excedrin (Migraine)

**Tablets:** 250 mg acetaminophen, 250 mg aspirin, 65 mg caffeine
**Usual adult dose:** 2 tablets PO at first sign of attack w/glass of water. No more than 2 tablets in 24 hr.

### ▶ ergotamine and caffeine
Cafergot, Migergot

**Tablets:** 1 mg ergotamine tartrate, 100 mg caffeine
**Suppositories:** 2 mg ergotamine tartrate, 100 mg caffeine
**Usual adult dose:** 2 tablets PO at first sign of attack, then 1 tablet q 30 min, if needed. Max, 6/attack, 10/wk. Or, 1 suppository at first sign of attack, then second dose after 1 hr, if needed. Max, 2/attack, 5/wk. Do not use w/ritonavir, nelfinavir, indinavir, erythromycin, clarithromycin, troleandomycin; serious vasospasm possible.

### ▶ SUMAtriptan and naproxen sodium
Treximet

**Tablets:** 85 mg sumatriptan, 500 mg naproxen
**Usual adult dose:** 1 tablet PO at onset of acute migraine. **BBW** Risk of CV thrombotic events and serious GI adverse events; contraindicated w/CABG surgery.

## *ANTINAUSEA DRUGS*

### ▶ doxylamine and pyridoxine
Diclegis

**DR tablets:** 10 mg doxylamine, 10 mg pyridoxine
**Usual adult dose:** 1 tablet PO at bedtime; max 4 tablets/d. Tx of n/v in preg in pts not responding to other tx.

### ▶ netupitant and palonosetron
Akynzeo

**Capsules:** 300 mg netupitant, 0.5 mg palonosetron
**Usual adult dose:** 1 capsule 1 hr before start of emetogenic chemotherapy. Avoid use w/severe renal/hepatic impairment.

## *ANTIPARKINSONIANS*

### ▶ levodopa and carbidopa
Duopa, Rytary, Sinemet, Sinemet CR

**Enteral suspension:** 20 mg levodopa, 4.63 mg carbidopa
**ER capsules (*Rytary*):** 23.75 mg carbidopa and 95 mg levodopa, 36.25 mg carbidopa and 145 mg levodopa, 48.75 mg carbidopa and 195 mg levodopa, 61.25 mg carbidopa and 245 mg levodopa
**Tablets:** 100 mg levodopa, 10 mg carbidopa; 100 mg levodopa, 25 mg carbidopa; 250 mg levodopa, 25 mg carbidopa
**Orally disintegrating tablets:** 100 mg levodopa, 10 mg carbidopa; 100 mg levodopa, 25 mg carbidopa; 250 mg levodopa, 25 mg carbidopa
**CR tablets:** 100 mg levodopa, 25 mg carbidopa; 200 mg levodopa, 50 mg carbidopa

**Usual adult dose:** Start w/lowest dose; titrate based on response, tolerance.

**▶ levodopa, carbidopa, and entacapone**
Stalevo 50, Stalevo 75, Stalevo 100, Stalevo 125, Stalevo 150, Stalevo 200

**Tablets:** 50 mg levodopa, 12.5 mg carbidopa, 200 mg entacapone; 75 mg levodopa, 18.75 mg carbidopa, 200 mg entacapone; 100 mg levodopa, 25 mg carbidopa, 200 mg entacapone; 125 mg levodopa, 31.25 mg carbidopa, 200 mg entacapone; 150 mg levodopa, 37.5 mg carbidopa, 200 mg entacapone; 200 mg levodopa, 50 mg carbidopa, 200 mg entacapone
**Usual adult dose:** 1 tablet PO q 3–8 hr.

*ANTIPLATELET DRUG*

**▶ aspirin and dipyridamole**
Aggrenox

**Capsules:** 25 mg aspirin, 200 mg dipyridamole
**Usual adult dose:** 1 capsule PO bid to decrease risk of stroke in pts w/ known cerebrovascular disease. Not interchangeable w/individual components of aspirin and dipyridamole tablets. Pt should not chew capsule.

*ANTIULCER DRUGS*

**▶ bismuth subcitrate potassium, metroNIDAZOLE, tetracycline hydrochloride**
Pylera

**Capsules:** 140 mg bismuth subcitrate potassium, 125 mg metronidazole, 125 mg tetracycline
**Usual adult dose (do not give to child ≤8 yr):** 3 capsules 4 ×/d (after meals and at bedtime) for 10 d.

**▶ lansoprazole, amoxicillin, and clarithromycin**
Generic

**Daily administration pack:** Two 30-mg lansoprazole capsules, four 500-mg amoxicillin capsules, two 500-mg clarithromycin tablets
**Usual adult dose:** Divide pack equally to take PO bid, a.m. and p.m., for 10–14 d.

**▶ omeprazole, clarithromycin, and amoxicillin**
Generic

**Capsules/tablets:** 20-mg omeprazole capsules, 500-mg clarithromycin tablets, 500 mg amoxicillin capsules
**Usual adult dose:** 20 mg omeprazole, 500 mg clarithromycin, and 100 mg amoxicillin PO bid before meals for 10 d.

*ANTIVIRALS*

**▶ abacavir and lamiVUDine**
Epzicom

**Tablets:** 600 mg abacavir w/300 mg lamivudine
**Usual adult dose, child ≥25 kg:** 1 tablet PO daily w/other antiretrovirals for tx of HIV infection. **BBW** Risk of severe hypersensitivity reactions, lactic acidosis, severe hepatomegaly, HBV exacerbation. Monitor pt accordingly.

### ▶ abacavir, zidovudine, and lamiVUDine
Trizivir

**Tablets:** 300 mg abacavir, 300 mg zidovudine, 150 mg lamivudine
**Usual adult dose, child ≥40 kg:** 1 tablet PO bid for tx of HIV infection. Carefully monitor for hypersensitivity reactions; potential increased risk of MI. **BBW** Risk of severe hypersensitivity reactions, bone marrow suppression, myopathy, lactic acidosis, severe hepatomegaly, HBV exacerbation. Monitor pt accordingly.

### ▶ atazanavir and cobicistat
Evotaz

**Tablets:** 300 mg atazanavir, 150 mg cobicistat
**Usual adult dose:** 1 tablet/d PO w/ food, other antiretrovirals for tx of HIV infection. Not recommended w/ severe hepatic/renal impairment. Many potentially serious drug interactions.

### ▶ bictegravir, emtricitabine, and tenofovir alafenamide
Biktarvy

**Tablets:** 50 mg bictegravir (equivalent to 52.5 mg of bictegravir sodium), 200 mg emtricitabine, 25 mg tenofovir alafenamide (equivalent to 28 mg of tenofovir alafenamide fumarate)
**Usual adult dose, child ≥25 kg:** 1 tablet PO daily for tx of HIV-1 infection. **BBW** Risk of severe HBV exacerbations; test pt for HBV before tx.

### ▶ darunavir and cobicistat
Prezcobix

**Tablets:** 800 mg darunavir, 150 mg cobicistat
**Usual adult dose:** 1 tablet/d PO w/ food for tx of HIV infection.

### ▶ darunavir, cobicistat, emtricitabine, and tenofovir alafenamide
Symtuza

**Tablets:** 800 mg darunavir, 150 mg cobicistat, 200 mg emtricitabine, 10 mg tenofovir alafenamide
**Usual adult dose:** 1 tablet/d PO w/ food for tx of HIV infection. **BBW** Risk of severe HBV exacerbations; test pt for HBV before tx.

### ▶ dolutegravir, abacavir, and lamiVUDin
Triumeq

**Tablets:** 50 mg dolutegravir, 600 mg abacavir, 300 mg lamivudine
**Usual adult dose:** 1 tablet/d. Many potentially serious drug interactions. **BBW** Risk of severe hypersensitivity reactions, lactic acidosis, hepatotoxicity, HBV exacerbation.

### ▶ dolutegravir and lamiVUDine
Dovato

**Tablets:** 50 mg dolutegravir, 300 mg lamivudine
**Usual adult dose:** 1 tablet PO q d w/ or w/o meal. If given w/carbamazepine or rifampin, 1 Dovato tablet once daily followed by additional dolutegravir 50-mg tablet about 12 hr later. **BBW** Risk of lamivudine-resistant HBV/HBV exacerbations in pts infected w/HBV and HIV-1.

### ▶ dolutegravir and rilpivirine
Juluca

**Tablets:** 50 mg dolutegravir, 25 mg rilpivirine
**Usual adult dose:** 1 tablet PO q d w/meal.

### ▶ doravirine, lamiVUDine, and tenofovir disoproxil fumarate
Delstrigo

**Tablets:** 100 mg doravirine, 300 mg lamivudine, 300 mg tenofovir disoproxil fumarate
**Usual adult dose:** 1 tablet PO q d w/ or w/o food. **BBW** Risk of severe acute HBV exacerbations in pts infected w/HIV-1 and HBV. Closely monitor hepatic function; start anti-HBV tx if needed.

### ▶ efavirenz, emtricitabine, and tenofovir
Atripla

**Tablets:** 600 mg efavirenz, 200 mg emtricitabine, 300 mg tenofovir
**Usual adult dose, child ≥40 kg:** 1 tablet PO at bedtime on empty stomach for tx of HIV infection. Not recommended w/moderate or severe renal impairment. Risk of rash, fetal harm, body fat redistribution, lactic acidosis, QTc prolongation, hepatotoxicity. **BBW** Not indicated for chronic HBV. Risk of severe exacerbations of HBV w/drug discontinuation; monitor hepatic function in these pts.

### ▶ efavirenz, lamiVUDine, and tenofovir disoproxil fumarate
Symfi

**Tablets:** 600 mg efavirenz, 300 mg lamivudine, 300 mg tenofovir disoproxil fumarate
**Usual adult dose, child ≥40 kg:** 1 tablet PO at bedtime on empty stomach for tx of HIV infection. Not recommended w/moderate, severe renal impairment. Risk of rash, fetal harm, body fat redistribution, lactic acidosis, prolonged QTc, hepatotoxicity. **BBW** Severe acute HBV exacerbations w/drug discontinuation in pts infected w/HBV and HIV-1. Monitor hepatic function; start anti-HBV tx if needed.

### ▶ elbasvir and grazoprevir
Zepatier

**Tablets:** 50 mg elbasvir w/100 mg grazoprevir
**Usual adult dose:** 1 tablet/d PO w/ or without ribavirin for 12–16 wk. Tx of chronic HCV genotypes 1 and 4. Monitor liver function. **BBW** Risk of HBV reactivation, sometimes fatal.

### ▶ elvitegravir, cobicistat, emtricitabine, and tenofovir alafenamide
Genvoya

**Tablets:** 150 mg elvitegravir, 150 mg cobicistat, 200 mg emtricitabine, 10 mg tenofovir alafenamide
**Usual adult dose, child ≥25 kg:** 1 tablet/d PO w/food. Tx of HIV-1 infection in adult/child. Risk of lactic acidosis, hepatomegaly, renal and/or hepatic impairment, redistribution of body fat. Many potentially dangerous drug interactions. **BBW** Not approved for tx of chronic HBV. Severe acute HBV exacerbations

w/drug discontinuation; monitor hepatic function closely in these pts.

### ▶ elvitegravir, cobicistat, emtricitabine, and tenofovir disoproxil fumarate
Stribild

**Tablets:** 150 mg elvitegravir, 150 mg cobicistat, 200 mg emtricitabine, 300 mg tenofovir
**Usual adult dose, child ≥12 yr, ≥35 kg:** 1 tablet PO/d for pts never treated for HIV. Many potentially serious drug interactions. Risk of lactic acidosis, severe hepatomegaly, renal impairment, decreased bone density. **BBW** Not approved for tx of chronic HBV. Severe acute HBV exacerbations w/drug discontinuation; monitor hepatic function closely in these pts.

### ▶ emtricitabine, rilpivirine, and tenofovir
Complera

**Tablets:** 200 mg emtricitabine, 25 mg rilpivirine, 300 mg tenofovir
**Usual adult dose, child ≥35 kg:** 1 tablet/d PO for tx of HIV infection in tx-naïve pts. Many potentially serious drug interactions, severe rash, risk of drug reaction w/eosinophilia and systemic symptoms. Risk of renal impairment, lactic acidosis, hepatomegaly. **BBW** Not approved for tx of chronic HBV. Severe acute HBV exacerbations w/drug discontinuation; monitor hepatic function closely in these pts.

### ▶ emtricitabine, rilpivirine, and tenofovir alafenamide
Odefsey

**Tablets:** 200 mg emtricitabine, 25 mg rilpivirine, 25 mg tenofovir
**Usual adult dose, child >35 kg:** Tx of HIV. 1 tablet/d PO. Not recommended w/renal impairment. Risk of lactic acidosis, hepatomegaly, severe skin reactions, renal impairment. **BBW** Not approved for tx of chronic HBV. Severe acute HBV exacerbations w/drug discontinuation; monitor hepatic function closely in these pts.

### ▶ emtricitabine and tenofovir alafenamide
Descovy

**Tablets:** 200 mg emtricitabine, 25 mg tenofovir
**Usual adult dose, child ≥25 kg:** 1 tablet PO daily w/other antiretrovirals for tx of HIV infection or HIV-1 preexposure px. Many potential drug interactions. Decrease dose if renal impairment. Risk of renal impairment, lactic acidosis, severe hepatomegaly, decreased bone mineral density. **BBW** Not approved for tx of chronic HBV. Severe acute HBV exacerbations w/drug discontinuation. Monitor hepatic function closely. Only approved for px if pt confirmed HIV-negative.

### ▶ emtricitabine and tenofovir disoproxil fumarate
Truvada

**Tablets:** 200 mg emtricitabine w/300 mg tenofovir; 167 mg emtricitabine w/250 mg tenofovir; 133 mg emtricitabine w/200 mg tenofovir; 100 mg emtricitabine w/150 mg tenofovir
**Usual adult dose, child ≥35 kg:** 1 tablet PO daily w/other antiretrovirals for tx of HIV infection or HIV-1 preexposure px. Many potential drug interactions. Decrease dose if renal impairment. Risk of renal impairment, lactic acidosis, severe hepatomegaly, decreased bone

mineral density. **BBW** Not approved for tx of chronic HBV. Severe acute HBV exacerbations w/drug discontinuation. Monitor hepatic function closely. Only approved for px if pt confirmed HIV-negative.

### ▶ glecaprevir and pibrentasvir
Mavyret

**Tablets:** 100 mg glecaprevir, 40 mg pibrentasvir
**Usual adult dose:** 3 tablets PO q d w/food for tx of chronic HCV genotype. **BBW** Risk of HBV reactivation in pts w/HCV and HBV.

### ▶ lamiVUDine and tenofovir disoproxil fumarate
Cimduo, Temixys

**Tablets:** 300 mg lamivudine, 300 mg tenofovir disoproxil fumarate
**Usual adult dose, child ≥35 kg:** 1 tablet PO daily for tx of HIV infection w/ or w/o food. Not recommended if CrCl <50 mL/min or if ESRD requiring hemodialysis. **BBW** Risk of severe acute HBV exacerbations in pts infected w/HIV-1 and HBV. Monitor hepatic function closely; start anti-HBV tx if needed.

### ▶ lamiVUDine and zidovudine
Combivir

**Tablets:** 150 mg lamivudine, 300 mg zidovudine
**Usual adult dose, child ≥30 kg:** 1 tablet PO bid for tx of HIV infection. Not recommended for adult, child <50 kg. **BBW** Risk of lactic acidosis, severe hepatomegaly, bone marrow suppression, myopathy, post-tx HBV exacerbation.

### ▶ ledipasvir and sofosbuvir
Harvoni

**Tablets:** 90 mg ledipasvir, 400 mg sofosbuvir
**Usual adult dose:** *Genotype 1:* 1 tablet/d PO w/food for 12 wk (tx-naïve) or 24 wk (tx-experienced). *Genotype 4, 5, 6:* 1 tablet/d PO w/ food for 12 wk. Tx of HCV. **BBW** Risk of severe cases of HBV reactivation.
**Child ≥3 yr:** Based on genotype and weight.

### ▶ lopinavir and ritonavir
Kaletra

**Tablets:** 200 mg lopinavir, 50 mg ritonavir; 100 mg lopinavir, 25 mg ritonavir. **Sol:** 80 mg/mL lopinavir, 20 mg/mL ritonavir
**Usual adult dose:** 800/200 mg daily either once a d or bid. **Preg adult:** 400/100 mg bid. **Child ≥14 d:** Base dose on BSA; give bid w/ or w/o food. Oral sol must be given w/food. Dose adjustments needed if used concomitantly.

### ▶ ombitasvir, paritaprevir, and ritonavir
Technivie

**Tablets:** 12.5 mg ombitasvir, 75 mg paritaprevir, 50 mg ritonavir
**Usual adult dose:** 2 tablets PO once daily in a.m. for 12 wk. Tx of genotype 4 chronic HCV. Many potential serious drug interactions. Not for use w/moderate hepatic impairment. Risk of serious to fatal liver injury. **BBW** Risk of severe cases of HBV reactivation.

### ▶ ombitasvir, paritaprevir, ritonavir, and dasabuvir
Viekira Pak

**Tablets:** 12.5 mg ombitasvir, 75 mg paritaprevir, 50 mg ritonavir; packaged w/250 mg dasabuvir
**ER tablets:** 8.33 mg ombitasvir, 50 mg paritaprevir, 33.33 mg ritonavir, 200 mg dasabuvir
**Usual adult dose:** 2 ombitasvir/paritaprevir/ritonavir tablets PO once daily in a.m. and 1 dasabuvir tablet PO bid (a.m. and p.m.) w/food. ER tablets: 3 tablets/d PO for 12–24 wk. Tx of HCV. Hepatic failure possible. Many potentially serious drug interactions. **BBW** Risk of severe cases of HBV reactivation.

### ▶ sofosbuvir and velpatasvir
Epclusa

**Tablets:** 400 mg sofosbuvir, 100 mg velpatasvir
**Usual adult dose:** Tx of HCV without cirrhosis, compensated cirrhosis: 1 tablet/d for 12 wk. Decompensated cirrhosis: 1 tablet/d plus ribavirin for 12 wk. Serious bradycardia w/amiodarone. **BBW** Risk of severe cases of HBV reactivation.

### ▶ sofosbuvir, velpatasvir, and voxilaprevir
Vosevi

**Tablets:** 400 mg sofosbuvir, 100 mg velpatasvir, 100 mg voxilaprevir
**Usual adult dose:** Tx of chronic HCV. 1 tablet PO q d w/food. **BBW** Risk of HBV reactivation in pts coinfected w/HCV and HBV.

## *BPH DRUG*

### ▶ dutasteride and tamsulosin
Jalyn

**Capsules:** 0.5 mg dutasteride, 0.4 mg tamsulosin
**Usual adult dose:** Tx of symptomatic BPH: 1 capsule/d PO about 30 min after same meal each d.

## *COLON CLEANSING DRUG*

### ▶ sodium picosulfate, magnesium oxide, and anhydrous citric acid
Clenpiq

**Oral sol:** 10 mg sodium picosulfate, 3.5 g magnesium oxide, 12 g anhydrous citric acid
**Usual adult dose, child ≥9 yr:** 1 bottle evening before and 1 bottle morning of colonoscopy as split-dose regimen for cleansing colon before colonoscopy. Pt must consume ≥5 8-oz cups of clear liquids before and after first and 4 8-oz cups after the second Clenpiq dose. Pt should not take oral drugs within 1 hr of start of each dose. Pt should take tetracyclines, fluoroquinolones, iron, digoxin, chlorpromazine, penicillamine at least 2 hr before and not less than 6 hr after Clenpiq administration if prescribed.

## *CYSTIC FIBROSIS DRUGS*

### ▶ elexacaftor, tezacaftor, and ivacaftor
Trikafta

**Tablets:** 100 mg elexacaftor, 50 mg tezacaftor, 75 mg ivacaftor w/75 mg ivacaftor

**Usual adult dose, child ≥12 yr:** 1 tablet in a.m. and ivacaftor 150-mg tablet in p.m. w/fat-containing food.

### ▶ lumacaftor and ivacaftor
Orkambi

**Tablets:** 100 mg lumacaftor, 125 mg ivacaftor; 200 mg lumacaftor, 125 mg ivacaftor
**Oral granules:** 100 mg lumacaftor, 125 mg ivacaftor; 150 mg lumacaftor, 188 mg ivacaftor
**Usual adult dose, child ≥12 yr:** 2 tablets (200 mg lumacaftor/125 mg ivacaftor) PO q 12 hr w/fat-containing food. **Child 6–11 yr:** 2 tablets (100 mg lumacaftor/125 mg ivacaftor) PO q 12 hr w/fat-containing food. **Child 2–5 yr ≥14 kg:** 1 packet granules (each containing 150 mg lumacaftor/188 mg ivacaftor) mixed w/1 tsp (5 mL) soft food or liquid and given PO q 12 hr w/fat-containing food. **Child 2–5 yr <14 kg:** 1 packet granules (each containing 100 mg lumacaftor/125 mg ivacaftor) mixed w/1 tsp (5 mL) soft food or liquid and given PO q 12 hr w/fat-containing food.

### ▶ tezacaftor and ivacaftor
Symdeko

**Tablets:** 50 mg tezacaftor, 75 mg ivacaftor w/75 mg ivacaftor; 100 mg tezacaftor, 150 mg ivacaftor w/150 mg ivacaftor
**Usual adult dose, child ≥12 yr or 6–<12 yr ≥30 kg:** 1 tablet (100 mg tezacaftor/150 mg ivacaftor) in a.m. and 1 tablet (150 mg ivacaftor) in p.m. about 12 hr apart w/fat-containing food. **Child 6–<12 yr <30 kg:** 1 tablet (50 mg tezacaftor/75 mg ivacaftor) in a.m. and 1 tablet (75 mg ivacaftor) in p.m. about 12 hr apart w/fat-containing food.

## *DIURETICS*

### ▶ aMILoride and hydroCHLOROthiazide
Generic

**Tablets:** 5 mg amiloride, 50 mg hydrochlorothiazide
**Usual adult dose:** 1 or 2 tablets/d PO w/meals.

### ▶ hydroCHLOROthiazide and triamterene
Dyazide

**Capsules:** 25 mg hydrochlorothiazide, 37.5 mg triamterene
**Usual adult dose:** 1 or 2 capsules PO once/d or bid after meals.

### ▶ hydroCHLOROthiazide and triamterene
Maxzide, Maxzide-25

**Tablets:** 25 mg hydrochlorothiazide, 37.5 mg triamterene; 50 mg hydrochlorothiazide, 75 mg triamterene
**Usual adult dose:** 1 or 2 tablets/d PO.

### ▶ spironolactone and hydroCHLOROthiazide
Aldactazide

**Tablets:** 25 mg spironolactone, 25 mg hydrochlorothiazide; 50 mg spironolactone, 50 mg hydrochlorothiazide
**Usual adult dose:** 1–8 tablets/d PO (25/25). 1–4 tablets/d PO (50/50).

## *ENZYME-DEFICIENCY DRUG*

### ▶ sodium phenylacetate and sodium benzoate
Ammonul

**Vials (single-use):** 50 mL sodium phenylacetate, sodium benzoate injection 10%/10%
**Usual adult dose, child >20 kg:** 55 mL/m². **0–20 kg:** 2.5 mL/kg. Give IV through central line w/arginine. Adjunct tx in hyperammonemia, encephalopathy in pts w/enzyme deficiencies associated w/urea cycle.

## *HF DRUGS*

### ▶ isosorbide dinitrate and hydrALAZINE hydrochloride
BiDil

**Tablets:** 20 mg isosorbide dinitrate, 37.5 mg hydralazine
**Usual adult dose:** 1 tablet PO tid; may increase to 2 tablets tid. For adjunct tx in self-identified black pts to improve functional survival. Not for use w/ED drugs.

### ▶ sacubitril and valsartan
Entresto

**Tablets:** 24 mg sacubitril, 26 mg valsartan; 49 mg sacubitril, 51 mg valsartan; 97 mg sacubitril, 103 mg valsartan
**Usual adult dose, child ≥50 kg:** Initially, 49/51 mg PO bid; titrate up q 2–4 wk if tolerated. **Child 40–<50 kg:** 24/26 mg PO bid; titrate q 2 wk if tolerated. **Child <40 kg:** 1.6 mg/kg PO bid; titrate up q 2 wk if tolerated. Give w/other HF tx in place of ACE I or ARB. Halve starting dose if pt not on ACE I or ARB or severe renal or moderate hepatic impairment. **BBW** High risk of fetal toxicity. Stop as soon as possible if pt preg.

## *LIPID-LOWERING DRUGS*

### ▶ ezetimibe and simvastatin
Vytorin

**Tablets:** 10 mg ezetimibe, 10 mg simvastatin; 10 mg ezetimibe, 20 mg simvastatin; 10 mg ezetimibe, 40 mg simvastatin; 10 mg ezetimibe, 80 mg simvastatin
**Usual adult dose:** 1 tablet/d PO in p.m. w/cholesterol-lowering diet/exercise. Must give at least 2 hr before or 4 hr after bile sequestrant (if used).

## *MENOPAUSE DRUGS*

### ▶ conjugated estrogen and bazedoxifene
Duavee

**Tablets:** 0.45 mg conjugated estrogen, 20 mg bazedoxifene
**Usual adult dose:** 1 tablet/d PO. **BBW** Risk of endometrial cancer, stroke, DVT, probable dementia. Not for use to decrease CAD.

### ▶ drospirenone and estradiol
Angeliq

**Tablets:** 0.5 mg drospirenone, 1 mg estradiol
**Usual adult dose:** 1 tablet/d PO. Monitor potassium level closely. **BBW** Risk of endometrial cancer, stroke, DVT, probable dementia.

### ▶ drospirenone and ethinyl estradiol
YAZ

**Tablets:** 3 mg drospirenone, 0.02 mg ethinyl estradiol
**Usual adult dose:** 1 tablet/d PO. Monitor potassium level closely.

**BBW** Risk of serious CV events in female smokers ≥35 yr.

### ▶ estradiol and norethindrone (transdermal)
CombiPatch

**Patch:** 0.05 mg/d estradiol, 0.14 mg/d norethindrone; 0.05 mg/d estradiol, 0.25 mg/d norethindrone
**Usual adult dose:** Change patch twice/wk. **BBW** Risk of endometrial cancer, stroke, DVT, probable dementia.

### ▶ estradiol and norethindrone (oral)
Activella, Amabelz, Aurovela, Blisovi

**Tablets:** 0.5 mg estradiol, 0.1 mg norethindrone; 1 mg estradiol, 0.5 mg norethindrone
**Usual adult dose:** 1 tablet/d PO. **BBW** Risk of endometrial cancer, stroke, DVT, probable dementia.

### ▶ estradiol and progesterone
Bijuva

**Capsules:** 1 mg/100 mg
**Usual adult dose:** 1 capsule PO q evening w/food for tx of pt w/uterus for moderate to severe vasomotor sx due to menopause. **BBW** Should not be used for px of CV disease or dementia; risk of stroke, DVT, PE, MI, breast cancer, dementia in females ≥65 yr.

### ▶ estrogens, conjugated, and medroxyPROGESTERone
Prempro

**Tablets:** 0.3 mg conjugated estrogen, 1.5 mg medroxyprogesterone; 0.45 mg conjugated estrogen, 1.5 mg medroxyprogesterone; 0.625 mg conjugated estrogen, 2.5 mg medroxyprogesterone; 0.625 mg conjugated estrogen, 5 mg medroxyprogesterone
**Usual adult dose:** 1 tablet/d PO. Use in women w/intact uterus. **BBW** Risk of endometrial cancer, stroke, DVT, probable dementia.

### ▶ ethinyl estradiol and norethindrone acetate
Femhrt, Fyavolv, Gildess, Hailey, Junel, Larin, Leribane, Taytulla

**Tablets:** 2.5 mcg ethinyl estradiol, 0.5 mg norethindrone acetate; 5 mcg ethinyl estradiol, 1 mg norethindrone acetate
**Usual adult dose:** 1 tablet/d PO. Use in women w/intact uterus. **BBW** Risk of endometrial cancer, stroke, DVT, probable dementia.

## *ONCOLOGY DRUGS*

### ▶ daunorubicin and cytarabine
Vyxeos

**Tablets:** 44 mg daunorubicin, 100 mg cytarabine
**Usual adult dose:** Induction: daunorubicin 44 mg/m$^2$ and cytarabine 100 mg/m$^2$ IV over 90 min on days 1, 3, and 5 and on days 1 and 3 for subsequent cycles of induction, if needed. Consolidation: daunorubicin 29 mg/m$^2$ and cytarabine 65 mg/m$^2$ liposome IV over 90 min on days 1 and 3. For tx of acute myeloid leukemia w/myelodysplasia. **BBW** Do not interchange w/ other daunorubicin and/or cytarabine-containing products.

### ▶ riTUXimab and hyaluronidase human
Rituxan Hycela

**Vials:** 1,400 mg rituximab, hyaluronidase human 23,400 units/11.7 mL

(120 mg/2,000 units/mL); 1,600 mg rituximab, hyaluronidase human 26,800 units/ 13.4 mL (120 mg/ 2,000 units/mL)
**Usual adult dose:** 1,400 mg/ 23,400 units subcut after rituximab, acetaminophen, and antihistamine for tx of follicular lymphoma and diffuse large B-cell lymphoma; 1,600 mg/26,800 units subcut after rituximab, acetaminophen, and antihistamine for tx of chronic lymphocytic leukemia. **BBW** Risk of severe mucocutaneous reactions, HBV reactivation, PML; all have risk of death.

**▶ trastuzumab and hyaluronidase-oysk**
Herceptin Hylecta

**Vials:** 600 mg trastuzumab, 10,000 units hyaluronidase
**Usual adult dose:** 1 vial subcut q 3 wk for 52 wk or disease progression/recurrence, w/other chemo regimens. **BBW** Risk of cardiomyopathy (HF including decreased LVEF), especially when given w/anthracyclines; stop if cardiomyopathy. Risk of pulmonary toxicity; stop if anaphylaxis, angioedema, interstitial pneumonitis, or acute respiratory distress syndrome. Risk of embryo-fetal toxicity; advise pt on effective contraception.

**▶ trifluridine and tipiracil**
Lonsurf

**Tablets:** 15 mg trifluridine, 6.14 mg tipiracil; 20 mg trifluridine, 8.19 mg tipiracil
**Usual adult dose:** 35 mg/m$^2$/dose PO bid on days 1–5, 8–12 of 28-d cycle within 1 hr of completing a.m. and p.m. meals. Tx of metastatic colorectal cancer after previous tx. Risk of severe bone marrow suppression, fetal toxicity.

## *OPIOID AGONISTS*

**▶ buprenorphine and naloxone**
CONTROLLED SUBSTANCE C-III
Bunavail

**Buccal film:** 2.1 mg buprenorphine, 0.3 mg naloxone; 4.2 mg buprenorphine, 0.7 mg naloxone; 6.3 mg buprenorphine, 1 mg naloxone
**Usual adult dose:** 8.4/1.4 mg as daily buccal dose for maint. Pts dependent on short-acting opioids and/ or in active withdrawal may need divided doses.

**▶ buprenorphine and naloxone**
CONTROLLED SUBSTANCE C-III
Suboxone

**SL tablets:** 2 mg buprenorphine, 0.5 mg naloxone; 8 mg buprenorphine, 2 mg naloxone
**Usual adult dose:** 12–16 mg/d by SL film after induction w/SL buprenorphine for tx of opioid dependence. Must taper to decrease risk of withdrawal. Risk of addiction, respiratory depression, neonatal opioid withdrawal syndrome.

**▶ buprenorphine and naloxone**
CONTROLLED SUBSTANCE C-III
Zubsolv

**SL tablets:** 0.7 mg buprenorphine, 0.18 mg naloxone; 1.4 mg buprenorphine, 0.36 mg naloxone; 2.9 mg buprenorphine, 0.71 mg naloxone; 5.7 mg buprenorphine, 1.4 mg naloxone; 8.6 mg buprenorphine, 2.1 naloxone; 11.4 mg buprenorphine, 2.9 mg naloxone
**Usual adult dose:** After induction, 1 tablet/d SL. Taper dose to avoid withdrawal. Risk of addiction, abuse,

withdrawal; respiratory depression, neonatal opioid withdrawal syndrome.

*PSYCHIATRIC DRUG*

**▶ dextromethorphan and quinidine**
Nuedexta

**Capsules:** 20 mg dextromethorphan, 10 mg quinidine
**Usual adult dose:** 1 capsule/d PO for 7 d; maint, 1 capsule PO q 12 hr. For tx of pseudobulbar affect associated w/neuro conditions.

*RESPIRATORY DRUGS*

**▶ aclidinium bromide and formoterol fumarate**
Duaklir Pressair

**Inhaled aerosol:** 400 mcg aclidinium bromide, 12 mcg formoterol fumarate
**Usual adult dose:** 2 oral inhalations bid. For COPD maint tx. Not for acute bronchospasm or asthma.

**▶ azelastine and fluticasone**
Dymista

**Nasal spray:** 137 mcg azelastine, 50 mcg fluticasone
**Usual dose in pts ≥6 yr:** 1 spray in each nostril bid for relief of sx of seasonal allergic rhinitis.

**▶ budesonide and formoterol fumarate**
Symbicort 80/4.5, Symbicort 160/4.5

**Inhalation:** 80 mcg budesonide, 4.5 mcg formoterol fumarate; 160 mcg budesonide, 4.5 mcg formoterol fumarate
**Usual dose in pts ≥12 yr:** Two inhalations bid, a.m. and p.m. For long-term maint of asthma/COPD; not for acute attacks.

**▶ fluticasone and salmeterol**
Advair Diskus, Advair HFA, AirDuo RespiClick, Wixela Inhub

**Inhalation:** 100 mcg fluticasone, 50 mcg salmeterol; 250 mcg fluticasone, 50 mcg salmeterol; 500 mcg fluticasone, 50 mcg salmeterol
**Inhalation (AirDuo RespiClick):** 55 mcg fluticasone, 14 mcg salmeterol; 113 mcg fluticasone, 14 mcg salmeterol; 232 mcg fluticasone, 14 mcg salmeterol
**Usual dose in pts ≥12 yr:** 1 inhalation bid to manage asthma/COPD. **Child 4–11 yr:** 1 inhalation (100 mcg fluticasone, 50 mcg salmeterol) bid, a.m. and p.m. about 12 hr apart. Not indicated for acute bronchospasm.

**▶ fluticasone, umeclidinium, and vilanterol**
Trelegy Ellipta

**Powder for inhalation:** 100 mcg fluticasone, 62.5 mcg umeclidinium, 25 mcg vilanterol
**Usual adult dose:** 1 inhalation daily to manage COPD. Not indicated for acute bronchospasm.

**▶ fluticasone and vilanterol**
Breo Ellipta

**Powder for inhalation:** 100 mcg fluticasone, 25 mcg vilanterol
**Usual adult dose:** One oral inhalation daily to manage asthma/COPD. Not indicated for acute bronchospasm.

**▶ glycopyrrolate and formoterol fumarate**
Bevespi Aerosphere

**Inhaled aerosol:** 9 mcg glycopyrrolate, 4.8 mcg formoterol
**Usual adult dose:** 2 oral inhalations bid. Not for acute bronchospasm or asthma

**▶ HYDROcodone and chlorpheniramine**
Vituz

**Oral sol:** 5 mg hydrocodone, 4 mg chlorpheniramine/5-mL sol
**Usual adult dose:** 5 mL PO q 4–6 hr; max, four doses/d for temporary relief of cough or allergy sx. **BBW** Risk of respiratory depression, coma, death when used w/ benzodiazepines or other CNS depressants; risk of neonatal opioid withdrawal syndrome.

**▶ HYDROcodone and pseudoephedrine**
Rezira

**Oral sol:** 5 mg hydrocodone, 60 mg pseudoephedrine/5-mL sol
**Usual adult dose:** 5 mL PO q 4–6 hr as needed; max, four doses in 24 hr. **BBW** Risk of respiratory depression, coma, death when used w/benzodiazepines or other CNS depressants; risk of neonatal withdrawal syndrome.

**▶ HYDROcodone and pseudoephedrine and chlorpheniramine**
Zutripro

**Oral sol:** 5 mg hydrocodone, 60 mg pseudoephedrine, 4 mg chlorpheniramine in 5-mL sol
**Usual adult dose:** 5 mL PO q 4–6 hr as needed; max, four doses in 24 hr. **BBW** Risk of respiratory depression, coma, death when used w/ benzodiazepines or other CNS depressants; risk of neonatal withdrawal syndrome.

**▶ indacaterol and glycopyrrolate**
Utibron Neohaler

**Powder for inhalation:** 27.5 mcg indacaterol, 15.6 mcg glycopyrrolate
**Usual adult dose:** Oral inhalation using *Neohaler* device, 1 capsule bid. Pt should not swallow capsules. For tx of COPD; not for asthma or acute bronchospasm.

**▶ ipratropium and albuterol**
Combivent Respimat

**Metered-dose inhaler:** 18 mcg ipratropium bromide, 90 mcg albuterol
**Usual adult dose:** 2 inhalations four times/d. Not for use during acute attack. Use caution w/known sensitivity to atropine, soybeans, soya lecithin, peanuts.

**▶ loratadine and pseudoephedrine**
Claritin-D

**ER tablets:** 5 mg loratadine, 120 mg pseudoephedrine
**Usual adult dose:** 1 tablet PO q 12 hr.

**▶ loratadine and pseudoephedrine**
Claritin-D 24 Hour

**ER tablets:** 10 mg loratadine, 240 mg pseudoephedrine
**Usual adult dose:** 1 tablet/d PO.

### ▶ mometasone and formoterol
Dulera 100/5, Dulera 200/5

**Metered aerosol inhaler:** 100 mcg mometasone, 5 mcg formoterol; 200 mcg mometasone, 5 mcg formoterol
**Usual adult dose:** For maint tx of asthma, 2 inhalations bid, a.m. and p.m. Rinse mouth after use. Not for children or for tx of acute bronchospasm.

### ▶ olodaterol and tiotropium
Stiolto Respimat

**Metered oral inhaler:** 2.5 mcg olodaterol, 2.5 mcg tiotropium
**Usual adult dose:** For long-term maint of COPD, 2 inhalations once a d at same time each d. Not for child. Risk of asthma-related deaths w/ long-acting beta agonists; must be combined w/inhaled corticosteroid. Not for use in asthma or acute deterioration of COPD.

### ▶ umeclidinium and vilanterol
Anoro Ellipta

**Inhalation powder:** 62.5 mcg umeclidinium, 25 mcg vilanterol
**Usual adult dose:** One oral inhalation/d for maint tx of COPD. Use of long-acting beta agonist without inhaled corticosteroid contraindicated in pts w/asthma.

## *TENSION HEADACHE DRUG*

### ▶ butalbital, acetaminophen, and caffeine
Generic

**Capsules:** 50 mg butalbital, 500 mg acetaminophen, 40 mg caffeine
**Usual adult dose:** 1 capsule, tablet, or sol PO q 4 hr as needed; max, 6/d. May be habit-forming; pt should avoid driving, dangerous tasks.

## *URINARY TRACT INFECTION DRUG*

### ▶ meropenem and vaborbactam
Vabomere

**Solution:** 1.4 g meropenem, 1 g vaborbactam
**Usual adult dose:** 4 g (meropenem 2 g, vaborbactam 2 g) IV q 8 hr over 3 hr for up to 14 d if estimated glomerular filtration rate (eGFR) ≥50 mL/min/1.73 $m^2$ for tx of complicated UTI. Adjust dose for lower eGFR.

## *WEIGHT-LOSS DRUGS*

### ▶ naltrexone and buPROPion
Contrave

**ER tablets:** 8 mg naltrexone, 90 mg bupropion
**Usual adult dose:** Wk 1, 1 tablet PO in a.m.; wk 2, 1 tablet PO in a.m. and 1 tablet PO in p.m.; wk 3, 2 tablets PO in a.m. and 1 tablet PO in p.m.; maint, 2 tablets PO in a.m. and 2 tablets PO in p.m. **BBW** Risk of suicidal thoughts/ behaviors. Not studied in children.

### ▶ phentermine and topiramate
Qsymia

**Capsules:** 3.75 mg phentermine, 23 mg topiramate; 7.5 mg phentermine, 46 mg topiramate; 11.25 mg phentermine, 69 mg topiramate; 15 mg phentermine, 92 mg topiramate
**Usual adult dose:** 1 capsule/d PO in a.m. w/diet/exercise. Hormonal contraceptives may be ineffective; cardiac issues, suicidality.

Appendix F

# Hormonal contraceptives

**IND & DOSE** Take 1 tablet PO daily for 21 d, starting within 5 d of first day of menstrual bleeding (day 1 of cycle is first d of menstrual bleeding). Take inert tablets or no tablets for next 7 d. Then start new course of 21 d. Sunday start: Take first tablet on first Sunday after menstruation begins.
**NC/PT** **Suggested measures for missed doses:** One tablet missed: Take tablet as soon as possible, or take 2 tablets next d. Two consecutive tablets missed: Take 2 tablets daily for next 2 d, then resume regular schedule. Three consecutive tablets missed: If Sunday starter, take 1 pill q d until Sunday; then discard pack and start new pack on that d. If day 1 starter, discard rest of pack and start new pack that same d. Use additional birth control method until start of next menstrual period. Increased risk of thromboembolic events if combined w/smoking.
**Postcoital contraception ("morning after" pills):** Safe, effective for emergency contraception. *Plan B:* 0.75 mg levonorgestrel; take 1 tablet within 72 hr of sexual intercourse, take second tablet 12 hr later. *Plan B One-Step, Her Style, Next Choice One Dose, My Way, Opcicon One-Step, Fallback Solo:* 1.5 mg levonorgestrel; take 1 tablet within 72 hr of unprotected sexual intercourse. Available OTC. *Ella* (ulipristal; progesterone agonist/antagonist): 30 mg tablet; take within 5 d of unprotected sexual intercourse.

## *ORAL CONTRACEPTIVES*

| *Trade name* | *Combination* |
|---|---|
| *MONOPHASIC* | |
| *Altavera, Introvale, Jolessa, Kurvelo, Levora 0.15/30, Marlissa, Portia, Quasense* | 30 mcg ethinyl estradiol/0.15 mg levonorgestrel |
| *Alyacen 1/35, Cyclafem 1/35, Dasetta 1/35, Necon 1/35, Norinyl 1 + 35, Nortrel 1/35, Ortho-Novum 1/35, Pirmella 1/35* | 35 mcg ethinyl estradiol/1 mg norethindrone |
| *Desogen, Emoquette, Enskyce, Isibloom, Ortho-Cept, Solia* | 30 mcg ethinyl estradiol/0.15 mg desogestrel |
| *Afirmelle, Aviane, Falmina, Lessina, Lutera, Orsythia, Sronyx* | 20 mcg ethinyl estradiol/0.10 mg levonorgestrel |
| *Balziva-28, Briellyn, Femcon Fe chewable tablets, Gildagia, Philith, Vyfemla, Wymzya FE, Zenchent* | 35 mcg ethinyl estradiol/0.4 mg norethindrone |

| *Trade name* | *Combination* |
|---|---|
| *Beyaz* | 3 mg drospirenone/20 mcg ethinyl estradiol/0.45 mg levomefolate; must monitor potassium levels |
| *Brevicon, Cyclafem 0.5/35, Cyonanz, Modicon, Necon 0.5/35, Nortrel 0.5/35, Wera* | 35 mcg ethinyl estradiol/0.5 mg norethindrone |
| *Cryselle, Elinest, Low-Ogestrel* | 30 mcg ethinyl estradiol/0.3 mg norgestrel |
| *Estarylla, Mononessa, Ortho-Cyclen, Previfem, Sprintec* | 35 mcg ethinyl estradiol/0.25 mg norgestimate |
| *Generess FE* | 25 mg ethinyl estradiol, 0.8 mg norethindrone |
| *Gianvi, Loryna, Melamisa, Nikki, Vestura, Yaz* | 3 mg drospirenone/20 mcg ethinyl estradiol |
| *Blisovi Fe 1/20, Blisovi 24 Fe, Gildess 1/20, Gildess Fe 1/20, Gildess 24 Fe, Junel Fe 1/20, Junel 21 Day 1/20, Larin 1/20, Larin FE 1/20, Loestrin 21 1/20, Loestrin Fe 21 1/20, Loestrin 24 Fe, Lomedia 24 FE, Mibelas 24 Fe, Microgestin Fe 1/20, Minastrin 24 FE* | 20 mcg ethinyl estradiol/1 mg norethindrone |
| *Blisovi Fe 1.5/30, Gildess 1.5/20, Gildess FE 1.5/30, Junel Fe 1.5/30, Junel 21 Day 1.5/30, FE 15/30, Larin Fe 1.5/30, Loestrin 21 1.5/30, Loestrin Fe 1.5/30, Microgestin Fe 1.5/30* | 30 mcg ethinyl estradiol/1.5 mg norethindrone acetate |
| *Kelnor 1/35, Norinyl 1/35, Ortho-Novum 1/35, Zovia 1/35E* | 35 mcg ethinyl estradiol/1 mg ethynodiol diacetate |
| *Necon 1/50, Norinyl 1 + 50* | 50 mcg mestranol/1 mg norethindrone |
| *Ocella, Safryal, Syeda, Yaela, Yasmin 28, Zarah* | 3 mg drospirenone/30 mcg ethinyl estradiol; must monitor potassium level |
| *Ogestrel 0.5/50* | 50 mcg ethinyl estradiol/0.5 mg norgestrel |
| *Ashlyna, Daysee, Quasense, Seasonale, Seasonique, Setlakin* | 0.15 levonorgestrel/30 mcg ethinyl estradiol taken as 84 days active tablets, 7 days inactive |

| *Trade name* | *Combination* |
|---|---|
| *Safyral* | 3 mg drospirenone/30 mcg ethinyl estradiol/45 mcg levomefolate |
| *Zovia 1/50E* | 50 mcg ethinyl estradiol/1 mg ethynodiol diacetate |
| ***Biphasic*** | |
| *Camrese, Daysee, Seasonique* | **phase 1:** 84 tablets, 0.15 mg levonorgestrel/30 mcg ethinyl estradiol **phase 2:** 7 tablets, 10 mcg ethinyl estradiol |
| *Amethia Lo* | **phase 1:** 84 tablets, 0.1 mg levonorgestrel/ 20 mcg ethinyl estradiol **phase 2:** 7 tablets, 10 mcg ethinyl estradiol |
| *Azurette, Bekyree, Kariva, Kimidess, Mircette, Pimtrea, Viorel, Volnea* | **phase 1:** 21 tablets, 0.15 mg desogestrel/ 20 mcg ethinyl estradiol **phase 2:** 5 tablets, 10 mcg ethinyl estradiol |
| *Camrese Lo, LoSeasonique* | **phase 1:** 84 tablets, 0.15 mg levonorgestrel/20 mcg ethinyl estradiol **phase 2:** 7 tablets, 10 mcg ethinyl estradiol |
| *Lo Loestrin Fe, Lo Minastrin Fe* | **phase 1:** 24 tablets, 1 mg norethindrone/ 10 mcg ethinyl estradiol **phase 2:** 2 tablets, 10 mcg ethinyl estradiol |
| *Necon 10/11* | **phase 1:** 10 tablets, 0.5 mg norethindrone/ 35 mcg ethinyl estradiol **phase 2:** 11 tablets, 1 mg norethindrone/ 35 mcg ethinyl estradiol |
| ***Triphasic*** | |
| *Alyacen 7/7/7, Cyclafem 7/7/7, Dasetta 7/7/7, Necon 7/7/7, Nortrel 7/7/7, Ortho-Novum 7/7/7, Pirmella 7/7/7* | **phase 1:** 7 tablets, 0.5 mg norethindrone (progestin)/35 mcg ethinyl estradiol (estrogen) **phase 2:** 7 tablets, 0.75 mg norethindrone (progestin)/35 mcg ethinyl estradiol (estrogen) **phase 3:** 7 tablets, 1 mg norethindrone (progestin)/35 mcg ethinyl estradiol (estrogen) |

| Trade name | Combination |
|---|---|
| Aranelle, Leena, Tri-Norinyl | **phase 1:** 7 tablets, 0.5 mg norethindrone (progestin)/35 mcg ethinyl estradiol (estrogen)<br>**phase 2:** 9 tablets, 1 mg norethindrone (progestin)/35 mcg ethinyl estradiol (estrogen)<br>**phase 3:** 5 tablets, 0.5 mg norethindrone (progestin)/35 mcg ethinyl estradiol (estrogen) |
| Caziant, Cyclessa, Velivet | **phase 1:** 7 tablets, 0.1 mg desogestrel/ 25 mcg ethinyl estradiol<br>**phase 2:** 7 tablets, 0.125 mg desogestrel/ 25 mcg ethinyl estradiol<br>**phase 3:** 7 tablets, 0.15 mg desogestrel/ 25 mcg ethinyl estradiol |
| Elifemme, Enpresse, Levonest, Myzilra, Trivora | **phase 1:** 6 tablets, 0.5 mg levonorgestrel (progestin)/30 mcg ethinyl estradiol (estrogen)<br>**phase 2:** 5 tablets, 0.075 mg levonorgestrel (progestin)/40 mcg ethinyl estradiol (estrogen)<br>**phase 3:** 10 tablets, 0.125 mg levonorgestrel (progestin)/30 mcg ethinyl estradiol (estrogen) |
| Estrostep Fe, Tilia Fe, Tri-Legest Fe | **phase 1:** 5 tablets, 1 mg norethindrone/ 20 mcg ethinyl estradiol; w/75 mg ferrous fumarate<br>**phase 2:** 7 tablets, 1 mg norethindrone/ 30 mcg ethinyl estradiol; w/75 mg ferrous fumarate<br>**phase 3:** 9 tablets, 1 mg norethindrone/ 35 mcg ethinyl estradiol; w/75 mg ferrous fumarate |
| Ortho Tri-Cyclen, Tri-Estarylla, Tri-Linyah, TriNessa, Tri-Previfem, Tri-Sprintec | **phase 1:** 7 tablets, 0.18 mg norgestimate/ 35 mcg ethinyl estradiol<br>**phase 2:** 7 tablets, 0.215 mg norgestimate/ 35 mcg ethinyl estradiol<br>**phase 3:** 7 tablets, 0.25 mg norgestimate/ 35 mcg ethinyl estradiol |
| Ortho Tri-Cyclen Lo | **phase 1:** 7 tablets, 0.18 mg norgestimate/ 25 mcg ethinyl estradiol<br>**phase 2:** 7 tablets, 0.215 mg norgestimate/ 25 mcg ethinyl estradiol<br>**phase 3:** 7 tablets, 0.25 mg norgestimate/ 25 mcg ethinyl estradiol |

| Trade name | Combination |
|---|---|
| *Tri-Legest* | **phase 1:** 5 tablets, 1 mg norethindrone/ 20 mcg ethinyl estradiol<br>**phase 2:** 7 tablets, 1 mg norethindrone/ 30 mcg ethinyl estradiol<br>**phase 3:** 9 tablets, 1 mg norethindrone/ 35 mcg ethinyl estradiol |
| ***4-PHASIC*** | |
| *Natazia* | **phase 1:** 2 tablets, 3 mg estradiol valerate<br>**phase 2:** 5 tablets, 2 mg estradiol valerate/ 2 mg dienogest<br>**phase 3:** 17 tablets, 2 mg estradiol valerate/3 mg dienogest<br>**phase 4:** 2 tablets, 1 mg estradiol valerate |
| *Fayosim, Leribane, Quartette* | **phase 1:** 42 tablets, 0.15 mg levonorgestrel, 0.02 mg ethinyl estradiol<br>**phase 2:** 21 tablets, 0.15 mg levonorgestrel, 0.025 mg ethinyl estradiol<br>**phase 3:** 21 tablets, 0.15 mg levonorgestrel, 0.03 mg ethinyl estradiol<br>**phase 4:** 7 tablets, 0.01 mg ethinyl estradiol |
| ***PROGESTIN ONLY*** | |
| *Camila, Errin, Heather, Jencycla, Nor-QD, Ortho Micronor* | 0.35 mg norethindrone |

### IMPLANTABLE SYSTEM

| Trade name | Combination |
|---|---|
| *Implanon, Nexplanon* | 68 mg etonogestrel implanted subdermally in inner aspect of nondominant upper arm. Left in place for no longer than 3 yr, then must be removed. May then insert new implants. |

### INJECTABLE CONTRACEPTIVES

| Trade name | Combination |
|---|---|
| *Depo-Provera* | 150, 400 mcg/mL medroxyprogesterone. Give 1-mL injection deep IM; repeat q 3 mo.<br>**BBW** Risk of significant bone loss. |
| *depo-sub Q provera 104* | 104 mg medroxyprogesterone. Give 0.65 mL subcut into anterior thigh, abdomen.<br>**BBW** Risk of significant bone loss. |

## INTRAUTERINE SYSTEM

| Trade name | Combination |
|---|---|
| *Liletta* | 52 mg levonorgestrel inserted into uterus for up to 6 yr. |
| *Mirena* | 52 mg levonorgestrel inserted into uterus for up to 5 yr. (Also approved to treat heavy menstrual bleeding in women using intrauterine system for contraception.) Releases 20 mcg/d. |
| *Skyla* | 13.5 mg levonorgestrel inserted into uterus for up to 3 yr. |

## TRANSDERMAL SYSTEM

| Trade name | Combination |
|---|---|
| *Ortho Evra, Xulane* | 6 mg norelgestromin/0.75 ethinyl estradiol in patch form; releases 150 mcg norelgestromin/20 mcg ethinyl estradiol each 24 hr for 1 wk. Patch applied on same d of wk for 3 consecutive wk, followed by patch-free wk. **BBW** Higher risk of thromboembolic events/death if combined w/smoking. |

## VAGINAL RING

| Trade name | Combination |
|---|---|
| *Annovera* | 0.15 mg segesterone acetate/0.013 mg ethinyl estradiol/d. Insert into vagina continuously for 21 d, followed by 7-d vaginal ring–free interval. One ring provides contraception for 13 28-d cycles (1 yr). **BBW** Higher risk of thromboembolic events/death if combined w/smoking, especially if pt >35 yr. |
| *NuvaRing* | 0.12 mg etonogestrel (progestin)/0.015 mg ethinyl estradiol (estrogen)/day. Insert into vagina on or before 5th d of menstrual period; remove after 3 wk. Insert new ring after 1-wk rest. **BBW** Higher risk of thromboembolic events/death if combined w/smoking, especially if pt >35 yr. |

Appendix G

# Commonly used biologicals

**IND & DOSE** Vaccines provide inactivated or attenuated antigens to stimulate production of antibodies; provides active immunity. Immune globulin provides acute, passive immunity by providing preformed antibodies to specific antigen; not long-term protection.
**ADV EFF** Anorexia, drowsiness, injection-area edema (w/redness, swelling, induration, pain that may persist for few d), fretfulness, generalized aches/pains, hypersensitivity reactions, malaise, transient fever, vomiting
**NC/PT** See individual labels for preg category/risk. Defer administration of routine immunizing or booster doses if acute infection present. Usually not indicated for pts on immunosuppressants or w/cancer, active infections. Have epinephrine 1:1,000 on hand during injection for hypersensitivity reactions. Provide comfort measures.

## ▶ adenovirus type 4 and 7 vaccine, live, oral

*Military population 17 through 50 yr:* Single oral dose consists of one adenovirus type 4 tablet and one adenovirus type 7 tablet. Not for use in preg. Postpone administration in pts w/vomiting and/or diarrhea. Indicated for active immunization for px of febrile acute respiratory disease caused by adenovirus type 4 and type 7. Pt should swallow tablets whole, not chew or crush.

## ▶ anthrax vaccine, absorbed
BioThrax

*Adult 18–65 yr, preexposure:* 0.5 mL IM at 0.1 and 6 mo, booster at 6 and 12 mo of primary series, then at 12-mo intervals. Or subcut at 0, 2, 4 wk and 6 mo, booster at 6 and 12 mo, then q 12 mo. *Adult 18–65 yr, postexposure:* 0.5 mL subcut at 0, 2, 4 wk w/antimicrobial therapy. Not for use in preg.

## ▶ cholera vaccine, live, oral
Vaxchora

*Adult 18–64 yr traveling to cholera-affected areas:* Single oral dose (1 packet active component, 1 packet buffer component) PO at least 10 d before potential exposure to cholera. Shed in stool for at least 7 d; use caution near immunocompromised. Must prepare in area equipped to dispose of medical waste. Do not give within 14 d of systemic antibiotics. Pt should avoid eating/drinking for 60 min before or after oral ingestion.

## ▶ diphtheria and tetanus toxoids, adsorbed
Decavac, Tenivac

*Adult, child:* Three 0.5-mL IM injections, first two at least 4 wk apart and third 6 mo later. Routine booster at 11–12 yr, then q 10 yr (*Decavac*). *Adult, child ≥7 yr:* Three 0.5-mL injections IM at 8-wk intervals, booster 6–8 mo later. Routine booster at 11–12 yr, then q 10 yr (*Tenivac*).

**▶ diphtheria and tetanus toxoids and acellular pertussis vaccine adsorbed (DtaP/Tdap)**
Adacel, Boostrix, Daptacel, Infanrix, Tripedia

*Primary immunization:* 3 IM doses of 0.5 mL at 4- to 8-wk intervals. Start doses by 6–8 wk of age; finish by 7th birthday. Use same vaccine for all three doses. *Fourth dose:* 0.5 mL IM at 15–20 mo at least 6 mo after previous dose. *Fifth dose:* 0.5 mL IM at 4–6 yr or preferably before entry into school (*Infanrix, Daptacel, Tripedia*). If fourth dose given after 4-yr birthday, may omit preschool dose. *Booster injections:* 11–64 yr (*Adacel*), 0.5 mL IM. ≥10 yr (*Boostrix*), 0.5 mL IM. Allow at least 5 yr between last of series and booster dose.

**▶ diphtheria and tetanus toxoids and acellular pertussis adsorbed, hepatitis B (recombinant), and inactivated poliovirus vaccine combined (DTaP-HePB-IPV)**
Pediarix

*Infants w/hepatitis B surface antigen (HBsAG)–negative mothers:* Three 0.5-mL doses IM at 6- to 8-wk intervals (preferably 8) stating at 2 mo. *Children previously vaccinated w/one dose of hepatitis B vaccine:* Should receive three-dose series. *Children previously vaccinated w/one or more doses of Infanrix or IPV:* May use *Pediarix* to complete series.

**▶ diphtheria and tetanus toxoids and acellular pertussis adsorbed and inactivated poliovirus vaccine (DTaP-IIPV)**
Kinrix

Fifth dose in diphtheria, tetanus, acellular pertussis series and fourth dose in inactivated poliovirus series in children 4–6 yr whose previous immunizations have been w/*Infanrix* or *Pediarix* for first three doses and *Infanrix* for fourth dose. One IM injection of 0.5 mL.

**▶ diphtheria and tetanus toxoids and acellular pertussis adsorbed, inactivated poliovirus vaccine, and *Haemophilus* b conjugate (tetanus toxoid conjugate) vaccine (DTaP-IPV/Hib)**
Pentacel

Four-dose series of IM injections of 0.5 mL at 2, 4, and 6 mo, followed by booster at 18 mo. Give between 6 wk and 4 yr.

**▶ Ebola Zaire vaccine, live**
Ervebo

*Adult ≥18 yr:* 1 mL IM single dose for px of disease caused by Zaire ebolavirus.

**▶ *Haemophilus* b conjugate vaccine**
ActHIB, Hiberix, Liquid PedvaxHIB

Active immunization of infants, children against *H. influenzae* b for primary immunization, routine recall; 2–71 mo (*PedvaxHIB*), 2–18 mo

(*ActHIB w/DPT*), or 15–18 mo (*ActHIB, Hiberix* w/ *Tripedia*). **ActHIB:** Reconstitute w/DTP, *Tripedia*, or saline. 2–6 mo, 3 IM injections of 0.5 mL at 2, 4, and 6 mo; 0.5 mL at 15–18 mo and DPT alone at 4–6 yr. 7–11 mo, 2 IM injections of 0.5 mL at 8-wk intervals; booster dose at 15–18 mo. 12–14 mo, 0.5 mL IM w/a booster 2 mo later. 15–18 mo, 0.5 mL IM, booster of *Tripedia* at 4–6 yr. **Hiberix:** 15 mo–4 yr, booster dose of 0.5 mL IM as single dose. Booster dose at ≥15 mo but not <2 mo from last dose. Unvaccinated children 15 71 mo, 0.5 mL IM **PedvaxHIB:** 2–14 mo, 2 IM injections of 0.5 mL at 2 mo and 2 mo later; 0.5-mL booster at 12 mo (if two doses complete before 12 mo, not <2 mo after last dose). ≥15 mo, 0.5 mL IM single injection.

## ▶ hepatitis A vaccine, inactivated
Havrix, Vaqta

**Adult:** *Havrix,* 1,440 ELISA units (1 mL) IM; same dose booster in 6–12 mo. *Vaqta,* 50 units (1 mL) IM; same dose booster in 6–18 mo. **Child 12 mo–18 yr:** *Vaqta,* 25 units/ 0.5 mL IM, w/repeat dose in 6–18 mo. *Havrix,* 720 ELISA units (0.5 mL) IM; repeat dose in 6–12 mo.

## ▶ hepatitis A inactivated and hepatitis B recombinant vaccine
Twinrix

Three doses (1 mL by IM injection) on 0-, 1-, and 6-mo schedule. *Accelerated dosage:* Four doses (1 mL by IM injection) on days 0, 7, 21, 30, followed by booster dose at 12 mo. Safety in pts <18 yr not established.

## ▶ hepatitis B immune globulin (HBIG)
HepaGam B, HyperHEP B S/D, Nabi-HB

*Perinatal exposure:* 0.5 mL IM within 12 hr of birth; repeat dose at 1 mo and 6 mo after initial dose. *Percutaneous exposure:* 0.06 mL/kg IM immediately (within 7 d); repeat 28–30 d after exposure. Usual adult dose, 3–5 mL. *Pts at high risk for infection:* 0.06 mL/kg IM at same time (but at different site) as hepatitis B vaccine is given. *HepaGam B after liver transplant:* 20,000 interna tional units IV at 2 mL/min. Give first dose w/liver transplant, then daily on days 1–7, q 2 wk from day 14 through 12 wk, and monthly from mo 4 onward. *Sexual exposure:* Single dose of 0.06 mL/kg IM within 14 d of last sexual contact.

## ▶ hepatitis B vaccine
Engerix-B, HEPLISAV-B, Recombivax HB

*Adults:* Initial dose, 1 mL IM, then 1 mL IM at 1 mo and 6 mo after initial dose *(Engerix-B, Recombivax HB)*; 0.5 mL IM, then 0.5 mL IM 1 mo after initial dose *(HEPLISAV-B)*. *Child 11–19 yr:* 1 mL IM, then 1 mL IM at 1 mo and 6 mo after initial dose *(Engerix-B, Recombivax HB)*. *Birth–10 yr:* Initial dose, 0.5 mL IM, then 0.5 mL IM at 1 mo and 6 mo after initial dose *(Engerix-B, Recombivax HB)*. *Dialysis, predialysis pts:* Initial dose, 40 mcg (2 mL) IM; repeat at 1, 2, and 6 mo after initial dose (*Engerix-B*). Or, 40 mcg (1 mL) IM; repeat at 1 and 6 mo (*Recombivax HB*). **Revaccination** (consider booster dose w/anti-HBs level under 10 milli-international units/mL 1–2 mo after third dose). *Adult, child >10 yr:* 20 mcg. *Child <10 yr:* 10 mcg. *Hemodialysis pts* *(when antibody testing indicates need):* Two 20-mcg doses.

**▶ human papillomavirus recombinant vaccine, bivalent types 16 and 18**
Cervarix

*Young girls, women 9–25 yr:* Three doses of 0.5 mL IM at 0, 1, and 6 mo.

**▶ human papillomavirus recombinant vaccine, quadrivalent**
Gardasil, Gardasil 9

*Pts 9–26 yr:* Three separate IM injections of 0.5 mL each, second dose 2 mo after initial dose, last dose 6 mo after first dose. For px of cervical cancer, precancerous genital lesions, genital warts, vaginal/vulvar/anal cancer in women; px of genital warts, anal cancer, precancerous lesions in males. *Pts 9–45 yr (Gardasil 9):* Two (9–14 yr) or three (9–45 yr) separate IM injections of 0.5 mL each, second dose 2 mo after initial dose, last dose 6 mo after first dose; if only two doses, second dose 6–12 mo after initial dose. For px of cervical, vulvar, vaginal, anal cancer, genital warts, precancerous lesions caused by multiple HPV types in females. For px of anal cancer, genital warts, precancerous lesions in males.

**▶ immune globulin intramuscular (IG; gamma globulin; IGIM)**
GamaSTAN S/D
**▶ immune globulin intravenous (IGIV)**
Carimune NF, Flebogamma 5%, Flebogamma 10%, Gammagard Liquid, Privigen
**▶ immune globulin subcutaneous (IGSC, SCIG)**
Cuvitru, Gamunex-C, Hizentra

**BBW** Risk of renal dysfx, renal failure, thrombosis, death; monitor accordingly.
*Hepatitis A:* 0.1 mL/kg IM for household, institutional contacts. Persons traveling to areas where hepatitis A common, 0.1 mL/kg IM if staying less than 1 mo; 0.2 mL/kg IM repeated q 2 mo for prolonged stay. *Measles (rubeola):* 0.25 mL/kg IM if exposed <6 d previously; immunocompromised child exposed to measles, 0.5 mL/kg to max 15 mL IM immediately. *Varicella:* 0.6–1.2 mL/kg IM promptly if zoster immune globulin unavailable. *Rubella:* 0.55 mL/kg IM to preg women exposed to rubella but not considering therapeutic abortion; may decrease likelihood of infection, fetal damage. *Immunoglobulin deficiency:* Initially, 1.3 mL/kg IM, followed in 3–4 wk by 0.66 mL/kg IM q 3–4 wk; some pts may need more frequent injections. *Carimune NF:* 0.4–0.8 g/kg by IV infusion q 3–4 wk. *Flebogamma:* 300–600 mg/kg IV q 3–4 wk. *Primary immune deficiency, idiopathic thrombocytopenic purpura, chronic inflammatory demyelinating polyneuropathy:* 100–200 mg/kg subcut q wk. Or initially, 1.37 × previous IGIV dose (grams)/number of wk between IGIV doses (*Gamunex-C*). Adjust based on response.

### ▶ influenza type A (H5N1) virus monovalent vaccine, adjuvanted
Generic

*Adult:* 0.5 mL IM into deltoid muscle; then 0.5 mL IM 21 d later. Prepare by mixing one vial AS03 adjuvant w/one vial H5N1 adjuvant just before administration; do not mix in syringe w/other vaccines. Virus grown in chicken eggs; use caution w/chicken allergies. Use caution in preg. Give pt written record.

### ▶ influenza type A and B virus vaccine
Afluria, Fluarix, Fluarix Quadrivalent, Flucelvax Quadrivalent, FluLaval, Fluvirin, Fluzone, Fluzone High Dose, Fluzone Quadrivalent

Do not give w/sensitivity to eggs, chicken, chicken feathers, chicken dander; hypersensitivity to vaccine components; hx of Guillain-Barré syndrome. Do not give to infants, children at same time as diphtheria, tetanus toxoid, pertussis vaccine (DTP) or within 14 d after measles virus vaccine. *6–35 mo:* 0.25 mL IM; repeat in 4 wk (*Afluria, Fluarix Quadrivalent, Fluzone*). *≥3 yr:* 0.5 mL IM (*Afluria, Fluarix, Fluarix Quadrivalent, Fluzone*). If <9 yr and receiving vaccine for first time or received only one dose last year, give repeat dose in 4 wk. *≥4 yr:* 0.5 mL IM (*Fluvirin*). If <8 yr and receiving vaccine for first time or received only one dose last year, give repeat dose in 4 wk. *≥18 yr:* 0.5 mL IM. Shake prefilled syringe before use (*Agriflu, Afluria, Fluarix, Fluarix Quadrivalent, FluLaval, Fluzone, Fluvirin*). *18–64 yr:* 0.1 mL intradermally (*Fluzone Intradermal*). *≥65 yr:* 0.5 mL IM (*Fluzone High Dose*).

### ▶ influenza type A and B virus vaccine, live, intranasal
FluMist Quadrivalent

*2–8 yr, not previously vaccinated:* Two doses (0.2 mL each) intranasally as one spray (0.1 mL)/nostril at least 1 mo apart. *2–8 yr, previously vaccinated:* One dose (0.2 mL) intranasally as one spray (0.1 mL)/nostril. *9–49 yr:* One dose of one spray (0.1 mL) in each nostril/flu season. *5–8 yr not previously vaccinated w/FluMist:* Two doses (0.5 mL each) 60 d apart ± 14 d. *5–8 yr previously vaccinated w/FluMist:* One dose (0.5 mL)/flu season. Not as effective as injected vaccine.

### ▶ influenza virus vaccine, H5N1
Audenz, H5N1

*For H5N1: adult ≥18 yr:* Two doses of 0.5 mL IM 21 d apart. *Child 6 mo–17 yr:* Two doses of 0.25 mL IM 21 d apart. Virus grown in chicken eggs; use caution in pts w/chicken allergy. *For Audenz: adult, child ≥6 mo:* 0.5 mL IM 21 d apart.

### ▶ measles, mumps, rubella vaccine, live (MMR)
M-M-R II

Inject 0.5 mL reconstituted vaccine subcut into outer aspect of upper arm. Dose same for all pts. Booster dose recommended on entry into elementary school. Use caution if giving to pt w/hx of sensitivity to eggs, chicken, chicken feathers. Do not give within 1 mo of immunization w/other live virus vaccines. Do not give for at least 3 mo after blood or plasma transfusions or serum immune globulin administration.

**▶ measles, mumps, rubella, and varicella virus vaccine, live**
ProQuad

*12 mo–12 yr:* 0.5 mL subcut. Allow 1 mo between administration of vaccines containing measles antigens and administration of *ProQuad*. If second varicella vaccine needed, allow 3 mo between administration of the two doses.

**▶ meningococcal groups C and Y, *Haemophilus* b tetanus toxoid conjugate vaccine**
MenHibrix

*Child 6 wk–18 mo:* Four doses, 0.5 mL IM each; first as early as 6 wk, 4th as late as 18 mo. Usual timing, 2, 4, 6, and 12–15 mo.

**▶ meningococcal vaccine**
Menactra, Menomune A/C/Y/W-135, Menveo

*Menactra:* 9 mo–55 yr, 0.5 mL IM in deltoid region as one dose. *Menomune:* 2–55 yr, 0.5 mL IM; may give booster in 3–5 yr. *Menveo:* 2 mo–55 yr, 0.5 mL IM as one dose. Children 2–5 yr may receive second dose 2 mo after first dose.

**▶ meningococcal vaccine, serotype B**
Bexsero, Trumenba

*Adult, child 10–25 yr:* Two doses, at least 1 mo apart, 0.5 mL IM (*Bexsero*). Three doses (0.5 mL IM each) on schedule of mos 0, 2, and 6 (*Trumenba*).

**▶ pneumococcal vaccine, polyvalent**
Pneumovax 23

*Adult ≥50 yr, child ≥2 yr who are at increased risk:* One 0.5-mL dose subcut, IM. Not recommended for child <2 yr. Give at least 2 wk before initiation of cancer chemo, other immunosuppressive therapy.

**▶ pneumococcal 13-valent conjugate vaccine (diphtheria CRM197 protein)**
Prevnar-13

0.5 mg IM, preferably in anterolateral aspect of thigh in infants, deltoid muscle of upper arm in older child. *6 wk–5 yr:* Four-dose series given 4–8 wk apart at 2, 4, 6 mo; then at 12–15 mo. *Catch-up schedule for child ≥7 mo:* 7–11 mo, three doses, first two doses at least 4 wk apart; third dose after first birthday. 12–23 mo, two doses at least 2 mo apart. 24 mo–5 yr, one dose (before 6th birthday). *Adult ≥50 yr:* One single dose.

**▶ poliovirus vaccine, inactivated (IPV, Salk)**
IPOL

Do not give w/known hypersensitivity to streptomycin, neomycin (each dose contains under 25 mcg of each). *Adult:* Not usually needed in adults in United States. Recommended if unimmunized adult is exposed, traveling to high-risk area, or household contact of child receiving IPV. Give 0.5 mL subcut: two doses at 1- to 2-mo intervals, third dose 6–12 mo later. Previously vaccinated adult at risk for exposure should receive 0.5-mL dose. *Child:* 0.5 mL subcut at 2, 4, and 6–18 mo. Booster dose needed at time of entry into elementary school.

**▶ RHo (D) immune globulin**
HyperRHO S/D Full Dose, RhoGAM Ultra-Filtered Plus
**▶ RHo (D) immune globulin micro-dose**
HyperRHO S/D minidose, MICRhoGAM Ultra-Filtered Plus
**▶ RHo (D) immune globulin IV (human) (RHo D IGIV)**
Rhophylac, WinRho SDF

**BBW** Risk of intravascular hemolysis, death when used for idiopathic thrombocytopenia purpura (ITP; *WinRho*). Monitor dipstick urinalysis at baseline, then at 2, 4, 8 hr. Ask pt to report back pain, chills, discolored urine.
*Postpartum px:* 1 vial IM, IV (*WinRho SDF*) within 72 hr of delivery. *Antepartum px:* 1 vial IM, IV (*WinRho SDF*) at 26–28 wk gestation; 1 vial within 72 hr after Rh-incompatible delivery to prevent Rh isoimmunization during preg. *After amniocentesis, miscarriage, abortion, ectopic pregnancy at or beyond 13 wk gestation:* 1 vial IM, IV. *Transfusion accident:* Multiply volume in mL of Rh-positive whole blood given by Hct of donor unit; divide this volume (in mL) by 15 to obtain number of vials to be given. If results of calculation are fraction, give next whole number of vials. *ITP:* 250 international units/kg IV at 2 mL/15–60 sec. *Spontaneous/induced abortion, termination of ectopic pregnancy up to and including 12 wk gestation (unless father Rh negative):* 1 vial microdose IM as soon as possible after preg termination.

**▶ rotavirus vaccine, live, oral pentavalent**
Rotarix, RotaTeq

Three ready-to-use liquid pouch doses (2 mL each) PO starting at age 6–12 wk, w/subsequent doses at 4- to 10-wk intervals (do not give third dose after age 32 wk) (*RotaTeq*). Two doses of 1 mL each PO starting at age 6 wk. Allow 4 wk before second dose. Must complete series by age 24 wk (*Rotarix*).

**▶ typhoid vaccine**
Typhim Vi, Vivotif Berna

Complete vaccine regimen 1–2 wk before potential exposure.
**Parenteral** *>10 yr:* Two doses of 0.5 mL subcut at intervals of 4 wk or longer. *≤10 yr:* Two doses of 0.25 mL subcut at intervals of 4 wk or longer. **Booster dose.** Given q 3 yr in cases of continued exposure. *>10 yr:* 0.5 mL subcut or 0.1 mL intradermally. *6 mo–10 yr:* 0.25 mL subcut or 0.1 mL intradermally.
**Parenteral (*Typhim Vi*).** *Child ≥2 yr:* 0.5 mL IM. Booster dose q 2 yr; 0.5 mL IM.
**Oral (*Vivotif Berna*).** *Pts >6 yr:* 1 capsule on days 1, 3, 5, 7 1 hr before meal w/cold, lukewarm drink. No data on need for booster dose; 4 capsules on alternating days once q 5 yr suggested.

**▶ varicella virus vaccine, live**
Varivax

*Adult, child ≥13 yr:* 0.5 mL subcut in deltoid area, then 0.5 mL 4–8 wk later. *Child 1–12 yr:* Single 0.5-mL dose subcut.

### ▶ zoster vaccine, live
Zostavax

*Adult ≥50 yr:* 1 injection of single-dose vaccine subcut in upper arm. Vaccine should be frozen and reconstituted, using supplied diluent, immediately after removal from freezer. Give immediately after reconstituting.

### ▶ zoster vaccine recombinant, adjuvanted
SHINGRIX

*Adult ≥50 yr:* Two doses (0.5 mL each) at 0 and 2–6 mo in deltoid region of upper arm. Administer immediately after reconstitution or store in refrigerator and use within 6 hr. Discard reconstituted vaccine if not used within 6 hr.

## *OTHER BIOLOGICALS*

| *Name* | *Indications* | *Instructions* |
|---|---|---|
| ***IMMUNE GLOBULINS*** | | |
| antithymocyte globulin (*Thymoglobulin*) | Tx of renal transplant acute rejection w/ immunosuppression | 1.5 mg/kg/d for 7–14 d as 6-hr IV infusion for first dose and at least 4 hr each subsequent dose. Give through 0.22-micron filter. Store in refrigerator; use within 4 hr of reconstitution. |
| botulism immune globulin (*BabyBIG*) | Tx of pts <1 yr w/ infant botulism caused by toxin A or B | 1 mL/kg as single IV infusion as soon as dx made. |
| cytomegalovirus immune globulin IV (CMV-IGIV) (*CytoGam*) | Px of CMV disease after renal, lung, liver, pancreas, heart transplant | 15 mg/kg IV over 30 min; increase to 30 mg/kg IV for 30 min, then 60 mg/kg IV to max 150 mg/kg. Infuse at 72 hr, 2 wk, then 4, 6, 8, 12, 16 wk. Monitor for allergic reactions. Use within 6 hr of entering vial. Give through IV line w/in-line filter (15 micron). |
| lymphocyte, immune globulin (*Atgam*) | Mgt of allograft rejection in renal transplant; tx of aplastic anemia | 10–30 mg/kg/d IV adult transplant; 5–25 mg/kg/d IV child transplant; 10–20 mg/kg/d IV for 8–14 days for aplastic anemia. Stable for up to 12 hr after reconstitution. Give skin test before first dose. |

| *Name* | *Indications* | *Instructions* |
| --- | --- | --- |
| rabies immune globulin (*HyperRab S/D, Imogam Rabies-HT, KEDRAB*) | Passive protection against rabies in non-immunized pts w/ exposure to rabies | 20 international units/kg IM as single dose at same time as rabies vaccine. Infuse wound area if possible. Never give in same site as vaccine. Refrigerate vial. |
| vaccinia immune globulin IV (*VIGIV*) | Tx, modification of vaccinia infections | 2 mL/kg (100 mg/kg) IV. |
| varicella zoster immune globulin (*VZIG*) | Decrease severity of chickenpox sx in high-risk pts | 125 units/10 kg IV or IM given within 96 hr of exposure. |
| ***Antitoxins, antivenins*** | | |
| antivenin (*Micrurus fulvius*) | Neutralization of venom of U.S. coral snakes | 3–5 vials by slow IV injection. Give first 1–2 mL over 3–5 min; observe for allergic reaction. Flush w/IV fluids after antivenin infused. May need up to 100 mL. |
| black widow spider species antivenin (Antivenin *Latrodectus mactans*) | Tx of sx of black widow spider bites | 2.5 mL IM. May give IV in 10–50 mL saline over 15 min. Ensure supportive tx, muscle relaxant use. |
| botulism antitoxin (*Botulism Antitoxin Heptavalent [HBAT]*) | Tx of suspected/ known exposure to botulinum neurotoxin | For pts ≥1 yr, base dose on CDC protocol and exposure. |
| centruroides (scorpion) immune fab (*Anascorp*) | Tx of scorpion stings | Initially, 3 vials infused IV over 10 min; then 1 vial at a time at intervals of 30–60 min until clinically stable. Begin as soon as possible after sting. Severe hypersensitivity reactions, delayed serum sickness reaction possible (contains equine proteins). |
| crotalidae immune fab (equine) (*Anavip*) | Tx of American rattlesnake bites | 10 vials IV over 60 min; may repeat in 60 min as needed. Give as soon as possible after bite. Reconstitute each vial w/10 mL NSS, then further dilute in 250 mL NSS. Monitor pt for at least 18 hr; re-emerging or late sx can be treated w/4 vials IV over 60 min. Monitor for possible allergic reactions. |

| *Name* | *Indications* | *Instructions* |
|---|---|---|
| crotalidae polyvalent immune fab (ovine) (*CroFab*) | Tx of rattlesnake bites | 4–6 vials IV; may repeat based on response. Dilute each vial w/10 mL sterile water, then w/250 mL 0.9% NSS. Give each 250 mL over 60 min. Contains specific antibody fragments that bind to four different rattlesnake toxins. Venom removal should be done at once. Monitor carefully for hypersensitivity reaction. Most effective if given within first 6 hr after snake bite. |
| ***Bacterial vaccines*** | | |
| BCG (*TICE BCG*) | Exposure to TB of skin test negative infants and child; tx of groups w/high rates of TB; travel to areas w/high endemic TB rates | 0.2–0.3 mL percutaneously using sterile multipuncture disc. Refrigerate, protect from light. Keep vaccination site clean until reaction disappears. |
| ***Viral vaccines*** | | |
| Japanese encephalitis vaccine (*generic*) | Active immunization in pts >1 yr who will reside, travel in endemic/epidemic areas | 3 subcut doses of 1 mL on days 0, 7, 30. Child 1–3 yr, 3 subcut doses of 0.5 mL. Refrigerate vial. Do not remove rubber stopper. Pt should not travel within 10 d of vaccination. |
| Japanese encephalitis virus (JEV) vaccine, inactivated, adsorbed (*Ixiaro*) | Active immunization in pts ≥17 yr | Two doses of 0.5 mL each IM 28 d apart. Should complete series at least 1 wk before exposure to JEV. Contains protamine sulfate. Use only if clearly needed in preg/breastfeeding. |
| rabies vaccine (*Imovax Rabies, RabAvert*) | Preexposure rabies immunization for pts in high-risk area; postexposure antirabies regimen w/rabies immunoglobulin | *Preexposure:* 1 mL IM on days 0, 7, and 21 or 28. *Postexposure:* 1 mL IM on days 0, 3, 7, 14, 28. Refrigerate. If titers low, may need booster. |
| yellow fever vaccine (*YF-Vax*) | Immunization of pts ≥9 mo living in or traveling to endemic areas | 0.5 mL subcut. Booster dose suggested q 10 yr. Use cautiously w/allergy to chicken, egg products. |

# Bibliography

Arcangelo, V. P., Peterson, A. M., Wilbur, V., & Reinhold, J. A. (2017). *Pharmacotherapeutics for advanced practice: A practical approach* (4th ed.). Philadelphia, PA: Wolters Kluwer.

Brunton, L., Hilal-Dandan, R., & Khollman, B. (2018). *Goodman and Gilman's The pharmacological basis of therapeutics* (13th ed.). New York, NY: McGraw-Hill.

Karch, A. M. (2020). *Focus on nursing pharmacology* (8th ed.). Philadelphia, PA: Lippincott Williams & Wilkins.

*Prescribers' Digital Reference.* (2018). Retrieved from http://www.pdr.net/

U.S. Department of Health and Human Services. (2020). *U.S. Food and Drug Administration.* Retrieved from https://www.fda.gov/default.htm

# Index



*Entries in* **boldface** *are drug classes.*

*Entries in* **boldface** *are drug classes.*

*Entries in* **boldface** *are drug classes.*

*Entries in* **boldface** *are drug classes.*

*Entries in* **boldface** *are drug classes.*

*Entries in* **boldface** *are drug classes.*

*Entries in* **boldface** *are drug classes.*

*Entries in* **boldface** *are drug classes.*

*Entries in* **boldface** *are drug classes.*

*Entries in* **boldface** *are drug classes.*

*Entries in* **boldface** *are drug classes.*

*Entries in* **boldface** *are drug classes.*

*Entries in* **boldface** *are drug classes.*

*Entries in* **boldface** *are drug classes.*

*Entries in* **boldface** *are drug classes.*

*Entries in* **boldface** *are drug classes.*

*Entries in* **boldface** *are drug classes.*

*Entries in* **boldface** *are drug classes.*

*Entries in* **boldface** *are drug classes.*

*Entries in* **boldface** *are drug classes.*

*Entries in* **boldface** *are drug classes.*

*Entries in* **boldface** *are drug classes.*

*Entries in* **boldface** *are drug classes.*

*Entries in* **boldface** *are drug classes.*

*Entries in* **boldface** *are drug classes.*

*Entries in* **boldface** *are drug classes.*

*Entries in* **boldface** *are drug classes.*

*Entries in* **boldface** *are drug classes.*

*Entries in* **boldface** *are drug classes.*

*Entries in* **boldface** *are drug classes.*